AAOS

Pharmacology Applications

Paramedic

Andrew N. Pollak, MD, FAAOS
Series Editor
Medical Director, Baltimore County Fire Department
Associate Professor
University of Maryland School of Medicine
Baltimore, MD

Bob Elling, MPA, REMT-P
Hudson Valley Community College
Andrew Jackson University
Colonie EMS Department
Schenectady, NY

Kirsten M. Elling
Hudson Valley Community College
Colonie EMS Department
Schenectady, NY

JONES AND BARTLETT PUBLISHERS
Sudbury, Massachusetts
BOSTON TORONTO LONDON SINGAPORE

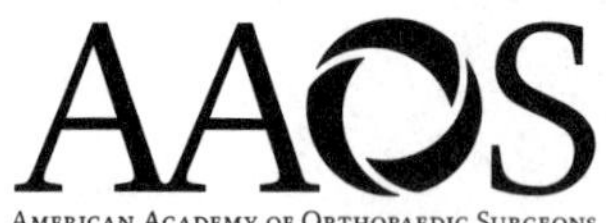

World Headquarters
Jones and Bartlett Publishers
40 Tall Pine Drive
Sudbury, MA 01776
978-443-5000
info@jbpub.com
www.jbpub.com

Jones and Bartlett Publishers Canada
6339 Ormindale Way
Mississauga, Ontario L5V 1J2
Canada

Jones and Bartlett Publishers International
Barb House, Barb Mews
London W6 7PA
United Kingdom

Jones and Bartlett's books and products are available through most bookstores and online booksellers. To contact Jones and Bartlett Publishers directly, call 800-832-0034, fax 978-443-8000, or visit our website www.jbpub.com.

Substantial discounts on bulk quantities of Jones and Bartlett's publications are available to corporations, professional associations, and other qualified organizations. For details and specific discount information, contact the special sales department at Jones and Bartlett via the above contact information or send an email to specialsales@jbpub.com.

This textbook is intended solely as a guide to the appropriate procedures to be employed when rendering emergency care to the sick and injured. It is not intended as a statement of the standards of care required in any particular situation, because circumstances and the patient's physical condition can vary widely from one emergency to another. Nor is it intended that this textbook shall in any way advise emergency personnel concerning legal authority to perform the activities or procedures discussed. Such local determination should be made only with the aid of legal counsel.

Production Credits

Chief Executive Officer: Clayton Jones
Chief Operating Officer: Don W. Jones, Jr.
President, Higher Education and Professional Publishing: Robert W. Holland, Jr.
V.P., Sales and Marketing: William J. Kane
V.P., Design and Production: Anne Spencer
V.P., Manufacturing and Inventory Control: Therese Connell
Publisher—Public Safety Group: Kimberly Brophy
Acquisitions Editor—EMS: Christine Emerton
Associate Managing Editor: Amanda J. Green
Senior Production Editor: Karen C. Ferreira
Composition: Shepherd, Inc.
Text Design: Anne Spencer
Cover Design: Kristin E. Ohlin
Photo Research Manager and Photographer: Kimberly Potvin
Photo Researcher: Lee Michelsen
Cover Image: © Jones and Bartlett Publishers. Courtesy of MIEMSS.
Printing and Binding: Malloy, Inc.
Cover Printing: Courier Stoughton

Library of Congress Cataloging-in-Publication Data

Paramedic : pharmacology applications / American Academy of Orthopaedic Surgeons ; Andrew N. Pollak, editor ; Bob Elling, Kirsten M. Elling.—1st ed.
p. ; cm.
Includes index.
ISBN 978-0-7637-5119-7 (alk. paper)
1. Pharmacology. 2. Medical emergencies. 3. Emergency medical technicians. I. Pollak, Andrew N. II. Elling, Bob. III. Elling, Kirsten M. IV. American Academy of Orthopaedic Surgeons.
[DNLM: 1. Drug Therapy. 2. Emergency Treatment. 3. Emergency Medical Services. 4. Emergency Medical Technicians. WB 105 P222 2009]
RM300.P28 2009
615'.1—dc22

2008020037

6048
Printed in the United States of America
12 11 10 09 08 10 9 8 7 6 5 4 3 2 1

Brief Contents

Contents

Chapter Resources

Paramedic: Pharmacology Applications is designed to give paramedic professionals the education and confidence they need to effectively treat patients with medications in the field. Features that reinforce and expand on essential information include:

Skill Drills

Step-by-step explanations including a visual summary of key medication administration skills and procedures are provided in Chapter 1 to enhance student comprehension.

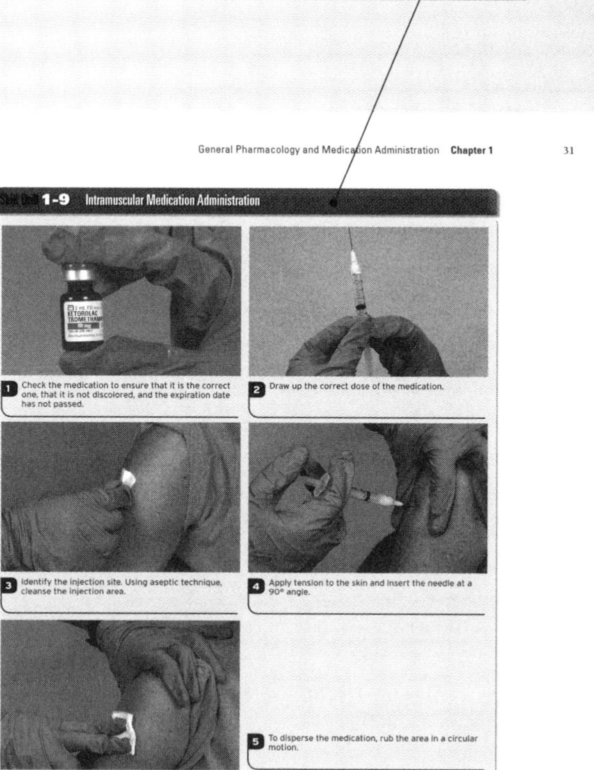

Progressive Case Studies

Each chapter contains a minimum of one progressive case study to encourage students to start thinking about what they might do if they encountered a similar case in the field. The case study introduces patients and follows their progress from dispatch to delivery at the emergency department. The case becomes progressively more detailed as new material is presented. This feature, which includes eight questions per case, is a valuable learning tool that encourages critical thinking skills. Answers and rationales for the case studies appear at the end of each chapter.

Case Study 1 Asthma Attack

Part 1

You unit has been dispatched to a gas station in town for a patient who is struggling to breathe. The attendant called because a car pulled into the station and almost crashed into the front of the mini-mart. When he ran out to see what was happening, he found the driver in the vehicle struggling to breathe.

Upon your arrival and although the police have just arrived, you make sure that the scene is safe. The patient is a man in his early forties who is sitting in the front seat of the vehicle. The driver's side door is open and he has both of his legs outside the vehicle. You do not need to be right next to the patient to hear he is wheezing or to see he is struggling. You quickly grab your first-in bag and proceed to begin the initial assessment on the patient (see **Table 1**). The police officer says the patient's name is Bill but he is barely able to speak more than a word or two at a time. You note that there are a couple of multiple dose inhalers sitting on the front seat of the vehicle.

Table 1 Initial Assessment

Initial Assessment	Recording Time: 1 Minute
General Impression/ Appearance	Middle-aged male, wearing a tee shirt and gym shorts, obviously struggling to breathe
Mental Status	"A" alert (oriented to person, place, and day)
Airway	Open, audible wheezing both inspiratory and expiratory
Breathing	Rapid and shallow, turning pale and blue and only able to speak a word or two at a time
Circulation	Rapid and thready radial pulse, no external bleeding
Priority/Plan	High priority due to severe respiratory distress

As you complete your initial assessment it is clear that this patient is in severe respiratory distress. Apparently he knew it and was attempting to drive himself to the hospital but felt he would not make it so he pulled into the gas station.

Your partner has already placed the patient on a nonrebreathing mask and supplemental oxygen and is getting an albuterol [Proventil, Ventolin] treatment ready. There is also an EMT-B on the scene who you ask to quickly get a set of baseline vital signs and hook up the pulse oximeter. The patient is able to nod his head and blurt out brief answers to your questions although it is clear he is getting very lightheaded and literally wearing himself out.

Question 1: When does a routine asthma attack become a life-threatening asthma attack?

Question 2: Why is this patient so dizzy and appears to be wearing out?

Part 2

A supervisor is now on the scene and has brought the stretcher over to the car where the patient is sitting. You and your partner gently lift the patient over to the stretcher which is now in the semi-Fowler's position. It seems that Bill had tried desperately to use his albuterol [Proventil, Ventolin] many times during his frantic ride in the car. Clearly it has not yet helped. Since Bill is a responsive medical patient, you begin a focused history and physical examination and start by listening to his chest (see **Table 2**). It is difficult to get the OPQRST questions answered because Bill is in so much distress.

You are able to determine that the breathing difficulty began about an hour ago and has gotten progressively worse. He has a history of asthma and a productive cough with green sputum. He thinks all of the coughing today has made him a lot worse.

Bill definitely has that sense of impending doom on his face and only speaks when spoken to. He is concentrating on his breathing, although it is not entirely successful.

Your partner begins getting a quick IV line into Bill as you listen once more to his lungs. He is getting quieter which is not always a good sign. In this

Table 2 Focused History and Physical Examination

Baseline Vital Signs	Recording Time: 5 Minutes
Skin CTC (color, temperature, condition)	Pale and cyanotic, warm, clammy
Pulse	Radial pulse of 136 beats/min, regular, and thready
Blood Pressure	146/88 mm Hg
Respirations	32 breaths/min, labored and shallow

Case Study ANSWERS

Case Study 1 Asthma Attack

Question 1: When does a routine asthma attack become a life-threatening asthma attack?

Answer 1: When it cannot be broken with simple bronchodilators and continues to exist causing the patient to become hypercarbic and/or hypoxic. The term "status asthmaticus" has been used in the past to refer to a life-threatening asthma attack.

Question 2: Why is this patient so dizzy and appears to be wearing out?

Answer 2: As the attack worsens the patient retains CO_2, becomes acidotic and hypoxic, and because of increased insensible water loss also becomes dehydrated. The patient will complain of lightheadedness or dizziness, with increasing fatigue. The work of breathing consumes all available energy and literally wears out the patient.

Question 3: Why do we sometimes ask the patient if they have ever required a "breathing tube" or to be intubated to treat their asthma?

Answer 3: If a patient has previously been intubated, that was definitely a significant and serious attack and the patient will remember the incident. They can also give you some subjective assessment of how today's symptoms compare to that prior event. Other significant historic points specifically related to understanding how severe an asthma attack is and how much therapy early on the patient may require include their last use of steroids to manage an attack, last ED visit for asthma, and last time hospitalized for asthma.

Question 4: How serious is the asthma problem in the US?

Answer 4: In the US, asthma is a disease that affects more than 17 million people, a third of whom are children. Asthma is the most common chronic disease in children, accounting for considerable school absences. Approximately 5,000 patients die from asthma yearly.

Question 5: What is the significance of the patient being on steroids for his disease?

Answer 5: Most physicians do not like to prescribe steroids, especially for lengthy periods of time. They are very effective at reducing the inflammation that comes with lower airway diseases. If the patient is on a steroid and has been for quite some time, that is a "red flag" that this patient has a very serious condition and should be handled as such. Remember, patients can and do die from asthma attacks!

Question 6: Why are you giving him additional steroids?

Answer 6: Because they are effective in fighting the inflammation and secretions that are clogging up his lower airways. Regardless of route of administration, they take time to work (anywhere from 2 to 24 hours), so starting to administer in the prehospital setting is an important part of this patient's care.

Question 7: What is the purpose of administering a steroid in the prehospital setting?

Answer 7: It is important to administer a steroid (glucocorticoid as opposed to mineralocorticoid) to deal with the attack. All steroids take some time to work so they should be started in the prehospital setting to get them "on-board." It really does not matter which specific steroid is used by your EMS system (ie, dexamethasone sodium phosphate [Decadron], methylprednisolone sodium succinate [Solu-Medrol], hydrocortisone sodium phosphate [Solu-Cortef], methylprednisolone acetate [Depo-Medrol], or prednisone [Prednisone Intensol, Sterapred, Sterapred DS]).

Question 8: If the patient was intubated, how does that affect their hospital care?

Answer 8: Asthmatics receiving mechanical ventilation are at serious risk of developing barotrauma. They tend to be very hyperinflated because of expiratory bronchiole collapse, and require careful attention to furnishing adequate expiratory time during the breathing cycle to allow for as complete an exhalation as possible. Failure to do so results in a phenomenon called "breath stacking" also known as "auto-peep." This puts the patient at exceptional risk of developing a pneumothorax, which would progress rapidly into tension given that the patient is also receiving positive-pressure ventilation. Respiratory patients who are serious enough to require prehospital intubation will need to be weaned off the respirator. This could take days to a week and there is always the possibility of pneumonia developing in the intubated patient.

Vital Vocabulary

Key terms are easily identified and defined. A comprehensive list follows each chapter.

Physiology Tips

Tie concepts into practice.

Endocrine Emergencies **Chapter 6**

adrenalin insufficiency is also referred to as Addison disease. Addison disease is a rare condition in which the adrenal glands produce an inadequate amount of adrenal hormones.

Cushing syndrome is hypersecretion of adrenal hormones and is caused by an excess of cortisol production by the adrenal glands or by excessive use of cortisol or other similar steroid hormones.

Neither of these conditions is managed with medications in the prehospital setting. Supportive care and consultation with Medical Direction are usually the most appropriate actions.

Conditions of the Pancreas

The pancreas is the gland that is responsible for secreting insulin. Insulin is the essential chemical that makes it possible for the glucose in the bloodstream to enter the cells of the body. Diabetes mellitus (DM) is a chronic endocrine disease caused by a decreased secretion action of the hormone insulin. Hyperglycemia is an elevation of the blood glucose level above normal. Hyperosmolar hyperglycemia nonketotic coma (HHNC) is insulin deficiency that leads to hyperglycemia without ketones and acidosis. Diabetic ketoacidosis (DKA) is a metabolic condition consisting of hyperglycemia, dehydration, and the accumulation of ketones and ketoacids. Hypoglycemia is a decrease in the blood glucose level to the point where it results in symptoms that can quickly become life-threatening. Because diabetic patients are often managed in both the prehospital as well as in the in-hospital setting, the entire next section of this text expands on the emergencies that can occur with a diabetic patient and how you should manage them in the field.

Diabetic Patients

When you encounter a patient with diabetes mellitus, you are expected to integrate the pathophysiological principals of this disease with your patient's assessment findings to help formulate a field impression. Once this is done, you should then proceed to implement a treatment plan for the patient having a diabetic emergency. Therefore, it is essential to understand the pathophysiology of the diabetic emergencies such as hypoglycemia, hyperosmolar hyperglycemia nonketotic coma (HHNC), hyperosmolar nonketotic coma (HONK), hyperglycemia, and diabetic ketoacidosis.

Diabetes mellitus is a disease with lifelong implications on the health of the patient. There are three forms of the disease that affect the body's ability to balance the carbohydrate needs of the cells with the endocrine hormone insulin. Insulin is manufactured in the pancreas and is responsible for helping carbohydrates in the form of glucose enter the cells (**Figure 6-1**). It works like the key to your car. Your car may be sitting in the driveway but without the key you simply cannot go any place with the car. Without a sufficient amount of functional insulin available, the glucose in a patient's bloodstream will not enter the cells. Insulin therefore works to keep blood glucose levels at a relatively stable and low level. By promoting carbohydrate metabolism, insulin also blocks fat metabolism, thereby preventing the breakdown of fat tissue in the body. Glucagon and epinephrine, so-called "stress hormones," have the opposite effect, resulting in increased circulating blood glucose. Glucagon, a protein hormone produced in the pancreas, stimulates an increase in glucose in the blood by stimulating the breakdown of glycogen to glucose. During a diabetic emergency, glucagon is often administered by a family member SC or IM prior to the arrival of EMS. It works by stimulating the liver to release glycogen stores which in turn results in increased blood glucose levels.

Types of Diabetes Mellitus

As mentioned above, there are three "types" of diabetes: type 1 (commonly referred to as juvenile-onset diabetes), type 2 (commonly referred to as adult-onset diabetes), and gestational diabetes. The type 1 (insulin-dependent DM) diabetic has a pancreas that cannot produce insulin. These patients have to monitor their blood glucose levels very closely throughout the day and inject themselves with insulin. The type 2 diabetic (non-insulin-dependent DM) has a pancreas that produces insulin but that is relatively nonfunctional, resulting in a state of so-called insulin resistance. Also, cell surface insulin receptors in a type 2 diabetic can, over time, develop resistance to one's own insulin, resulting in the progression of non-insulin-dependence. The net effect is the same as in the case of a type 1 patient. Most of the time a patient with type 2 diabetes can control his or her glucose/insulin balance through a combination of oral antidiabetic medications and an appropriate diet. Many times insulin resistance is a function of advancing age and/or obesity. The patient with gestational diabetes mellitus (GDM) is a pregnant woman who develops all the symptoms of diabetes during pregnancy. In most

A hypoglycemic patient may experience permanent cell damage from remaining unconscious, with an altered LOC, for an extended period of time. Be ready to act quickly.

Renal and Urologic Emergencies **Chapter 8** 267

Physiology Tip

Because patients in chronic renal failure already have serum electrolyte imbalances, be conservative with the treatment plan.

Chronic Renal Failure

Chronic renal failure is progressive and irreversible inadequate kidney function due to permanent loss of nephrons, the structural and functional units of the kidneys that form urine. Chronic renal failure can occur from any renal dysfunction, most commonly diabetic neuropathy. Uremia, severe hyperkalemia, and CHF are life-threatening conditions associated with chronic renal failure. Uremia is a toxic condition that occurs when nitrogenous substances that are normally excreted in the urine are retained owing to renal insufficiency. Hyperkalemia is caused by the failure of the kidneys to excrete potassium adequately. This condition can develop in end-stage renal failure when a scheduled dialysis is delayed. When severe hyperkalemia develops, ECG findings include peaked T waves, prolonged P-R interval, QRS widening, and, eventually, ventricular fibrillation. CHF is most commonly a result of sodium and fluid retention.

Management of Chronic Renal Failure

Uremia requires renal dialysis or kidney transplantation. Calcium chloride or calcium gluconate may be helpful to treat severe hyperkalemia before dialysis to counteract toxic effects of the excessive potassium to the cardiac membrane. Diuretics are usually effective, and angiotensin-converting enzyme (ACE) inhibitors can be used if left ventricular function is depressed. The treatment of chronic renal failure is similar to that for ARF in that it includes management of the ABCs, administration of high-flow oxygen, and provision of ventilatory support with a bag-mask device as needed. Consider administration of an IV bolus of normal saline if there are signs of shock but no signs of pulmonary edema. Treatment should focus on the regulation of fluid imbalances and cardiovascular function. If hypotension occurs, a vasopressor may be administered or medical control may order the administration of sodium bicarbonate. Patients with chronic renal failure will ultimately require dialysis (**Table 8-2**).

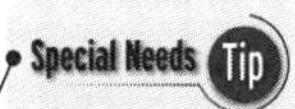

Be prepared to adjust the dose and frequency of medication administration for elderly people. Because the kidneys and the liver are the primary routes of drug elimination, age-related changes in the functions of these organs can have a major impact on the effects of the drugs.

Table 8-2 Medical Emergencies in Dialysis Patients

Problem	Prehospital Management
Problems related to dialysis itself:	
Hypotension	Give 50 mL of normal saline IV
Hemorrhage from the shunt	If the shunt cannot be reconnected, clamp it off; check for signs of shock
Potassium imbalance	For hypokalemia: treat bradycardia with atropine For hyperkalemia: calcium and bicarbonate may be considered
Disequilibrium syndrome	Supportive treatment only
Air embolism	Left lateral recumbent position in about 10° of head-down tilt
Machine dysfunction	Turn off machine; clamp ends of shunt; disconnect patient from machine; transport
Problems to which dialysis patients are more vulnerable:	
Congestive heart failure	Oxygen; sitting position; rapid transport to dialysis facility
Myocardial infarction and cardiac dysrhythmias	Treat as any other patient, but use caution in administering any medications
Hypertension	Transport only; the treatment is dialysis
Pericardial tamponade	Emergency transport as soon as detected
Uremic pericarditis	Oxygen; position of comfort; transport
Subdural hematoma	Oxygen; urgent transport

Safety Tips

Reinforce safety concerns for both the paramedic and the patient.

Special Needs Tips

Highlight specific concerns for the elderly and/or pediatric patient.

Medication Review

The indications, contraindications, and dosage and administration information is provided at the end of each chapter for the drugs discussed within the chapter.

Prep Kit

End of chapter resources reinforce important concepts with a chapter summary and a comprehensive list of vital vocabulary.

Medication Review

Albuterol (Proventil, Ventolin)

Indications Treatment of bronchospasm in patients with reversible obstructive airway disease (COPD/asthma). Prevention of exercise-induced bronchospasm.

Contraindications Known prior hypersensitivity reactions to albuterol. Tachycardia arrhythmias, especially those caused by digitalis. Synergistic with other sympathomimetics.

Dosage and administration Adult: Administer 2.5 mg (0.5 mL of the 0.5% solution) added to 2 mL of normal saline for inhalation by nebulizer treatment and administer over 10–15 minutes. May repeat every 20 minutes up to three times. MDI: 1–2 inhalations (90–180 µg). Five minutes between inhalations. Pediatric: (between the ages of 2 and 12) administer 2.5 mg (0.5 mL of the 0.083% solution) added to 2 mL of normal saline for inhalation by nebulizer treatment and administer over 10–15 minutes. May repeat every 20 minutes up to three times.

Dexamethasone Sodium Phosphate (Decadron, Hexadrol)

Indications Anaphylaxis, asthma, croup.

Contraindications Hypersensitivity to product, systemic sepsis, bacterial infection.

Dosage and administration Adult: 10–100 mg IV (1 mg/kg slow IV bolus) (considerable variance through medical control). Pediatric: 0.25–1.0 mg/kg/dose IV, IO, IM.

Diphenhydramine (Benadryl)

Indications Symptomatic relief of allergies, allergic reactions, anaphylaxis, acute dystonic reactions (phenothiazines). Blood administration reactions; used for motion sickness, hay fever.

Contraindications Asthma, glaucoma, pregnancy, hypertension, narrow-angle glaucoma, infants, patients taking monoamine oxidase inhibitors (MAOIs).

Dosage and administration Adult: 25–50 mg IM or IV or PO. Pediatric: 1–2 mg/kg IV, IO slowly or IM. If given PO, 5 mg/kg/24 hours.

Dopamine (Intropin)

Indications Cardiogenic, septic, or spinal shock, hypotension with low cardiac output states, distributive shock.

Contraindications Hypovolemic shock, pheochromocytoma, tachyarrhythmias, V-fib.

Dosage and administration Adult: 2–20 µg/kg/min titrated to patient response. Pediatric: 2–20 µg/kg/min titrated to patient response.

Epinephrine (Adrenalin)

Indications Cardiac arrest (V-fib/pulseless V-tach, asystole, PEA), symptomatic bradycardia as an alternative infusion to dopamine, severe hypotension secondary to bradycardia when atropine and transcutaneous pacing are unsuccessful, allergic reactions, anaphylaxis, asthma.

Contraindications Hypertension, hypothermia, pulmonary edema, myocardial ischemia, hypovolemic shock.

Dosage and administration Adult: Mild allergic reactions and asthma: 0.3–0.5 mg (0.3–0.5 mL of 1:1,000) SC. Anaphylaxis: 0.1 mg (1 mL of 1:10,000) IV/IO over 5 minutes. Cardiac arrest: IV/IO dose: 1 mg (10 mL of 1:10,000 solution) every 3–5 minutes during resuscitation. Follow each dose with 20 mL flush and elevate arm for 10 to 20 seconds after dose. Higher dose: Higher doses (up to 0.2 mg/kg) may be used for specific indications (beta-blocker or calcium channel blocker overdose). Continuous infusion: Add 1 mg (1 mL of 1:1,000 solution) to 500 mL normal saline or D_5W. Initial infusion rate of 1 µg/min titrated to effect (typical dose: 2–10 µg/min). Endotracheal (ET) dose: 2–2.5 mg diluted in 10 mL normal saline. Profound bradycardia or hypotension: 2–10 µg/min; titrate to patient response. Pediatric: Mild allergic reactions and asthma: 0.01 mg/kg (0.01 mL/kg) of 1:1,000 solution SC (maximum of 0.3 mL). Cardiac arrest: IV/IO dose: 0.01 mg/kg (0.1 mL/kg) of 1:10,000 solution every 3–5 minutes during arrest. All endotracheal (ET) doses: 0.1 mg/kg (0.1 mL/kg) of 1:1,000 solution. Symptomatic bradycardia: IV/IO dose: 0.01 mg/kg (0.1 mL/kg) of 1:10,000 solution. Continuous IV/IO infusion: Begin with rapid infusion, then titrate to response. Typical initial infusion: 0.1–1 µg/min. Higher doses may be effective.

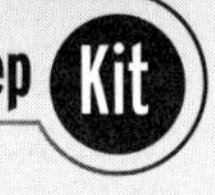

Prep Kit

Chapter Summary

- Assessment of the patient having an allergic reaction will reveal various signs and symptoms from mild to severe.
- Signs that indicate that a patient may be experiencing a mild allergic reaction include localized itching or swelling, redness, or rash.
- The key signs that can indicate a patient may be having a severe, or anaphylactic, reaction are altered mental status; respiratory distress often involving airway swelling, wheezing, and chest tightness; and/or hypoperfusion.
- The primary treatment in anaphylaxis is the injection of the hormone epinephrine [Adrenalin].
- The SAMPLE history includes "allergies" and "medications." An example of a home medication many patients take that may precipitate an adverse reaction is cimetidine [Tagamet], commonly taken for GI disorders.
- Cimetidine [Tagamet] has an extensive drug interaction list, particularly with antiarrhythmics (ie, amiodarone, lidocaine, phenytoin, procainamide hydrochloride, and quinidine) and may also increase the likelihood of toxic effects of theophylline and cyclosporine.
- Patients with known allergies are treated in three ways. First, they are educated about how to avoid exposure; second, they may be given a variety of medications to use at home, including oral and intranasal antihistamines, inhaled bronchodilators, and inhaled or intranasal steroids; and third, immunotherapy via desensitization is performed by gradually increasing the amount of offending allergen the body receives so that the immune system can learn to defend itself against that specific allergen.
- The common causes of anaphylactic reactions include animals, insect stings, foods, latex, immunotherapy (such as in skin testing), and drugs.

Vital Vocabulary

Allergic reaction A hypersensitivity reaction to an antigen.

Anaphylactic reaction Also called anaphylaxis; an IgE-medicated hypersensitivity reaction involving bronchoconstriction and cardiovascular collapse in the case of anaphylactic shock.

Angioedema Localized tissue edema caused by an allergic-like process.

Antibodies Substances that destroy or neutralize antigens.

Antigen A substance that produces an immune response.

Desensitization Also called hyposensitization; a process of exposing a patient to the offending antigen in small increments in an effort to minimize systemic immune response to the antigen.

Histamine A chemical substance that causes blood vessels to dilate and become leaky and promotes increased production of mucus in the respiratory tract.

Immunoglobulins A family of proteins with specific functions in the immune system.

Immunoglobulin E (IgE) One of the five major classes of immunoglobulins that is present primarily in the skin and mucous membranes.

Mast cells Basophils that are located in the tissues.

Instructor Resources

Instructor's ToolKit CD-ROM

ISBN: 0-7637-5211-8

Preparing for class is easy with the resources found on this CD-ROM, including:

- **PowerPoint Presentations**—Providing you with a powerful way to make presentations that are educational and engaging to your students. The slides can be modified to meet your needs.
- **Lecture Outlines**—Providing you with complete, ready-to-use lesson plans that outline all of the topics covered in the text. The lesson plans can be modified to meet your needs.
- **Image Bank**—Providing you with a selection of images found in the text. You can use them to incorporate more images into the PowerPoint presentation, make handouts, or enlarge a specific image for further discussion.
- **Test Bank**—Providing you with multiple-choice general knowledge and critical thinking questions similar to those found on national certification exams.

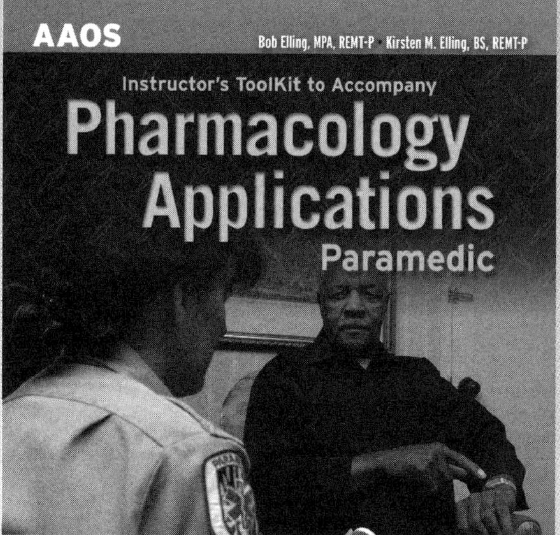

The resources on the Instructor's ToolKit CD-ROM that accompanies this text have been formatted so that instructors can seamlessly integrate them into the most popular course administration tools. Please feel free to contact Jones and Bartlett technical support at any time with questions.

Student Resources

PharmaFlash Cards

ISBN: 978-0-7637-6913-0

These handy flash cards will help paramedic students learn the pertinent information about each medication they will use in the field. The front of each card features the name of the medication along with a pronunciation key. On the back of each card, students will find indications, contraindications, and doses for that drug.

Technology Resources

Paramedic.EMSzone.com

- **Online Chapter Pretests**—Prepare students for training with instant results and feedback on incorrect answers.
- **Vocabulary Explorer**—Interactive online glossary to expand student's medical vocabulary.
- **Animated Flash Cards**—Review vital vocabulary and key concepts.

Acknowledgments

Series Editor

Andrew N. Pollak, MD, FAAOS
Medical Director, Baltimore County Fire Department
Associate Professor, University of Maryland School of Medicine
Baltimore, Maryland

Medical Reviewer

Jonathan S. Halpert, MD, FACEP, REMT-P
Medical Director
Prime Care Physicians PLLC
Albany, New York

Reviewers

Rick Anderson, MS, EMT-P
Mid-State Technical College
Wisconsin Rapids, Wisconsin

Robert Bernini, REMT-P
Harrisburg Area Community College
Harrisburg, Pennsylvania

Christopher Black, Division Chief
Gila River Emergency Medical Services
Sacaton, Arizona

Art Breault, RN, NREMT-P
Albany Medical Center Hospital—Department of Emergency Medicine
Albany, New York

Deborah A. Clapp, BA, I/C, EMT-P
Massachusetts Department of Public Health—EMS for Children Project
Boston, Massachusetts

Heather Davis, MS, NREMT-P
UCLA-Daniel Freeman Paramedic Education Program
Inglewood, California

Daryl Doering, BA, EMT-P
Inver Hills Community College
Inver Grove Heights, Minnesota

Andy Fox, NREMT-P
Bulverde-Spring Branch Emergency Medical Services
Kerrville, Texas

Lee Gillum, MPH, LP, EMS-CC
Montgomery County Hospital District Emergency Medical Services
Conroe, Texas

John Gosford
Lake City Community College
Lake City, Florida

Rick Hilinski, BA, EMT-P
Community College of Allegheny County—Public Safety Institute
Pittsburgh, Pennsylvania

Jonathan Hockman, EMSIC, NREMT-P, AHA-Instructor
Goldrush Consulting Services
Livonia, Michigan

Jay Keefauver, President
National Academy for Prehospital Care, LLC
Fremont, Nebraska

Richard T. Koch Sr., NREMT-P
Cecil County Department of Emergency Services
Elkton, Maryland

Jon Levine, EMT-P, I/C
EMS Training LTD
South Weymouth, Massachusetts

Judy Levy, BSN, RN, NREMT-P, EMSI
TriHealth—Bethesda Paramedic Training Program
Cincinnati, Ohio

John Lewis, M.ED, NREMT-P
Brigham Young University—Idaho
Rexburg, Idaho

Brittany Ann Martinelli, MHSC, BSRT-NPS, NREMT-P
Sante Fe College
Gainesville, Florida

Dr. Chris Nollette, NREMT-P, LP
Riverside Community College District—Ben Clark Public Safety Training Center
Moreno Valley, California

Frank S. Nuqui, EMT-P, CIC
LaGuardia Community College
Long Island City, New York

Guy Peifer, BS, NREMT-P, CIC/RF
Borough of Manhattan Community College
New York, New York

Timothy J. Perkins, BS, EMT-P
Virginia Department of Health—Office of Emergency Medical Services
Richmond, Virginia

Robert C. Salinas, MD (CAQ-G)
The University of Oklahoma—College of Medicine
Oklahoma City, Oklahoma

Kent R. Spitler, RN, MSEd, NREMT-P, CPP
Gaston College—Department for Emergency Medical Services Education
Dallas, North Carolina

William Sugiyama, NREMT-P, RN, BSL
Alameda County Emergency Medical Services
San Leandro, California

Sherm Syverson, BS, NREMT-P
F-M Ambulance Service—Emergency Medical Education Center
Fargo, North Dakota

Lance Villers, PhD, EMT-P
The University of Texas Health Science Center at San Antonio—Department of Emergency Health Sciences
San Antonio, Texas

Matt Zukosky, MA, NREMT-P
Suffolk County Community College
Selden, New York

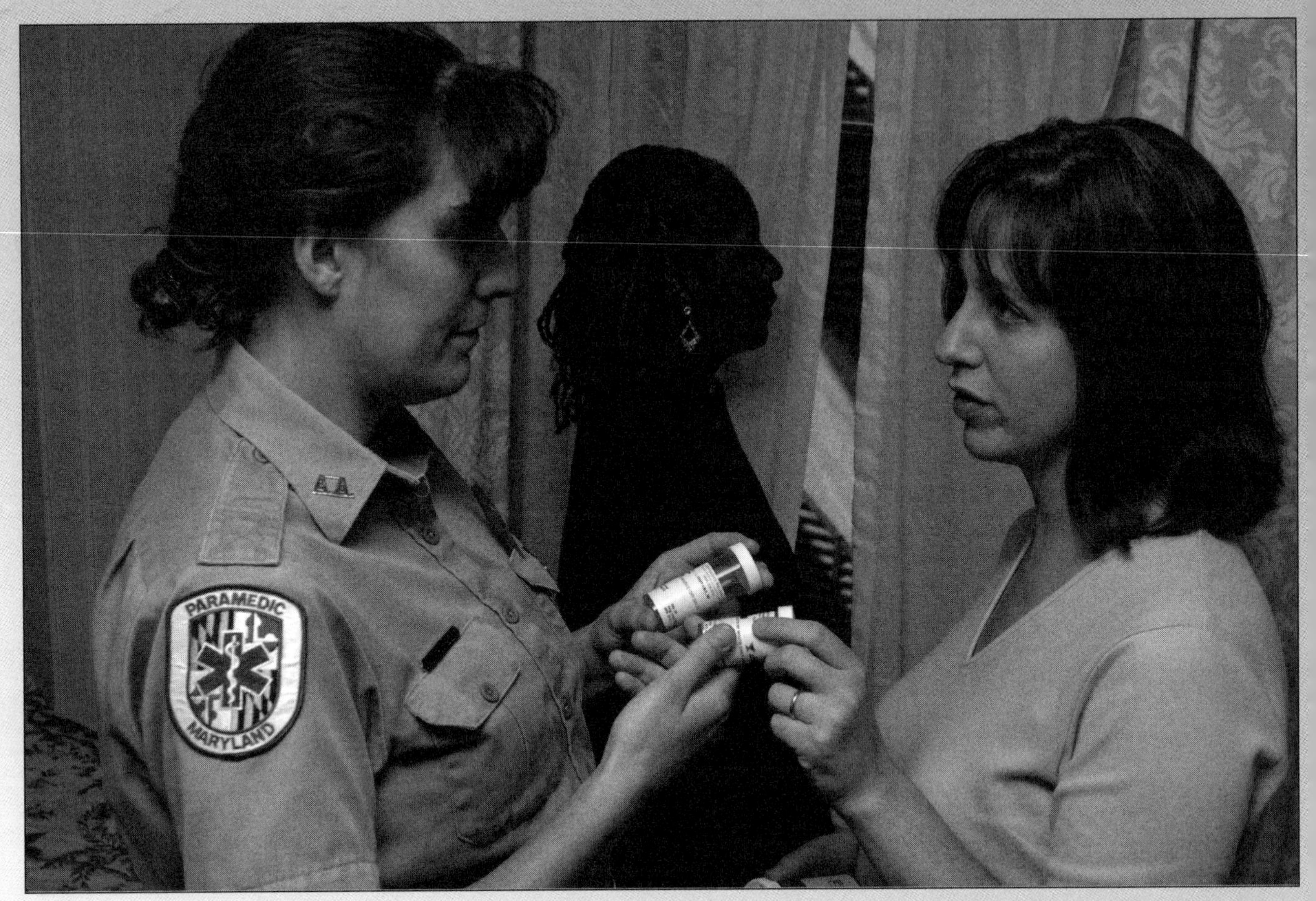
PARAMEDIC
MARYLAND

General Pharmacology and Medication Administration

1

Objectives

Cognitive

1-7.1 Describe historical trends in pharmacology. (page 5)

1-7.2 Differentiate among the chemical, generic (nonproprietary), and trade (proprietary) names of a drug. (page 8)

1-7.3 List the four main sources of drug products. (pages 8–9)

1-7.4 Describe how drugs are classified. (page 9)

1-7.5 List the authoritative sources for drug information. (page 10)

1-7.6 List legislative acts controlling drug use and abuse in the United States. (page 5)

1-7.7 Differentiate among Schedule I, II, III, IV, and V substances. (pages 5–6)

1-7.8 List examples of substances in each schedule. (page 6)

1-7.9 Discuss standardization of drugs. (pages 6–7)

1-7.10 Discuss investigational drugs, including the Food and Drug Administration (FDA) approval process and the FDA classifications for newly approved drugs. (pages 6–8)

1-7.11 Discuss special consideration in drug treatment with regard to pregnant, pediatric and geriatric patients. (pages 16–17)

1-7.12 Discuss the paramedic's responsibilities and scope of management pertinent to the administration of medications. (pages 17–18)

1-7.13 Review the specific anatomy and physiology pertinent to pharmacology with additional attention to autonomic pharmacology. (pages 10–22)

1-7.14 List and describe general properties of drugs. (pages 10–11)

1-7.15 List and describe liquid and solid drug forms. (page 15)

1-7.16 List and differentiate routes of drug administration. (pages 15–16)

1-7.17 Differentiate between enteral and parenteral routes of drug administration. (page 15)

1-7.18 Describe mechanisms of drug action. (page 11)

1-7.19 List and differentiate the phases of drug activity, including the pharmaceutical, pharmacokinetic, and pharmacodynamic phases. (pages 10–11)

1-7.20 Describe the process called pharmacokinetics, pharmacodynamics, including theories of drug action, drug-response relationship, factors altering drug responses, predictable drug responses, iatrogenic drug responses, and unpredictable adverse drug responses. (pages 10–15)

1-7.21 Differentiate among drug interactions. (pages 13–15)

1-7.22 Discuss considerations for storing and securing medications. (pages 17–18)

1-7.23 List the component of a drug profile by classification. (pages 8–10)

1-7.24 List and describe drugs that the paramedic may administer according to local protocol. (page 17)

1-7.25 Integrate pathophysiological principles of pharmacology with patient assessment. (pages 10–22)

1-7.26 Synthesize patient history information and assessment findings to form a field impression. (page 18)

1-7.27 Synthesize a field impression to implement a pharmacologic management plan. (page 18)

1-7.28 Assess the pathophysiology of a patient's condition by identifying classifications of drugs. (pages 8–10)

1-8.1 Review the specific anatomy and physiology pertinent to medication administration. (pages 8–15)

1-8.8 Describe the indications, equipment needed, technique used, precautions, and general principles of peripheral venous or external jugular cannulation. (page 21)

1-8.9 Describe the indications, equipment needed, technique used, precautions, and general principles of intraosseous needle placement and infusion. (pages 21–22, 27–28)

1-8.10 Discuss legal aspects affecting medication administration. (pages 34–35)

1-8.11 Discuss the "six rights" of drug administration and correlate these with the principles of medication administration. (pages 34–35)

1-8.12 Discuss medical asepsis and the differences between clean and sterile techniques. (pages 36–37)

1-8.13 Describe use of antiseptics and disinfectants. (pages 36–37)

1-8.14 Describe the use of universal precautions and body substance isolation (BSI) procedures when administering a medication. (pages 36–37)

1-8.15 Differentiate among the different dosage forms of oral medications. (page 19)

1-8.16 Describe the equipment needed and general principles of administering oral medications. (page 19)

1-8.17 Describe the indications, equipment needed, techniques used, precautions, and general principles of administering medications by the inhalation route. (pages 15–16, 33–34)

1-8.18 Describe the indications, equipment needed, techniques used, precautions, and general principles of administering medications by the gastric tube. (pages 19, 23–25)

1-8.19 Describe the indications, equipment needed, techniques used, precautions, and general principles of rectal medication administration. (pages 19, 25)

1-8.20 Differentiate among the different parenteral routes of medication administration. (pages 19, 25–30)

1-8.21 Describe the equipment needed, techniques used, complications, and general principles for the preparation and administration of parenteral medications. (pages 19, 25–30)

1-8.22 Differentiate among the different percutaneous routes of medication administration. (pages 30–32)

1-8.23 Describe the purpose, equipment needed, techniques used, complications, and general principles for obtaining a blood sample. (page 23)

1-8.24 Describe disposal of contaminated items and sharps. (pages 36–37)

1-8.25 Synthesize a pharmacologic management plan including medication administration. (pages 17–22)

1-8.26 Integrate pathophysiological principles of medication administration with patient management. (pages 17–22)

Affective

1-7.29 Serve as a model for obtaining a history by identifying classifications of drugs. (pages 35–36)

1-7.30 Defend the administration of drugs by a paramedic to affect positive therapeutic affects. (page 37)

1-7.31 Advocate drug education through identification of drug classifications. (pages 8–10)

1-8.27 Comply with paramedic standards of medication administration. (pages 17–18)

1-8.28 Comply with universal precautions and body substance isolation (BSI). (pages 36–37)

1-8.29 Defend a pharmacologic management plan for medication administration. (page 37)

1-8.30 Serve as a model for medical asepsis. (pages 36–37)

1-8.31 Serve as a model for advocacy while performing medication administration. (page 37)

1-8.32 Serve as a model for disposing contaminated items and sharps. (pages 36–37)

Psychomotor

1-8.33 Use universal precautions and body substance isolation (BSI) procedures during medication administration. (pages 36–37)

1-8.34 Demonstrate cannulation of peripheral or external jugular veins. (pages 25–30)

1-8.35 Demonstrate intraosseous needle placement and infusion. (pages 27–28)

1-8.36 Demonstrate clean technique during medication administration. (pages 36–37)

1-8.37 Demonstrate administration of oral medications. (page 23)

1-8.38 Demonstrate administration of medications by the inhalation route. (pages 33–34)

1-8.39 Demonstrate administration of medications by the gastric tube. (pages 23–25)

1-8.40 Demonstrate rectal administration of medications. (page 25)

1-8.41 Demonstrate preparation and administration of parenteral medications. (pages 25–30)

1-8.42 Demonstrate preparation and techniques for obtaining a blood sample. (page 23)

1-8.43 Perfect disposal of contaminated items and sharps. (pages 36–37)

Additional Objectives

1-1 List ILCOR's five classifications of recommendations. (pages 9–10)

1-2 Discuss the types of drug receptors. (pages 10–15)

1-3 Define the terms routinely used to describe the effects of drugs such as: hypersensitivity, half-life, habituation, cumulative effect, adverse reaction, side effect, idiosyncracy, and tolerance. (pages 13–15)

1-4 List the steps in the procedure for the following parenteral medication administration routes: IV, IO, SC, IM, and intranasal. (pages 25–30)

1-5 List the steps in the procedure for the following enteral medication administration routes: oral, gastric, and rectal. (pages 23–25)

Historical Milestones and Standards for Drugs

Pharmacology is the study of (*ology*) of drugs or medications (*pharm*). In the minds of the general public, the term "drugs" often conjures up negative images; the term tends to be associated with societal ills that result from "street" drugs or those that are illicitly manufactured. This is why paramedics usually do not ask an elderly patient, when taking a SAMPLE history, "Do you take drugs?" Health care providers typically use the terms "medications," "medicines," or "meds" to describe the over-the-counter (OTC) or prescribed (Rx) medications a patient may be taking. **Medication** is a licensed drug taken to cure or reduce symptoms of an illness or medical condition or as an aid in diagnosis, treatment, or prevention of a disease or other abnormal condition. To be complete, the history of a patient's medication or drug use should include each of the following five types:

1. Over-the-counter remedies
2. Prescribed medications
3. Herbals
4. Vitamins
5. Illicit or "recreational drugs"

Because this text is directed at EMS professionals and other health care providers, the terms drugs, medicines, and medications will be used interchangeably, and readers should presume that all five types of drugs are included.

New drugs are coming on the market all the time that offer health benefits and successful treatments of medical conditions. EMS providers need to be aware of the dangers of drug use—such as with patients who have good intentions but who use their medications inappropriately and thus experience a harmful effect. In these instances, the patient is using the medication contrary to its desired use or indications. Thus every drug has its *indications* as well as its *contraindications*, which will be discussed in detail throughout this text as well as in the paramedic formulary in the appendix. The history of pharmacology includes many legislative milestones put in place to control, regulate, and make substances safer for the users. The following is a brief history, including a list of legislative acts and manufacturing related regulations that were intended to help control the inappropriate use of drugs and to standardize the forms of drugs that are available in the United States:

- Prior to the 1900s, many people were injured by, became addicted to, or died because of certain ingredients contained in medications and remedies.
- The *Pure Food and Drug Act* of 1906 was the first law to protect the public from impure or mislabeled drugs. It did not deal with safety or effectiveness issues. The *U.S. Pharmacopeia (USP)* and the *National Formulary (NF)* were designated as the official standards, which the federal government had the authority to enforce.
- The *Shirley Amendment* of 1912 prohibited fraudulent **therapeutic** claims.
- The *Harrison Narcotic Act* of 1914 was the first law passed that controlled the sales of narcotics and drugs causing dependence.
- The *Federal Food, Drug, and Cosmetic Act* of 1938 was designed to ensure drug testing, safety, and accuracy of the list of ingredients and a drug's directions for use.
- The *Kefauver-Harris Amendment* of 1962 required proof of safety and efficacy prior to a new drug being approved for use.
- The *Comprehensive Drug Abuse Prevention and Control Act* of 1970 superseded the *Harrison Narcotic Act* and set forth the rules for the manufacture and distribution of drugs with the potential for abuse. This *Controlled Substances Act* is the legal foundation of the government's fight against the abuse of drugs and other substances. This law is a consolidation of numerous laws that regulate the manufacture and distribution of narcotics, **stimulants**, depressants, hallucinogens, anabolic steroids, and chemicals used in the illicit production of controlled substances. The regulatory agency is the DEA (Drug Enforcement Agency). Drugs are classified into five categories or "schedules" (**Table 1-1 ▸**).
- The *Orphan Drug Act* of 1983 was enacted by the Food and Drug Administration (FDA) to provide incentives for drug companies to research drugs to treat rare or chronic diseases.
- In 2006, the Institute of Medicine's (IOM) report discussed the culture of patient safety in America. Medication administration is a fundamental tenet of that important discussion and this document is likely to be the catalyst for improvements in the rules, regulations, and policies over the next decade.

Each of the enacted laws, and their respective regulations, have helped to standardize the units, packaging, and information provided about the drugs that are available in the U.S. Legislation has helped to guarantee the standardization of doses so that when a patient is given a specific amount or dose of a medication with a stated amount of active ingredient, they will in fact receive that actual amount, no more or no less. The Consumer Product Safety Commission, as well as the FDA, have been partners or advocates in the most progressive legislation.

Table 1-1 Controlled Substance Schedules

Schedule	Specifics about Substances that Fit this Schedule	Examples
I	■ High abuse potential. ■ No currently accepted medical use in treatment in the United States. ■ Lack of accepted safety for use of the drug or other substance under medical supervision.	Heroin, LSD, marijuana, methaqualone, and psychedelics
II	■ High abuse potential. ■ Currently accepted medical use in treatment in the United States or a currently accepted medical use with severe restrictions. ■ Abuse may lead to severe psychological or physical dependence.	Morphine, PCP, cocaine, codeine, methadone, methamphetamine, **barbiturates**, **opioids**, and stimulants
III	■ Less abuse potential than the Schedule I and II drugs. ■ Currently accepted medical use in treatment in the United States. ■ Abuse may lead to moderate or low physical dependence or high psychological dependence.	Anabolic steroids, aspirin or Tylenol combined with codeine or hydrocodone, some barbiturates, stimulants, and preparations containing limited opioids
IV	■ Less abuse potential than Schedule III drugs. ■ Currently accepted medical use in treatment in the United States. ■ Abuse may lead to limited physical dependence or psychological dependence relative to the drugs or other substances in Schedule III.	Darvon, Talwin, Equanil, Valium, Xanax, barbiturates, **benzodiazepines**, steroids, stimulants, and others
V	■ Lower abuse potential than Schedule IV drugs. ■ Currently accepted medical use in treatment in the United States. ■ Abuse may lead to limited physical dependence or psychological dependence relative to the drugs or other substances in Schedule IV.	OTC cough medicines and anti-diarrheal medications containing limited quantities of opioids, such as dextromethorphan

The Role of the Food and Drug Administration (FDA)

In the United States, if a substance is considered a drug, it falls under the regulation of the Food and Drug Administration (FDA). The mission statement of the FDA on its website is: "The FDA is responsible for protecting the public health by assuring the safety, efficacy, and security of human and veterinary drugs, biological products, medical devices, our nation's food supply, cosmetics, and products that emit radiation. The FDA is also responsible for advancing the public health by helping to speed innovations that make medicines and foods more effective, safer, and more affordable; and helping the public get the accurate, science-based information they need to use medicines and foods to improve their health."

The FDA does not actually develop, manufacture, or test drugs. Drug manufacturers must submit reports of a drug's studies so that the FDA's Center for Drug Evaluation and Research (CDER) can evaluate its data. The studies must answer the question: "Does this drug work for the proposed use?" By analyzing the data, CDER reviewers assess the benefit-to-risk relationship and determine if the drug will be approved.

The FDA works with pharmaceutical companies to ensure that all drugs marketed in the United States meet specifications for identity, strength, quality, purity, and potency. Before approving a **generic drug** product, or a medication that is not patented, CDER requires many rigorous tests and procedures to ensure that the generic versions of a drug can be substituted for the brand or trade name drug.

In 2004, the FDA announced a series of steps designed to strengthen and improve the management of drug safety issues. In fact, safety is the central focus of the FDA's regulatory work. This effort is of vital importance to the health of the public and to the mission of the FDA. Each year, approximately 300,000 preventable adverse events occur in the hospital setting, and many of these events are a result of confusing medical information. Currently there is no database that tracks adverse events that have occurred in the field setting. The FDA has made significant strides

Table 1-2 The FDA Approval Phases

Phase	Clinical Phase Trials
I Pre-clinical Trials (1–3 yrs, aver 18 mo) Basic science research, initial synthesis, cultures, and animal testing designed to determine pharmacological and metabolic actions of the drug in mammals.	Phase I: Human trials of an investigational drug. These studies, often conducted with healthy volunteer subjects, are designed to determine pharmacokinetics and toxicity in humans.
II Clinical Investigation (1–10 yrs, aver 5 yrs) Involves three Clinical Phase Trials	Phase II: Involving several hundred subjects with established illness, this phase is designed to establish therapeutic levels and side effects of the drug.
III New Drug Application Review (2 mo – 7 yrs, aver 2 yrs) FDA reviews research and issues approval to market by manufacturer	Phase III: Involving several hundred to several thousand subjects, this phase is designed to obtain data about the overall safety and effectiveness so the benefit to risk of the drug may be evaluated.
IV Post-Marketing Surveillance	Phase IV: Involves the drug's post-marketing surveillance to monitor the new drug through voluntary information reported by health care providers, consumer surveys, and inspections.

in reducing the complexity of prescription drug information, thus making it more useful for physicians, paramedics, and patients.

Enforcement of drug laws comes under the responsibility of the Drug Enforcement Agency (DEA). The mission of the DEA is to enforce the U.S. controlled substance laws and regulations. The DEA targets organizations and principal members of organizations that are involved in the growing, manufacture, or distribution of controlled substances in the United States. The agency also works with other groups to support non-enforcement (ie, voluntary best practices) programs aimed at reducing the availability of illicit controlled substances both within the United States and in other countries.

Before a new drug enters the market, the "investigational drug" must undergo an extensive testing process that has been developed by the FDA. Some pharmaceutical companies contend that the validation process is too costly and time-consuming; the FDA counters that it is designed to ensure that the new drug is safe and effective for consumers. The FDA approval process has multiple steps for approval of investigational drugs. The drug has to complete four phases to ensure its safety and efficacy (**Table 1-2**▲). This process can take 20 or more years and cost millions of dollars. Pharmaceutical companies have only a few years to recoup their investment before a drug can be manufactured as a generic—a fact that they often use to justify the high cost of drugs. The FDA's Orphan Drug Act has provided incentives for research for diseases that are extremely rare or for drugs on which they would likely not recoup investment costs.

Additional Resources on Newly Approved Drugs

The FDA classifies newly approved drugs, as well as maintains a database of information on FDA-approved brand name and generic drugs and therapeutic biological products. This resource is called Drugs@FDA and is accessible on the CDER website [http://www.accessdata.fda.gov/scripts/cder/drugsatfda/]. The Drugs@FDA database allows you to search for official information about FDA-approved brand name and generic drugs and therapeutic biological products. At this site the paramedic can find the following information: labels for approved drug products, generic drug products for a brand name drug product, therapeutically equivalent drug products for a brand name or generic drug product, consumer information for drugs approved from 1998 on, all drugs with a specific active ingredient, and view the approval history, since 1939, of drugs.

The specific drugs that are in the database are prescription and over-the-counter human drugs and therapeutic biologicals currently approved for sale in the U.S. Therapeutic biological products would include: monoclonal antibodies, cytokines, growth factors, enzymes, immunomodulators; and thrombolytics, proteins intended for therapeutic use that are extracted from animals or microorganisms, including recombinant versions of these products (except clotting factors), and other non-vaccine therapeutic immunotherapies.

The Drugs@FDA database does not include the following: OTC products approved for marketing through a process other than submission of a New

Drug Application or Biologic License Application, drugs sold outside the U.S. that are not approved for marketing in the U.S., drugs not approved by the FDA, drugs under review at the FDA for which no action (approved or not approved) has occurred yet, dietary supplements, which do not require FDA approval to be sold in the U.S., biological products regulated by the Center for Biologic Evaluation and Research, and animal drugs, which are regulated by the Center for Veterinary Medicine.

Drug Profile

Every medication must include a drug profile in the packaging of the medication. The drug profile includes all of the information for the medication including:

- Drug name—includes the generic name and trade name
- Classification—determined based on its effect on the patient and its mechanism of action
- **Mechanism of action**—describes how the medication causes the intended effect
- Indications—reasons or conditions why the medication is given
- Pharmacokinetics—describes how the medication is absorbed, distributed, and eliminated from the body
- Side and adverse effects—lists the undesired effects that are found during the development of the drug
- Routes of administration—lists the route of administration for that drug
- Drug forms—lists available forms and their concentrations
- Doses—amount of medication that should be administered for a particular condition
- Contraindications—conditions under which it is inappropriate to administer the medication
- Special considerations—information necessary to administer the medication to pediatric, pregnant, or geriatric patients, and any other special groups defined for the drug

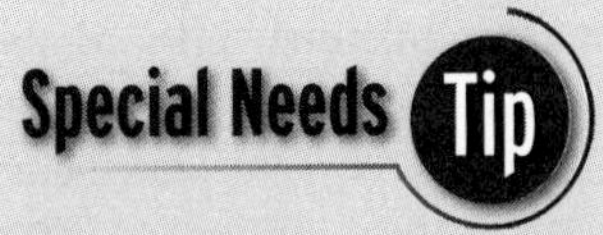

You may need to modify a dose given to a pediatric or geriatric patient due to slow absorption and elimination times.

Drugs: Names, Sources, Classes, and References

When a new drug is developed, it is given a name by the manufacturer who invested in its development and conducted the extensive research on the drug to meet the rigorous requirements of the FDA. The manufacturer usually picks a proprietary or **trade name**. The trade name is capitalized and the registered (®) or trademark (™) symbol follows the name of the drug. The chemical is actually the first name given to the drug and is generally not used in EMS. It would be of interest to a chemist as it is a precise description of the formula, such as the chemical name for water would be dihydroxide (H_2O). The **generic name** is the nonproprietary name, or the name given to the drug by the original manufacturer. An example would be a chemical name of N-(4-hydroxypheny) acetamide. The generic name is acetaminophen, the official name is acetaminophen USP, and the trade or brand name is Tylenol. Each drug also has an **official name**, which is the one that is listed in the U.S. Pharmacopeia once the generic name has been approved by the United States Adopted Name Council and the drug has been approved by the FDA. The official name is followed by the initials *USP* or *NF* for National Formulary.

Typically the manufacturer will register the trade name for a specific number of years during which the drug will not be manufactured by other companies. After this time has expired the drug can be produced by other companies and sold in the generic form with the generic name (**Table 1-3▼**). Some prescription plans will only pay for generic drugs because they are considerably less expensive.

Drug Sources and Classifications

Drugs are developed from four main sources: plants (ie, digitalis, atropine, etc), animals and humans (ie, insulin, epinephrine, etc), minerals (ie, iodine, iron, etc), and synthetic or chemicals (ie, heptavox, etc) (**Figure 1-1▶**).

Table 1-3 Commonly Used Drug Names

Generic Name	Trade or Brand Name
Furosemide	Lasix
Dopamine	Intropin
Epinephrine	Adrenalin
Nitroglycerin	Nitro Stat
Naloxone	Narcan
Midazolam	Versed

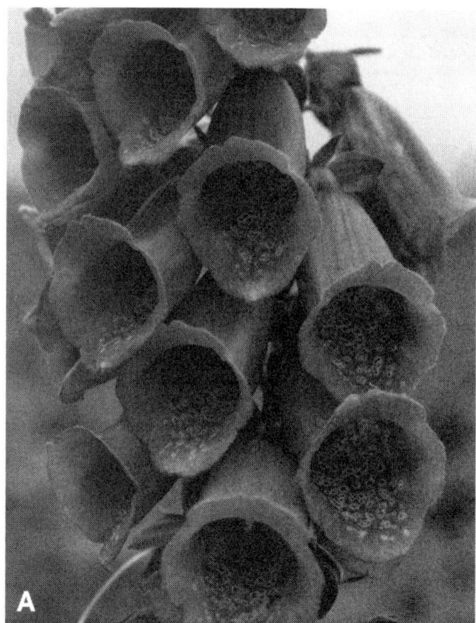

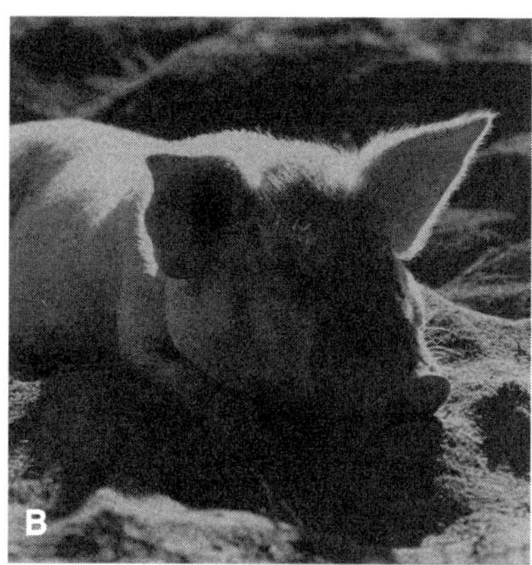

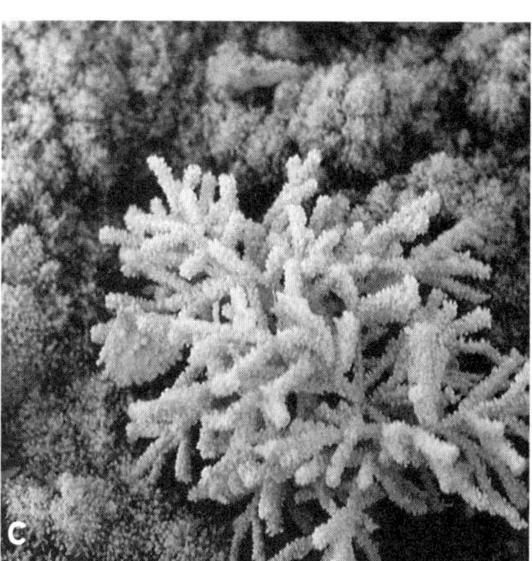

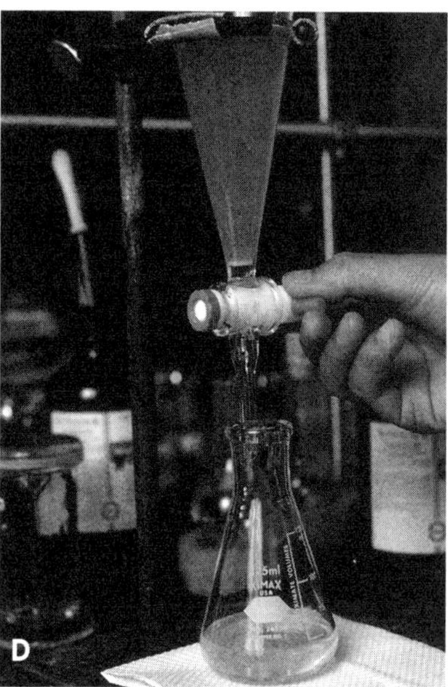

Figure 1-1 Drug sources and examples. A. Plant source. B. Animal source. C. Mineral source. D. Laboratory source.

Drugs are classified in a number of ways and many drugs fit into multiple classifications. The most common classifications are based on the effect that the drug has on a specific part of the body or specific condition. The drug classifications that will be included throughout this book, whether actually administered by the paramedic and included in the paramedic formulary (Appendix C) or medications that patients may be taking, include the following:

- **Analgesics** (opiate and nonopiate)
- **Antagonists**
- **Anesthetics**
- Antianxiety medications
- Sedatives
- Hypnotics
- **Anticonvulsants**
- **Central nervous system (CNS) stimulants**
- Psychotherapeutics
- Drugs for specific CNS and peripheral nervous system (PNS) dysfunctions
- Drugs affecting the parasympathetic nervous system (ie, **cholinergic** and **anticholinergic**)
- Drugs affecting the sympathetic nervous system (**sympathomimetics**)
- **Skeletal muscle relaxants**
- Drugs affecting the cardiovascular system (ie, **antihypertensives**, **anticoagulants**, **fibrinolytic agents**, and **antiplatelet agents**)
- **Antihyperlipidemics**
- Drugs affecting the respiratory system (ie, **mucokinetics**, bronchodilators, oxygen)
- Drugs affecting the gastrointestinal system (**Table 1-4**)
- Eye and ear medications
- Drugs affecting the endocrine system (ie, parathyroid and thyroid glands, pituitary gland, adrenal cortex and pancreas)
- Drugs for labor and delivery
- Drugs affecting the reproductive system
- **Antineoplastic medications**
- Drugs used in infectious disease and inflammation (ie, HIV meds, **antibiotics**, antifungal, antiviral, antiparasitic meds, **nonsteroidal anti-inflammatory drugs (NSAIDs)**)
- **Uricosuric medications**
- **Immunobiologic medications** (ie, serums, **vaccines**, and other immunizing agents)
- **Immunosuppressant medications**
- Dermatological medications
- Vitamins and minerals
- Fluids and electrolytes

Drugs and other interventions are also classified by the strength of scientific research and evidence that supports recommending their use. The International

Table 1-4 Gastrointestinal Agents

Agent(s)	Action
Antacids	Neutralize stomach acid, used to relieve acid indigestion, upset stomach, "sour stomach," and heartburn; typically are OTC preparations, for example, Mylanta, Tums, Maalox, and milk of magnesia
Antiflatulents	Prevent or are used to treat excessive gas in the intestinal tract, for example, Gas-X and simethicone
Digestants	Used to aid in or stimulate the digestive process; for example, lactase, used by people who are intolerant to dairy products
Antiemetics	Prevent or arrest vomiting, for example, include promethazine (Phenergan), prochlorperazine (Compazine), metoclopramide (Reglan), trimethobenzamide (Tigan), and ondansetron (Zofran)
Cannabinoids	Provide relief to people whose chemotherapy drug causes minimal nausea and vomiting; believed to work in an area of the brain thought to be partly responsible for causing nausea and vomiting; mild drowsiness, dizziness, and euphoria are common side effects
Emetics	Used to promote or cause vomiting, for example, syrup of ipecac
Cytoprotective agents	Predominantly used to treat peptic ulcer disease; provide protection to the lining of the stomach and the duodenum to allow ulcers to heal H2-receptor antagonists Reduce acid production in the stomach; act by blocking acid-producing cells in the stomach, for example, include cimetidine (Tagamet) and esomeprazole (Nexium)
Laxatives	Stimulate loosening, relaxation, or evacuation of the bowels; sometimes abused by patients with eating disorders and can lead to profound dehydration if taken improperly; often used for in-hospital management of acute coronary syndrome (ACS) patients to avoid vagal stimulation during bowel movements

Table 1-5 ILCOR Classes of Drug Recommendations

Class	Description
I	Excellent evidence, widely accepted, little or no risk. Recommended use. This drug should be utilized.
IIa	Good research evidence, benefit outweighs risk. Acceptable use. This drug is reasonable to utilize.
IIb	Fair evidence, benefit ~ risk. Optional alternative. Treatment with this drug may be considered.
Indeterminate	Insufficient evidence. May be used. Because the research is either just starting or ongoing, at this point there is no final recommendation until further research is conducted. Neither for nor against.
III	Risk exceeds benefit. Harmful. This drug should not be administered. It is not helpful and may be harmful.

Liaison Committee on Resuscitation (ILCOR) uses the five "classes" of drug recommendations (**Table 1-5▲**).

Drug References

There are a number of information resources for drugs. Most paramedics carry a pocket reference or pocket guide that contains limited useful information to refer to including a drug formulary and a list of the top most-prescribed medications. Typically there is a more extensive drug book carried on the medic unit that can be used to look up important information about drugs. *The Physician's Desk Reference (PDR)* is one of the most widely used and respected sources of drug information. Other excellent sources include the Emergency Cardiovascular Care (ECC) Handbook/Guidelines (an ILCOR publication), Epocrates, and Tarascon's Pharmacopeia interactive websites that provide downloads and updates every time your PDA is synchronized with their website. Additionally, there are numerous websites with good drug information such as Rxlist.com and Medlineplus.gov. Poison control centers, pharmacists, and professional journals are also useful sources to learn more about medications. The telephone number of the nearest poison control center should always be kept available in the EMS provider's compendium of important professional reference information.

Drug: Physiology, Receptors, Actions, and Interactions

There are three phases of drug activity. **Pharmaceutics** is the science of preparing and dispersing drugs, the various drug forms, and how they affect the pharmacokinetic and pharmacodynamic stages. As you will learn later in this chapter, different forms of the same drug are absorbed into the patient's bloodstream at different rates. Researchers look for the best method for specific circumstances to administer a drug. For example, great strides are being made in this area with newly released inhaled insulin, saving the patient the pain of having to inject themselves multiple times a day, as well as the inconvenience and responsibility of managing a large number of contaminated "sharps" on a regular basis.

Researchers who study **pharmacokinetics** are interested in how a medication is altered as it travels through the patient's body. Once in the body, a drug goes through the following four stages:

1. In the **absorption stage** the drug enters the body and reaches the bloodstream.
2. In the **distribution stage** the drug moves through the bloodstream to the target organ. There are two methods by which drugs cross the cell membrane. Most cross through by **passive transport** which includes: diffusion, facilitated diffusion, osmosis, and filtration. **Active transport** moves via pumps that require energy and move the drug from an area of low concentration to an area of high concentration.
3. In the metabolism or **biotransformation stage**, the drug is altered chemically or broken down. Many of these processes occur in the liver.
4. In the **elimination stage** or excretion stage, the drug, or its metabolites, are removed from the body.

In **pharmacodynamics** researchers investigate biochemical and physiological effects and interactions with the target organs or tissues.

Medications are administered to achieve a therapeutic effect, a preventive effect, or a diagnostic effect. The interaction between a drug and the end organ or tissue in the body, which it is designed to have an effect upon, is only a physiologic modification because drugs are not designed to produce new functions. The body's building blocks range from cells to tissues to organs to organ systems to the organism itself (human). To exert its effect, a drug must interact with the cells and tissues of the body and will typically work through several mechanisms. When a medication is administered to have a positive effect on the cells or tissues, it ultimately affects each level of the body's building blocks. As you should have learned in the pathophysiology of shock, conditions that impact on the organism, such as hemorrhaging, ultimately have an effect on each level of the body's building blocks. For example, drug-induced physiologic changes in body function such as that produced by acetaminophen [Tylenol] resets the body's thermostat to relieve fever and its associated symptoms. This would be construed as the drug's action. The drug action is the desired effect, such as relief of pain, relief of nausea, relief of a fever, or a decrease in swelling or bronchodilation. Medications usually affect more than one tissue, organ, and/or body system. They also vary in the degree of desired and undesired effects. There are several ways in which a drug affects a body's organs (mechanism of action). In most cases the drug may bind to a receptor site or trigger a stimulus. In some cases the chemical properties of the cells or tissues may change to ultimately alter the metabolic functions of the cells or tissues. The key mechanism by which a medication affects the body is by working with the receptors on the target organs or tissues. Receptors are specialized target molecules on the surface of cells or within the cell. A medication that stimulates a response in a receptor site is called an **agonist**. The strength of the effect of an agonist is often related to the dose of the drug administered, the drug's rate of absorption, distribution, and metabolism, all concepts which will be discussed later in this chapter. Most of the time medications work in a fairly predictable fashion. This is true of side effects as well. A dictum that all health care providers should always keep in mind is that ***any medicine can do anything to any patient at any time***; so it is possible that a patient will occasionally manifest an unusual or untoward response to a medication that was not predicted or does not make sense as a usual side effect.

Pharmacology and the Nervous System

Since the nervous system controls the functions of the body, many drugs are designed to alter or affect specific receptors within the nervous system. As you have learned in your EMS training, the nervous system is anatomically broken into the **central nervous system (CNS)** (ie, brain and spinal cord) and the **peripheral nervous system (PNS)** controlling the sensory (**afferent nerves**) and motor (**efferent nerves**) functions of the body (**Figure 1-2 ▸**). The PNS provides a communication between the muscles of the body and the patient's brain, and its "wiring" consists of the pairs of nerves that exit between each of the spinal vertebrae. There are also pairs of cranial nerves that exit the brain and help with sensation and movement from the shoulder up. The functions of the nervous system that you do not need to constantly think about (ie, blood vessels, the heart, and organs of the chest, abdomen, and pelvis) are controlled by the

In order to avoid potentially dangerous drug interactions, be knowledgeable about the medications that your patients take daily. Most medications used in the prehospital setting interact with other medications.

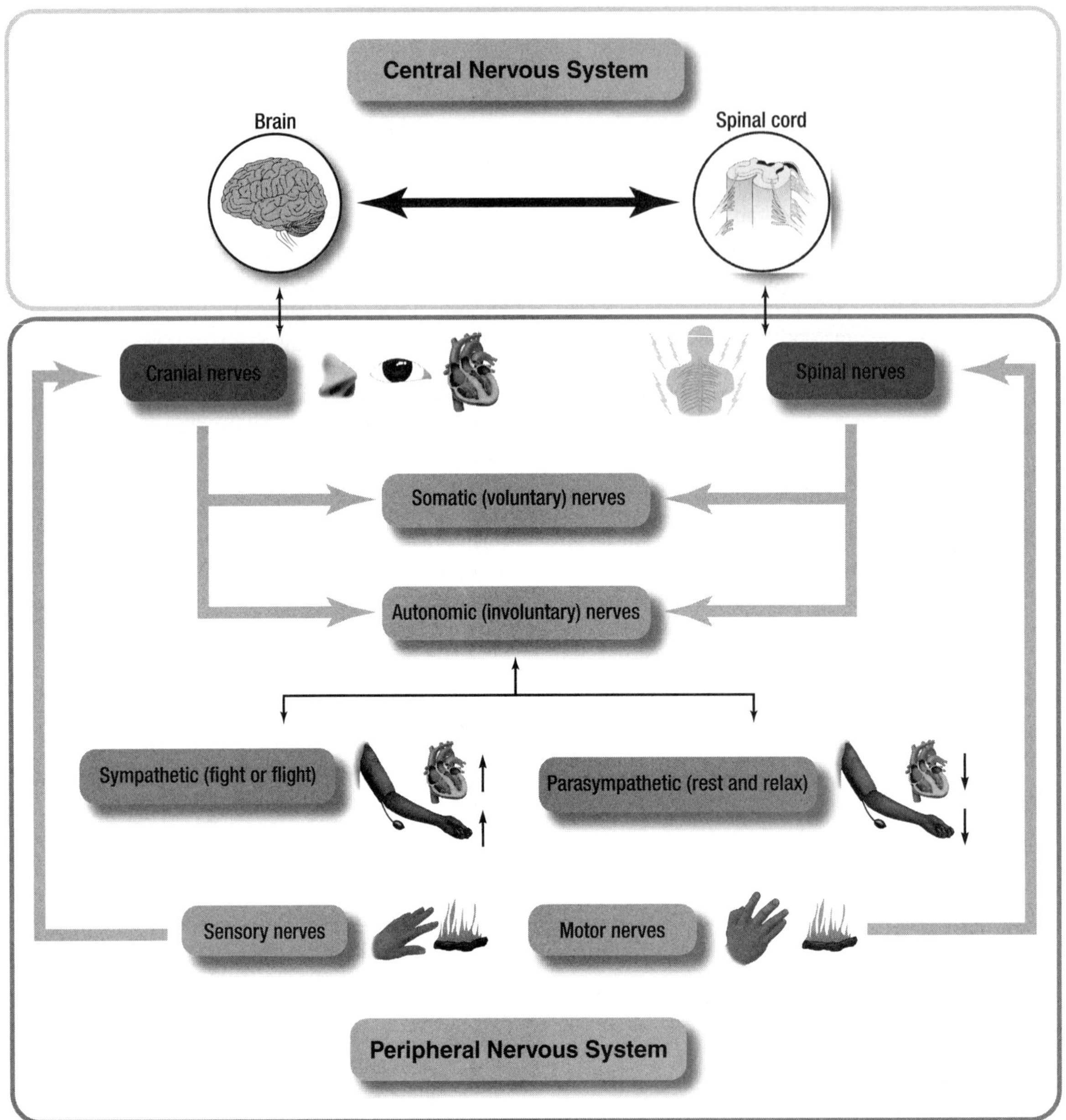

Figure 1-2 Organization of the nervous system.

autonomic nervous system, which is actually a subdivision of the PNS. It is these autonomic functions that many of the medications used in prehospital care seek to affect.

The autonomic nervous system is further divided into the sympathetic nervous system and the parasympathetic nervous system. The **sympathetic nervous system** is responsible for the "fight or flight" responses and is dominant during times of stress. It is responsible for the signs and symptoms that develop in AMI, trauma, and hypoglycemia. The **parasympathetic nervous system**, on the other hand, is dominant during periods of rest and relaxation and has been called the "rest and digest" system. The nerves from the brain stem pass through four of the cranial nerves (ie, oculomotor (III), facial (IV), pharyngeal (IX), and vagus (X)). These nerves innervate most of the body including the eyes, salivary glands, ears, lungs, and abdominal organs. The two systems of the autonomic nervous system have opposing effects on the body and are in a constant tug-of-war to control the functions of the body.

There are two types of receptors within the autonomic nervous system that drugs often stimulate: the cholinergic and the **adrenergic**. Cholinergic receptors respond to the neurotransmitter acetylcholine and the adrenergic receptors respond to the neurotransmitters epinephrine and norepinephrine. Drugs that block

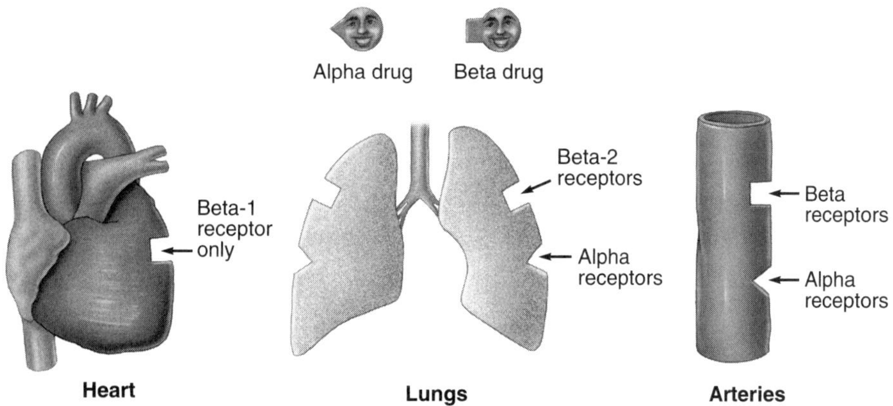

Figure 1-3 Receptor sites of the sympathetic nervous system in the heart, lungs, and arteries.

the cholinergic receptor response (parasympathetic response) are called parasympatholytics. The drug atropine is a good example. In effect, atropine "allows the heart to speed up" by blocking the brakes (blocks increased vagal tone) instead of pressing on the gas pedal that controls the heart rate.

When stimulated, the adrenergic receptors elicit a response of the sympathetic nervous system. In fact, the medications that mimic the functions of the sympathetic nervous system are referred to as sympathomimetic drugs. A number of the medications used in the prehospital setting for Advanced Cardiac Life Support (ACLS) fit in this category (ie, dobutamine [Dobutrex], dopamine [Intropin], epinephrine [Adrenalin], and norepinephrine [Levophed]).

When a drug blocks the function of the sympathetic nervous system, it is referred to as antiadrenergic or sympatholytic. Although used less frequently in the prehospital setting, there are still a few such as labetalol [Normodyne or Trandate] and metoprolol [Lopressor]. Other medications in this category that patients may be taking, and should be found in a paramedic's formulary, would include: atenolol [Tenormin], esmolol [Brevibloc], propranolol [Inderal], and timolol [Blocadren].

There are actually two types of the sympathetic receptors: the dopaminergic receptors and the adrenergic receptors. Dopaminergic receptors affect the dilation of the cerebral, coronary, and renal arteries. Manipulation of these receptor sites has limited utility in the prehospital setting and therefore will not be addressed further in this text (aside from discussing the administration of the medication dopamine [Intropin]). There are four subgroups of adrenergic receptors: the alpha 1 and 2 and the beta 1 and 2 (**Figure 1-3▲**). The effects of stimulating these receptors are listed in **Table 1-6▶**. Manipulation of the alpha-2 receptor sites has limited utility in the prehospital setting and therefore will not be addressed further in this text.

Table 1-6 The Adrenergic Receptors

Receptor type	Effect when stimulated
Alpha 1	Smooth muscle vasoconstriction
Beta 1	Increase the rate, contraction, automaticity, and conduction of the heart
Beta 2	Bronchodilation and mild vasodilation

Drug Response on the Body

Each drug is distinctive in relation to the rate of absorption, distribution, metabolism, and elimination. The drug response relationship is the expectation that the administration of a drug will produce a desired or therapeutic effect on a target organ or tissue. Entire body systems may be affected as well. There are many factors that can alter the drug response including: age, body mass, gender, environment, time of administration, pathologic state, and genetic and physiologic factors. The minimum amount of drug required to produce the desired response is called a drug's **therapeutic threshold**. The **therapeutic index** is the difference between the therapeutic threshold and the amount of the drug considered to produce unwanted and possibly dangerous side effects. The therapeutic index is used to understand the margin of safety that exists for the use of a drug. Medications are described as having a wide or narrow therapeutic index or window. Those with a narrow window are more difficult to dose and administer and may require therapeutic drug monitoring (ie, coumadin, digoxin). Therapeutic drug monitoring measures the drug levels in the blood, specifically plasma levels. **Half-life** refers to the amount of time that a drug remains at a therapeutic level to produce a desired effect and the time it takes the body to metabolize or reduce a drug's concentration by 50%. The administration of a **loading dose** is considered to be a single dose or the accumulation of several closely repeated single doses (**bolus**) used to obtain the therapeutic level to achieve a desired effect. As a drug loses its therapeutic effect as a result of its half-life, additional administration may be given as a single dose or as an IV drip to maintain the desired effect. This is called a **maintenance dose**.

A number of terms are used to describe the interactions and pharmacology of drugs. When a drug is given, its effect on the body may be local, systemic, or both. A drug interaction is the combined effect of drugs taken concurrently or simultaneously which then alters the effect of at least one of the drug's therapeutic effects. This is important to understand since many of our patients may already be taking certain medications prior to the introduction of any medications during the course of our care.

The following is a list of terms used throughout this text that describe the various kinds of effects and reactions that patients can experience as a result of medication interactions.

- Addiction—the state of being enslaved to a habit or practice or to something that is psychologically or physically habit-forming, as narcotics, to such an extent that its cessation causes severe trauma.
- **Additive effect** (also known as the **summation effect**)—when two drugs work together to produce an effect a single drug would not produce alone.
- **Adverse reaction**—an undesirable response to a drug that may be either sudden or take days to occur.
- Allergy—a reaction to a medication that causes local and systemic symptoms (ie, itching, rash, watery eyes, swelling, wheezing).
- Anaphylactic reaction—the most severe allergic reaction which involves cardiovascular collapse (ie, hypotension, airway constriction, and altered mental status).
- Antagonist—when one drug prevents or reverses the reaction of another. This may be chemical (ie, two effects that are opposite of each other such as barbiturates and amphetamines), competitive (ie, naloxone [Narcan] preventing the effects of a narcotic by competing for and occupying available narcotic receptor sites), or physiologic (ie, atropine to block vagal tone to raise the heart rate).
- **Cross tolerance**—the resistance to the effect or effects of a drug as a result of tolerance previously developed to another drug having a similar pharmacologic action.
- **Cumulative effect**—develops with repeated doses prior to the initial dose being metabolized/excreted by the body. If excessive, this can lead to toxicity and is a particular problem in either the very young or very old, and in patients with liver or kidney failure.
- Delayed reaction—a reaction that takes an extended amount of time to appear. Usually involves an inappropriate reaction (ie, serum sickness).
- Dependence—physical "need" or psychological "desire" for a medication.
- Desired action—based on the reason why you are giving the drug to the patient, the effect you would expect to occur.
- **Habituation**—the emotional or psychological dependence on a drug after repeated use (ie, narcotics or analgesics).
- Half-life—the amount of time that a drug remains at a therapeutic level to continue to produce the desired effect and the time it takes the body to metabolize the drug's concentration by 50%. This is important to know when planning repeated dosing.
- **Hypersensitivity**—an exaggerated response to a drug such as an allergic reaction to an antibiotic (ie, itching, rash, or shortness of breath).
- **Iatrogenic response**—an adverse effect, condition, or disorder that is unintentionally produced by the administration of a drug.
- **Idiosyncratic reaction**—an abnormal reaction that is unpredictable and unique to a specific patient rather than a group of patients.
- Interference—some classes of medications may interfere with specific body processes. A classic type of medication interference occurs with blood perfusion at a wound site. Steroids and chemotherapy agents can interfere with wound healing.
- Loading dose—a single dose or accumulation of several closely repeated doses used to obtain the therapeutic level that achieves the desired effect.
- Maintenance dose—additional doses of a medication, administered after the loading dose, added to keep the medication at the therapeutic level.
- **Potentiation**—a combination reaction where one drug enhances the effect of the other (ie, use of codeine and alcohol together).
- **Side effect**—a response to a drug that is not the desired effect but seems to occur in many patients (ie, headache with nitroglycerin).
- **Synergistic effect**—the effect of two drugs working together in an additive manner that results in an effect that is greater than the sum of their effects if taken individually.

- Tolerance—a decrease in the expected reaction to a drug with repeated doses. This is common in patients who are taking analgesics.

It is very important for the paramedic to become familiar with all of the drug action and interaction terms. Knowing the classifications of drugs can provide helpful clues to the patient's past medical history, as well as the presenting problem, especially when the patient cannot speak for himself or herself. If the patient is on a beta-blocker this could explain why he or she is deeply in shock yet still has a slow pulse rate. If the patient normally takes insulin and has not eaten today this could explain why he or she has an altered mental status and the blood glucose is low. If the patient with a history of COPD presents with a fever and you find he or she is taking large doses of bronchodilators and steroids, this may help you better understand that the recent respiratory infection is probably overwhelming for this patient whose physician has been treating already very aggressively. In this case an understanding of the drugs the patient is taking and the pathophysiology of the patient's condition should help alert you that this patient is likely to decompensate quickly and requires aggressive airway measures!

Drug Forms and Routes of Drug Administration

Medication formulations vary depending upon their route of administration. Drugs come in many forms and each form has advantages and disadvantages. Most are subdivided into solids, liquids, or gases. Solid forms of drugs include:

- Capsule
- Pulvule
- Pill
- Powder
- Suppository
- Tablet
- Lozenge
- Medication patch

Liquid forms of drugs include:

- Solution
- Elixir
- Emulsion
- Suspension
- Syrup
- Tincture
- Topical cream

Gas forms of drugs include:

- Oxygen and nitrous oxide
- Other assorted anesthetics

The route of administration may vary considerably. Most patients take their daily medications orally by drinking a fluid or swallowing a pill. The oral route may be referred to as PO or "per os" (Latin—by mouth) in a physician's prescription. Forms of liquid or solid medications taken PO would include: elixirs, emulsions, suspensions, syrups, capsules, timed-release capsules, pills, lozenges, and tablets. Other patients may allow a medication to be absorbed or dissolved under the tongue using the **sublingual (SL) route**, or via the inhalation route by administration of a mist or spray into the lungs using a **small-volume nebulizer** or a **metered-dose inhaler (MDI)**. There are a number of other routes of administration for medications (**Table 1-7 ▸**). These include: nasal, rectal or "per rectum" (PR), intravenous (IV), subcutaneous (SC or SQ), intramuscular (IM), endotracheal (ET), intraosseous (IO), transdermal, epidural, gastric, or buccal. The intracardiac route was previously used, but was abandoned many years ago in the prehospital setting.

The absorption rates of the various routes of medication differ considerably. **Enteral routes** are those where the drug is absorbed via some aspect of the gastrointestinal tract (mouth to anus). Drugs administered via this route tend to be absorbed slower and are therefore not commonly used in an emergency setting. **Parenteral routes** include those in which medications are administered via any route other than the digestive tract, skin, and mucous membranes. They are generally administered via syringes and needles. Medications are absorbed much more quickly into the patient's central circulation and tend to offer more predictable and more immediately measurable responses. The **percutaneous route** includes those routes where medication is absorbed through the skin or mucous membrane (ie, transdermal route, sublingual route, aural route, buccal route, ocular route, and nasal route). The administration of medications intranasally is accomplished using a **mucosal atomizer device (MAD)** and syringe (**Figure 1-4 ▸**).

The speed in which a medication is absorbed is a function of the route of administration. Drugs given by the parenteral routes are absorbed faster than those

Patients frequently experience significant complications due to duplicated drug types with multiple physician specialists.

Table 1-7 Routes of Administration

Route	Route Meaning	Example of Medication
Sublingual (SL) route	Under the tongue	nitroglycerin [Nitrostat]
Inhalation route	Into the lungs	albuterol [Ventolin]
Intranasal route	Within the nose	midazolam [Versed]
Intravenous (IV) route	Into the vein	furosemide [Lasix]
Intramuscular (IM) route	Within the muscle	Glucagon
Subcutaneous (SC or SQ) route	Between the dermis and the muscle layer	epinephrine [Adrenalin]
Endotracheal (ET) route	Via an ET tube	atropine
Oral route	By mouth	activated charcoal [Liqui-Char]
Buccal route	Between the cheek and gum	Glucose
Rectal route (PR)	Rectum, urethra, or vagina	diazepam [Diastat]
Transdermal route	Applied topically to the skin (as in a patch)	nitroglycerin [Transderm-Nitro]
Aural route	Ear	levofloxacin [Levaquin]
Intradermal route	Within the dermal layer of the skin	PPD (tuberculosis testing)
Ocular route	Drops in the eye	betaxolol ophthalmic solution [Betoptic]
Gastric route	Via a gastric tube	activated charcoal [Liqui-Char] (most common in the prehospital setting)
Intraosseous (IO) route	Marrow cavity of the bone (when quick IV access is not practical)	furosemide [Lasix] (any drug that can be administered intravenously can be administered intraosseously)

administered by enteral routes because they do not have to be absorbed through the GI tract to achieve their therapeutic effect. Also, medications absorbed enterally enter into the bloodstream after passing through the liver, which slows down and can fundamentally alter a drug's properties. There are many differences in the rates of absorption (**Table 1-8** ▸). It is important to note that the endotracheal route that has traditionally been used in cardiac arrest patients is now rarely recommended due to poor absorption rates and subsequent unpredictability of effect.

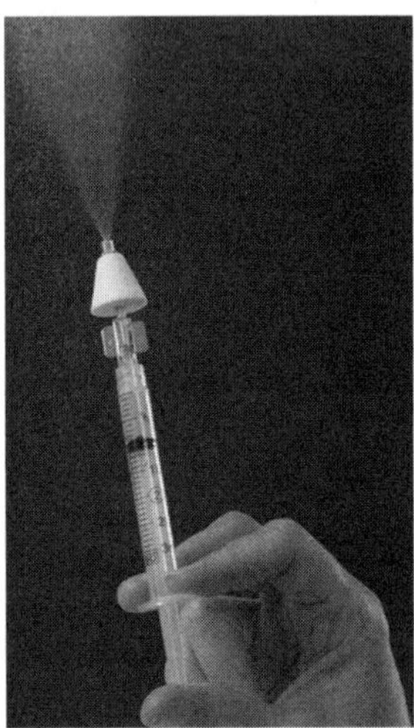
Figure 1-4 The mucosal atomizer device (MAD).

Finally, realize that the rate of absorption does not always translate into rate of effect onset at the intended physiologic target. In some circumstances, one route is preferred over another because of patient factors. Consider the case of an asthmatic in the midst of a severe exacerbation of their disease. Administering a dose of corticosteroids might be useful to help alleviate the attack. An intravenous dose of methylprednisolone (Solu-Medrol) could be used, but at the cellular level we know that it will not have a faster or better effect than an equal amount of oral prednisone. Health care providers may choose to use the IV formulation because the patient may be too sick to tolerate oral dosing, but physiologically there is no benefit to the patient in using that particular medication in the IV versus an oral preparation.

Table 1-8 Rates of Absorption by Different Routes

Route	Rate of Absorption
IV	30–60 seconds
IO	60 seconds
Inhalation	3 minutes
Sublingual tablet	3–5 minutes
Rectal	5–30 minutes (unpredictable)
IM injection	10–20 minutes
SC or SQ	15–30 minutes
Oral	30–90 minutes
Transdermal	Minutes to hours

Special Considerations: the Very Old, the Very Young, and Pregnancy

There are a number of special considerations in the administration of drugs with regard to the geriatric, pediatric, or pregnant patient. The manner in which a drug is absorbed and processed by the body differs in the very old and very young patient. This could make them prone to developing cumulative effect problems. The patient's age can be a factor that influences

Table 1-9 Pregnancy Category Ratings for Drugs

Category	Pregnancy Safety of Drug Reveals
A	Controlled studies in women fail to demonstrate a risk to the fetus in the first trimester, and there is no evidence of risk in later trimesters; the possibility of fetal harm appears to be remote.
B	Either: (1) animal reproductive studies have not demonstrated a fetal risk but there are no controlled studies in women, or (2) animal reproductive studies have shown an adverse effect (other than decreased fertility) that was not confirmed in controlled studies on women in the first trimester and there is no evidence of risk in later trimesters.
C	Either: (1) studies in animals have revealed adverse effects on the fetus and there are no controlled studies in women, or (2) studies in women and animals are not available. Drugs in this category should be given only if the potential benefit justifies the risk to the fetus.
D	There is positive evidence of human fetal risk, but the benefits for pregnant women may be acceptable despite the risk, as in life-threatening diseases for which safer drugs cannot be used or are ineffective. An appropriate statement must appear in the "Warnings" section of the labeling of drugs in this category.
X	Studies in animals and humans have demonstrated fetal abnormalities, there is evidence of fetal risk based on human experience, or both; the risk of using the drug in pregnant women clearly outweighs any possible benefit. The drug is contraindicated in women who are or may become pregnant. An appropriate statement must appear in the "Contraindications" section of the labeling of drugs in this category.

the action of a drug. Geriatric and pediatric patients have a higher risk of adverse reactions. The liver and kidney are responsible for metabolizing and eliminating most drugs. An elderly patient with physiologically decreased renal or hepatic function, or a person with underlying liver or kidney disease will process medications differently from someone without those underlying issues. Similarly, neonates, infants, and toddlers may have immature liver and kidney functions, and will also potentially metabolize and excrete drugs differently from adults.

Medications are designed to work in relation to the patient's total body weight. The average adult dose is based on the amount of drug that would produce a specific effect in 50% of the patients who are between 18 and 65 years of age and 150 lb. (Some medications have no pediatric recommendations so they should be administered according to weight and medical direction.)

When dealing with a patient who is pregnant, there should be concern about potential medication effects on the fetus. The FDA categorizes all drugs according to the level of risk to the fetus (**Table 1-9▲**). The five categories are A, B, C, D, and X. Though we always try to use the least amount of medication possible during pregnancy, realize that it is entirely appropriate to employ category A and B medications when necessary. Categories C and D are used if absolutely necessary and typically after expert consultation. Generally speaking, the same is true regarding medication use in lactating patients, and pregnancy safety categories can be roughly translated to that class of patients as well.

Paramedic Responsibilities and Pharmacology

The paramedic is responsible for the assessment and management of patients in the prehospital setting. This management often involves interventions such as the administration of medications. In some cases this may involve advocating for the needs of the patient by conveying your findings to medical control for their authorization to administer the needed medicine. For the paramedic to be prepared to administer medications and serve as an example for one's peers, the paramedic needs to know all of the medications in the formulary that their regional protocols include. We have included an example of a paramedic level prehospital formulary, which will be used throughout this book, in Appendix C.

Many drugs can become ineffective or unsafe due to their age, storage temperature, or prolonged exposure to light. All drugs have a shelf life and are clearly marked with an expiration date. It is the responsibility of the paramedic to check the drug box each shift for those medications that are soon to expire so they can be either used or replaced. It is also important

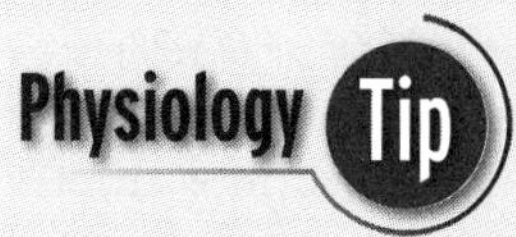

Pregnancy limits the types of medications that can be used because of possible risk to the fetus.

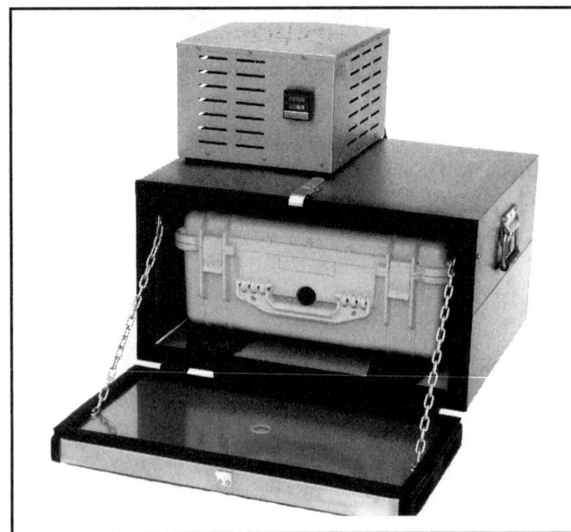

Figure 1-5 A heated drug box used in EMS medic units that work in colder climates.

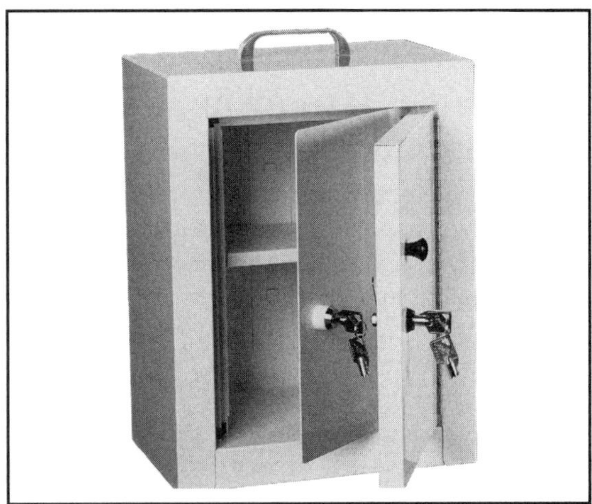

Figure 1-6 An example of a locking narcotics box.

to make sure that if the weather is extreme (very hot or very cold), the drug box is stored appropriately (**Figure 1-5**▲). State controlled substance regulations may require that narcotics and similar medications be double locked, in a box within a box (**Figure 1-6**▲).

Throughout each chapter of the text we will integrate the pathophysiological principles of pharmacology with patient assessment by using the case review technique. We feel this is a helpful way to learn about medications so that the paramedic does not simply memorize a long list of drugs. Rather, this method helps you to remember each drug as it relates to a real world situation as it is commonly found in the field. As the information is revealed in each of the progressive cases, the paramedic will be given the opportunity to synthesize patient history and assessment findings to form a working clinical impression. This "working diagnosis" will be used to implement a treatment plan that includes any appropriate pharmacologic interventions.

Table 1-10 Types of Medications as Clues to Medical History

Type of Medication	Patient History
Antihypertensive	Hypertension
Anticonvulsant	Seizure disorder
Antianxiety or Antidepressant	Behavioral disorder
Antihistamine	Allergies
Antiarrhythmic	Irregular cardiac rhythms
Antidiabetic	Diabetes
Antianginal	Angina
Anti-inflammatory	Arthritis, injury, infection, fever
Antiemetic	Nausea and gastrointestinal disorders
Analgesic	Acute or chronic pain
Bronchodilator	Asthmatic, reactive airway disease, chronic lung disease
Anticoagulant or Fibrinolytics	TIA, ischemic stroke, blood clots, ACS
CNS stimulants	Attention deficit disorder

An understanding of the types of medications that patients take can be helpful to the paramedic in providing clues to their medical history, especially in those situations where the patient cannot speak for him- or herself. Let's say you find an elderly woman with an altered level of consciousness lying on the ground in a public restroom. If a police officer, who is going through her pocketbook looking for identification, locates an anticonvulsant medication, that could be a clue that she may have had a seizure. Perhaps insulin and a syringe were found which could provide a clue the patient is a diabetic, or maybe she has taken most of a vial of sedatives. Examples of medications and the clues they may give about the patient's medical history are shown in **Table 1-10**▲.

We strongly suggest that all paramedics carry a reliable and easy-to-use pocket reference to refer to from time to time. It should contain commonly used drugs, as well as protocols and reference charts, and it should be periodically updated.

Medication Administration: Anatomy, Physiology, Equipment, and Techniques

It is important for the paramedic to understand the specific anatomy and physiology involved in medication utilization. Your pharmaceutical management plan for the patient will need to take into consideration the specific administration techniques that are most appropriate for the specific medication that the patient needs. Let's review the different ways in which medicines can be administered to our patients.

Oral medications are drugs that are taken by mouth. Forms of solid and liquid oral medications include pills, capsules, timed-release capsules, lozenges, tablets, elixirs, emulsions, syrups, and suspensions. Drugs taken by mouth will follow the GI tract and be absorbed into the bloodstream as nutrients in food are. As we have pointed out, this tends to be a slow process, usually somewhere between 30 and 90 minutes. If the medication is chewed, such as aspirin in the acute coronary syndrome patient, it is absorbed into the bloodstream not only via the GI tract but also through the oral mucosa. To administer liquid oral medications, you may use a medicine cup, a medicine dropper, a teaspoon, an oral syringe, or a nipple.

No equipment is needed when a patient is given a medication to swallow or chew. It may be important that you wear gloves when handing a patient a pill, as in the case of nitroglycerin, since the powder that collects in the bottle from partially crushed pills can easily be absorbed through the skin on your fingers. The best advice is if you want the patient to get the medicine and not take some yourself, wear disposable gloves. It is also important to note the specific dose of oral medications. This is particularly important when obtaining an exchange for medication given to the patient to restock your drug box. For example, sometimes the hospital may supply the medicine in different doses. Aspirin is supplied in chewable tablets: 81 mg; Caplets and tablets: 160 mg and 325 mg. Be sure to select the appropriate dose and form as specified in your protocols.

If an oral medication is the desired route, make sure your patient's mental status is up to the task of swallowing safely without posing a potential hazard to their own airway. In general, if a patient is not alert enough to follow directions and is specifically unable to swallow on command, then they should not be given medication by mouth. When a patient is not alert, it is not advisable to place items like medication in the mouth that may ultimately become an airway obstruction.

An enteral medication that may be given in the prehospital setting by the gastric tube route is activated charcoal [Liqui-Char] for the management of certain poisons. This involves passing either a nasal or oral gastric tube first, and tends to be uncomfortable for the patient. Another route of enteral medication administration that is often used with great success is via the rectal mucosa. In the prehospital setting this is used to manage the patient with seizures where rapid safe intravenous access can be problematic. Use of this route typically involves a specialized medication-

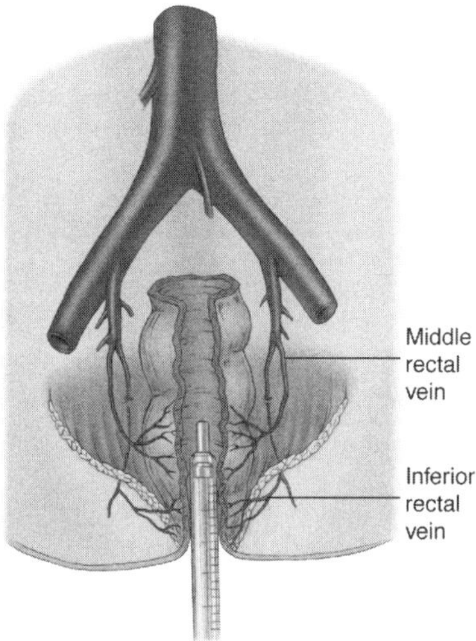

Figure 1-7 The rectal route of administration can be used for diazepam [Valium, Diastat].

containing suppository or a small bore syringe (without needle) along with a water soluble lubricant (**Figure 1-7**▲).

Parenteral medications, such as those given by the SC or SQ, IV, IO, IM, and inhalation routes require specific devices for administration. Needles are usually from 3/8″ to 3″ in length and can range from 16- to 28-gauge in diameter. Syringes are measured by volume, and commonly vary from 1 to 60 mL. When giving any injection, properly prepping the site and proper disposal of the sharps are essential steps. The typical subcutaneous needle is on the short side and injected at a 45° angle to the skin. The subcutaneous tissue covering the deltoid muscle site of the shoulder and the anterior thigh are the most common injection sites. The lateral abdomen is also a common site used by diabetic patients. SC or SQ injections should be 1 mL or less; therefore, a very small syringe can be used (½″ to 1″ in length and ranging from 24- to 26-gauge in diameter). Subcutaneous absorption is faster than that of enteral absorption, but depending on the patient's perfusion status, absorption can be erratic and delayed. This route is rarely used in the prehospital setting. An example would be SC epinephrine that may be administered to the patient experiencing an allergic reaction. The intradermal route is rarely used in prehospital care. An example of a medication that would be given by the intradermal route would be the Mantoux test the paramedic has to take every 6 to 12 months to test for tuberculosis.

The intramuscular (IM) route involves a longer needle and can involve volumes of up to 5 mL. Typically smaller volumes (1 to 3 mL) are given in the deltoid, vastus lateralis, or rectus femoris muscles. The

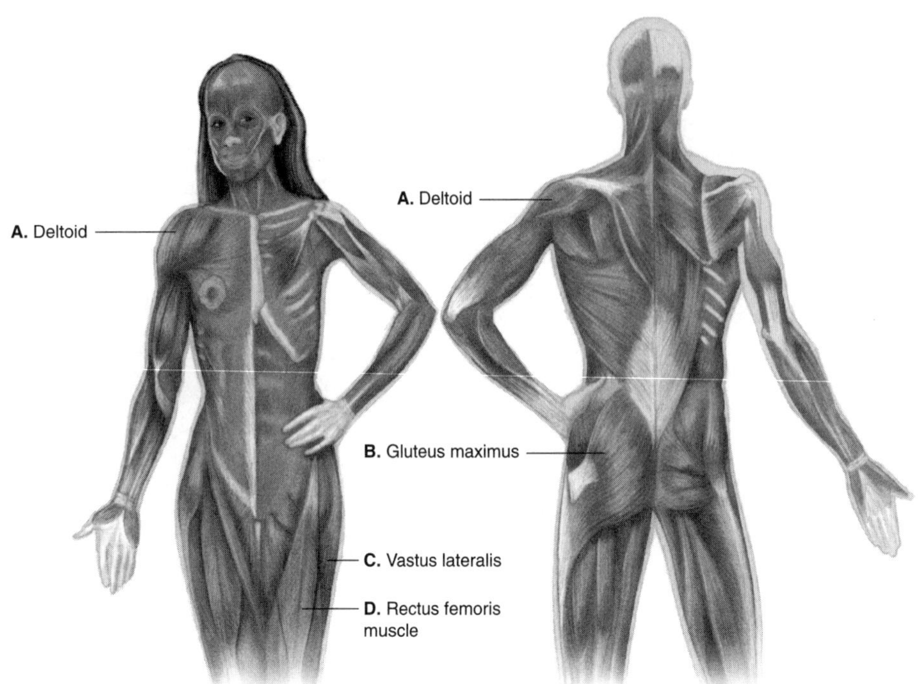

Figure 1-8 Common sites for intramuscular injections. A. Deltoid muscle. B. Gluteal area. C. Vastus lateralis muscle. D. Rectus femoris muscle.

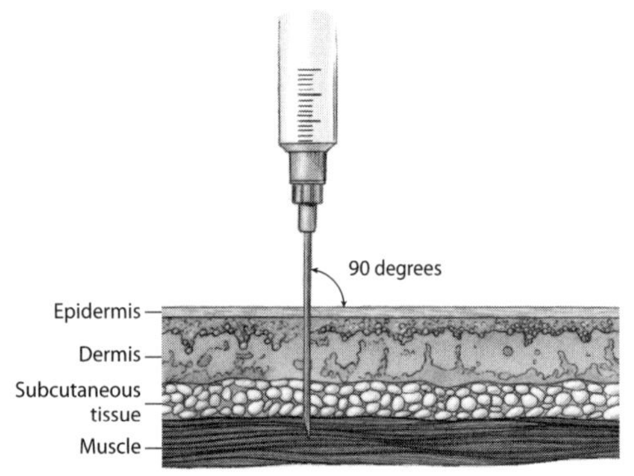

Figure 1-9 An intramuscular injection is below the dermis and subcutaneous layer and into the muscle.

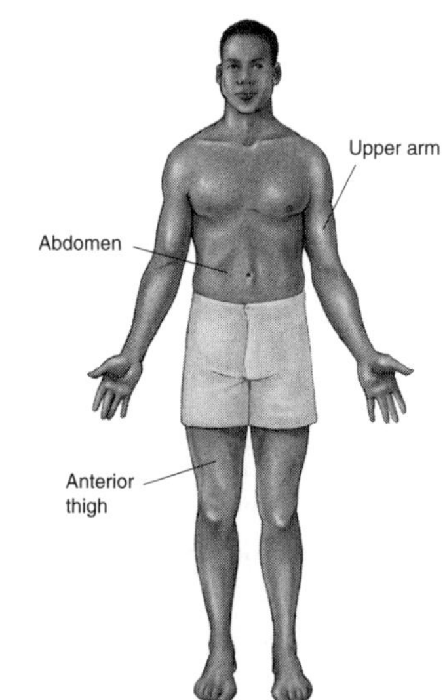

Figure 1-10 Common sites for subcutaneous injections.

5-mL IM injection is generally given in the upper outer quadrant of the buttocks (gluteus maximus) to avoid coming in contact with the sciatic nerve (**Figure 1-8▲**). The needle used is a 21-gauge 1″ to 3″ needle on a 3- to 5-mL syringe. When injecting into the muscle, the needle is held at 90°, or perpendicular to the skin (**Figure 1-9▲**). Prior to injecting the drug it is important to aspirate back on the syringe's plunger to be sure the needle has not unintentionally entered a blood vessel.

Common sites for subcutaneous injections include the upper arms, anterior thighs, and the abdomen (**Figure 1-10▶**).

Subcutaneous injections are given into the loose connective tissue between the dermis and the muscle layer (**Figure 1-11▶**).

If a medication is given by an injection, it is directly absorbed into the bloodstream (most medications end up in the bloodstream regardless of the administration route), or the medication can be injected directly into the blood vessels themselves as

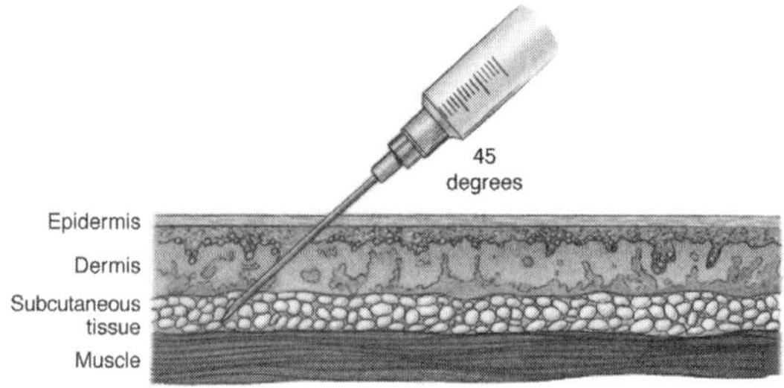

Figure 1-11 A subcutaneous injection is below the dermis and above the muscle.

in an intravenous administration. It is important for the paramedic to use the correct length needle and to use the correct technique and location. Otherwise, an intended subcutaneous injection could become an intramuscular injection or intravenous injection.

Sites for intravenous insertion and subsequent IV medication injection often include peripheral veins such as: the dorsal hands, radial wrist, folds of the elbow (antecubital fossa, median cubital vein), upper arm (median cephalic vein, median basilic vein, basilic vein, cephalic vein, axillary vein), and the neck (external jugular (EJ)) vein. The internal jugular (IJ) vein and under the clavicle (subclavian vein) are considered central IV sites and are rarely started by paramedics in the field. The leg veins are not commonly used but they are certainly available if needed, including the dorsum of the foot, anterior medial malleolus of the ankle (long saphenous vein), and the lower and upper leg (great saphenous vein, common femoral vein). To place an IV on the forearm, locate a section of veins that have a straight appearance (**Figure 1-12 ▸**).

In the past, paramedics would have attempted access on numerous veins and occasionally used a leg vein or an external jugular vein in a critical situation. Currently, the availability of equipment has made intraosseous access considerably easier and quicker to accomplish. During critical patient management, paramedics make one or two attempts at peripheral IV placement and then consider switching to an IO device. ACLS algorithms issued as a part of the 2005 Guidelines (*2005 American Heart Association Guidelines for Cardiopulmonary Resuscitation and Emergency Cardiovascular Care, Circulation: Journal of the American Heart Association (Volume 112, Number 24), December 13, 2005*) specifically endorse the use of both IV and IO routes for administration of drugs (vasopressors and antiarrhythmics) to the pulseless patient.

The intraosseous (IO) technique has been known to be a very effective route for many years. The marrow cavity found within long bones is an exceptionally vascular space, and it provides one of the fastest routes for access to the central circulation. The sternal route has recently proven to be rapid and effec-

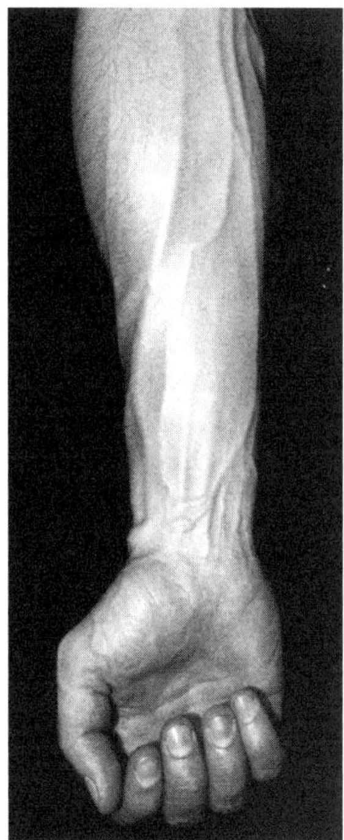

Figure 1-12 Look for veins that are relatively straight on the forearm.

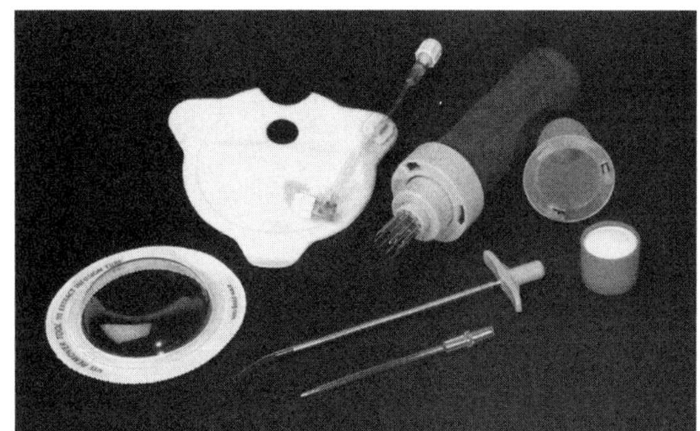

Figure 1-13 The F.A.S.T.1 device.

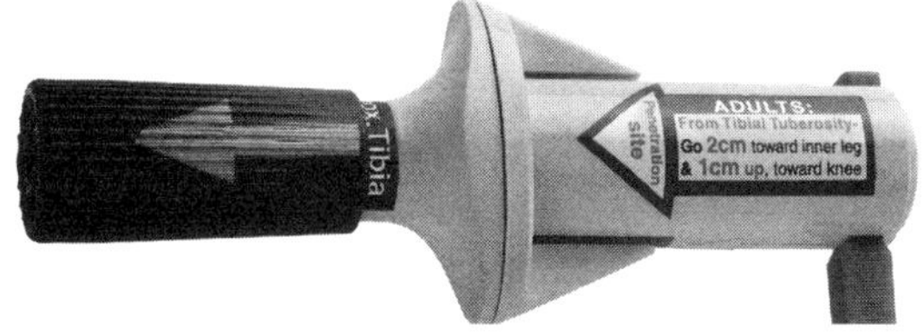

Figure 1-14 The BIG device.

tive in adult patients when using the F.A.S.T.1 (First Access for Shock and Trauma) device (**Figure 1-13 ▴**). IO access into the tibia has become easier with the introduction of both the adult and pediatric versions of the Bone Injection Gun (BIG) and the EZ-IO (**Figure 1-14 ▴ and Figure 1-15 ▸**). The EZ-IO is actually a battery-powered bone drill, and is FDA-approved for

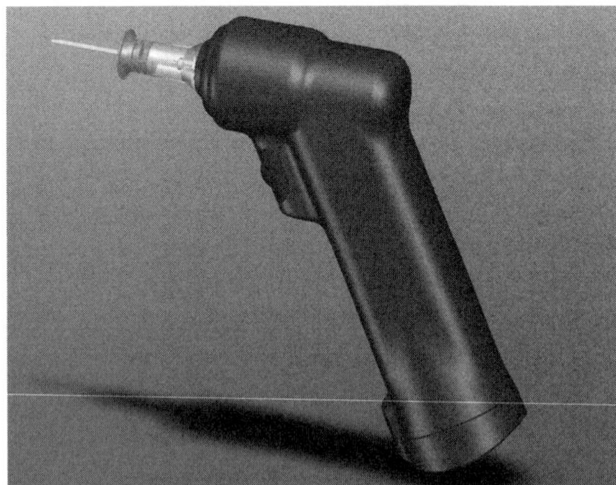

Figure 1-15 The EZ-IO device.

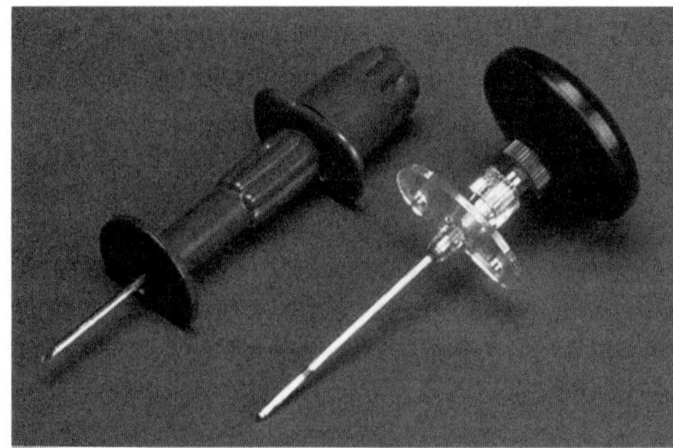

Figure 1-16 The Jamshedi IO needle is used for manual insertion.

accessing sites on both the tibia and the humerus. The Jamshedi needle is the original device used for adult and pediatric manual insertion of the IO needle. The Jamshedi needle is still used in the prehospital setting (**Figure 1-16 ▸**).

Paramedics should make a point of obtaining and maintaining competence in IO insertion techniques.

Once medications have been absorbed into the bloodstream, carried to their target organ, and performed their function, they are eliminated from the body. This is usually accomplished by either the liver or kidney, either working individually or in concert with each other to metabolize and/or excrete the medications or their by-products.

Metabolism and Excretion

The liver is a critically important organ, responsible for a wide variety of metabolic processes. It is a huge source of biosynthesis, and also works to break down and process various substances as they enter the body. Specific enzymes produce various chemical reactions, which are responsible for metabolizing drugs. These enzymes are located in various body tissues, but a large number of them are concentrated within the liver (cytochromes). How well the liver can metabolize and clear a drug from the body depends on how well the liver is functioning. Some individuals can metabolize and clear drugs so fast that the drug does not have the desired effect, while others may metabolize drugs so slowly that the drug accumulates in the body and produces an unwanted toxic effect. When liver disease is present, there will be complicated effects on medication biotransformation, pharmacokinetics, and drug clearance. As almost all drugs pass through the liver, drugs can be a significant source of liver disease. Damage can occur when a drug causes directly toxic or dose-related effects, or there is a hypersensitivity to the drug.

As stated earlier, newborns and elderly patients do not metabolize many drugs well. Newborns have immature liver enzyme systems, which makes it difficult to metabolize many drugs. How well an elderly patient metabolizes a drug will vary depending on the condition of the liver, concurrent diseases, and concomitant medication use.

The body excretes most medications or the by-products of their metabolism via the renal system. The kidneys are major organs of excretion. Within each kidney the renal cortex contains in excess of 1 million nephrons. The nephron is the primary unit of blood filtration within the kidney and it uses three discrete processes to do this. Each nephron consists of two parts. The glomeruli is a bed of capillaries and surrounds the renal tubule, a relatively long and twisted tube where blood plasma expressed from the glomerulus is ultra-filtered through the four segments (Bowman's capsule, proximal convoluted tubule, loop of Henle, distal convoluted tube) of the renal tubule. Together, all of the glomerulus filter approximately 45 gallons (180 L) of blood each day removing and/or conserving excess water, sodium, glucose, and waste products, including drugs. Only 1% of glomerular filtration produces urine, leaving the rest to be reabsorbed through the renal tubule (tubular reabsorption) back into circulation. Tubular reabsorption takes back the water, sodium, and glucose whereas the waste products are excreted in the urine. Certain waste products may be resistant to glomerular filtration. In that case, an additional process known as tubular secretion occurs and its responsibility is to eliminate wastes not initially filtered out. Filtration occurs when wastes pass from capillary walls in renal arteries to the nephrons. Tubular secretion also helps regulate the acid concentration and pH balance of the blood.

Obtaining Blood Samples

Often the paramedic draws a blood sample upon which tests will be done by the lab on arrival at the hospital. This can be done as a part of the process of starting an IV or separately to draw blood with a vacutainer or syringe to fill blood tubes. Sometimes it is necessary to obtain the samples prior to treating the patient as in the case of a diabetic patient whose blood glucose is tested and it is decided that you will be administering dextrose because the patient is hypoglycemic. In other cases bloods are drawn to save time or save the patient the discomfort of an additional stick on arrival at the hospital. Finally, in patients who are critical it may become even more difficult to obtain a blood sample as their condition deteriorates; the blood drawn in the field can be very important. Always label the blood per the requirements of your EMS system (ie, patient's name, date, etc); otherwise some hospitals may not be able to run tests on the blood.

Each regional system may have some differences in the number and types of blood tubes that are delivered with the patient to the emergency department. Examples of the types of tubes and their purpose are shown in **Table 1-11**.

Table 1-11 Blood Tubes

Tube Top Color	Tube Purpose
Red/grey speckled	Any test where serum is required
Yellow	Paternity testing, DNA, blood banking
Red	Blood banking and when serum is required for testing
Green	Ammonia, tissue typing, ionized calcium
Lavender	Complete blood count (CBC), platelet count
Blue	Sodium citrate for clotting functions

Enteral Medication Administration Techniques

Procedures for enteral medication administration routes are discussed in this section.

Oral Medication Administration

Follow these steps to perform oral medication administration (**Skill Drill 1-1**).

1. Take BSI precautions.
2. Obtain a focused history and physical examination, and confirm any patient medication allergies.
3. Follow standing orders, or contact medical control for permission.
4. Check the medication to be sure it is the right medication, it is not cloudy or discolored, and its expiration date has not passed. (**Step 1**)
5. Determine the appropriate dose. If using a liquid medication, pour the desired amount into a calibrated cup.
6. Instruct the patient to chew (if appropriate) and swallow the medication with water, if administering a pill or tablet. (**Step 2**)
7. Monitor the patient's condition, and document the medication given, route, time of administration, and response of the patient.

Administering Medication via the Gastric Tube

Follow these steps to administer medication via a gastric tube (**Skill Drill 1-2**).

1. Take BSI precautions.
2. Obtain a focused history and physical examination, and confirm any patient medication allergies.

Skill Drill 1-1 Oral Medication Administration

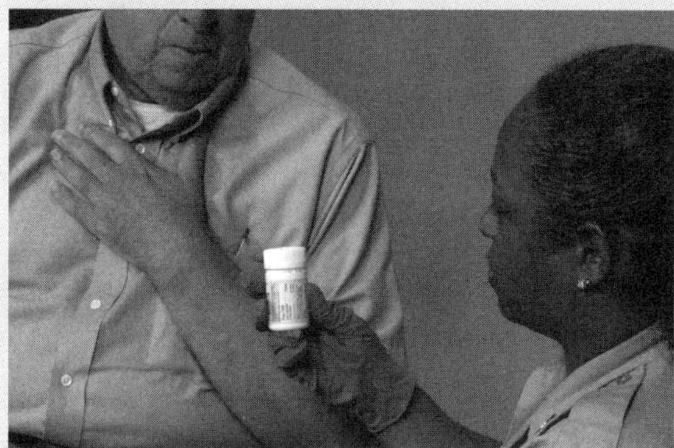

1 Check the medication to be sure it is the right medication, it is not cloudy or discolored, and its expiration date has not passed.

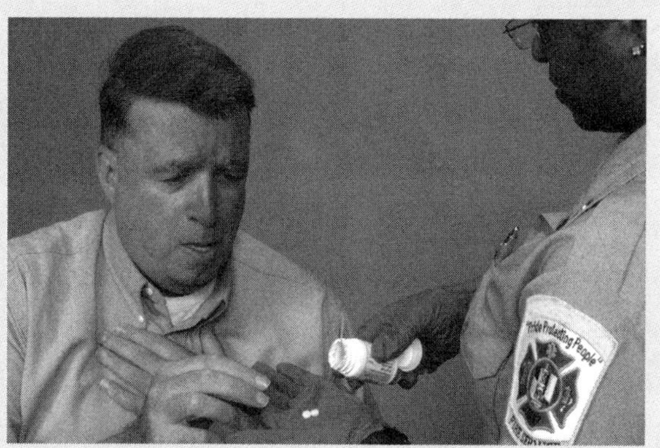

2 Instruct the patient to chew (if appropriate) and swallow the medication with water, if administering a pill or tablet.

3. Follow standing orders, or contact medical control for permission.

4. Attach a 60-mL syringe (this may require a Cath Tip syringe and not a conventional Luer-Lok

Skill Drill 1-2 Administering Medication via the Gastric Tube

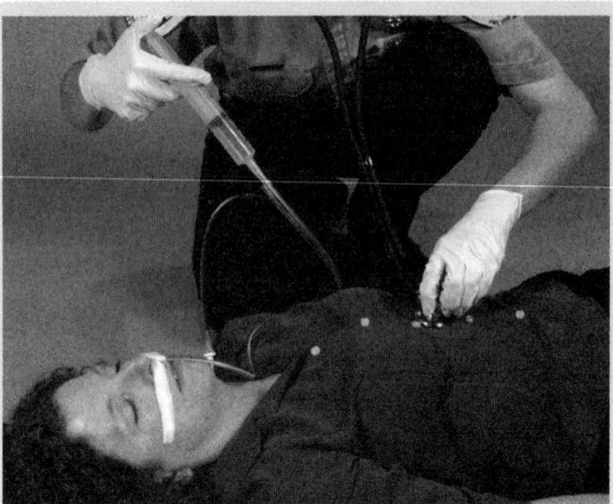

1 Attach a 60-mL syringe to the proximal end of the gastric tube and slowly inject air into the tube while auscultating over the epigastrium to confirm proper placement.

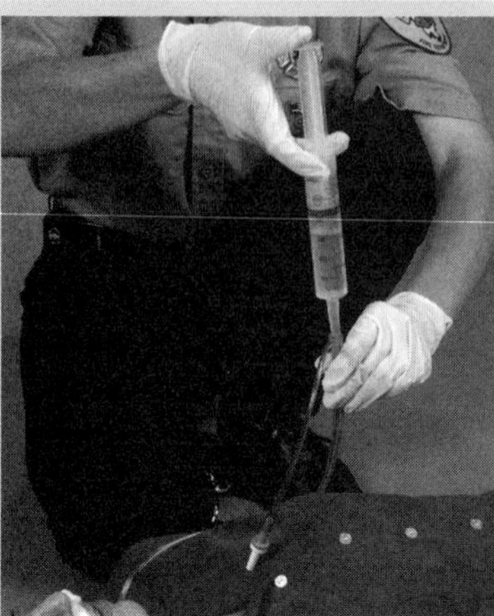

2 Inject 30 to 60 mL of normal saline into the gastric tube to irrigate the tube.

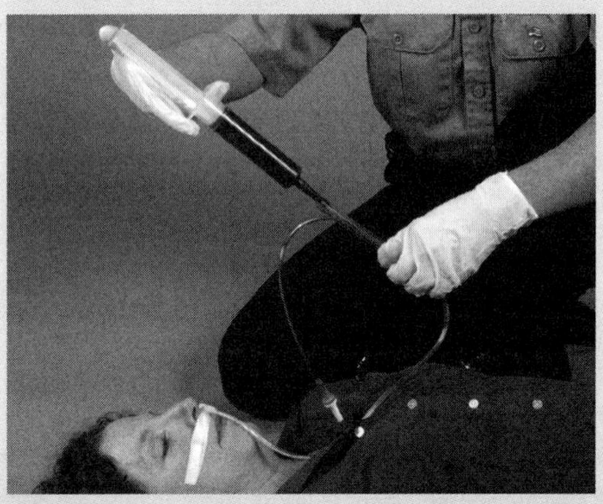

3 Inject the appropriate amount of medication into the gastric tube.

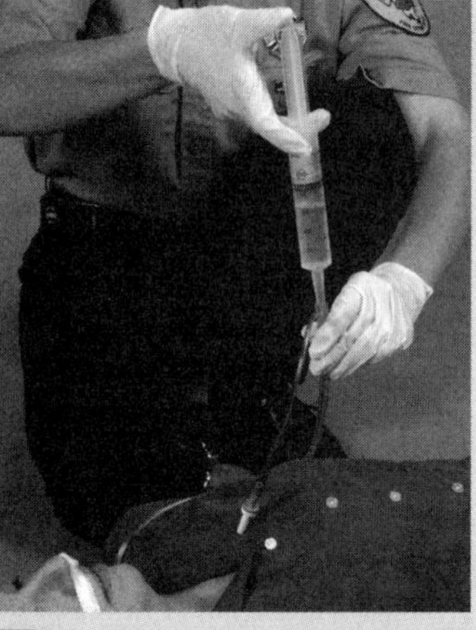

4 Flush the gastric tube with 30 to 60 mL of normal saline to ensure dispersal of the drug into the stomach.

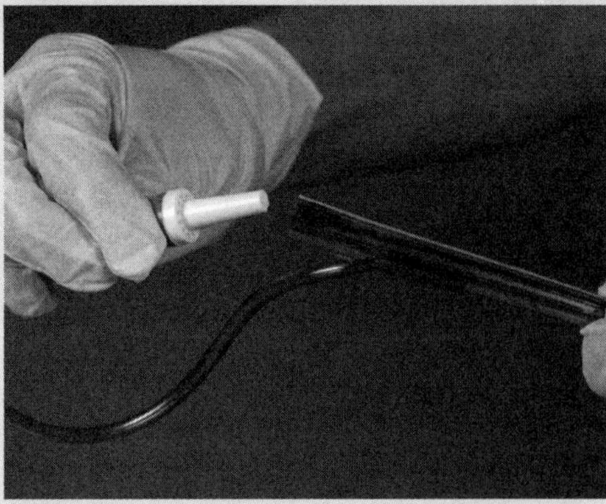

5 Clamp off the proximal end of the gastric tube.

60-mL syringe to perform) to the proximal end of the gastric tube and slowly inject air into the tube while auscultating over the epigastrium to confirm proper placement. (**Step 1**)
5. To further confirm correct tube placement, aspirate with the syringe and observe for gastric contents.
6. Inject 30 to 60 mL of normal saline into the gastric tube to irrigate the tube. (**Step 2**) If you meet resistance, ensure that the tube is not kinked.
7. Inject the appropriate amount of medication into the gastric tube. (**Step 3**)
8. Flush the gastric tube with 30 to 60 mL of normal saline to ensure dispersal of the drug into the stomach. (**Step 4**)
9. Clamp off the proximal end of the gastric tube. (**Step 5**)
10. Monitor the patient's condition and document on the PCR the medication given, route, time of administration, and response of the patient.

Rectal Medication Administration

Follow these steps to administer medication via the rectal route (**Skill Drill 1-3▼**).

1. Take BSI precautions.
2. Obtain a focused history and physical examination, and confirm any patient medication allergies.
3. Follow standing orders, or contact medical control for permission.
4. Determine the appropriate dose, and check that the medication is the right medication, there is no cloudiness or discoloration, and the expiration date has not passed.
5. Attempt to place the patient in a laterally recumbent position with the knees and hips flexed. Explain to the patient or any available responsible parties what you are doing prior to the procedure. When inserting a suppository, use a water-soluble gel for lubrication. Using a gloved finger, insert the suppository into the rectum approximately 1" to 1½" while instructing the patient to not bear down.
   Note: For medication in a liquid or gel form, it may be necessary to use a small nasopharyngeal airway or a small endotracheal tube as the delivery device. (**Step 1**)
6. Monitor the patient's condition and document the medication given, route, time of administration, and response of the patient.

Skill Drill 1-3 Rectal Medication Administration

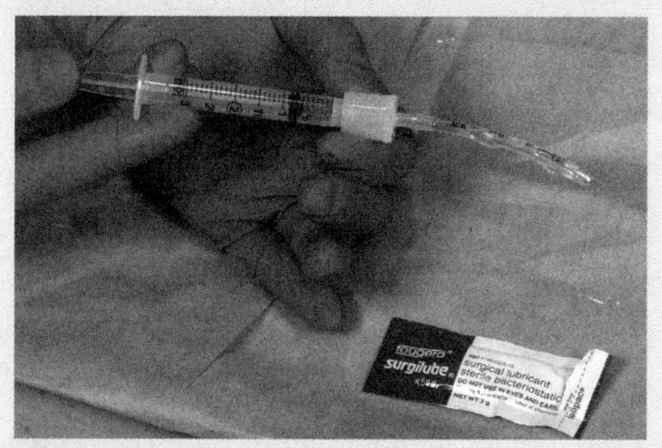

1 For medication in a liquid or gel form, it may be necessary to use a small nasopharyngeal airway or a small endotracheal tube as the delivery device.

Parenteral Medication Administration Techniques

The procedures for the parenteral medication administration routes are discussed in this section. Some medications are run in through an IV line or prepared in a second IV bag and then run into the administration port of the existing IV line by piggybacking the medication line into the original KVO line through a needle at the end of the administration set. When a medication is to be added to an IV bag (ie, a 100 mL, 500 mL, or 1,000 mL), it is essential that the paramedic prepare the mixture of the medication and fluid in the IV bag prior to attaching the administration set. If this is not done, the patient will not actually begin to receive the medication until the fluid in the tubing runs through into the patient and may delay the start of a life-saving medication.

Adding Medication to an IV Bag

Follow these steps to prepare an IV bag with medicine mixed in for infusion into the patient (**Skill Drill 1-4 ▸**).

1. Take BSI precautions.
2. Obtain a focused history and physical examination, and confirm any patient medication allergies.
3. Follow standing orders, or contact medical control for permission.
4. Check the solution (IV bag) as well as the medication that will be injected into the solution (IV bag) to ensure that they are correct per your orders, that they are not cloudy or discolored, and that the expiration date has not passed on either the IV solution bag or the medicine to be mixed into the IV bag. Reconfirm your orders for the appropriate solution, volume bag, and the amount of medicine that will be injected into the IV bag as well as the desired concentration after the medicine is mixed with the IV solution.
5. Assemble and check the supplies (needle, syringe, alcohol prep, sharps container). Draw

Skill Drill 1-4 Adding Medication to an IV Bag

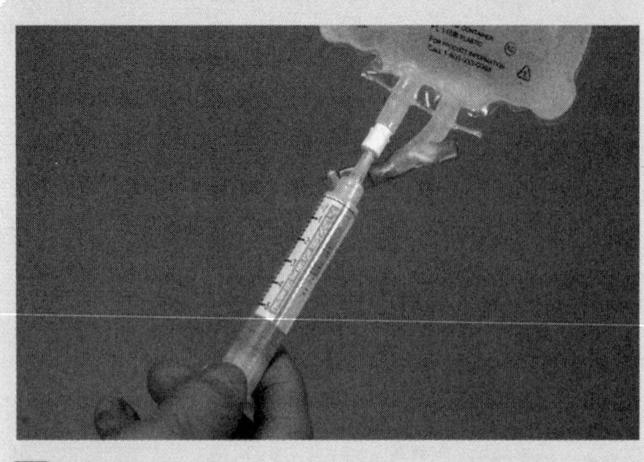

1 Cleanse the injection port and administer the correct dose of medication at the correct rate into the IV bag.

up the volume (ie, mL) that contains the correct dose (ie, mg) of the medication. Expel any air in the syringe.

6. Cleanse the medication injection port with an alcohol swab. If using a needleless system you will need to remove the protective cap.
7. Inject the desired volume of medication into the IV bag, withdraw the syringe, and dispose of the needle in a sharps container. (**Step 1**)
8. Gently shake the IV bag to mix the medication into the fluid.
9. Always label the IV bag with the name of the medication added, the amount added, the concentration in the IV bag (ie, mg/mL), the date, the time, and your name.
10. Attach the IV administration set, run through the line, and set the drip rate to administer the dose that your order calls for.
11. Monitor the patient's condition and document the medication given, IV drip rate, route, time of administration, and response of the patient.

Administering Medication via the Intravenous Bolus Route

Follow these steps to administer medication via the IV bolus route (**Skill Drill 1-5 ▸**).

1. Take BSI precautions.
2. Obtain a focused history and physical examination, and confirm any patient medication allergies.
3. Follow standing orders, or contact medical control for permission.
4. Check the medication to ensure that it is the correct one, that it is not cloudy or discolored, that the expiration date has not passed, and determine the appropriate dose to administer (ie, mg/mL).
5. Explain the procedure to the patient and the need for medication.
6. Assemble the needle onto the syringe, and draw up medication. Expel any air from the syringe. Some medications may require you to draw up 20 mL of normal saline in a separate syringe to use as a flush for the medication.
7. Cleanse the injection port nearest the patient with an alcohol prep, or remove the protective cap if using the needleless system. (**Step 1**)
8. Insert the needle into the port, and pinch off the IV tubing proximal to the administration port. Failure to shut off the line will result in the medication taking the pathway of least resistance and flowing up the line (toward the IV bag) instead of into the patient.
9. Administer the correct dose of the medication at the appropriate rate (ie, slow, fast). Some medications must be administered very quickly while others must be pushed slowly to prevent adverse effects. (**Step 2**)
10. Place the needle and syringe into a sharps container.
11. Unpinch the IV line to flush the medication into the vein. Allow it to run briefly wide open, or flush with a 20-mL bolus of normal saline.
12. Readjust the IV flow rate to the original setting. (**Step 3**)
13. Properly store and label any unused medication.
14. Monitor the patient's condition, and document the medication given, route, time of administration, and response of the patient.

Administering an IV Drip "Piggyback" into an Already Running IV Line

Follow these steps to administer an IV drip into an already running IV line via the piggyback method into a port (**Skill Drill 1-6**).

1. Take BSI precautions.
2. Follow the steps for Skill Drill 1-4 to prepare the IV bag with the correct medication solution.
3. Obtain a focused history and physical examination, and confirm any patient medication allergies.
4. Follow standing orders, or contact medical control for permission.
5. Cleanse the injection port with an alcohol prep, or remove the protective cap if using the needleless system.
6. Remove the cap on the end of the administration tubing and attach a needle.
7. Carefully insert the needle into the IV injection port closest to the patient.

Skill Drill 1-5 Administering Medication via the Intravenous Bolus Route

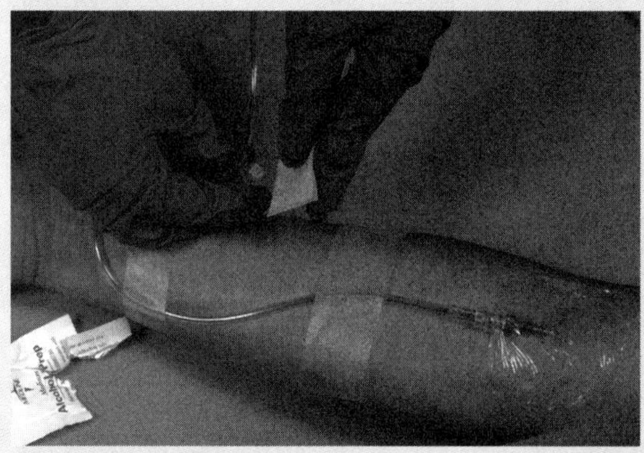

1 Assemble and check the supplies. Cleanse the injection port, or remove the protective cap if using the needleless system.

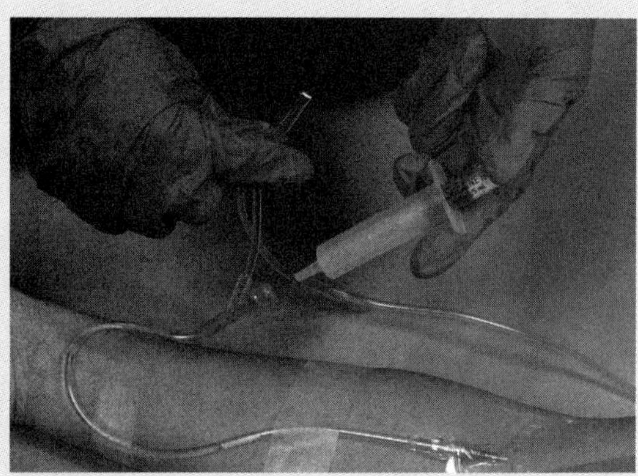

2 Insert the needle into the port closest to the patient, and pinch off the IV tubing clamp proximal to the administration port. Administer the correct dose at the appropriate rate (ie, slow, fast).

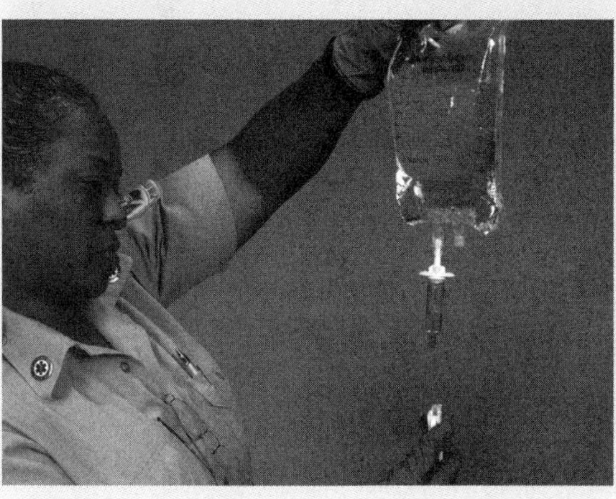

3 Unpinch the IV line to flush the medication into the vein, allowing it to run briefly wide open, or flush with a 20-mL bolus of normal saline. Readjust the IV flow rate to the original setting, and monitor the patient's condition.

8. Clamp off the original IV line to stop it from flowing/dripping.
9. Adjust the drip rate of the now piggybacked medication line to comply with your orders.
10. Monitor the patient's condition, and document the medication given, route, time of administration, and response of the patient.

Intraosseous Medication Administration

Follow these steps to administer medication via the IO route (**Skill Drill 1-7** ▸).

1. Take BSI precautions.
2. Obtain a focused history and physical examination, and confirm any patient medication allergies.
3. Follow standing orders, or contact medical control for permission.
4. Check the medication for proper fluid, clarity, and expiration date. (**Step 1**)
5. Select appropriate equipment, including IO needle (Illinois Trocar, F.A.S.T.1, EZ-IO, BIG, Jamshedi), syringe, and extension tubing/ 3-way stopcock.
6. Draw up the medication and 20 mL of normal saline for a flush.
7. Identify the proper anatomic site for IO puncture.
8. Cleanse the injection port appropriately. (**Step 2**)
9. Stabilize the tibia and insert the needle at a 90° angle, advance the Jamshedi with a twisting motion until a "pop" is felt. The F.A.S.T.1 is placed similarly but on the sternum. The BIG is placed at a 90° angle firmly against the leg while a rapid-fire mechanism is discharged similar to a hammer gun. The EZ-IO is a drill-type device. (**Step 3**)

Skill Drill 1-7 Intraosseous Medication Administration

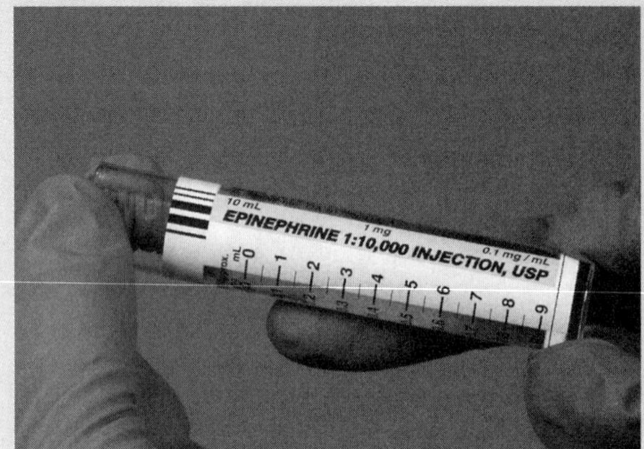

1 Check the medication for proper fluid, clarity, and expiration date.

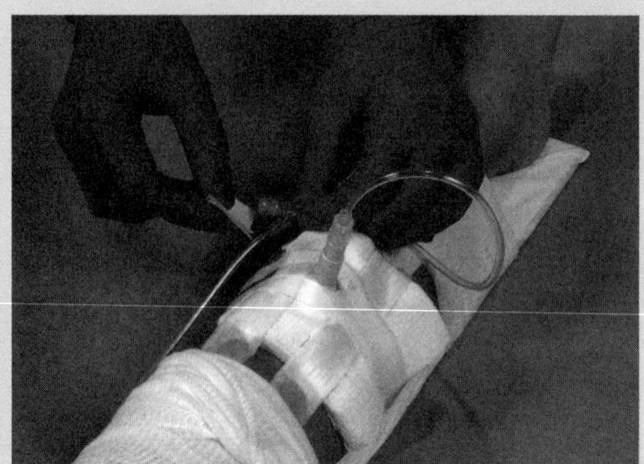

2 Identify proper site and cleanse the injection port appropriately.

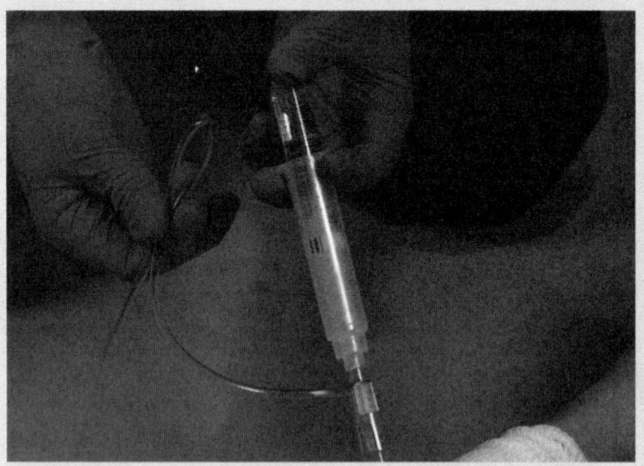

3 Stabilize the tibia and insert the needle at a 90° angle. Advance the needle with a twisting motion until a "pop" is felt.

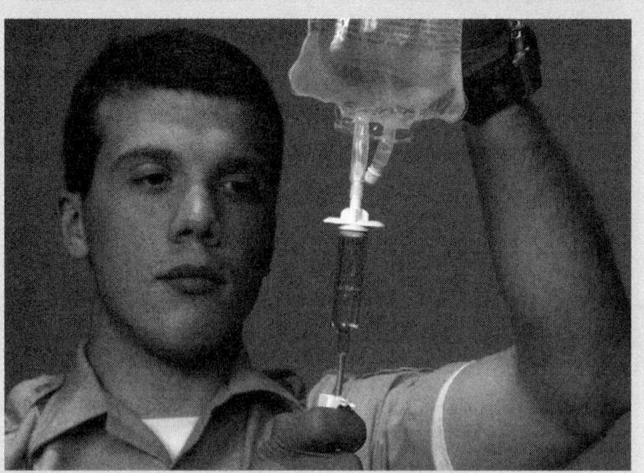

4 Attach the syringe and extension set/3-way stopcock to the IO needle. Pull back on syringe and slowly inject saline to ensure proper placement of the needle.

10. Unscrew the cap and remove the stylet from the needle.
11. Immediately dispose of the sharp stylet.
12. Attach the syringe and extension set/3-way stopcock to the IO needle.
13. Pull back on the syringe to aspirate blood and particles of bone marrow to ensure proper placement.
14. Slowly inject saline to ensure proper placement of the needle. (**Step 4**)
15. Watch for extravasation, and stop the infusion immediately if it is noted.
16. Connect the administration set, and adjust the flow rate as appropriate. Often IV pressure infusion is required as the flow is not as rapid as in vascular access.
17. Monitor the patient's condition and document the medication given, route, time of administration, and response of the patient.

Subcutaneous Medication Administration

Follow these steps to administer medication via the subcutaneous route (**Skill Drill 1-8 ▸**).

1. Take BSI precautions.
2. Obtain a focused history and physical examination, and confirm any patient medication allergies.
3. Follow standing orders, or contact medical control for permission.

Reassess the insertion site if the patient complains of pain or you have a difficult time maintaining an infusion rate.

Skill Drill 1-8 Subcutaneous Medication Administration

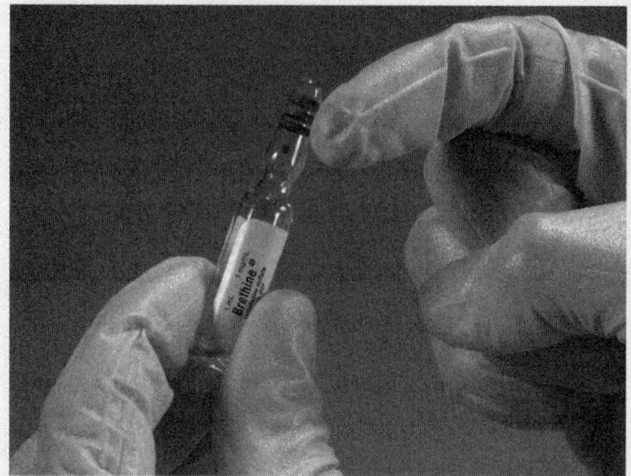

1 Check the medication to ensure that it is the correct one, that it is not discolored, and the expiration date has not passed.

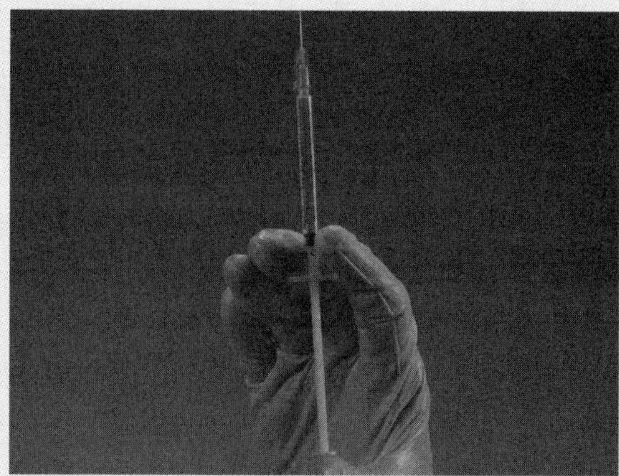

2 Draw up the correct dose of the medication.

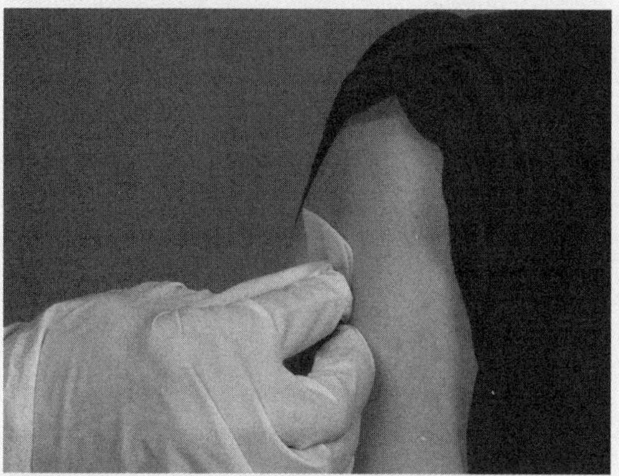

3 Using aseptic technique, cleanse the injection area.

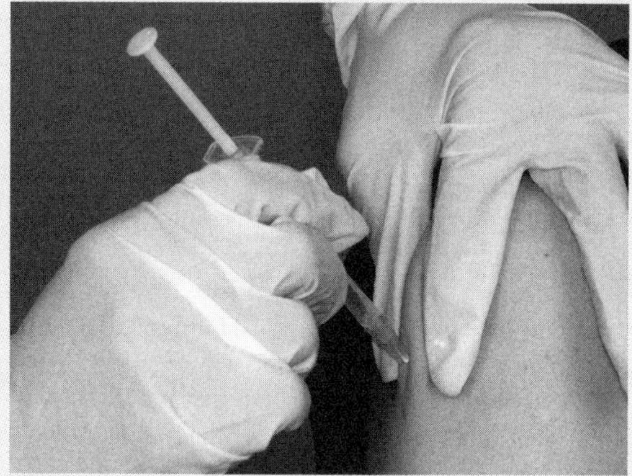

4 Pinch the skin, insert the needle at a 45° angle, and pull back on the plunger to aspirate for blood. If there is no blood in the syringe, inject the medication, remove the needle, and hold pressure over the area.

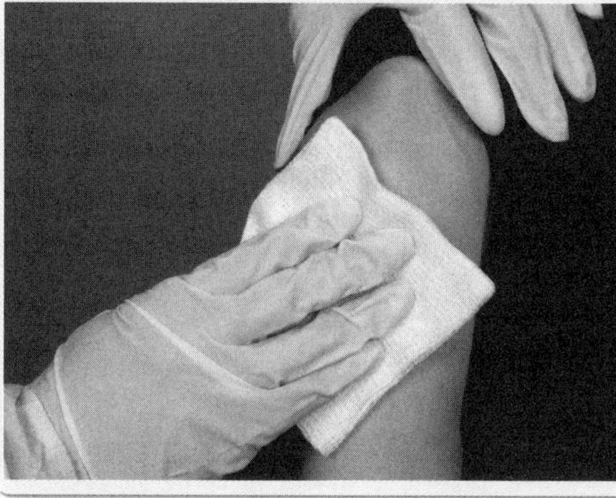

5 To disperse the medication, rub the area in a circular motion.

4. Check the medication to ensure that it is the correct one, that it is not discolored, and the expiration date has not passed. (**Step 1**)
5. Assemble and check the equipment.
6. Draw up the correct dose of the medication. (**Step 2**)
7. Using aseptic technique, cleanse the injection area. (**Step 3**)

8. Pinch the skin surrounding the area and insert the needle at a 45° angle.
9. Pull back on the plunger to aspirate for blood. If there is no blood in the syringe, inject the medication, remove the needle, and hold pressure over the area. (**Step 4**)
   Note: If blood is present, this indicates that you may have entered a blood vessel. In such a case, remove the needle, hold pressure on the site, prepare a new syringe and needle, and select another site.
10. Immediately dispose of the needle and syringe in a sharps container.
11. To disperse the medication, rub the area in a circular motion. (**Step 5**)
12. Monitor the patient's condition and document the medication given, route, time of administration, and response of the patient.

Intramuscular Medication Administration

Follow these steps to administer medication via the intramuscular route (**Skill Drill 1-9** ▸).

1. Take BSI precautions.
2. Obtain a focused history and physical examination, and confirm any patient medication allergies.
3. Follow standing orders, or contact medical control for permission.
4. Check the medication to ensure that it is the correct one, that it is not discolored, and the expiration date has not passed. (**Step 1**)
5. Assemble and check the equipment.
6. Draw up the correct dose of the medication. (**Step 2**)
7. Identify the injection site. The deltoid muscle of the shoulder and upper arm and the upper outside quadrant of the gluteus muscle are commonly used.
8. Using aseptic technique, cleanse the injection area. (**Step 3**)
9. Apply tension to the skin.
10. Insert the needle at a 90° angle. (**Step 4**)
11. Pull back on the plunger to aspirate for blood. If there is no blood, inject the medication, remove the needle, and hold pressure over the area.
    Note: If blood is present, this indicates that you may have entered a blood vessel. In such a case, remove the needle, hold pressure on the site, prepare a new syringe and needle, and select another site.
12. Immediately dispose of the needle and syringe in a sharps container.
13. To disperse the medication, rub the area in a circular motion. (**Step 5**)
14. Monitor the patient's condition and document the medication given, route, time of administration, and response of the patient.

Percutaneous Medication Administration Techniques

The procedures for the percutaneous medication administration routes are discussed in this section.

Intranasal Medication Administration

Follow these steps to administer medication via the intranasal route (**Skill Drill 1-10** ▸).

1. Take BSI precautions.
2. Obtain a focused history and physical examination, and confirm any patient medication allergies.
3. Follow standing orders, or contact medical control for permission.
4. Check the medication to ensure that it is the correct one, that it is not cloudy or discolored, and that the expiration date has not passed.
5. Draw up the appropriate dose of medication in the syringe.
6. Attach the mucosal atomizer device (MAD) to the syringe. (**Step 1**)
7. Explain the procedure to the patient and the need for the medication.
8. Spray half of the medication dose into each nostril.
9. Dispose of the atomizer device and syringe in the appropriate container.
10. Monitor the patient's condition and document the medication given, route, time of administration, and response of the patient.

Sublingual Drug Administration

Follow these steps to administer medication via the sublingual route (**Skill Drill 1-11** ▸).

1. Take BSI precautions.
2. Obtain a focused history and physical examination, and confirm any patient medication allergies.
3. Follow standing orders, or contact medical control for permission.

Skill Drill 1-9 Intramuscular Medication Administration

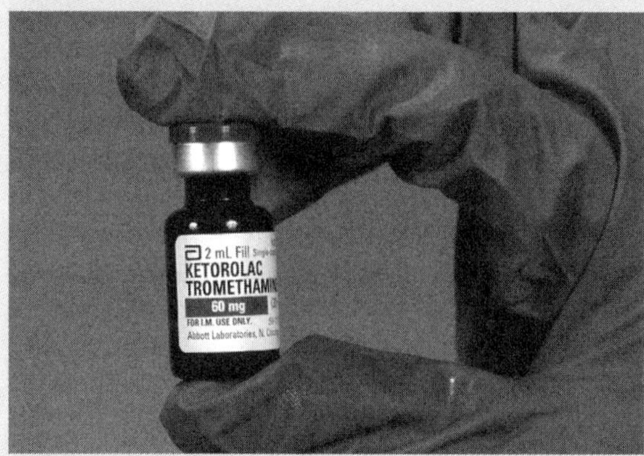

1 Check the medication to ensure that it is the correct one, that it is not discolored, and the expiration date has not passed.

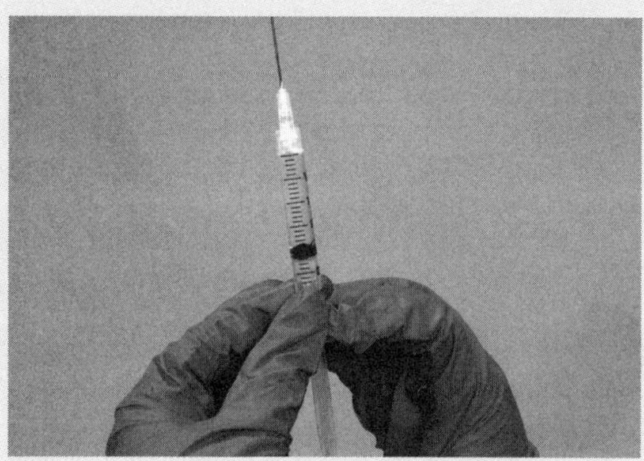

2 Draw up the correct dose of the medication.

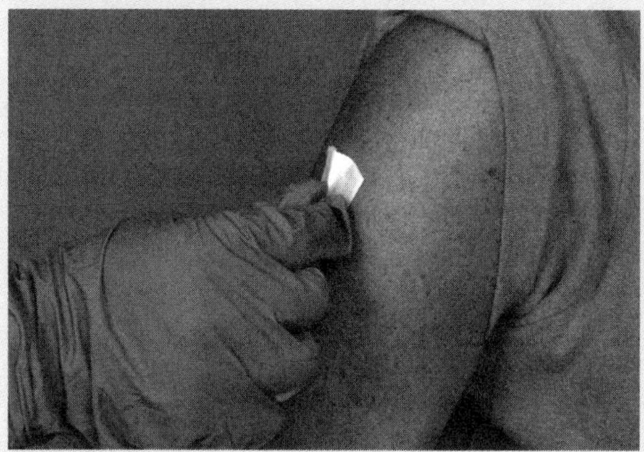

3 Identify the injection site. Using aseptic technique, cleanse the injection area.

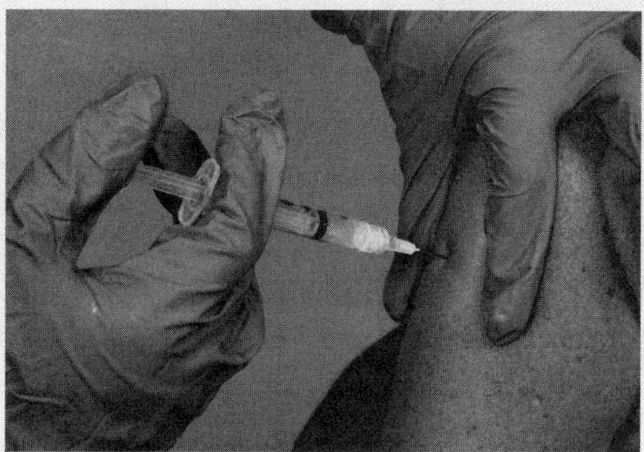

4 Apply tension to the skin and insert the needle at a 90° angle.

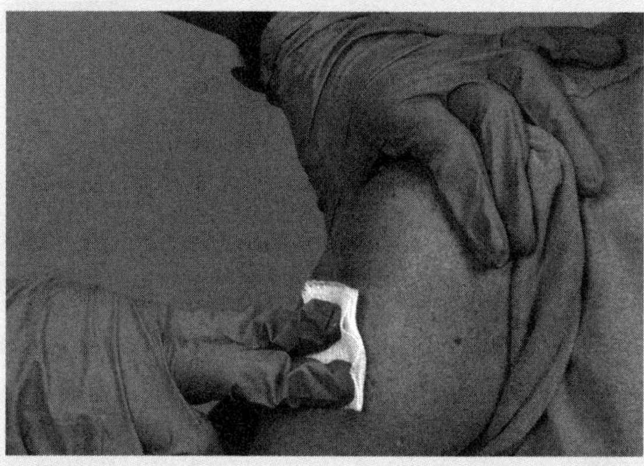

5 To disperse the medication, rub the area in a circular motion.

4. Check the medication to ensure that it is the correct one and that its expiration date has not passed, and determine the appropriate amount for the correct dose. (**Step 1**)
5. Ask the patient to rinse his or her mouth with a little water if the mucous membranes are dry.
6. Explain the procedure, and ask the patient to lift his or her tongue. Place the tablet or spray the dose under the tongue, or ask the patient to do so. (**Step 2**)
7. Advise the patient not to chew or swallow the tablet, but to let it dissolve slowly.
8. Monitor the patient's condition and document the medication given, route, time of administration, and response of the patient.

Skill Drill 1-10 Intranasal Medication Administration

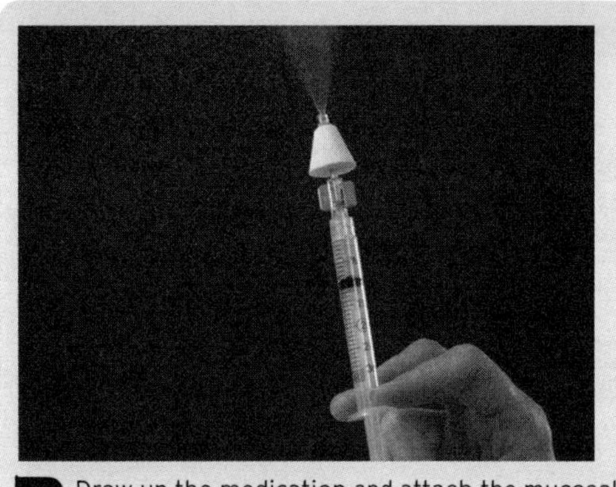

1 Draw up the medication and attach the mucosal atomizer device (MAD) to the syringe.

Buccal Drug Administration

Follow these steps to administer medication via the buccal route (**Skill Drill 1-12**).

1. Take BSI precautions.
2. Obtain a focused history and physical examination, and confirm any patient medication allergies.
3. Follow standing orders, or contact medical control for permission.
4. Check the medication to ensure that it is the correct one and that its expiration date has not passed, and determine the appropriate amount for the correct dose.
5. Place the medication in between the patient's cheek and gum, or ask the patient to do so.
6. Advise the patient not to chew or swallow the tablet, but to let it dissolve slowly.
7. Monitor the patient's condition and document the medication given, route, time of administration, and response of the patient.

Skill Drill 1-11 Sublingual Drug Administration

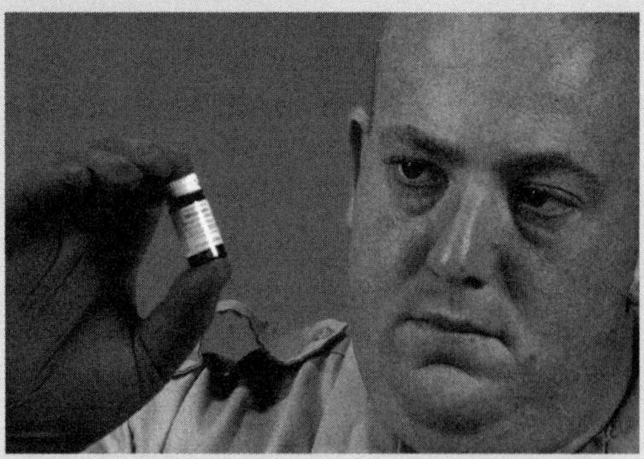

1 Check the medication for drug type and its expiration date, and determine the appropriate amount for the correct dose.

Have the patient rinse his or her mouth with a little water if the mucous membranes are dry.

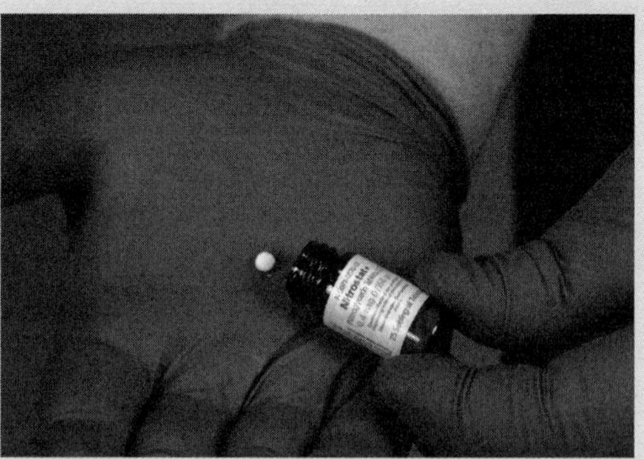

2 Explain the procedure to the patient, and ask the patient to lift his or her tongue. Place the tablet or spray the dose underneath the tongue, or have the patient do so.

Advise the patient not to chew or swallow the tablet, but to let it dissolve slowly.

Monitor the patient, and document the medication given, the route, administration time, and the response of the patient.

Inhalation Medication Administration Techniques

The procedures for inhalation medication administration are discussed in this section.

Small-Volume Nebulizer Medication Administration

Follow these steps to administer medication with a small-volume nebulizer (**Skill Drill 1-13**).

1. Take BSI precautions.
2. Determine the need for an inhaled bronchodilator based on patient presentation.
3. Obtain a focused history and physical examination, and confirm any patient medication allergies.
4. Follow standing orders, or contact medical control for permission.
5. Check the medication and its expiration date. Make sure you have the right medication and that it is not cloudy or discolored. (**Step 1**)
6. Add premixed medication to the bowl of the nebulizer. (**Step 2**)
   Note: If the medication is not premixed, add the medication to the bowl and mix it with the specified amount of normal saline (usually 3 mL).
7. Connect the T piece with the mouthpiece to the top of the bowl, connect it to the oxygen tubing, and set the flowmeter to 6 L/min. (**Step 3**)
8. With the nebulizer in position, instruct the patient to breathe as deeply as possible and hold his or her breath for 3 to 5 seconds before exhaling.
9. Monitor the patient's condition and document the medication given, route, time of administration, and response of the patient. (**Step 4**)

When a medication is given by the inhalation route, the paramedic has a few specific options: the multiple-use metered-dose inhaler (MDI), a

Skill Drill 1-13 Small-Volume Nebulizer Medication Administration

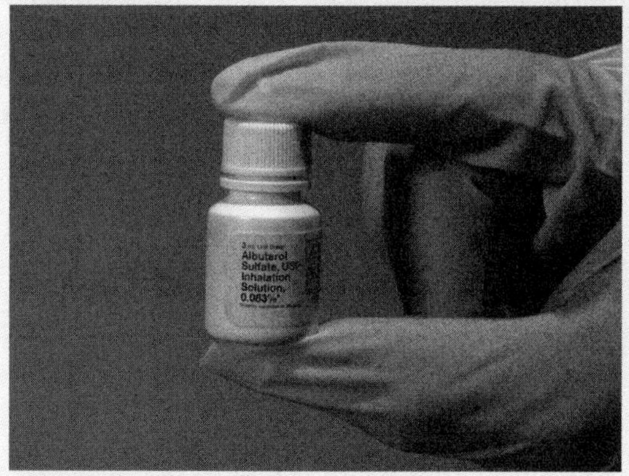

1 Check the medication and its expiration date. Make sure you have the right medication and that it is not cloudy or discolored.

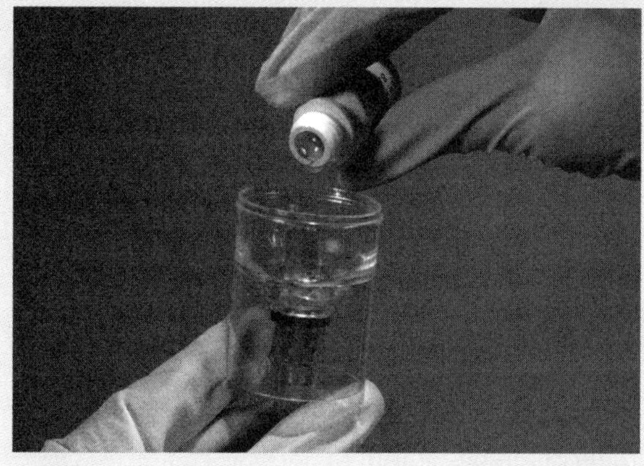

2 Add premixed medication to the bowl of the nebulizer.

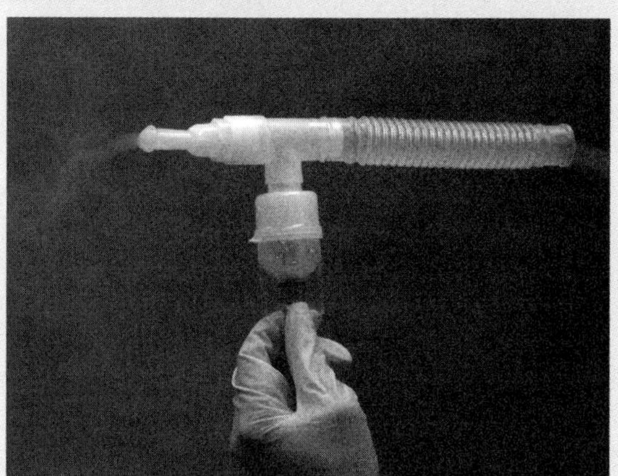

3 Connect the T piece with the mouthpiece to the top of the bowl, connect it to the oxygen tubing, and set the flowmeter to 6 L/min.

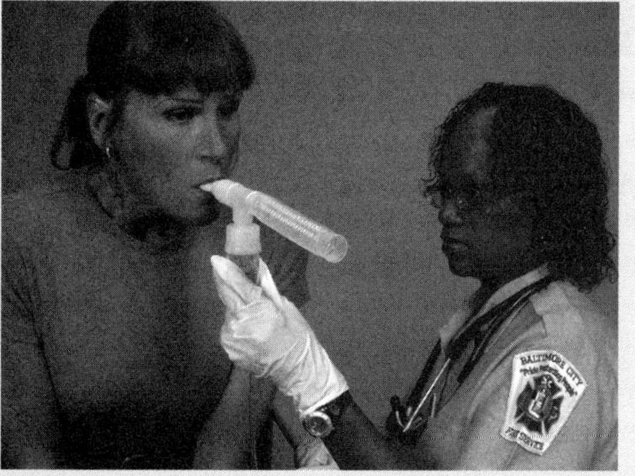

4 Monitor patient's condition and document the medication given, route, time of administration, and response of the patient.

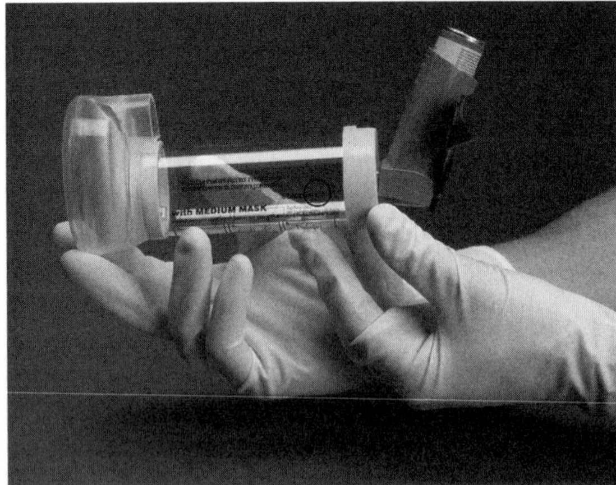

Figure 1-17 An MDI and a spacer can be used with or without a mask.

nebulizer, an Aerochamber or spacer device, or ventilated in with the assistance of a bag-mask device. Most patients with reactive airway disease have a prescribed bronchodilator that they administer to themselves through an MDI or home nebulizer. Some of these patients may also have a spacer device that makes it easier for them to take full advantage of the medication and not rely on proper timing to inhale the medication deep down into their lungs (**Figure 1-17▲**). It is helpful to observe the new MDI user with their device as some patients in distress who are not well practiced with their device have been known to get the timing off, not hold the medication in their lungs, or simply spray the medication on the inside of their mouth. In this case, physicians often prescribe a spacer device that holds the dose in the Aerochamber until the patient inhales it. The nebulizer primarily for home use delivers the medication continuously until the dose is complete. The drug is aerosolized using room air pumps or "oxygen machines" unlike the nebulizers used by paramedics which are connected to a traditional oxygen source.

Drugs: The Legal Issues and the "Drug Rights"

When a paramedic carries a box full of drugs into the patient's home, there is a tremendous responsibility carried along with that box. Some of the medications, if given inappropriately, can cause harmful or even deadly effects. Simple steps can help to reduce the potential for medication mistakes (ie, always check and double check the medication and the dose, write it down, always label mixtures you prepare right away, administer the medication yourself, and do not let someone else administer the medication you drew up, etc). To prepare for this challenge, paramedics need to learn a lot of information about each of the drugs they may ultimately administer. They also need to know the "six rights" of drug administration and practice them every time a medication is administered. Prior to giving any medication, the paramedic must review the following "six rights":

- Right patient
- Right drug
- Right dose
- Right route
- Right time
- Right documentation and reporting

Throughout each of the cases involving pharmacological interventions in this book, we will be emphasizing the six rights because they are so very important to practice in the prehospital setting.

Prior to administering a medication the paramedic should consider, "Is this the right patient for this medication?" If you were in the hospital setting you might have multiple medications to administer to multiple patients, so it would be essential to ensure the right medication went to the specific patient it was prescribed for. In the prehospital setting this is rare, but with all you will learn about patients, their conditions, your treatment protocols, and the SAMPLE medical history a patient presents with, it is always important to know that this is definitely the right medication to be administering to this specific patient.

In many cases there are choices of two or more medications that are indicated and would accomplish what you would like to do. Consider the question, "Is this the right drug?" For example, in your SAMPLE history you find out that the patient has allergic reactions to the "caine drugs" and he learned this when he was administered his first shot of novacaine in the dentist office. If this specific patient needs an antiarrhythmic medication, it would be a smart decision to pick an alternate drug to lidocaine [Xylocaine] such as amiodarone [Cordarone] which is less likely to cause an allergic reaction.

You are responsible for knowing the right dose of every medication. Consider the question, "Is this the correct dose of this medication?" Some of the medications carried in the paramedic's drug box are in different concentrations. For example, lidocaine [Xylocaine] may be carried in the 2% and 20% concentrations. The 2% is for an IV bolus administration and the 20% is used to set up a drip. The manufacturers had to create a specialized needle cover to make it clear that the 20% concentration was not to be used directly into an IV administration port. There have been cases where the wrong concentration was given directly into the IV administration port and the patient received 10 times the appropriate dose, had a seizure, and died. Always calculate the appropriate dose and then check your math prior to proceeding with the administration of the drug. Many paramedic services have charts based on estimated patient weight which already have the calculations done for drugs that are weight-based, such as dopamine [Intropin] drips.

You are responsible for knowing the right route for the administration of the medication. It does not help the patient to swallow aspirin when it is supposed to be chewed, nor is a swallowed nitroglycerin pill effective at relieving the angina patient's chest pain. If a patient is in extremis with poor peripheral circulation, medications like epinephrine are better administered by the IV route rather than the SC or IM route.

You are responsible for knowing the right timing for medication administration. Some medications need to be a fast IV bolus, while others are administered slowly. The actions of the medication can be altered if administered inappropriately.

Documentation is a very important final step in the administration of any medication. Make sure your documentation is clear and that it states who gave what to the patient, in what dose, by what route, for what reason, at what time, and indicate if it worked or not. The paramedic is responsible for monitoring the patient and performing an ongoing assessment to include reassessment of vital signs and appropriate physical examination. Always go back and reassess to see if the interventions, specifically the drug given in this situation, have had an effect on the patient.

The administration of medications by the paramedic requires medical control authorization. Medical control can come in the form of direct or on-line medical control or indirect or off-line medical control. Typically, a committee of physicians at the state, regional, or local level meet to discuss and develop treatment protocols that the paramedics in their jurisdiction must follow. Drug therapy, just like specific ALS modalities (ie, advanced airway placement, cardioversion, etc) must be specified in the treatment protocols so that it is clear which medications the paramedic should consider in specific patient situations. Some drugs will come under a standing order in the protocol which means that the paramedic is authorized by the written treatment protocol to administer that specific medication by the specific route and dose prescribed in the circumstance that protocol calls for. An example would be a standing order to administer an IM injection of epinephrine using an EpiPen auto-injector in the circumstance of a patient who is exhibiting the signs and symptoms of anaphylaxis. Provided the patient fits the criteria, when there is a standing order the paramedic does not need to call in for an order to administer the medication. In other circumstances the physicians may create a series of medical control options where the paramedic has to call in (by radio or telephone) to the medical control physician to present the case and receive authorization to administer one of the drug options. Either way, on-line or off-line, the paramedic always needs authorization and should clearly document which physician authorized the order for the medication.

Consider the scenario where a patron walks into a first aid tent at a rock concert. The tent is manned by an EMT-B and a paramedic. The patron is looking for medicine because he has a splitting headache and stomach pain. The provider who supplies those pills in the absence of a medical authorization would be dispensing medications without a license. To be on the safe side, it is always more appropriate to discuss the development of standing orders authorized by your Medical Director for situations that could come up.

Throughout this text we will discuss cases and treatment. There are certainly differences between the treatment provided in urban and rural settings as well as regional differences. It is not our intent to get into heated discussion on the most appropriate regional variances in treatment; rather, we will illustrate our cases with typical treatment. If your service has a treatment protocol that differs from those listed in our cases, always follow local medical control protocols because it is your local medical control treatment protocols that you are authorized to follow. Since we needed to follow some standard, we have chosen to use the ILCOR Algorithms and Guidelines where they apply, as well as the drugs listed in the paramedic's formulary (found in Appendix C). Remember, as a paramedic it is your responsibility to know your treatment protocols and the drug formulary for your region. Most paramedics carry a pocket-sized version of these protocols to refer to in those situations that are not common.

Patient Management Pharmaceutical Plan

As we proceed through this book, you will note that the pharmaceutical intervention plan has been incorporated right into the management plan for each of the cases discussed. Drug therapy is not something that occurs as an aside, but rather it is part of the patient management plan and just like skills such as placing an advanced airway or inserting an IV line, the administration of a drug can, in many cases, be an important step in the patient's management. Within each case you will see we have introduced the medications that are often referred to in the paramedic's formulary for prehospital interventions. Of course the decision of whether a patient is given a particular medication is always in the context of the situation, and as such, this involves an assessment of the patient and a determination if they are symptomatic of a particular condition. When the patient is complaining of cardiac chest pain, nitroglycerin is typically indicated. However, it should not be given prior to an assessment, including vital signs. In the circumstance when the blood pressure is below 90 mm Hg systolic, nitroglycerin is not indicated because it could make the condition worse by inducing vasodilatory hypotension.

The pathophysiological principles of medication administration also should be taken into consideration since medication makes changes to the patient's condition. Once again in the patient with cardiac chest pain where nitroglycerin is indicated, a full assessment including diagnostics must be completed and interpreted correctly or the patient's condition could be made critically worse. In a patient who is having a myocardial infarction in the right ventricle, administering nitroglycerin can result in the blood pressure dropping so low as to produce cardiogenic shock or death. Nitrates relax vascular smooth muscle, resulting in peripheral vasodilation. In acute right heart failure due to myocardial infarction, the cardiac output decreases and can lead to cardiogenic shock or death if the damage is severe enough. Nitrates can rapidly accelerate this process.

Infection Control During Medication Administration

Medication administration in the prehospital setting poses a potentially high risk of exposure to infection for the paramedic, primarily because most medications are administered parenterally using needles, syringes, and glass medication containers. Often an IV must be started prior to administering a drug and this involves the use of additional sharps, including angiocatheters and glass blood tubes. The prehospital setting is often referred to as an *uncontrolled* setting as opposed to the *controlled* clinical setting. The uncontrolled setting represents situations such as poor lighting, challenging areas in which to work, demanding conditions, and often hurried circumstances. For example, handling needles and glass in the back of a moving ambulance is a task that carries an inherently high risk for an inadvertent puncture or laceration.

Each year many health care providers both in and out of the hospital setting experience exposures from accidental punctures or cuts from various sharps. Sharps are any medical instrument that can break through the skin and include: needles, syringes, scalpels, suture needles, and medical glassware such as ampules, vials, and blood tubes. The proper disposal of sharps requires the use of a sharps container. This container is a rigid puncture-proof container that is available in various sizes and carries a label marked "Biohazard" (**Figure 1-18**). Sharps containers should be placed as close as practical to the area where the sharps are used.

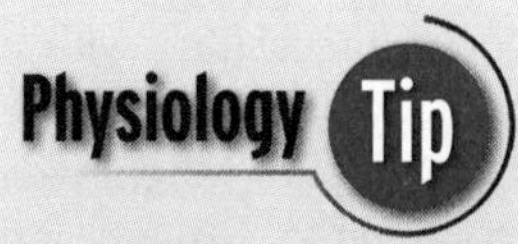

Look for medication patches during the assessment of your patient. Narcotic and nitroglycerin patches can result in hypotension.

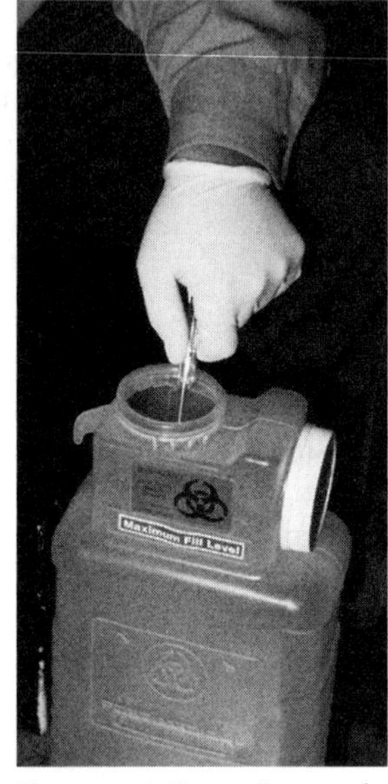

Figure 1-18 Always dispose of sharp objects or blood-filled items in a puncture-proof sharps container.

Universal precautions are the practices used by health care providers to ensure specific safety practices are taken with each patient contact. These practices take into consideration that there is the chance for exposure with each patient contact; therefore, steps must be taken to avoid the potential to be exposed to blood or any potentially infectious body fluid. Body substance isolation (BSI) is the process of using personal protective equipment (PPE) such as gloves, masks, and gowns while caring for patients to prevent an exposure. In 1996, the Center for Disease Control and Prevention (CDC) revised and enhanced these guidelines and replaced both terms with **standard precautions**. Many needlestick accidents could have been avoided had recommended precautions been followed.

The standard precautions guidelines for preventing needlestick injury include:

- Training and continuing education on the proper handling and disposal of sharps.
- Training and continuing education on infection protection and what to do when an injury occurs.

- Wearing gloves and additional PPE as needed.
- Avoid opening needles until a sharps container is immediately available.
- Using devices with safety features as often as possible (ie, needleless access ports and self-sheathing needles).
- Avoid recapping needles.

Medication administration is performed using a very clean technique with sterile and clean equipment. Parenteral medication administration has the potential to expose the patient to pathogens. The last thing a sick or injured patient needs is iatrogenic infection caused by the paramedic who used a poor technique starting an IV or administering a drug. Sterile technique is the method used in the operating room (OR) to prevent contamination of a wound. This cannot be achieved outside of the OR; therefore, a very clean or aseptic technique is what should be strived for with medication administration in the prehospital setting.

Clean or **aseptic technique** entails wearing gloves, cleansing the area of skin to be punctured using an **antiseptic** product such as alcohol and iodine preparations, and careful handling of sterile equipment (ie, needle, syringes, containers) used for drug administration. If a port is accessed, it must also be cleaned prior to inserting the needle. Once the package is opened, the needle should not touch anything except the cleansed area. If the needle does touch anything other than the cleansed area (ie, your glove, any surface, other equipment), it should be discarded immediately and replaced with another sterile needle.

Properly dispose of all sharps into a sharps container immediately after use without bending, breaking, or removing needles from syringes, and do not attempt to recap needles. The cleanup of any surfaces and reusable equipment should be done using the appropriate **disinfectant**. Most disinfectants are designed to destroy pathogens on nonliving objects such as surfaces and equipment. They are not intended to be used to disinfect the skin. Examples include Virex, Cidex, and Microcide.

Developing Paramedic Pharmacology Best Practices

Throughout this book, as in your practice in the streets as a paramedic, it is essential that you always comply with the highest standards of medication administration. That is to say that all medications are always handled with a serious sense of responsibility and prior to their administration the six rights for the specific medication are taken into consideration. If at any point you are not clear if this is the right medication for this patient in this situation, then do not proceed without first looking it up, referring to a reference or protocol, or consulting with your medical control. Mistakes made with medications can be tragic, life-threatening, and career-ending for the paramedic. Always know the rights before proceeding.

Since the administration of medications is linked hand-in-hand with the necessity for taking the appropriate standard precautions, the paramedic must be very familiar with their service's exposure control plan. This includes the engineering controls in place to keep the job a safe work environment such as not recapping needles and using sharps containers at the patient's side. If at any point you are not entirely clear on the disposal procedure for sharps, the cleanup procedures for a blood spill, disinfection procedures, or the follow-up procedure for a needlestick injury or potential exposure, you should review the procedure in question with your medical director or infection control officer before an incident occurs.

If the treatment plan involves a pharmacological intervention, the paramedic should be able to defend the drug choices that are being incorporated into the patient's management plan. Medications are not given because we have a box full of them. They are given in the prehospital setting because they will help the patient in specific situations and because the administration should not be delayed until arrival at the hospital.

The best paramedics serve as "models" for medical asepsis, advocate while performing medication administration, and properly dispose of contaminated items and sharps. Disinfecting reusable equipment and work surfaces after each use helps to reduce the spread of pathogens to the next patient or coworker. Employing infection control protects both the patient and the health care provider. Using good technique with every patient and all procedures helps to ensure the health and safety for both you and the patient.

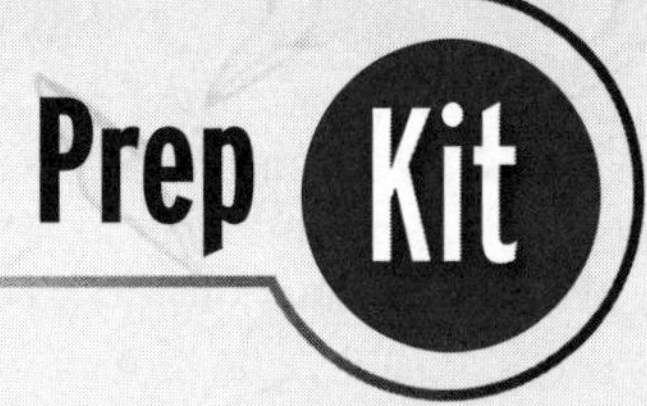

Chapter Summary

- Pharmacology is the study of (*ology*) drugs or medications (*pharm*).
- The history of a patient's medication or drug use should include each of the following five types of medications: over-the-counter remedies, prescribed medications, herbals, vitamins, and illicit or "recreational drugs."
- In the United States, if a substance is considered a drug, it falls under the regulation of the Food and Drug Administration (FDA).
- The drug profile includes all of the information for the medication including: drug name, classification, mechanism of action, indications, pharmacokinetics, side and adverse effects, routes of administration, drug forms, doses, contraindications, and special considerations.
- Drugs are developed from four main sources: plants, animals and humans, minerals, and synthetics and chemicals.
- There are three phases of drug activity: pharmaceutics, pharmacokinetics, and pharmacodynamics.
- Each drug is distinctive in relation to the rate of absorption, distribution, metabolism, and elimination.
- Drugs come in many forms and each form has advantages and disadvantages. Most are subdivided into solids or liquids.
- The routes of administration are classified into three categories: the enteral route (absorbed via some aspect of the gastrointestinal tract [mouth to anus]), the parenteral route (those given by any means other than the enteric system), and the percutaneous route (absorbed through the skin or mucous membrane).
- There are a number of special considerations in the administration of drugs with regard to the pregnant, pediatric, or geriatric patient.
- To be prepared to administer medications, every paramedic needs to know all of the medications in the formulary that their general and particular protocols include.
- It is important for the paramedic to understand the specific anatomy and physiology involved in medication utilization.
- Prior to giving any medication the paramedic must review the following "six rights" of drug administration: Right patient, Right drug, Right dose, Right route, Right time, and Right documentation.
- Medication should not be given prior to an assessment, including vital signs. The pathophysiological principles of medication administration should also be taken into consideration since medication makes changes to the patient's condition.
- The best paramedics serve as "models" for medical asepsis, advocate while performing medication administration, and properly dispose of contaminated items and sharps.

Vital Vocabulary

Absorption stage The stage when a drug enters the body and reaches the bloodstream.

Active transport There are two general methods by which drugs cross the cell membrane: by active or passive transport. Active transport moves via pumps that require energy and move the drug from an area of low concentration to an area of high concentration.

Additive effect When two drugs work together to produce an effect a single drug would not produce. This is also referred to as summation.

Adrenergic Pertaining to nerves that release the neurotransmitter norepinephrine or noradrenaline (such as adrenergic nerves, adrenergic response). The term also pertains to the receptors acted on by norepinephrine, that is, the adrenergic receptors.

Adverse reaction An undesirable response to a drug that may be sudden or take days to occur.

Afferent nerves The nerves that carry sensory impulses from all parts of the body to the brain.

Agonist A substance that mimics the actions of a specific neurotransmitter or hormone by binding to the specific receptor of the naturally occurring substance.

Analgesics A classification for medications that relieve pain, or induce analgesia.

Anesthetics A type of medication intended to induce a loss of sensation to touch or pain.

Antagonist When one drug prevents or reverses the reaction of another. This may be chemical, competitive, or physiologic.

Antibiotics The medications that fight bacterial infection by killing the bacteria or by preventing multiplication of the bacteria to allow the body's immune system to overcome them.

Anticholinergic Of or pertaining to the blocking of acetylcholine receptors, resulting in inhibition of transmission of parasympathetic nerve impulses.

Anticoagulants The medications used to prevent intravascular thrombosis by preventing blood coagulation in the vascular system.

Anticonvulsants The medications used to treat seizures, which are believed to work by inhibiting the influx of sodium into cells.

Antihyperlipidemics Medications that help to lower cholesterol.

Antihypertensives The medications used to control blood pressure.

Antineoplastic medications The medications designed to combat cancer.

Antiplatelet agents The medications that interfere with the collection of platelets.

Antiseptic An agent designed to prevent growth of caustic microorganisms.

Aseptic technique A method of cleansing used to prevent contamination of a site when performing an invasive procedure, such as starting an IV.

Aural route Medication given into the patient's ear.

Autonomic nervous system The component of the peripheral nervous system that sends sensory impulses from internal structures (such as blood vessels, the heart, and organs of the chest, abdomen, and pelvis) through afferent autonomic nerves to the brain.

Barbiturates Any medications of a group of barbituric acid derivatives that act as central nervous system depressants and are used as sedatives and hypnotics.

Benzodiazepines Any medications of a group of psychotropic agents used as antianxiety, muscle relaxants, sedatives, and hypnotics.

Biotransformation stage The stage when a drug is altered chemically or broken down. Many of these processes occur in the liver.

Bolus A single dose (small or large) given by the IV or IO route.

Buccal route Medication given to be absorbed between the cheek and the gum.

Capsule A cylindrical gelatin container enclosing a dose of medication.

Central nervous system (CNS) The system containing the brain and spinal cord.

Central nervous system (CNS) stimulants Any medications or agents that increase brain activity.

Cholinergic Fibers in the parasympathetic nervous system that release a chemical called acetylcholine.

Cross tolerance The resistance to the effect or effects of a drug as a result of tolerance previously developed to another drug having a similar pharmacologic action.

Cumulative effect An effect that occurs when several successive doses of a medication are administered or when absorption of a medication occurs faster than excretion or metabolism.

Disinfectant A chemical or physical agent designed to destroy pathogenic microorganisms on nonliving objects such as surfaces or equipment.

Distribution stage The stage when a drug moves through the bloodstream to the target organ.

Efferent nerves The nerves that carry messages from the brain to the muscles and all other organs of the body.

Elimination stage The stage when a drug, or its metabolites, are removed from the body.

Elixir A syrup with alcohol and flavoring added.

Emulsion A preparation of one liquid (usually an oil) distributed in small globules in another liquid (usually water).

Endotracheal (ET) route Medication administered down the tube inserted in the trachea.

Enteral route The introduction of medication to the body through the gastrointestinal tract.

Fibrinolytic agents The only medications available to dissolve blood clots after they have already formed; the drugs promote the digestion of fibrin.

Gastric route Medication given through a gastric tube which is commonly inserted in patients in the prehospital setting to decompress the stomach.

Generic drug A medication that is not patented.

Generic name A general name for a drug that is not manufacturer-specific; usually the name given to the drug by the company that first manufactures it.

Habituation The emotional or psychological dependence on a drug after repeated use (ie, narcotics or analgesics).

Half-life The amount of time that a drug remains at a therapeutic level to continue to produce the desired effect and the time it takes the body to metabolize the drug's concentration by 50%.

Hypersensitivity An exaggerated response to a drug such as an allergic reaction to an antibiotic (ie, itching, a rash, or shortness of breath).

Iatrogenic response An adverse effect, condition (mental or physical), or disorder that is induced inadvertently by the health care provider.

Idiosyncratic reaction An abnormal reaction that is unpredictable and unique to a specific patient rather than a group of patients.

Immunobiologic medications The medications that include serums, vaccines, and other immunizing agents.

Immunosuppressant medications The medications intended to inhibit the body's ability to attack the "foreign" organ, or in the case of autoimmune diseases, the medications that inhibit the body's attack on itself.

Intradermal route An injection of a small quantity (≤ 1 mL) of a medication into the dermal layer of the skin.

Intramuscular (IM) route An injection of 3 to 5 mL of a medication into the muscle (ie, deltoid or gluteus maximus).

Intranasal route Medication given by spraying into the patient's nose.

Intraosseous (IO) route Administration of medication into the marrow cavity of the bone. Any drug that can be administered intravenously can be administered intraosseously.

Intravenous (IV) route Medication that is given directly into the patient's vein, usually through an already flowing IV line by injecting the injection port on the administration set.

Loading dose A single dose or accumulation of several closely repeated doses used to obtain the therapeutic level that achieves the desired effect.

Maintenance dose After the loading dose is administered, additional doses are administered to keep the medication at the therapeutic level.

Mechanism of action The way in which a drug works to achieve its intended result.

Medication A licensed drug taken to cure or reduce symptoms of an illness or medical condition or as an aid in diagnosis, treatment, or prevention of a disease or other abnormal condition.

Medication patch A solid medication impregnated into a membrane or adhesive that is applied to the surface of the skin.

Metered-dose inhaler (MDI) Medication given by the inhalation route in a device that the patient can easily administer in a single dose.

Mucokinetics Drugs that increase and aid the clearance of respiratory tract secretions.

Mucosal atomizer device (MAD) A device that is attached to the end of a syringe for the purpose of spraying (atomized) medication into the nose.

Nonsteroidal anti-inflammatory drugs (NSAIDs) Medications with analgesic and fever-reducing properties.

Ocular route Medication that is given by drops into the eye.

Official name The name listed in the United States Pharmacopeia (USP) once the generic name has been approved by the United States Adopted Name Council and the drug has been approved by the US Food and Drug Administration.

Opioid A medication that has opiate-like qualities but is not actually derived from the opium plant.

Oral route Medication, such as a pill or liquid, that is swallowed and taken into the patient's gastrointestinal tract.

Parasympathetic nervous system A subdivision of the autonomic nervous system that is involved in control of involuntary, vegetative functions, mediated largely by the vagus nerve through the chemical acetylcholine.

Parenteral route The introduction of medication to the body outside of the GI tract.

Passive transport There are two general methods by which drugs cross the cell membrane: by active or passive transport. Most cross through by passive transport which includes diffusion, facilitated diffusion, osmosis, and filtration.

Percutaneous route Administration of medicine through the skin or mucous membrane.

Peripheral nervous system (PNS) Consists of all nervous tissue outside of the brain and spinal cord and is subdivided into two divisions, the somatic and autonomic nervous systems.

Pharmaceutics The science of preparing and dispersing drugs, the various drug forms, and how they affect pharmacokinetics and pharmacodynamics.

Pharmacodynamics Branch of pharmacology that investigates biochemical and physiological effects and interactions with the target organs or tissues.

Pharmacokinetics Branch of pharmacology that studies metabolism and the action of a medication as it travels through the patient's body.

Pharmacology The branch of medicine dealing with the actions of drugs in the body—therapeutic and toxic effects—and development and testing of new drugs and new uses of existing drugs.

Pill A drug shaped into a ball or oval to be swallowed; often coated to disguise an unpleasant taste.

Potentiation A combination reaction where one drug enhances the effect of the other (ie, codeine and alcohol).

Powder A drug that has been ground into pulverized form.

Pulvule A solid medication form that resembles a capsule but it is not made of gelatin and it does not separate.

Rectal route Medication that is absorbed through the rectal mucosa and usually given by a suppository designed to melt at body temperature. This is a common route used for infants.

Side effect A response to a drug which is not the desired effect but seems to occur in most patients (ie, headache with nitroglycerin).

Skeletal muscle relaxants Medications that provide relief of skeletal muscle spasms.

Small-volume nebulizer A device that produces a fine spray or mist administration of a medication.

Solution A liquid containing one or more chemical substances entirely dissolved, usually in water.

Standard precautions Guidelines recommended by the Centers for Disease Control (CDC) to reduce the risk of the spread of infection between patients and health care providers.

Stimulants An agent that increases the level of body activity.

Subcutaneous (SC or SQ) route Medication administered into the tissue between the skin and muscle.

Sublingual (SL) route Medication administered under the tongue.

Summation effect The process whereby multiple medications can produce a response that the individual medications alone do not produce.

Suppository A drug mixed in a firm base that melts at body temperature and is shaped to fit the rectum, urethra, or vagina.

Suspension A preparation of a finely divided drug intended to be (or already) incorporated in a suitable liquid.

Sympathetic nervous system Subdivision of the autonomic nervous system that governs the body's fight-or-flight reactions by inducing smooth muscle contraction or relaxation of the blood vessels and bronchioles.

Sympathomimetics The medications administered to stimulate the sympathetic nervous system.

Synergistic effect The effect of two drugs working together in an additive manner that result in an effect that is greater than the sum of their effects if taken individually.

Syrup A drug suspended in sugar and water to improve its taste.

Tablet A powdered drug that has been molded or compressed into a small disk.

Therapeutic The desired or intended action of a medication.

Therapeutic index The difference between the therapeutic threshold and the amount of the drug considered to produce unwanted and possible dangerous side effects.

Therapeutic threshold The minimum amount of drug required to produce the desired response.

Tincture A dilute alcoholic extract of a drug.

Tolerance A decrease in the expected reaction to a drug with repeated doses. This is common in patients who are taking analgesics.

Trade name The brand name registered to a specific manufacturer or owner; also called proprietary name.

Transdermal route Medication administration applied topically to the skin, as in a patch.

Uricosuric medications The medications designed to lower the uric acid level in the blood by increasing the excretion by the kidneys into the urine.

Vaccine A suspension of whole (live or inactivated) or fractionated bacteria or viruses that have been made nonpathogenic; given to induce an immune response and prevent disease.

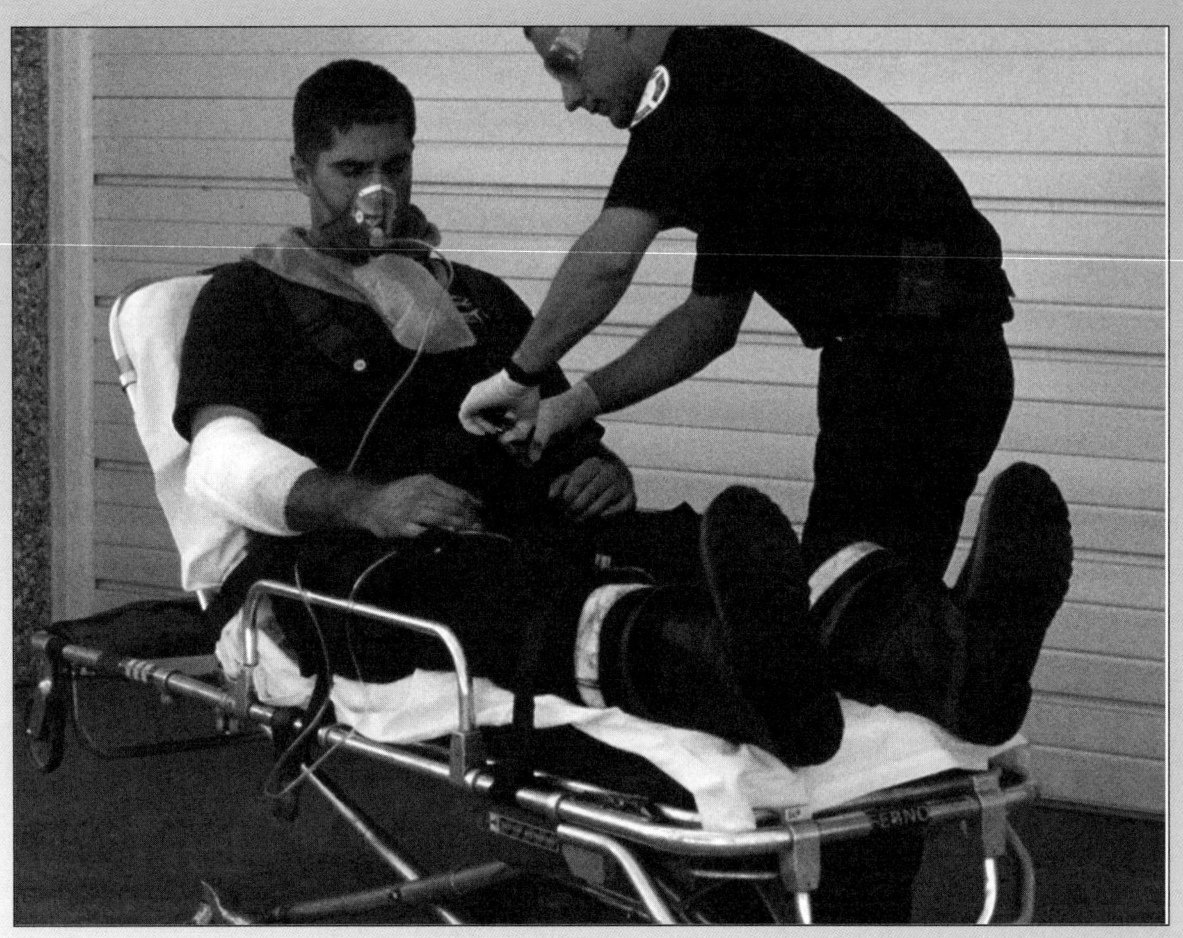

Trauma 2

Objectives

Cognitive

4-4.13 Describe the management of a burn injury, including airway and ventilation, circulation, pharmacological, non-pharmacological, transport considerations, psychological support/ communication strategies, and other management described by local protocol. (pages 44–52)

4-4.21 Describe the management of a thermal burn injury, including airway and ventilation, circulation, pharmacological, non-pharmacological, transport considerations, psychological support/ communication strategies, and other management described by local protocol. (pages 44–45, 52)

4-4.30 Describe the management of an inhalation burn injury, including airway and ventilation, circulation, pharmacological, non-pharmacological, transport considerations, and psychological support/ communication strategies. (pages 45, 52)

4-4.38 Describe the management of a chemical burn injury and a chemical burn injury to the eye, including airway and ventilation, circulation, pharmacological, non-pharmacological, transport considerations, and psychological support/ communication strategies. (pages 45–46, 52)

4-4.46 Describe the management of an electrical burn injury, including airway and ventilation, circulation, pharmacological, non-pharmacological, transport considerations, and psychological support/ communication strategies. (pages 46, 52)

4-4.55 Describe the management of a radiation exposure, including airway and ventilation, circulation, pharmacological, non-pharmacological, transport considerations, and psychological support/ communication strategies. (pages 46, 52)

4-5.46 Describe and explain the general management of the head/brain injury patient, including pharmacological and non-pharmacological treatment. (pages 52–59)

Affective

4-9.42 Advocate for the use of pain management in the treatment of musculoskeletal injuries. (pages 65–70)

Psychomotor

4-4.80 Perform management of a thermal burn injury, including airway and ventilation, circulation, pharmacological, non-pharmacological, transport considerations, psychological support/ communication strategies, and other management described by local protocol. (pages 44–45, 52)

4-4.81 Perform management of an inhalation burn injury, including airway and ventilation, circulation, pharmacological, non-pharmacological, transport considerations, psychological support/ communication strategies, and other management described by local protocol. (pages 45, 52)

4-4.82 Perform management of a chemical burn injury, including airway and ventilation, circulation, pharmacological, non-pharmacological, transport considerations, psychological support/ communication strategies, and other management described by local protocol. (pages 45–46, 52)

4-4.83 Perform management of an electrical burn injury, including airway and ventilation, circulation, pharmacological, non-pharmacological, transport considerations, psychological support/ communication strategies, and other management described by local protocol. (pages 46, 52)

4-4.84 Perform management of a radiation exposure, including airway and ventilation, circulation, pharmacological, non-pharmacological, transport considerations, psychological support/ communication strategies, and other management described by local protocol. (pages 46, 52)

Additional Objectives

2-1 Discuss the following medications used in the prehospital setting for the management of trauma patients: oxygen; morphine sulfate [Astramorph/PF]—for pain; Methylprednisolone sodium succinate [Solu-Medrol]. (pages 50–51, 62)

2-2 Discuss the following medications used in the prehospital setting for the management of eye injury patients: using the Morgan lens with tetracaine HCL ophthalmic solution [Pontocaine] to irrigate an eye injury. (pages 45, 59)

2-3 Discuss the following medication that may be used in the prehospital and/or in-hospital setting: mannitol [Osmitrol]. (pages 57–58)

Pharmacologic Agents and Trauma

Pharmacologic agents have a limited role in the treatment of trauma patients. Generally, the only drugs currently used for prehospital trauma patients, aside from fluids for resuscitation, are agents for pain and nausea management, and oxygen for hypoxemia. Narcotic and nonnarcotic analgesics are considered essential components when providing appropriate and compassionate treatment of any trauma patient. In this chapter we will discuss a number of cases that emphasize medications as well as the nonpharmaceutical management of the trauma patient.

Burn Trauma

The skin is composed of two principle layers: the epidermis and the dermis (**Figure 2-1** ▼).

The epidermis is the outermost layer of the skin that provides a protective covering against the environment. The outermost layer of cells is a layer of dead cells that are constantly being shed. This process of shedding cells is referred to as desquamation. The next three layers are constantly dividing in order to push up additional dead cells. Below the epidermis is the dermis layer which is a thick, highly elastic connective tissue layer composed mostly of collagen fibers, elastin fibers, and a mucopolysaccharide gel. The blood vessels and nerve endings are found in this layer and play a key role in sensation as well as regulating body temperature. Below the dermis is the subcutaneous layer which is mostly a fat layer that provides insulation.

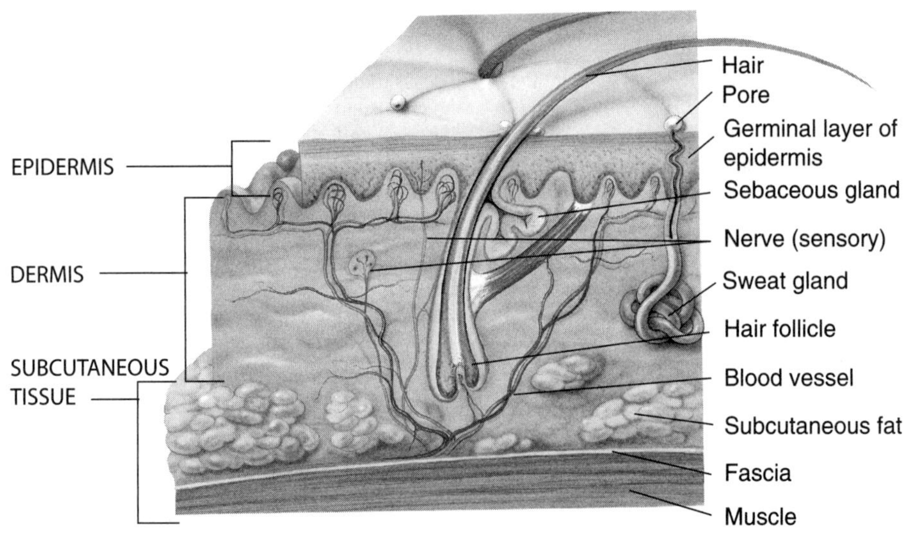

Figure 2-1 The anatomy of the skin.

Your assessment of a burned patient involves determining the cause of the burn, establishing the extent and total body surface area (TBSA) of the burn, and classifying the thickness of the burn (ie, superficial, partial-thickness, or full-thickness). You should also check to see if there is anything that would immediately categorize the burn as a critical burn (ie, circumferential, hands or feet, electrical, respiratory, genital, or complicated by other trauma or preexisting medical conditions).

Causes of Burns

Burns are categorized by their cause. The categories include: thermal, inhalation, chemical, electrical, and radiation.

Thermal Burns

Thermal burns involve a heat source coming in contact with the patient's skin. This can involve a scald, flame, contact, steam, or flash burn. Significant damage can occur to the skin and its underlying structures from a thermal burn. Initially the body transfers large amounts of fluids to the burn site. This can easily lead to the development of shock and is why the management of a burn injury involves a significant volume of fluids. A scald burn commonly occurs in a situation where a toddler reaches up and grabs a pot handle of boiling soup that was placed on a front burner of the stove. The hot, boiling liquid can cause a very serious burn injury to the toddler, resulting in lifelong scars. When someone is caught in a house fire, or a smoker falls asleep in bed and the bed catches on fire, the flame burns can quickly destroy the layers of the skin (**Figure 2-2** ▶). Most people have experienced the sensation of a contact burn by touching a hot surface such as a heat element in the oven or on the backyard grill. The general management of all critical burns should include the drug oxygen! Burn patients go into shock and with the resultant poor perfusion to the tissues they become hypoxic at the cellular level. Early administration of high concentration supplemental oxygen may be helpful

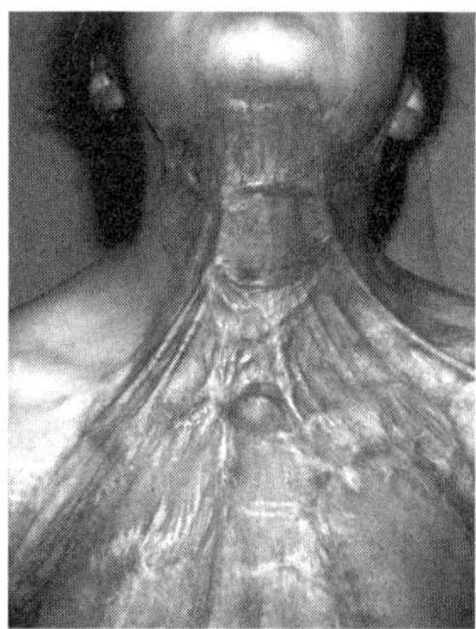

Figure 2-2 Flame burns are usually very deep, leaving horrific scars.

in improving the oxygenation at the cellular level.

Inhalation Burns

When a patient is caught in a confined space and there is a fire or superheated air that is breathed in, there is an increased chance of a respiratory burn or inhalation burn. According to the American Burn Association 2005 National Burn Repository, 6.5% of the patients admitted to burn centers had an inhalation injury, and the mortality rates associated with these injuries are high. A clue to inhalation burns is soot on the face around the nose and mouth as well as singed nasal hairs and thick black sputum. When a room and its contents are on fire, the temperature at the floor is cooler than the temperature at the ceiling because heat rises. The air close to the ceiling can reach temperatures of over 1,000° F. When a patient stands up, just breathing in this superheated air can cause a life-threatening burn to the upper respiratory tract. With rapid accumulation of airway edema, the patient's airway can acutely narrow and become occluded. Patients with respiratory burns will need to be taken to a burn center. If the need for intubation arises, it is strongly suggested that the most experienced provider do the intubation because a patient with inhalation or respiratory burns is likely to be a difficult intubation. As always, the largest sized tube should be inserted but also have smaller sizes readily available because it may be necessary to use a smaller tube due to the airway swelling.

Another condition to watch out for in the inhalation burn patient, as well as any patient with a headache, chest pain, and nausea, is toxic inhalation. The most likely toxic inhalation associated with a burn is carbon monoxide (CO). Portable devices are now available to measure the blood concentration of CO. Inhalation of CO causes a problem because there are a limited number of receptor sites on the hemoglobin on the patient's red blood cells. Normally oxygen molecules bind to these receptor sites to allow the oxygen to travel to each of the cells, tissues, and organs of the body. In CO poisoning, the CO has a greater affinity (about 250 times better) than oxygen to bind to the hemoglobin's receptor sites so the patient ends up with red blood cells that are well saturated with the wrong chemical. The patient literally suffocates at the cellular level. There is also a possibility that the patient may also have cyanide poisoning. If CO poisoning is suspected, the patient may be treated in a hyperbaric chamber if one is available.

Chemical Burns

Chemical burns are caused by acids, bases, phenols, and dry chemicals such as cement powder. Most of these burn injuries occur in an industrial manufacturing setting. If you find a patient who has been burned with a dry chemical, the first priority is to identify the chemical and be sure that water is the most appropriate substance to use to irrigate with. Keep in mind that some chemicals develop into toxic substances if water is applied to them. If possible, the patient should remove the clothing that has the chemical on it and if possible, brush off any excess powder. Lime, a dry powder form that is most often sold as calcium oxide, should be washed off using copious amounts of water for about 20 minutes. While minor amounts of heat will be generated in most cases, the appropriate action is to wash quickly and thoroughly. To avoid being exposed to the chemical, you should always wear the appropriate PPE for the chemical involved. In the industrial setting it is not uncommon for paramedics to arrive on the scene and find emergency medical responders already showering the patient. If the eyes have been involved, flush them, making sure that you direct the flow from the bridge of the nose to the chemically burned eye, taking care to prevent the chemical from getting into the other eye during the flushing (**Figure 2-3**▼).

If the patient has contact lenses, they should be removed. It is possible to irrigate the eyes using a device called a Morgan lens but this will require a local anesthetic to be used. Another example of a chemical that burns the eyes is the pepper spray used by law

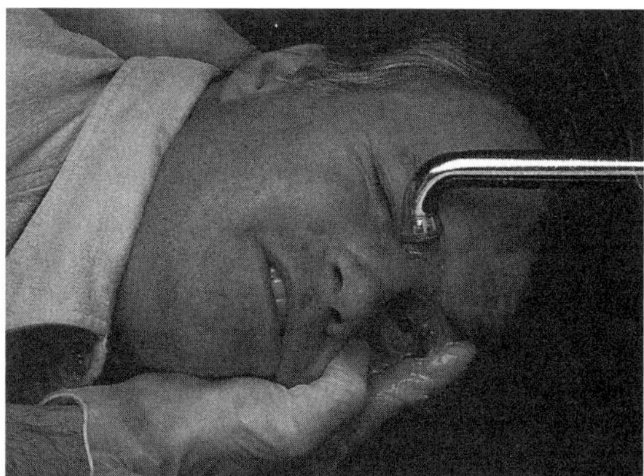

Figure 2-3 Irrigating the chemically burned eye.

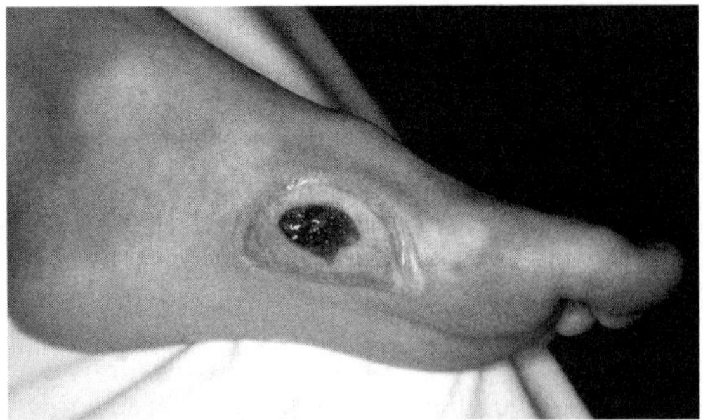

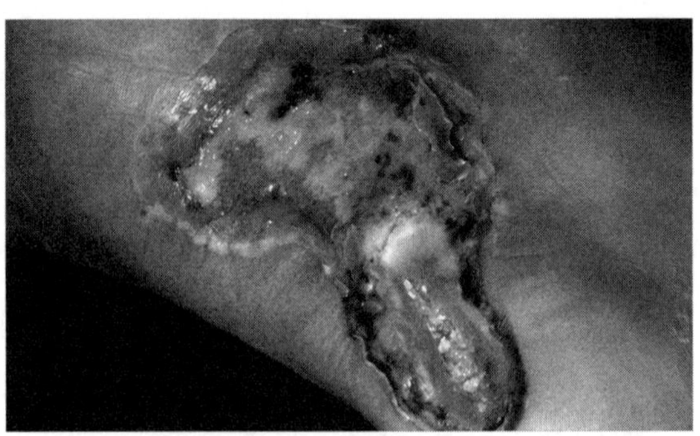

Figure 2-4 Electrical burns have an entrance and an exit wound.

enforcement personnel. The residue left behind after being sprayed is an oil that can be removed by using mineral oil on the skin. Do not put mineral oil into the eyes, rather continue flushing with large quantities of water.

Electrical Burns

Electrical burns are considered to be another critical type of burn because it is often difficult to determine the extent of the burn's effect on the internal organs of the body. In most patients there is an entry wound and an exit wound and in some cases the pathway of electricity may have crossed the heart causing a lethal arrhythmia to occur (**Figure 2-4▲**).

A small number of patients who receive electrical burns receive them from lightning strikes. In the U.S. there are about 90 people who die each year from lightning strikes. Before assessing a potential lightning strike injury make sure the scene is safe for the rescuers! This may involve rapidly moving the patient to a safe place out of the storm. Patients who have been struck by lightning have been known to stop breathing so the priority is to complete your initial assessment and resuscitate their ABCs. Some patients may be found in ventricular fibrillation. Have your AED handy and be ready to perform CPR. A lightning burn injury is different than the electrical burn injury because a lightning injury is usually not the result of a direct hit, but rather by lightning striking nearby the patient. If the patient is actually struck, there are also rarely exit wounds and a lot less internal muscle damage (myoglobulinuria) due to the very quick duration of the current traveling through the skin. Once you have managed the initial assessment priorities, the patient's burn should be treated as you would other burn injuries. However, do not underestimate the extent of damage and make sure all lightning strike patients are treated in the ED.

Radiation Burns

If you have reason to suspect that your patient has sustained a radiation burn, you should first consider the scene safety issues and you may need to consult with the local hazmat team before proceeding. It may be necessary for you to wait for properly protected personnel with the proper training to decontaminate the patient prior to your management and transportation. The priority in this situation is to avoid the rescuers getting contaminated also.

Fortunately, radiation injury follows the "inverse square law," meaning that exposure drops exponentially as distance is increased. It is best to stay back until the substance is identified. The patient may be exposed to the radiation source or have had actual contact with the source. Most of the "burning" and its extent is difficult to determine in the prehospital setting. With contact radiation, decontamination should be performed in the same manner as a chemical burn. If there are open wounds, carefully flush them and be sure to notify the ED that you will be transporting the patient to. As far as medications, your treatment plan may involve IV therapy if the patient is in shock and analgesia with the consultation of medical control.

Personal safety should be your concern when treating a patient during a storm that has produced hazards.

Total Body Surface Area

As a part of the assessment of the burn injury you will need to estimate the total body surface area (TBSA) that has been burned. This is, of course, just an estimation and is likely to change in the hospital setting when the patient is evaluated under the bright lights and closer view, but the methods used in the prehospital setting work well for management and triage, and determining the most appropriate facility. The most common way to calculate the TBSA burned is using the "rule of nines" (**Figure 2-5▸**).

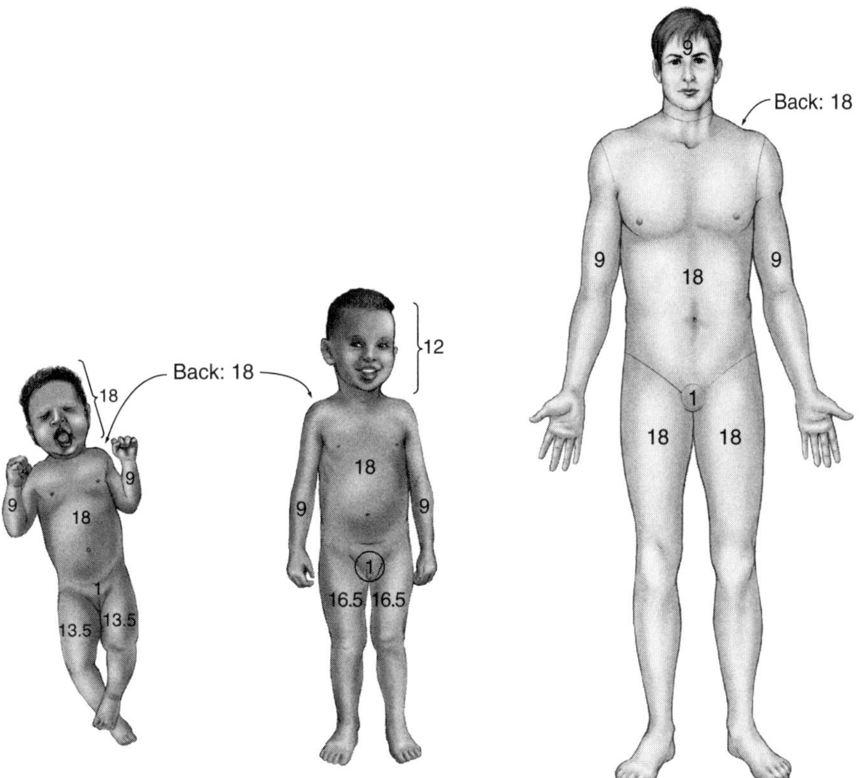

Figure 2-5 The rule of nines divides the body into sections each representing approximately 9% of the total body surface area.

The rule of nines is based on dividing the body into nine segments. For example, the toddler discussed previously received a thermal burn by grabbing a pot of hot soup. He received a scald burn over most of his head, his entire right arm, and down the front of the torso. His TBSA burned would be 39%.

12 (head) + 9 (arm) + 18 (torso) = approximately 39% TBSA burned.

A patient can also have a relatively minor burn that covers a large TBSA burned. A sunburn would be a perfect example.

Burn Thickness

Burns are classified by their extent or thickness such as superficial (first-degree), partial-thickness (second-degree), and full-thickness (third-degree) (**Figure 2-6 ▸**).

Superficial Burns

A superficial, or first-degree burn involves red skin, usually without the presence of blisters. A superficial burn involves the epidermis and exposes the nerve endings to air which causes pain. A sunburn is an example of a superficial burn.

Partial-Thickness Burns

Partial-thickness, or second-degree, burns involve the epidermis and various degrees of the dermis. This can be very painful due to the presence of blisters and moisture on the skin. Analgesics, or medications that relieve pain may be needed to treat the patient provided the vital signs are stable. Patients in severe pain expend too much energy that could be better used in their fight to live or compensate for their condition or begin the healing process. It is also inhumane to allow patients to continue to be in extreme pain if the means exist to manage that pain.

Full-Thickness Burns

When a patient sustains a burn injury that involves destruction of both the epidermis and the dermal layers of skin, this is referred to as a full-thickness, or third-degree burn. Capillaries and sensory nerves are destroyed. Pain will vary because patients have mixed depths of burns. These patients may require fluid resuscitation, surgery, and skin grafting in order to heal.

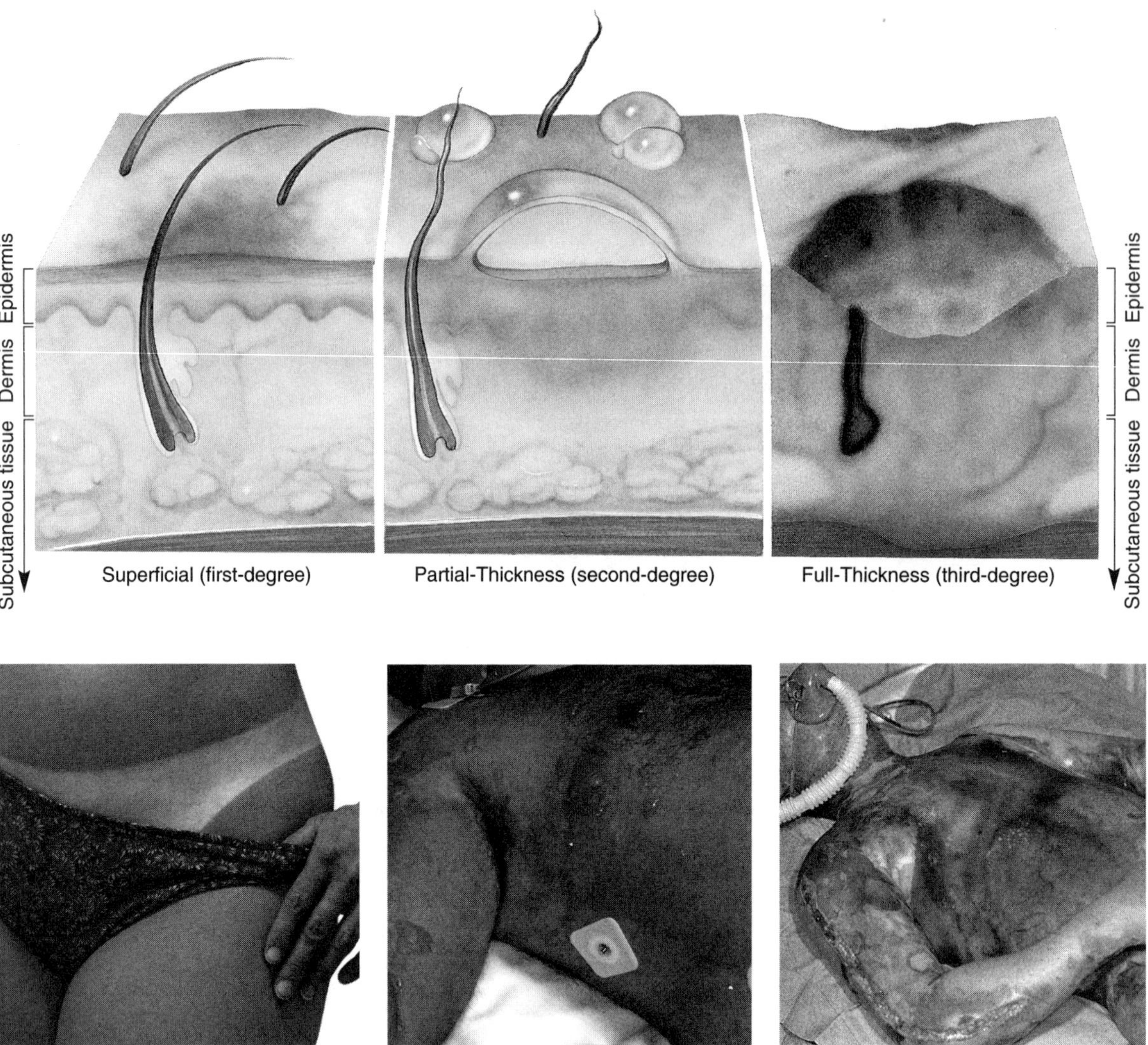

Figure 2-6 Classification of burns.

Circumferential Burns

A number of injuries are automatically considered a critical burn injury, including burns of the hands or feet, an electrical burn, a respiratory burn, burns of the genitals, or burns that are complicated by multiple trauma or preexisting medical conditions (ie, ACS, stroke, or diabetes). Circumferential burns are also considered to be a critical burn injury. A circumferential burn is very serious because it involves a burn around an entire extremity or the torso. Interstitial fluid accumulations at or near the site of a burn is known as edema. Edema that builds up in a circumferentially burned extremity can result in marked increases in pressure within the fascial compartments of the extremities. If the outer layers of the skin are burned, a leathery ring of tissue can form around the injured part that does not allow for expansion from all the edema. In this case, the pressure within the tissue increases tremendously and can cause tissue necrosis, secondary to a compartment syndrome. If the patient is not attended to quickly and properly, amputation of the extremity ultimately could be required. In some situations emergency medical staff may need to provide an incision into the leather-like tissue (eschar) to allow the underlying injured extremity to expand. The procedure is called an escharotomy. This can be a life-threatening event when a patient has a circumferential burn around the chest wall that restricts their ability to breathe.

Case Study I Full-Thickness Burns

Part 1

Your unit has been dispatched to a fire scene in a residential neighborhood where the Fire Department has been fighting a two-alarm blaze. The family is outside the house and a firefighter has just carried out the badly burned body of a 10-year-old boy who they suspect was playing with matches and caused the inferno.

Table 1 Initial Assessment

Initial Assessment	Recording Time: 1 Minute
General Impression/ Appearance	Young male, upper body badly burnt, crying, in severe pain
Mental Status	"A" alert
Airway	Open but soot around the mouth and nose
Breathing	Rapid and shallow, sounds are hoarse and raspy
Circulation	Rapid and thready radial pulse, no external bleeding
Priority/Plan	High due to respiratory burns

The scene is safe. As you don your protective equipment, you note there are no electrical or structural hazards in the location that the child has been brought out to. You quickly grab your bag and begin your initial assessment on the young boy (see **Table 1**). His parents are nearby, anxious but very helpful. The boy's name is Jake.

After completing the initial assessment and ensuring that ample help is on the way, you proceed with applying supplemental oxygen before you begin the examination for a trauma patient with a significant mechanism of injury (MOI).

Question 1: Why is this injury considered a significant MOI?

Question 2: What is the significance of the hoarse and raspy sounding voice?

Part 2

Because Jake has a significant MOI, you begin assessing him using the rapid trauma assessment which takes a quick look at the major body regions (ie, head, neck, chest, abdomen, pelvis, back, buttocks, and four extremities). You begin to tally up the percentage of TBSA burned. The child has full-thickness burns to the chest and both arms as well as partial-thickness burns to the neck and chin. Next, you will ask relevant questions to elaborate on the chief complaint of critical burns using the OPQRST pneumonic. Your partner obtains a set of baseline vital signs during the focused history and physical examination (see **Table 2**).

Table 2 Focused History and Physical Examination

Baseline Vital Signs	Recording Time: 5 Minutes
Skin CTC (color, temperature, condition)	Aside from the burned areas, the skin is pale, cool, clammy, and damp
Pulse	Radial pulse of 110 beats/min, regular and thready
Blood Pressure	Blood pressure is 98/70 mm Hg
Respirations	26 breaths/min, regular and shallow

It is clear that Jake has also inhaled heated gas that may have damaged his upper airway. He is able to answer your questions accurately but he is obviously in a considerable amount of pain.

Question 3: The first drug of choice for this patient was oxygen. Why?

Question 4: Would a medication for pain relief be appropriate to administer?

Case Study I Continued

Part 3

From the rapid trauma assessment you learned that Jake had no other injuries aside from the very serious burns. You have estimated approximately 36% TBSA, full-thickness burns including circumferential burns of both arms. Due to the availability of a landing zone and helicopter, you decide that this patient should be taken by helicopter directly to the regional burn center.

Table 3 SAMPLE History

SAMPLE History	Comments
Signs/symptoms	Thermal burn injury, respiratory burn, nausea, severe pain
Allergies	None known
Medications	Only taking a multi-vitamin
Pertinent past medical history	Patient states, "I have an old fracture to my right wrist that took a long time to heal. The doctor told me I have problems healing and may have diabetes."
Last oral intake	Dinner 4 hours ago
Events leading up to the incident	Playing with matches, lighting candles, the curtains caught on fire, and he tried to put them out by hand

In preparation for the transfer, the airway is further evaluated and an IO is considered for fluid infusion since the burns to the arms are severe. The SAMPLE history reveals some important information (see **Table 3**).

Treatment Plan

This patient will receive preparation for a rapid transport.

1. Verify that the child has a properly managed airway (which could include both basic and advanced procedures) and is well oxygenated (see **Table 4**).
2. Ensure the patient has a good site for normal saline fluid administration (IV or IO).
3. Wrap the patient in a dry sterile burn sheet or dressing.
4. If the serial vital signs remain stable, it would be appropriate to consider administration of morphine sulfate as an analgesic to control the severe pain (see **Table 5**). Some EMS systems also offer fentanyl citrate [Sublimase] as an alternative to morphine, especially if the patient is allergic to morphine. (Fentanyl citrate is discussed in detail in Chapter 10.) The patient should be kept warm since burned patients have difficulty maintaining their body temperature.

Table 4 Oxygen

Do you know?	Comments
Right drug? Generic name: **[Oxygen]** Trade name: [Oxygen]	Helps improve tissue hypoxia.
Right patient?	Any patient who is potentially hypoxic, anoxic, or in shock.
Right dose?	10 to 15 liters per minute (L/min) of supplemental oxygen, humidified if possible, to avoid further compromise of the potentially burned airway. Note that some services routinely administer 4 L/min by nasal cannula and let the SpO_2 guide the need (< 97%) for a nonrebreathing mask. Consult your state or regional protocols or the medical director for further advice.
Right route?	Inhalation via nonrebreathing (NRB) mask if the patient continues to breathe adequately on his own. Otherwise assist ventilations with a bag-mask device.
Right time?	For duration of the prehospital patient encounter.
Right documentation?	The time, route, dose, and duration of administration.
Expected action	Increase tissue oxygenation. The tissue oxygen saturation (SpO_2) should improve.
Side effects	Oxygen can dry out the airway structures.
Contraindications	High percentages may cause drowsiness and respiratory arrest in the end-stage COPD patient. If this patient needs oxygen, administer it and watch closely for the need to switch to bag-mask ventilation.
Precautions	None in this age child or an adult.

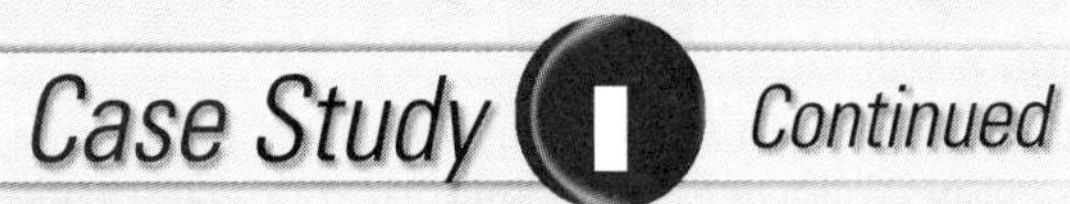

Table 5 **Morphine Sulfate**

Do you know?	Comments
Right drug? Generic name: [**Morphine Sulfate**] Trade name: [Astramorph/PF]	Helps to alleviate extreme pain.
Right patient?	Any patient who is in extreme pain with an adequate blood pressure and no allergy to the medicine.
Right dose?	Initial pediatric dose of 0.1 to 0.2 mg/kg. Burn patients often require high doses to relieve the pain so additional medication is likely to be given in the hospital setting.
Right route?	IV, IM, IO.
Right time?	After baseline vital signs as soon as it is clear that the blood pressure is stable.
Right documentation?	The route, dose, and duration of administration as well as any changes in the respirations or blood pressure.
Expected action	Pain relief, reduced anxiety, and the patient should become less concerned about the pain.
Side effects	Nausea/vomiting; may want to consider **antiemetic** coadministration. Hypotension or drop in blood pressure—place patient in Trendelenburg position and **titrate** IV fluids as indicated. Excessive sedation.
Contraindications	Low blood pressure, allergy, other medications.
Precautions	Respiratory depression may occur. Be prepared to assist ventilations. Titrating naloxone hydrochloride [Narcan] would be effective, though it should be used as a last resort as it would eliminate the effects of the morphine.

Question 5: How might an end-stage COPD patient, who you suspect is on hypoxic drive, alter your oxygen administration?

Question 6: If the patient's respiratory effort becomes depressed after the administration of morphine, what action should you take and why?

Part 4

A reassessment and an ongoing assessment of the patient is performed en route (see **Table 6**).

Question 7: If the patient had a sudden drop in blood pressure, what should you do?

Question 8: If the patient had rales, rhonchi, or crackles in both lungs (ie, pulmonary edema), what should you consider and are there any medications that may be useful?

Table 6 **Reassessment and Ongoing Assessment of the Patient**

Serial Vital Signs and Relevant Data	Recording Time: 10 Minutes
Skin CTC	Pale, cool, clammy
Pulse	Radial 120 beats/min, regular and thready
Blood Pressure	100/72 mm Hg
Respirations	26 breaths/min and regular
Mental Status	"A" alert
ECG	Sinus tachycardia with no ectopy
SpO_2	92%
Lung Sounds	Clear bilateral but a lot of upper airway noise
Other (ie, glucose, core temperature)	Cool to touch

Part 5

Fortunately Jake remains a candidate for the morphine sulfate which helps to relieve his pain. This in turn helps slow his pulse and calms him down. In the first days of managing the care of burn patients, they will need a tremendous amount of fluid and require significant energy just to survive. As a general rule, the elderly and the very young do not fair well with critical burns. Some paramedics may opt to take control of the airway immediately by performing Rapid Sequence Intubation because of the potential of losing airway patency due to swelling while en route to the ED. In this case that was not done and Jake was transported to the regional burn center. They have a team of well trained and experienced health care providers prepared to deal with his injuries, pain, skin grafts, and multiple surgeries, as well as the emotional support he will need.

Management of Specific Types of Burn Injuries

The specific management of each of the five categories of burns (thermal, inhalation, chemical, electrical, and radiation) involves care of the airway, ventilation, circulation, pharmacological and non-pharmacological strategies, as well as transport, psychological support or communication strategies, and other management such as local protocols. The following is a brief review of the management:

- The thermal burn—If it is a partial- or full-thickness burn, apply dry, sterile dressings or sheets to the injury. Keep in mind that your regional burn center is the authority on this subject. In some areas the burn center recommends the use of a Water-Jel burn dressing.
- The inhalation burn—Involves supplemental oxygen, IV fluids, and airway management. These are critical patients who should be treated in a regional burn center.
- The chemical burn—Flush the burn with copious amounts of water. In chemical powder burns, the actual substance should be identified first because some substances may react with water.
- The electrical burn—Turn the power off. The treatment of an electrical burn often requires airway, breathing, and circulation resuscitation. Some patients may be found in cardiac arrest, requiring high-quality compressions and defibrillation. The treatment should also include supplemental oxygen and IV fluid therapy. The patient will require an analgesic such as morphine sulfate for intense pain.
- The radiation burn—Protect the rescuer from secondary contamination and exposure to the radiation. Once the scene is safe, try to determine what the patient was exposed to and the length of the exposure. When a patient has a burn that encompasses more than 30% TBSA and was exposed to a radioactive source that caused the burn, they are critical and may not survive. It is very difficult to assess these patients in the field as they are often seriously injured from the inside out. The treatment for a radiation burn involves initial decontamination, irrigation of open wounds, and transportation to a facility that can handle patients in need of further decontamination. If the patient is "dirty" or was in contact with the radioactive source, they should be decontaminated by the appropriate hazmat team members in the appropriate protective gear.

Fluid Resuscitation

Patients can lose a tremendous volume of fluid in the first hours following a burn injury. An IV is normally inserted in the prehospital setting by the paramedic for the purpose of beginning fluid resuscitation as well as providing a route for administration of an analgesic such as morphine sulfate. Of course, this presumes the patient is stable enough to handle a medication that has effects on the respirations and blood pressure. During the assessment, you would have calculated the total TBSA that was burned. The TBSA is part of the formula for fluid resuscitation of the burned patient. The **Parkland formula** states that during the first 24 hours, the burned patient will need:

4 mL × body weight (in kg) × percentage of body surface burned

The Parkland formula gives you an idea of how aggressively the patient will need to be fluid resuscitated (provided the patient's lungs stay dry).

In case study I the patient is a 25 kg, 10-year-old boy and the TBSA burned is estimated to be 36%, with full-thickness burns. He is considered critical because of the potential respiratory involvement and your fluid calculation would be as follows:

$$4 \text{ mL} \times 25 \text{ kg} \times 36\% = 3{,}600 \text{ mL}$$

Half of that fluid volume will be administered within the first 8 hours of care for this patient. Since this is a child, you should consider medical direction in guiding your fluid therapy.

Head and Face Trauma

When a patient falls and strikes his or her head or injures his or her face this can cause a very serious, sometimes life-threatening injury. There are over 2 million brain injuries every year in the U.S. Since the head and face are very vascular, open injuries often bleed considerably and can be quite distracting to the paramedic. Remember the priority is to perform the initial assessment and not be immediately drawn to the bloody injury unless it is a potential life-threat that needs immediate management. Closed injuries to the face may involve a hematoma or a contusion indicating that a more serious internal injury to the brain is present (**Figure 2-7 ▸**).

Types of Head Trauma

The types of brain injury and their pathophysiology include:

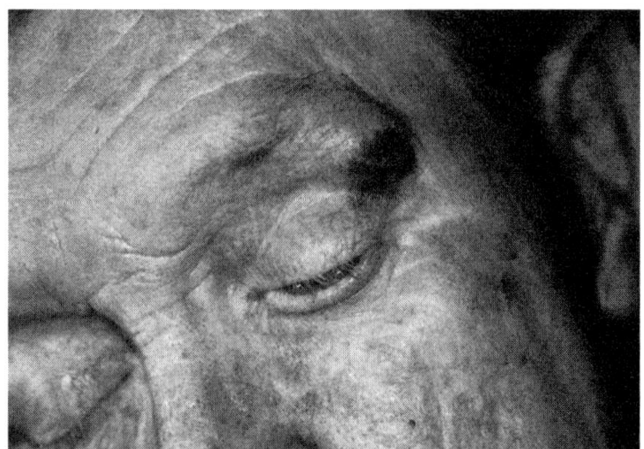

Figure 2-7 Closed soft-tissue injury to the face may indicate more serious underlying injuries.

- Concussion—a mild closed head injury that results in a transient loss of brain function that may or may not result in a loss of consciousness. The symptoms include: headache, memory loss, and irritability lasting for 1 or more days. There is no evidence of visible injury on neurologic imaging studies.
- Contusion—bruising of the brain tissue is seen on imaging; it is considered a moderately severe closed head injury with small bleeds and cerebral edema. The signs and symptoms can include a longer period of unconsciousness as well as amnesia, aphasia, and slight paralysis on one side of the body (hemiparesis).
- Intracranial Hemorrhage—when bleeding occurs inside the skull it increases intracranial pressure. The collection of blood, usually clotted, is also known as a hematoma. Brain hematomas often can be fatal if not recognized and attended to promptly. The type of brain hematoma is named by its location in relationship to the three meninges (ie, dura mater, arachnoid, and pia mater layers). The most common brain hematomas are epidural (outside the dura mater) and subdural (beneath the dura mater) (**Figure 2-8 ▸**).

Development of Brain Hematomas

When a hematoma develops within the skull, it may displace the brain in a downward direction in the most serious cases causing the brain to herniate through the ligaments that help to compartmentalize it within the skull (ie, the falx cerebri and the tentorium) as if to attempt to push the base of the brain out the foramen magnum (the large hole at the base of the skull in which the spinal cord exits). Of course the brain cannot really squeeze out the foramen magnum but the hematoma can put a lot of pressure on the base of the brain (medulla). As the pressure increases within the head from swelling and cerebral edema, the blood supply is limited and the body attempts to compensate by increasing the blood pressure to help force the blood up into the head. At the same time the pulse rate drops and the combination of these two vital sign changes are the hallmark of the Cushing's reflex. As the brain reaches its point of decompensation, the blood pressure suddenly drops and the pulse rises just before the impending cardiac arrest. This point of decompensation is usually about the same time that the medulla is squeezed to the point of being rendered inoperable and the patient loses the ability to control the vital signs and other involuntary actions.

You can make a tremendous difference in the care of the traumatic brain injury (TBI) patient if the signs and symptoms of a hematoma are recognized, early transport is provided to the most appropriate facility, and early notification is made so the personnel are ready to treat this often critical patient. Let's review the classic presentations of the two most common hematomas. The epidural hematoma is often caused when the side of the head is struck by a blunt object, such as a bat or ball. In the temporal/parietal area of the skull the bone is at its thinnest and is most susceptible to injury. In this area also lies the middle meningeal artery which is often lacerated by an injury to the temporal bone. If arterial injury occurs, the potential for a rapid accumulation of blood within a very confined space can result in hematoma formation. The classic presentation of the epidural hematoma is a patient who was struck on the side of the head, rendered unconscious, then regains consciousness, and is a bit confused. There is a lucid interval or period of consciousness that is followed by a rapid deterioration of brain function due to the rapidly expanding hematoma. Recognition of this injury, merely by the mechanism of injury and location, can help save the patient's life. This patient needs to go directly to a facility that has the resources for CT scanning and neurosurgery so that an intracranial clot can be rapidly identified and evacuated.

Always consider the mechanism of injury and monitor the mental status for subtle changes if head injury is suspected.

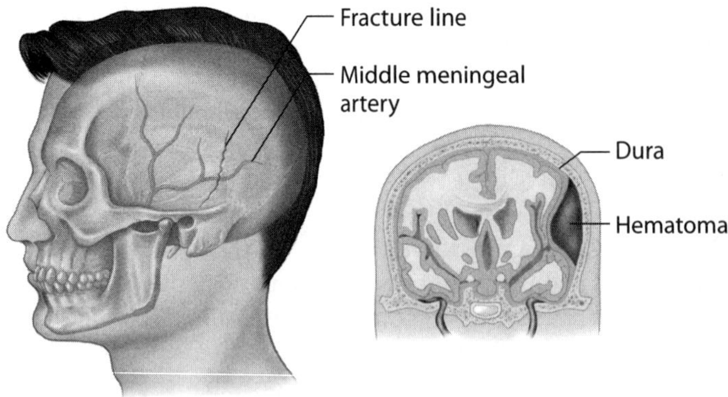

Figure 2-8 An epidural hematoma.

The patient who has a subdural hematoma has venous bleeding, often from the veins that bridge the cerebral cortex and the dura, frequently as a result of a rapid deceleration of the skull and brain. The signs of increased intracranial pressure (ICP) typically develop at a slower rate than an epidural hematoma (hours to weeks), yet the injury caused by this kind of bleeding can still be very significant. The patient will experience changes in mental status, focal neurologic signs, and slurred speech. Subdural hematomas are categorized either as acute or chronic, based on the onset of clinical signs. In an acute subdural, the patient experiences signs within a day whereas the chronic subdural may take as long as 2 weeks to occur. The homeless as well as the elderly are at a high risk for delayed subdurals. The onset of signs for a head injury is typically delayed in the elderly patient since as we age the brain shrinks. Therefore there is actually more room in the skull for a hematoma to develop prior to the impact of brain herniation being observed by the paramedic. Always consider the mechanism of injury and monitor the mental status for subtle changes if head injury is suspected.

In the case of a patient with a TBI, the earliest sign of increasing ICP is subtle changes in the patient's mental status. If you can observe and document subtle changes in the patient's mental status, significant changes in the patient's condition are being observed. If one of the patient's pupils becomes dilated and sluggish, this is considered a late indication of a developing TBI.

Vomiting also indicates unacceptable elevations in ICP, and also poses the distinct threat of airway compromise. This can be especially worrisome if a patient has been immobilized for transport as it will require moving the patient and board on its side to maintain a clear airway.

Case Study II Epidural Hematoma

Part 1

Your unit responds to a local ball field where a high school junior varsity team is playing baseball. You are met by a coach who is very excited and begins to relay this story. During the top of the fifth inning the batter, Mike Kelly, was struck on the side of the head with a wild pitch that caused a crack in his helmet. He was immediately knocked unconscious and sustained a ½″ laceration to the side of his head. After a few moments he sat up and was a little confused. The coach walked him to the dugout where he was bandaged and ice was applied. In about 10 minutes, during the sixth inning, a teammate noticed that Mike was sitting slumped over on the bench. That is when the local EMS was alerted. You quickly grab the first-in bag along with the stretcher and long backboard. With a scene that appears safe, you and your partner proceed to the patient's side to perform the initial assessment (see **Table 1**).

Table 1 Initial Assessment

Initial Assessment	Recording Time: 1 Minute
General Impression/ Appearance	Unconscious teenage male
Mental Status	Responds to pain by withdrawal
Airway	Open and clear
Breathing	Fast and shallow
Circulation	Minor bleeding to head, slow, strong radial pulse
Priority/Plan	High due to the MOI and altered mental status

Realizing that the presenting problem is that of trauma with a significant mechanism of injury (MOI), you know that a rapid trauma assessment (RTA) will need to be done on Mike. You begin to start your RTA to quickly evaluate the head, neck, chest, abdomen, back, buttocks, and the four extremities.

Case Study II Continued

Question 1: What is the significance of the location of the injury being on the side of the head?

Question 2: Why is the assessment of the mental status so important to this patient?

Part 2

Realizing that the RTA has no significant findings other than the injury to the side of the head, you decide the changes in Mike's mental status are most likely due to a traumatic brain injury (TBI).

Other findings of significance include a dilated pupil (on the injury side). Periorbital ecchymosis (raccoon eyes) and Battle's sign (discoloration behind the ears) are not present.

As you quickly place Mike on a long backboard and stabilize the head and neck with a rigid cervical collar, your partner applies supplemental oxygen via a nonrebreathing mask. As part of your focused history and physical examination, a set of baseline vital signs are taken, paying close attention to the mental status (see **Table 2**). At this point it is clear he will need surgery and there should be no delays on the scene. The IV will be started en route and ventilatory status will be reevaluated. The coach advises you that Mike is 16 years old and that his mother has been notified and is already on the way to the local ED.

Table 2 **Focused History and Physical Examination**

Baseline Vital Signs	Recording Time: 5 Minutes
Skin CTC (color, temperature, condition)	Pale, normal temperature, dry
Pulse	56 beats/min, strong and regular
Blood Pressure	182/98 mm Hg
Respirations	28 breaths/min and shallow

Question 3: Although Mike has been quiet, had he become suddenly violent and combative, what would be the most likely cause of this change in affect?

Question 4: Why is it important to be prepared for vomiting when treating a patient who was struck in the head?

Part 3

With all the information you have so far, your partner advises the coach to call the mother's cell phone and redirect her to the regional trauma center as that facility will be the most appropriate to transport her son to. The patient has vomited and his airway is being managed by manual techniques as well as suctioning. You are considering the possibility of manually assisting ventilations, in an effort to optimize both oxygenation and CO_2 retention. Considering that there is no reason to delay on the scene, you and your partner load him into the ambulance. In the meantime, a first responder unit has arrived on the scene so you will be able to take another crew member with you for the transport. There will be much to do en route to the hospital so you definitely can use the help.

Meanwhile a SAMPLE history reveals necessary information, mostly attained from the coach and from a friend of Mike's (see **Table 3**).

Just prior to heading off to the hospital, the Glasgow Coma Scale (GCS) is evaluated and Mike rates an 8. The IV is easily placed. When response to pain is reassessed, you note he pulls his arms to the core of his body and flexes his legs slightly. This is a definite change that you will be notifying the ED of in a couple of minutes.

Table 3 **SAMPLE History**

SAMPLE History	Comments
Signs/symptoms	Blown pupil, altered mental status followed by lucid interval and then rapidly deteriorating mental status
Allergies	Penicillin and "sulfa drugs" (sulfonamides)
Medications	Just takes a multi-vitamin
Pertinent past medical history	Fractured right humerus 2 years ago
Last oral intake	Light lunch 3 hours ago and a sports drink 20 minutes ago
Events leading up to the incident	Struck on the side of the head in the area overlying the temporoparietal scalp

Treatment Plan

This patient needs a rapid transport to the regional trauma center. You remember your paramedic instructor telling you, "Sometimes the patient needs you to realize the best drugs are oxygen and gasoline (transport)!"

1. Focus your attention on the ABCs.
2. His neck and spine should be immobilized and if he is not hypotensive, consider elevating the head of the long backboard about 12″ to 18″.

Case Study II Continued

3. An IV of normal saline is helpful and it would not be unreasonable to consider checking blood glucose as part of a standard approach to assessment of altered mental status. Do not administer glucose unless his blood glucose is documented as low.
4. Selection of the destination hospital is very important. The ED selected must have the appropriate medical personnel, an available CT scanner to confirm the hematoma, a neurosurgeon, and an intensive care unit capable of handling neurosurgical patients. This care is best provided in a regional trauma center. Transport decisions may also involve aeromedical evacuation from the scene if the conditions permit and your local protocols allow, as the prognosis of this condition is extraordinarily time-sensitive.
5. Aggressively treat hypoxemia (ie, pulse oximetry < 90%) and hypotension (ie, systolic blood pressure below 90 mm Hg) because they are both associated with poor outcomes in the TBI patient.
6. Assess oxygenation and end-tidal carbon dioxide. Consider the need for placing an advanced airway in this patient. If signs of brain herniation are present (as they are in this case with a dilated pupil and neurologic posturing), certainly consider intubation if the GCS score is less than 8 or is rapidly declining.
7. If he becomes combative it may be necessary to consider sedation and analgesia.
8. Monitor him continuously and call the ED or regional trauma center to give them a report on his condition and what has changed in the short time he has been in your care.

Question 5: How would you define and manage hypoxia and hypotension in the field?

Question 6: Can a head-injured patient have hypotension and what would be examples of hypotension for children in the field?

Part 4

En route to the hospital, after inserting an IV and beginning ventilations of the patient, you begin a reassessment of the patient (see **Table 4**).

Mike continues to respond only to painful stimuli. He vomited once more and was quickly suctioned.

Question 7: Why is it so important that the ED be informed as early as possible of your arrival and the patient's condition?

Question 8: What do you expect is likely to be done to treat this patient?

Part 5

As you arrive at the hospital and give a verbal report to the staff, you think to yourself that it seemed like it was just a couple of minutes ago you were arriving on the scene and meeting the coach. Mike Kelly was in the wrong place at the wrong time and was struck in the side of the head with a fastball. His life has just taken a very serious turn and at this point he is struggling to survive. You suspect he has an epidural hematoma that will soon be confirmed by the CT scan he will be receiving just prior to his surgery. The neurosurgeon is already up in the operating room scrubbing as the result of your early notification and a quick report from the physician. Mike has a tough day ahead of him and his recovery will be a long, hard road. However, he would not have had this second chance if it was not for the rapid recognition of the MOI, and some very quick assessment and management en route to the most appropriate hospital in the region. This was a classic epidural hematoma and the lesson can be translated to future calls you will go on. The day will come when you will see the same situation again.

Table 4 Reassessment and Ongoing Assessment of the Patient

Serial Vital Signs and Relevant Data	Recording Time: 10 Minutes
Skin CTC	Pale, normal temperature, dry skin
Pulse	52 beats/min, regular and strong
Blood Pressure	160/88 mm Hg
Respirations	8 breaths/min assisted by bag-mask device with supplemental oxygen
Mental Status	"P" responds with decorticate posturing to painful stimuli
ECG	Sinus bradycardia
SpO_2	95%
Lung Sounds	Clear bilaterally
Other (ie, glucose, core body temperature)	Glucose and body temperature are both within normal range

Management of Head Trauma

The prehospital management of the head-injured patient involves assessment and management of the ABCs, cervical spine immobilization, supplemental oxygen, ventilatory assistance, and rapid transport to the trauma center. The in-hospital management includes prompt resuscitation, CT scanning, prompt evacuation of significant intracranial hematomas, and ICP monitoring and treatment. In years past some EMS systems employed intravenous steroids (dexamethasone was commonly used) as part of an attempt at managing significant closed head injury while en route to the hospital. That strategy was never found to have been of any benefit, and is no longer done. Mannitol [Osmitrol] is occasionally used to assist with management of severe intracranial injury when there is a risk of herniation syndrome, and you may certainly be called on to manage its infusion while performing an interfacility patient transfer. We have included some additional information on mannitol [Osmitrol] so you understand why it is given in hospitalized and closely monitored situations. Some systems deploy medication-facilitated intubation (MFI) to help manage securing the airway of a patient with a significant head injury.

One of the symptoms of moderate to severe or traumatic brain injury (TBI) can be agitation and violence due to brain hypoxia and stimulation of the frontal and/or temporal lobes of the brain. The ability to chemically sedate and restrain patients while providing analgesia can be beneficial to both patients and providers by ensuring the transport will be a safe one. Benzodiazepines and phenothiazines are two categories of drugs with a tranquilizing effect, and are commonly used to manage the combative traumatic brain-injured patient. Specific examples of these drugs (ie, diazepam [Valium]) are discussed throughout this book.

Initial mental status assessment is typically done via the AVPU method. This is a very useful tool for determining if the patient is **A**lert (oriented to person, place, and day), **V**erbally responsive (either appropriate or inappropriate responses to verbal stimuli), **P**ainful response (responds with withdrawal, or neurologic posturing, or no response), and finally **U**nresponsive (pain was applied and there was no response by the patient to the pain). Classifying the patient's mental status into one of the four categories is helpful, yet describing the specific response is even more useful in describing the exact mental status that was observed. An example would be the comparison between a patient who is verbally responsive but not responding appropriately to questions being asked and a patient who is verbally responsive and knows his name but is confused about what day it is and where he is. Another example would be the difference between the patient who is responsive to pain and withdraws from a pain source as compared to the patient who is responsive to pain and who postures every time pain is applied. Neurologic posturing in response to a painful stimuli falls into either decorticate posturing which involves flexion of the arms and extension of the legs, or decerebrate posturing which involves extension of both the arms and legs. The Glasgow Coma Scale (GCS) score, originally developed as a prognostic tool for the head-injured patient, is also used to further define the patient's mental status and how he or she is responding (**Table 2-1** ▾).

Many EMS systems use the GCS for triage to the trauma center and other interventions. A GCS score of 11 to 13 is considered moderate to severe TBI and a GCS score of 3 to 10 is considered severe TBI. Both should be transported to the regional trauma center if this is possible. Most of the research being conducted on the TBI patient takes into consideration the GCS so it is important that a GCS score be calculated for every TBI patient and reassessed as other serial assessments and vital signs are reassessed.

Is There Still a Role for Hyperventilation?

The role of hyperventilation has changed over the past two decades. Initially we were all taught that there was a vicious cycle of brain swelling causing CO_2 retention, causing swelling of brain tissue, causing less blood flow into the brain, which in turn leads to hypoxemia,

Table 2-1 The Glasgow Coma Scale

Eye Opening		Best Verbal Response		Best Motor Response	
Spontaneous	4	Oriented and converses	5	Follows commands	6
To verbal command	3	Disoriented conversation	4	Localizes pain	5
To pain	2	Speaking but nonsensical	3	Withdraws to pain	4
No response	1	Moans or makes unintelligible sounds	2	Decorticate flexion	3
		No response	1	Decerebrate extension	2
				No response	1

Scores:
14–15: Mild dysfunction
11–13: Moderate to severe dysfunction
10 or less: Severe dysfunction (The lowest possible score is 3.)

CO_2 retention, and more brain tissue swelling. We were also told to simply blow off the CO_2 by hyperventilating the patient. This in turn would decrease the brain swelling. In the 1990s, we were told to stop hyperventilating head-injured patients as it may be dangerous. Studies have questioned the value of hyperventilating the patient and even suggested that it produces a marked reduction in the cerebral blood flow, exacerbating the brain's developing ischemia. If hyperventilation was to be used, the experts stated it should only be used with arterial blood gasses to follow the patient's response, as well as ICP monitoring. These tests are not available in the prehospital setting.

Today the Brain Trauma Foundation has taken a more refined view of this topic. Clearly hypoxemia (< 90% arterial hemoglobin oxygen saturation) is associated with poor patient outcome in the severely head-injured patient. A pulse oximeter is now routinely used on all critical patients by paramedics in the field so hypoxemia can be assessed objectively. In cases where the mechanism of injury (MOI) leads you to suspect that the patient has a serious TBI and there are already signs of an elevated ICP from brain herniation, the field use of increased ventilations with supplemental oxygen would be appropriate. Today experts agree that in the context of active monitoring of end-tidal carbon dioxide ($EtCO_2$) levels, ventilation should be directed toward keeping the $EtCO_2$ between 30 and 35 mm Hg. Note that these are patients who are not in cardiac arrest. Should they become pulseless, you should always resort to the latest guidelines for resuscitation from ILCOR which consist of much slower rates.

Other Drugs for Consideration

The patient with a head injury may have symptoms that mimic hypoglycemia. If you suspect the patient has hypoglycemia, check the blood glucose level using a drop of blood and a glucometer. Do not automatically administer D_5W because a high concentration of glucose given to the patient with a neurological problem, such as a stroke or TBI, could be harmful to the brain. However, if the patient is found to have a low blood glucose, then administer D_5W into a large bore, very secure, IV site.

As stated previously, some patients who are transported to a local or community hospital may then be transferred to a trauma center by ground or air. Therefore, it is possible that these patients are on a mannitol [Osmitrol] drip as well as sedation, analgesics, and paralytics. Mannitol [Osmitrol] is not recommended for use in the prehospital setting, but in interfacility transfers you may come in contact with a patient receiving this drug. In the 1970s and 1980s, a number of EMS systems were studying the use of mannitol [Osmitrol] for prehospital use. Most found the drug too controversial and have removed it from the formulary. It is given for TBI due to its immediate plasma-expanding properties and delayed osmotic diuresis actions. The immediate effects reduce hematocrit and blood viscosity, which in turn increases the cerebral blood flow and oxygen delivery. The gradient created by the osmotic effect of mannitol [Osmitrol] produces a fluid gradient and shifting of water from the intracellular to extracellular compartments, resulting in both a local and systemic diuresis. This process works to initially decrease intracellular edema and ICP, beginning about 30 minutes after administration of the drug and lasting up to 6 hours. Patients will have a dramatically increased urine output. Mannitol [Osmitrol] is administered via either IV bolus or drip, and must be monitored very closely in the ICU as it can accumulate in the brain tissue and has been shown to have a reverse effect of causing cerebral edema. It has also been known to cause renal failure in patients with kidney diseases.

Types of Face Trauma

Patients can sustain a number of facial injuries. Examples would include:

- Injuries to the ears or nose—these are usually soft-tissue injuries that bleed considerably.
- Injuries to the mid-face such as fractures—the types of facial fractures have been classified as Le Fort I, II, and III fractures (**Figure 2-9**▾).

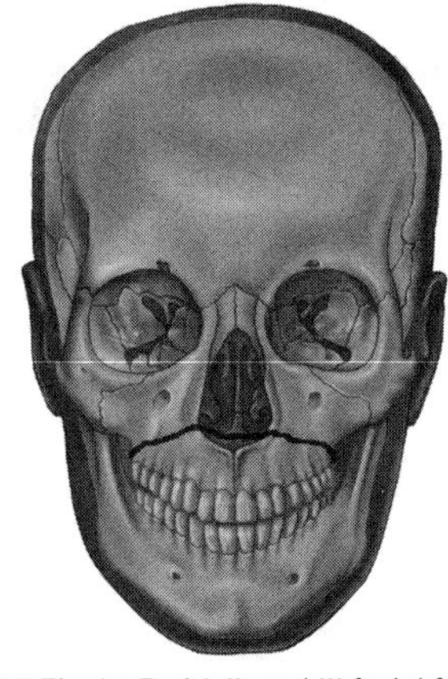

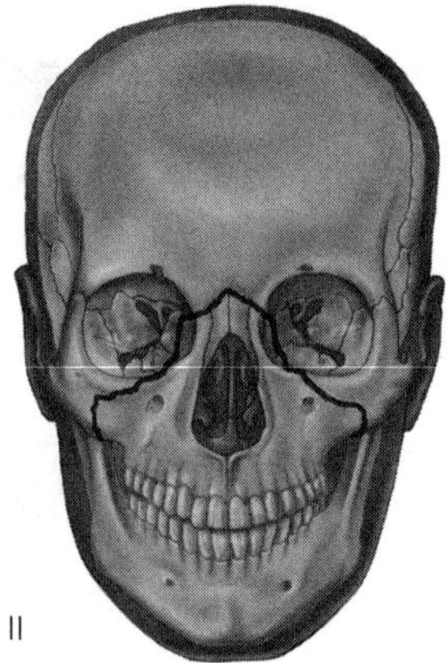

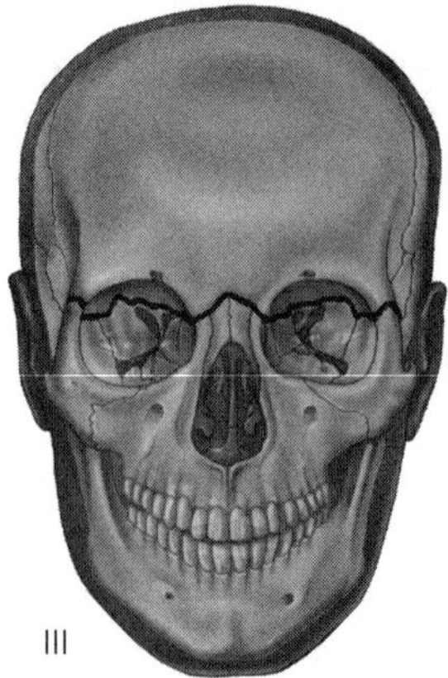

Figure 2-9 The Le Fort I, II, and III facial fractures.

Table 2-2 Tetracaine HCL

Do you know?	Comments
Right drug? Generic name: [**Tetracaine HCL**] Trade name: [Pontocaine]	Use prior to the insertion of the Morgan lens when irrigation of the eye is needed.
Right patient?	Patients who need a local anesthetic so that an ophthalmic procedure can be done.
Right dose?	0.5% solution is used and 1 or 2 drops provided into each eye.
Right route?	Drops into the eye.
Right time?	Just prior to an ophthalmic procedure.
Right documentation?	Make sure you document the dose and route given as well as the time on your patient care report.
Expected action	Decreases the pain of an ophthalmic procedure such as insertion of the Morgan lens or irrigation of the eye.
Side effects	Tearing, stinging, sensitivity to light, and swelling may occur in the patient's eyes.
Contraindications	Do not use the medication if it contains particles or is cloudy.
Precautions	Beware of allergies to this medication, medical history of heart or liver disease, thyroid problems, or myasthenia gravis.

- Injuries to the scalp—actually can bleed considerably but are easily controlled by bandaging.
- Injuries to the eyes—can be very serious and threaten the patient's sight. If the eye is sprayed with a chemical or needs to be flushed, many services use the Morgan lens. Insertion of the lens requires the use of a local anesthetic such as tetracaine HCL [Pontocaine] (**Table 2-2▲**).

Whenever dealing with facial injuries, always perform an assessment of the ABCs before being distracted by the bleeding. Consider that the injury may have caused a potential injury to the cervical spine and ensure manual stabilization of the head and neck at all times.

Spinal, Thoracic, and Abdominal Trauma

The Spinal Cord

The spinal cord is the major group of nerve tissues that are bundled together originating at the base of the brain and extending down the spinal column (approximately 15″ to 18″ depending on the individual's height) and ending typically at the level of the second lumbar vertebrae. The spine is made up of 33 interconnecting bones called vertebra, muscles, tendons, and ligaments, which are supported with blood vessels and nerves. Thirty-one pairs of spinal nerves (peripheral nerves) originate from the spinal cord and exit between each vertebra (actually spinal nerves are not classified as "peripheral" until they exit the spinal column foramina—prior to that they are still a part of the CNS so they are technically "central" nerves). These peripheral nerves provide motor and sensory function and carry two-way communication between the spinal cord and the rest of the body. Injury to the spinal cord can occur acutely with trauma and progressively over time with age and disease.

Spinal Cord Injuries

It is estimated that each year 10,000 to 12,000 people sustain a spinal cord injury (SCI). The most common are acute spinal cord injuries (ASCIs) and they occur when the neck or spine is bent or compressed as can happen with:

- Falls
- Motor vehicle collisions
- Sports
- Violence (gunshot wounds or stabbing)
- Diving accidents
- Trampoline accidents
- Birth injuries

ASCI has two phases, the primary and the secondary. The primary injury to the spinal cord occurs at the time of impact, when the force involved causes cord compression, fractures of the bone, dislocation of the structures of the spinal column, and disruption of blood supply. Neurologic function may be lost temporarily as seen with cord contusion or last longer as seen with cord compression and contusion with bleeding. Or, the injury can be permanent due to lacerations or transection.

Secondary injuries follow primary injuries and are caused by swelling and ischemia in and around the cord, vasospasm, thrombosis, electrolyte derangements, neurotransmitter accumulation, oxidative free radical formation, or when additional movement of unstable bone fragments occurs. Secondary damage can continue for days and weeks after the primary injury, increasing the damaged area.

As with so many traumatic injuries, the normal response is swelling and bleeding at the site of injury. The diameter of the spinal cord is approximately 10 mm. The diameter of the spinal column is not much larger, approximately 15 mm. This leaves very limited room for swelling. Within minutes of the injury the spinal cord swells within the spinal cavity at the level of the injury, thus cutting off the blood supply to the spinal cord tissue.

In addition to a temporary or permanent loss of motor function and sensation, ASCI can result in loss of temperature regulation, weakness, bladder dysfunction, paralysis, and death. The specific types of spinal cord injuries include: cord contusion, cord concussion, cord compression, cord transection, laceration, hemorrhage, neurogenic shock, and spinal shock. The severity and lasting effects a patient experiences will vary depending on the extent of injury and how the patient is managed following the injury.

Case Study III Spinal Cord Injury

Part 1

It is a sunny and warm Saturday afternoon when your ambulance is dispatched to a residence for a diving accident. En route to the call you consider the possibilities associated with a diving accident: submersion, traumatic brain injury, spinal cord injury, paralysis, and death. You know that this type of injury could be devastating and if the patient is not handled properly his or her condition could be made worse. Not far after turning on to the street of the residence you see many vehicles parked and get the impression that there is a gathering that could be a picnic or barbeque. There are a couple of men waving at you and they look upset. You pull over. Your partner grabs a long backboard and head stabilizer while you get the stretcher and equipment.

Table 1 Initial Assessment

Initial Assessment	Recording Time: 1 Minute
General Impression/ Appearance	Conscious in a pool with friends supporting his head out of the water
Mental Status	Alert and panic-stricken
Airway	Open and shouting
Breathing	Adequate for now
Circulation	Adequate for now
Priority/Plan	High priority due to the MOI and the unstable neck injury

You are led to the back yard where there is an in-ground pool. It is a pool party, with an entire youth baseball team and their parents who have come to celebrate after a game. Three men call to you from in the pool; they are holding up another man in the shallow end of the pool. One of the men tells you that Jim was floating face down after jumping into the pool, and he is unable to move. The man is holding Jim's head and neck in a neutral position while two other men are supporting Jim's body. Jim is conscious and is shouting "my neck is broken." He is nearly hysterical and continues to shout "Get the children inside, I don't want them to see me like this." Jim has an airway and is breathing adequate for now. Now you want to know exactly what happened and how serious the injury is. Your partner takes off his shoes and jumps into the pool to help with stabilization and to perform an initial assessment (see **Table 1**). He determines that Jim's arms are limp and that Jim is unable to feel any sensation below his clavicles. Jim explains that when he did a flip into the pool from the side, he immediately heard and felt his neck snap when his head struck the bottom of the pool. Then he floated face down to the surface because he was unable to move. Fortunately, someone saw him right away and helped him get his head above water.

Question 1: Why are spinal cord injuries so devastating?

Question 2: What single factor in the prehospital setting can make the most difference in the patient's prognosis?

Part 2

More emergency responders arrive and one of them knows Jim because Jim was a coach for his son's team last year. There are a lot of excited and emotionally charged people at this scene and things are escalating. Some of Jim's friends at the party are also coworkers who are police. They are anxious to help in any way. Tasks are assigned to gain control of the scene. The priority is to get Jim out of the pool without causing further injury. One responder is going to clear a

Case Study III Continued

path for the stretcher to get back to the ambulance. Another one is going to get the children and their parents inside and out of sight. This will help keep Jim from getting more upset. Keeping Jim calm is important now because physical and mental agitation will not help his situation.

Next the extrication out of the pool with the long backboard is organized and carried out as you practiced in your EMT course. Jim is loaded on the stretcher, but he is very agitated and is trying to move his head. You decide to get him into the ambulance right away and begin transport to the trauma center. Greg, the responder who knows Jim, will come with you to help calm him. Joan is Jim's wife and she will ride up front. Once in the ambulance Jim is dried, vital signs are obtained, and a neurologic examination is performed.

Jim tells you that he is not a drinker, but today at the party he had a few wine coolers. He says he knows he should not have attempted the flip in the shallow end of the pool and that the alcohol impaired his judgment. He is inconsolable and says he knows that his paralysis is permanent. Jim says he remembers everything and did not swallow too much water. You do not think he had a loss of consciousness.

Jim has use of his respiratory muscles for now but cannot move his arms or legs. He has no sense of touch below the clavicle, potentially indicating a cervical fracture/dislocation of C5 or C6. You draw a line on his chest to establish a baseline. His vital signs are stable with respirations of 24 breaths/min and regular, lung sounds remain clear although he could have aspirated some water, pulse is 88 beats/min strong and regular, blood pressure is 126/66 mm Hg, and skin signs are warm, with good color (see **Table 2**). There is no evidence of injury to the mouth, facial bones, or skull, and no bleeding from the nose or ears. There is however tenderness over the lower cervical spine.

Table 2 Focused History and Physical Examination

Baseline Vital Signs	Recording Time: 5 Minutes
Skin CTC (color, temperature, condition)	Warm and dry with good color
Pulse	88 beats/min, strong and regular
Blood Pressure	126/66 mm Hg
Respirations	24 breaths/min and regular with good effort

Question 3: At what level of the cervical spine do you estimate the primary injury has occurred?

Question 4: What is the body's initial response to a spinal cord injury?

Part 3

In the front of the ambulance your partner is providing emotional support for Joan while at the same time attempting to get some SAMPLE history about Jim (see **Table 3**). Jim is 29 years old and he is physically fit and active. He has no allergies to medications and his only medication is omeprazole [Prilosec] for gastritis. Each year Jim's work requires a physical and he had one last month with no issues. There has been food available all afternoon at the party and she is not aware of Jim having any alcohol to drink. She was in the house when the accident occurred.

Treatment Plan

Jim will need rapid transport to a trauma center.

1. Maintain complete spinal immobilization.
2. Provide supportive psychological care.

Table 3 SAMPLE History

SAMPLE History	Comments
Signs/symptoms	Loss of motor and sensory functions below the clavicles after diving into the pool
Allergies	No known drug allergies
Medications	Omeprazole (Prilosec)
Pertinent past medical history	Gastritis, otherwise healthy, fit and active
Last oral intake	Wine coolers; unknown how much and could have been continuous over the afternoon
Events leading up to the incident	Pool party with alcohol ingestion reported by the patient who did a flip into the pool

Case Study III Continued

3. Provide high-flow supplemental oxygen. Serial neurologic examinations will ensure that Jim's respiratory effort remains adequate and any changes in his condition are monitored.
4. Establish an IV of normal saline.
5. Draw blood samples.
6. Keep the patient warm.
7. Notify the trauma center with Jim's status.
8. There is no recommended pharmacologic treatment for the ASCI patient in the prehospital setting. Methylprednisolone sodium succinate may be administered in the hospital setting (see **Table 4**).

Question 5: Why is methylprednisolone sodium succinate [Solu-Medrol] not administered in the prehospital setting for the ASCI patient?

Question 6: What changes in vital signs should you be alert for with severe ASCI?

Table 4 **Methylprednisolone Sodium Succinate**

Do you know?	Comments
Right drug? Generic name: [**Methylprednisolone Sodium Succinate**] Trade name: [Solu-Medrol]	For possible use in the ASCI patient in the hospital setting to help decrease the swelling in the spinal cord. Use is controversial, *and is rarely used in the prehospital setting* because of the many risks associated with its high dose use in this situation.
Right patient?	ASCI if started within 8 hours following the primary blunt ASCI.
Right dose?	High dose 30 mg/kg IV administered over the first hour followed by 5.4 mg/kg/h for the next 23 hours may be considered if started within 8 hours following the primary blunt ASCI.
Right route?	IV drip.
Right time?	In the hospital less than 8 hours following the primary injury and using ASCI treatment protocols.
Right documentation?	Dose and route given as well as the time.
Expected action	Decreased swelling of the spinal cord tissue.
Side effects	Increased incidence of sepsis and pneumonia, also marked glycemic, wound healing, and gastrointestinal complications.
Contraindications	Correlate with preexisting conditions that could be exacerbated by its side effects.
Precautions	Age, overall health, extent of ASCI, tolerance, and expectations for the course of treatment.

Part 4

The 20-minute transport to the trauma center has been a long and difficult ongoing assessment (see **Table 5**). Despite all efforts to get Jim settled down, he remains terribly upset. He has three young children and is devastated that he is not going to recover from this injury. Jim knows he can still move his head and attempts to do so even though you have explained how dangerous it is. You have Greg help you to check to make sure he is secured within the immobilization device and stays that way. The oxygen mask is agitating Jim so you ask Greg to hold it near his face for the blow-by effect. An IV is established, blood is drawn, a blood glucose reading is obtained, and axillary temperature is taken. Serial vital signs are stable; however, there are crackles in the bases of the lungs now. The neurologic examinations are similar to the baseline examinations. The trauma center has been notified.

Case Study III Continued

Table 5 Reassessment and Ongoing Assessment of the Patient

Serial Vital Signs and Relevant Data	Recording Time: 8 Minutes
Skin CTC	Warm and dry with good color
Pulse	76 beats/min, strong and regular
Blood Pressure	116/68 mm Hg
Respirations	28 breaths/min, shallow
Mental Status	Conscious and panic-stricken
ECG	Normal sinus rhythm
SpO_2	99%
Lung Sounds	Crackles in the bases of the lungs now
Other (ie, glucose, core body temperature)	Axillary temp 97.9°F, glucose 96 mg/dL

Question 7: What two factors may be contributing to the change in lung sounds?

Question 8: Why does Jim try to move his head even though it could make the injury worse?

Part 5

Once in the emergency department, you are directed into trauma room one. The early notification to the hospital gave the staff time to clear the room and get the necessary personnel ready for your patient. You give the report while Greg helps Joan to get Jim registered. Jim is a young man. He and his family have a challenging life ahead. Patients with ASCI are likely to have medical complications such as respiratory and heart problems, chronic pain, bladder and bowel dysfunction, spasticity, and reproductive and sexual dysfunction. Successful recovery will depend on how well these chronic conditions are managed day to day.

Classification, Location, and Effects of Spinal Cord Injuries

Spinal cord injuries are classified as either complete or incomplete, depending on how much cord width is injured. A complete injury is characterized by the total loss of sensory and motor function below the level of injury. An incomplete injury means that the ability of the spinal cord to convey messages to or from the brain is not completely lost. Patients with incomplete injuries retain some motor or sensory function below the injury because the nerves are compressed rather than severed or degenerated as seen in a complete injury.

Injuries can occur at any level of the spinal cord and deficits produced by SCI will be distal to the point of injury. The level of injury is very helpful in predicting what parts of the body might be affected by loss of function and paralysis. Paralysis affecting the lower half of the body is called paraplegia and quadriplegia involves loss of function in all four limbs, as well as the chest muscles and occasionally requires a ventilator for the patient.

The following are the landmark dermatomes that should be evaluated in the patient with a SCI as they relate to the location of injury on the cord (**Table 2-3** ▸).

Table 2-3 The Landmark Spinal Dermatomes

Nerve	Anatomic Location
Root	
C2	Occipital protuberance
C3	Supraclavicular fossa
C5	Lateral side of the antecubital fossa
C6	Thumb and medial index finger
C7	Middle finger
C8	Little finger
T2	Apex of axilla
T4	Nipple line
T10	Umbilicus
L1	Inguinal line
L2	Mid anterior thigh
L3	Medial aspect of the knee
L5	Dorsum of the foot
S1–S3	Back of the leg
S4–S5	Perianal area

Neurogenic Shock with Spinal Cord Injury

Spinal cord injury can produce neurogenic shock, also called vascular shock, due to the loss of sympathetic nervous system tone and vasodilation. When the muscles in the blood vessels are cut off from their impulses to contract, the vessels dilate widely, increasing the size and capacity of the vascular system. The blood in the body can no longer fill the enlarged vessels. The massive vasodilation often results in fluid-refractory hypotension. Loss of thermoregulation and the vasodilation produces shock with skin that is pink, warm, and dry and the loss of sympathetic tone causes bradycardia. Together these signs, hypotension, bradycardia, and skin that is pink, warm and dry, are the hallmark signs of neurogenic shock.

Treatment of Spinal Cord Injury

Currently there is no way to repair an injured spinal cord, though researchers are vigorously looking for ways of stimulating spinal cord regeneration. Recovery requires long-term hospitalization and rehabilitation. Rehabilitation focuses on preventing muscle wasting and contraction, as well as retraining the patient to use other muscles to aid in movement and mobility.

Remember that SCIs are not always obvious, so the MOI is a significant factor when considering how to manage a trauma patient. Any injury involving the head, pelvis, or penetrating injuries near the spine should be managed as an ASCI. Placing the body in a neutral position is the most stable position for the spinal column and helps to reduce excess pressure and cord hypoxia. Respiratory compromise is an indication of the severity of SCI and nearly one third of patients with spinal cord injuries involving the cervical area will need at least temporary mechanical ventilation.

Medical management and observation in the intensive care unit may include a ventilator, indwelling urinary catheter, feeding tube, and medications such as corticosteroids or nonsteroidal anti-inflammatory drugs (NSAIDs) to reduce swelling, analgesics for pain, and medicines to protect the stomach lining during periods of poor GI utilization.

Surgery may be an option if the spinal cord is compressed or when the spine requires stabilization. The timing of this option is controversial as some argue that surgery, when required, has a better outcome when performed within 8 hours following the injury. Others argue that delaying or avoiding surgery is better. The use of large doses of corticosteroids is also controversial. This option may only be considered if started within 8 hours following the primary blunt ASCI and most likely only when there is some evidence of preserved distal neurologic function to start with. Methylprednisoline sodium succinate 30 mg/kg IV administered over the first hour followed by 5.4 mg/kg/h for the next 23 hours has been used in ASCI treatment protocols. There are many problems associated with the use of high dose steroids and their use is controversial. Risks involve increased incidence of sepsis and pneumonia, as well as significant problems with hyperglycemia, poor wound healing, and gastrointestinal bleeding complications.

When the spine is stable and there is no significant neurologic involvement, injuries are managed with ice, rest, stretching, and physical therapy. Medications for acute cases involving the back and spine will typically include a course of NSAIDs such as ibuprofen and its various cousins. For cases refractory to more conventional therapy, a course of oral or locally injected steroids is sometimes used.

Treating pain is necessary in almost two thirds of patients with SCI. This area also has no universal treatment plan. Analgesics such as acetaminophen may be an option and for severe pain could be compounded with a narcotic (ie, codeine, hydrocodone, oxycodone). Occasionally so-called "muscle-relaxers" are prescribed to help manage discomfort associated with the acute phase of these injuries. These include medications such as cyclobenzaprine [Flexeril], metaxalone [Skelaxin], and diazepam [Valium]. The treatment of neuropathic pain may also include the use of antidepressants and anticonvulsants although they are not uniformly effective. Alternative nonpharmacologic therapies such as acupuncture, massage, and chiropractic may be useful as well.

Many patients with ASCIs have associated injuries in the chest and abdomen. Injuries at the level of C3-C5 can impair the phrenic nerve and paralyze the diaphragm so the patient stops breathing. Injuries at the level of C5 and below may not affect the diaphragm, but the thoracic muscles will become weak. The patient may have shallow respirations and experience difficulty coughing and clearing secretions from the lungs. Lung capacity is impaired and the patient is vulnerable to pneumonia and sepsis. Pneumonia is the leading cause of death in patients with SCI.

A MOI that produces blunt or penetrating force to the chest can result in injuries such as:

- Fractures (ribs, sternum, spinal column)
- Lung injuries (pneumothorax, pulmonary contusion, hemothorax, tension pneumothorax)
- Cardiac injuries (cardiac contusion, cardiac tamponade)
- Diaphragm injuries (rupture, herniation, phrenic nerve impairment)
- Esophageal injuries (tears, perforation)
- Aortic injuries (dissection, rupture)

Advances in stem cell research are giving patients and doctors hope that spinal cord injuries will eventually be repairable. Researchers in neurology and cell biology are working with several types of possible treatments in an effort to help victims with SCI. One of the most promising research areas is the use of stem cells for regeneration. Stem cells are the body's master cells, sparingly found throughout the tissue and blood. In animal studies, stem cells have grown new nerve fibers and structures that allow the new fibers to reconnect with other parts of the spinal cord restoring some functions that had been lost.

Stem cell research, whether from embryos or adults, has provided increased knowledge about how cells communicate with each other and someday may be used to find treatments for debilitating diseases such as diabetes, cancer, amyotrophic lateral sclerosis (ALS), cerebral palsy, multiple sclerosis, Parkinson's, and other devastating diseases as well as stroke and SCI.

Spinal Cord Injury in Children

Spinal cord injury without evidence of radiologic (such as CT, MRI, or electromyelography) abnormality (SCIWORA) is an injury that may include spinal cord concussion, traction, or vascular injury to the cord. This type of SCI injury occurs in children because of the shape of their vertebrae. Children have flat vertebrae as compared to the adult vertebrae which are more curved-shaped. In rapid acceleration or deceleration, the child's vertebrae can easily dislocate and quickly relocate back into their normal position causing the cord to become injured by compression or traction.

Musculoskeletal Trauma

In the United States alone, complaints related to the musculoskeletal system are estimated at approximately 60 million a year. It is further estimated that 1 in every 7 Americans will experience musculoskeletal impairment. Although a great many of the patients paramedics treat who have multiple trauma also have musculoskeletal injuries, usually there are not that many multiple trauma patients in most communities. On the other hand, there are plenty of isolated, painful, swollen, and deformed extremity injuries. When these injuries occur as single injuries, they are not generally life-threatening. However, they can be very painful with a lengthy rehabilitation.

The bones provide the framework and protection for internal organs while the muscles provide the bulk and strength of the body. There are a number of different shapes of bones in the human body (**Table 2-4**▼).

The bone is a living structure with its own blood supply. We have already learned the usefulness of this vascular cavity in the long bone in which fluids administered by the IO route can be rapidly transported to the patient's central circulation (**Figure 2-10**▶).

The bones articulate at the joints. There are a number of different types of joints (**Table 2-5**▶). They each have specific functions allowing for movement and the body's range of motion.

Table 2-4 The Shapes of Human Bones

Shape	Examples
Long bones	Femur, humerus, tibia, radius, ulna
Short bones	Phalanges, metacarpals, metatarsals
Flat bones	Sternum, ribs, scapula, skull bones
Irregular bones	Vertebrae, mandible
Round bones	Patella

There is always a chance that blood will be splashed when working with open fractures. Always use the appropriate body substance isolation (BSI) techniques.

The skeleton and muscles are held together and supported by connective tissue. The specific tissues include the tendons, ligaments, and cartilage. The tendons connect muscle to bones. Ligaments are designed to connect bones to bones, and cartilage provides a cushioning surface over the ends of the bones so they can articulate over each other at the joints. Cartilage is also found in soft spots such as the ears and tip of the nose.

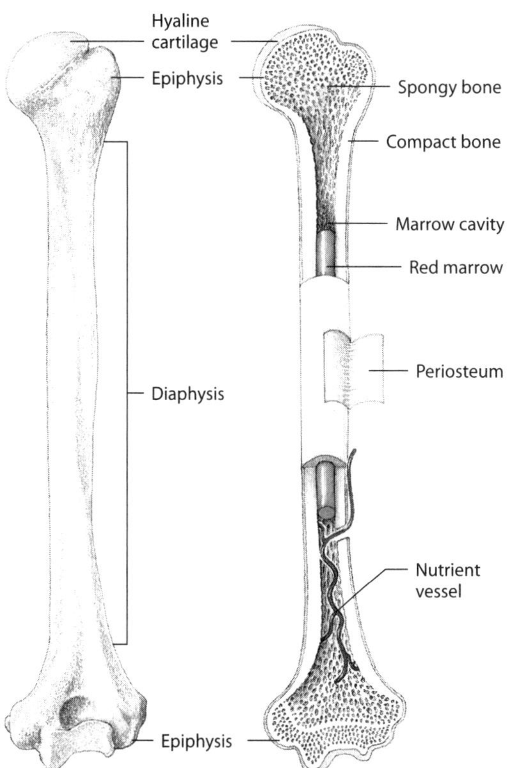

Figure 2-10 Anatomy of a long bone.

Case Study IV Musculoskeletal Injury

Part 1

Your unit has been dispatched to the local high school soccer field where an athlete is down on the side of the field. On arrival you are met by a member of the coaching staff. Apparently a 17-year-old girl must have caught a cleat in the ground, pinning her right leg as the rest of her body continued to move sideways. This movement forced her right knee laterally past its normal range of motion leaving the knee joint torn apart.

Table 1 Initial Assessment

Initial Assessment	Recording Time: 1 Minute
General Impression/ Appearance	Teenage female quietly crying in pain
Mental Status	Alert and oriented to person, place, and day
Airway	Open and clear
Breathing	24 breaths/min and rapid but normal volume
Circulation	Tachycardia and strong at the radius, no external bleeding
Priority/Plan	High due to the patient being in considerable pain

The scene is safe and the patient was moved to the sidelines so they could continue playing the game. You and your partner grab the stretcher along with the first-in bag and a knee splint. Fortunately someone has already applied ice to the very swollen knee joint. The patient is anxious, yet introduces herself as Shelly. As part of your initial assessment you note that she is well-oriented to the day and place so you note her mental status as alert (see **Table 1**).

You proceed to begin the rapid trauma assessment with an evaluation from head-to-toe of the major body regions (ie, head, neck, chest, abdomen, back/buttocks, extremities) using the pneumonic DCAP-BTLS. Aside from the obviously deformed knee and a few contusions from yesterday's practice, you find no other injury. Shelly states that she did not pass out from the pain. When asked to rate the pain on a scale of 1 to 10, she says it is a 7. She can describe exactly how and when the injury occurred and is especially upset because she previously had ACL surgery 2 years ago on her left knee. She understands that a knee injury can have a devastating impact on her chances of an athletic scholarship next year.

Question 1: What type of joint is the knee?

Question 2: Why is the knee easily injured when it is forced laterally?

Part 2

Shelly continues to talk about her sports career and the season coming to an end as the tears flow down her cheeks. It is obvious she is in a lot of pain from the injury. She denies any other associated symptoms (ie, nausea, dizziness) at this time. After completing the initial assessment, you begin to inquire about Shelly's past medical history. She has been on aspirin (which a friend told her to take every day) and nonsteroidal anti-inflammatory drugs since her previous knee surgery. Because she is so pale and a bit tachycardic you suspect she is having a lot more pain than she is telling you.

Table 2 Focused History and Physical Examination

Baseline Vital Signs	Recording Time: 5 Minutes
Skin CTC (color, temperature, condition)	Pale, cool, clammy
Pulse	110 beats/min which is fast for the patient at rest
Blood Pressure	110/72 mm Hg
Respirations	20 breaths/min and regular

Prior to providing pain medication and splinting the knee in the most comfortable position, you closely assess distal pulses, motor function, and sensation (PMS). Fortunately Shelly has good PMS in the ankles and toes at this point. Remember the six "Ps" of musculoskeletal assessment which include: pain, paralysis, paresthesia, pulselessness, pallor, and pressure. As you continue your focused history and physical examination your partner gets a set of vital signs (see **Table 2**). You realize the treatment will focus on pain relief and proper splinting.

Question 3: Can a patient with a closed fracture be in shock and likely require fluid resuscitation and analgesia?

Question 4: Which comes first, the pain relief or the splinting of a painful long bone or joint injury?

Case Study IV Continued

Part 3

Based on the patient's vitals being stable at this point, you opt for IM morphine sulfate [Astramorph PF] and then get her splinted up using the triangulation technique which you learned years ago in EMT-Basic school. You may also administer an antiemetic. Another cold pack is applied to keep the knee swelling down and you reassess the distal PMS after the splint is applied. You obtain additional information through the SAMPLE history (see **Table 3**).

Table 3 SAMPLE History

SAMPLE History	Comments
Signs/symptoms	Pain, discoloration, and swelling of the knee
Allergies	Denies any
Medications	Aspirin and ibuprofen (Motrin) daily
Pertinent past medical history	Prior injury to other knee with ACL surgery, appendicitis 5 years ago
Last oral intake	Sports drink 20 minutes ago
Events leading up to the incident	Playing soccer and caught a cleat forcing the knee laterally out of its normal range of motion

Treatment Plan

The coach tells you that Shelly's father has been notified and is already en route to the local hospital ED. Shelly uses a cell phone to talk to him and is surprisingly very calm. You think to yourself she would make a great health care provider!

1. Assess and manage the ABCs.
2. Consider administration of analgesic once stable vitals are established.
3. Splint and apply ice to minimize pain and swelling. Assess PMS before and after applying the splint.
4. Administer supplemental oxygen as needed.
5. Keep the patient warm, reassess and monitor the patient en route.
6. Contact medical control for additional analgesia if there is a long transport time.

Question 5: What other pain medication could be considered if the patient has an allergy to morphine sulfate?

Question 6: If the patient starts to complain of nausea, should an antiemetic be considered?

Part 4

En route to the hospital you hear all about the soccer team's season from Shelly. It is clear she has less pain from the medication you gave her. On reassessment she states she is a 2 out of 10 on the pain scale but still feels every bump in the road. You reassess her vital signs, check the splint and distal PMS, as well as change the cold pack on her knee (see **Table 4**). You give the hospital a quick call on the radio and they state she will be going to trauma room 2 and that her father has already arrived.

The rest of the ride is a nice conversation about other sports-related professions and you mention that athletic training would be worth investigating for someone who loves sports and can handle the orthopaedic injuries. The conversation switches to the World Cup as you arrive at the ED.

Table 4 Reassessment and Ongoing Assessment of the Patient

Serial Vital Signs and Relevant Data	Recording Time: 15 Minutes
Skin CTC	Pale, normal, dry
Pulse	100 beats/min and regular
Blood Pressure	108/74 mm Hg
Respirations	16 breaths/min and regular
Mental Status	Alert (oriented to person, place, and day)
ECG	Sinus tachycardia with no ectopy
SpO_2	99% on nonrebreathing mask
Lung Sounds	Clear in all lung fields
Other (ie, glucose, core temperature)	None

Question 7: Why is it helpful to have a concerned conversation with the patient?

Question 8: Will Shelly be back this season and if asked, how should you answer that question?

Case Study IV Continued

Part 5

This case was a simple knee injury that commonly occurs. Yet for Shelley, it is very painful and possibly the end of her run as a competitive soccer player. Knee injuries can be devastating and most athletes would agree they would much rather break a bone than tear a ligament in their knee. The rehabilitation is lengthy and in many situations they may have to wear a knee brace when and if allowed to go back to certain stressing physical activities. Just take a look at many of the experienced ski patrollers who still enjoy the sport yet wear knee braces.

In this case the actions you took, proper assessment, management, and calming conversation, will go a long way in helping Shelly begin to deal with her injury. A lot of what the best paramedics and EMT-Bs do is help patients calm down and make it through some very stressful and painful situations.

About 2 months later you are back at the high school for another injury and see Shelly still on crutches sitting on the sideline. You stop to say hello and she is all excited to see you and tell you that she just got accepted to a college that has an excellent athletic trainer curriculum!

Table 2-5 Types of Joints

Type	Example	Purpose
Pivot	Joint between first two vertebrae	Side-to-side movement
Ball and socket	Hip and shoulder	Movement in most directions
Hinge	Knee and elbow	Similar to a door hinge
Plane or Gliding	Intervertebral processes	Sliding in many directions
Saddle	Thumb	Movement at right angles
Ellipsoidal	Between skull and 1st vertebrae and between radius and carpals	Restricted hinge-like movement
Slightly movable	Between adjacent vertebrae, between radius and ulna	Small amount of movement
Immovable	Sutures in cranium, teeth within the jaw; first pair of ribs and breast bone	No movement, basically fused together

When a patient sustains a musculoskeletal injury, it falls into one or more of the following types of injuries: sprain, strain, dislocation, or a fracture. A sprain is an injury to the ligament from excessive movement and it involves pain, swelling, and disfiguration of the skin over the joint. It is often difficult to determine in the field if an injured ankle is a sprain or a small bone break but fortunately the treatment in the prehospital setting is the same (splinting, cold application, and pain relief). A strain is an injury to either a muscle or a tendon usually from overuse or excessive stretching of the muscle without adequate prior preparation. A dislocation is the movement of the bone end out of its normal location in the joint. The integrity of the joint has been disrupted and sometimes the patient may be found in a strange position such as with a shoulder dislocation. These injuries often look grotesque yet are rarely a life-threatening high priority. The exceptions would be a knee dislocation, where the tibia has been forced backward, often compressing (occasionally tearing) the popliteal artery behind the knee. This can easily be a limb-threatening injury without prompt intervention. Another high priority dislocation is the elbow dislocation due to the blood supply of the lower arm traveling through the elbow joint.

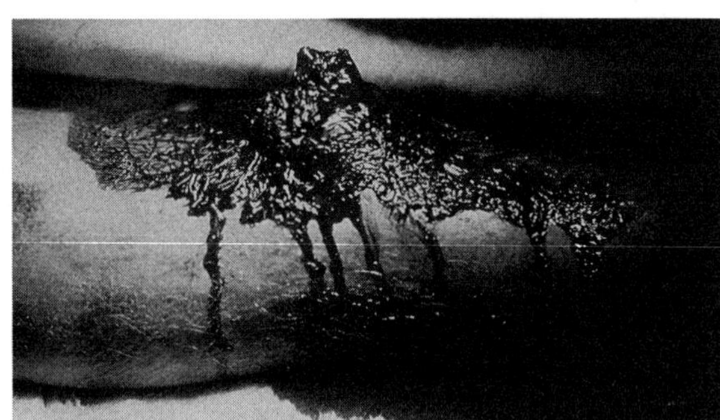

Figure 2-11 An open fracture.

There are two general types of fractures: open and closed. An open fracture has a break in the overlying skin (**Figure 2-11** ▲). In a closed fracture, the skin over the fracture site remains intact (**Figure 2-12** ▶).

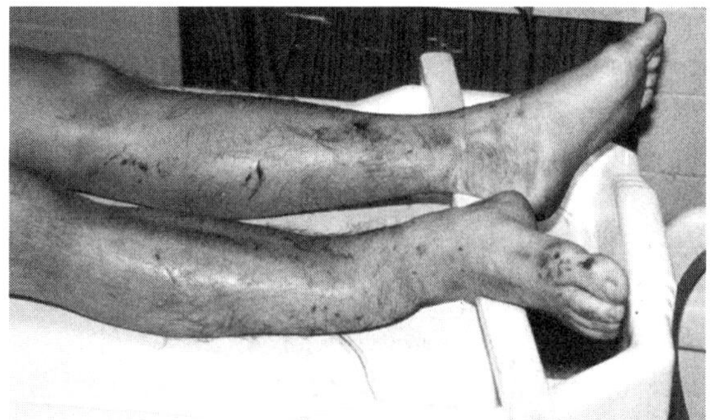

Figure 2-12 Obvious deformity is seen in a closed fracture.

The care of open fractures involves surgery so the bone ends can be exposed, debrided, cleaned, and realigned. Often pins, screws, and plates are used to set the fracture on its course for proper healing. Closed fractures are sometimes simpler to repair and do not always involve surgery or a hospital stay.

The physician manipulates and applies traction to the extremity to realign it and ensures it is properly aligned with a radiograph. Then a cast is applied to allow for several weeks of healing. Sometimes patients do not feel the pain from all of their injuries at the same time. In this situation, or if the patient is intoxicated, you may arrive on the scene to find a patient moving a fractured extremity excessively. Assign someone to hold the extremity still while you conduct your assessment. In this way, a closed fracture will not turn into an open fracture while you are on the scene! That will hopefully reduce the risks of long-term complications. A complicated fracture is considered to be a fracture that has a laceration to an artery that could cause exsanguination. Any fracture involving decreased or absent distal pulse, motor function, or sensory function (PMS) is considered to be a complication associated with the fracture. Other complications of a fracture would include the injuries sustained from a crushing injury.

When a patient has a musculoskeletal injury, the associated injuries may involve hemorrhage, loss of tissue, contamination of the wound, instability, and an interruption of the blood vessels or nerves as well as potential long-term disability.

The principles of musculoskeletal injury management include the following key points:

- If a joint does not have a distal pulse, it is acceptable to gently realign the joint once to see if a pulse returns.
- Long bones should be gently straightened so they fit into a splint. Remember that splints are basically straight.
- Open fractures should be covered to minimize contamination.

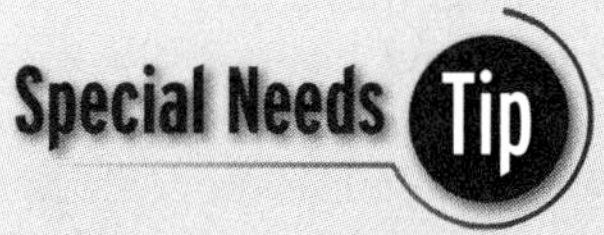

Special Needs Tip

Straightening the injured extremity in older patients may not be possible and may cause further injury. You may have to splint the limb in the position in which it is found.

- Your splint should immobilize the bone ends and the two adjacent joints.

Cold packs are useful to reduce the swelling of a musculoskeletal injury and for the first 48 hours. Thereafter, when the initial swelling has subsided, heat can be helpful in improving the circulation in the injured area. Pain management is important and should not be an afterthought! Most EMS systems have traditionally used morphine sulfate which has its limitations in the patient who has a borderline BP. Some EMS systems also use fentanyl citrate [Sublimase] because it has a faster onset of effect and time to peak effect than morphine sulfate [Astramorph PF]. This makes it easier to titrate to effect than morphine sulfate [Astramorph PF] as well as less masking of the effects of any yet undiagnosed injuries or conditions.

Age-Associated Changes to Bones

The aging process has an impact on our bones. These changes are likely to increase the chances of fractures occurring. The bones become more porous and brittle as we age. The development of osteoporosis, which is a thinning of the density of the bones, leads to an increased frequency of fractures. This disease is more common in elderly women. The water content of the intervertebral disks decreases, which in turn makes the spine stiffer. This accounts, in part, to the decrease in the overall height of the patient. Arthritis is an inflammation of the joint and is a common ailment in the older patient. Many of these patients will be on medications specific to their condition (ie, rheumatoid arthritis, gout, or osteoarthritis) which are designed to relieve chronic pain and decrease the inflammation. Some examples would include: nonsteroidal anti-inflammatory drugs, methotrexate [Trexall], tramadol hydrochloride [Ultram], and allupurinol [Zyloprim]. (Tramadol hydrochloride tends to be used more in the management of chronic pain problems, especially as an adjunct to other pain medications and with more neuropathic pain problems.)

Osteoporosis is a disease that causes bones to lose density, become fragile, and break easily. It is a major health threat that can strike at any age and if not prevented or if left untreated can progress painlessly until a bone breaks. Any bone can be affected and the fractures of most concern include the spine, hip, and wrist. Not only do fractures cause pain, but serious fractures such as the hip and spine can cause permanent deformity and disability, loss of independence, and death.

There are two types of osteoporosis, primary and secondary. Primary osteoporosis is caused by age-related bone loss or the cause may be unknown. In secondary osteoporosis, bone loss occurs because of chronic disease, certain medication use, or certain lifestyle behaviors.

Osteoporosis begins with low bone density or osteopenia; however, osteopenia does not always lead to osteoporosis. Osteopenia can be caused by:

- Inadequate bone mass development during adolescence
- Medical conditions or treatments that affect bones
- Genetics

Causes of osteoporosis include those that cause osteopenia and more:

- Aging
- Decreased levels of estrogen and progesterone (post-menopause or removal of ovaries)
- Inadequate amounts of physical activity
- Diets that are deficient in calcium, vitamin D, and phosphorous (critical building blocks for bone)
- Medications that affect or interfere with calcium absorption (anticoagulants, cortisone, corticosteroids, thyroid supplements)
- Chronic diseases (diabetes, rheumatoid arthritis, hyperthyroidism)

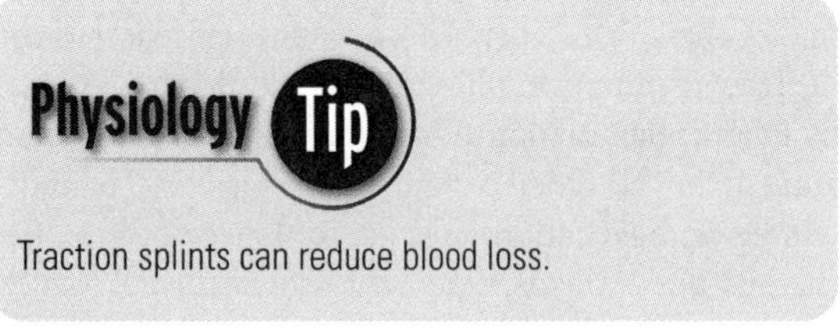

Traction splints can reduce blood loss.

Osteoporosis is not inevitable but it is frequently irreversible. Our bodies are designed to regulate the metabolic process of bone loss with proper nutrients, hormonal balance, and weight-bearing exercises.

When Traction Is Part of the Treatment

The muscles surrounding the femur are the strongest muscles in the body and can easily go into a spasm. Normally they are tethered to the proximal femur and proximal tibia. When fracture of the femur occurs, the muscles are allowed to contract and produce a significant, painful, and unrelenting spasm. When this happens, the fractured femur bone ends rub against each other and injure the surrounding soft tissue, nerves, and blood vessels. A traction splint is used to help with bone end realignment, minimize tissue damage, and reduce pain. In the prehospital setting, EMT-Basics and paramedics have been trained to apply the unipolar or Sager-type traction splint and the bipolar or Hare-type traction splint (**Figure 2-13**▼). The traction splint is designed for use with a midshaft femur fracture and not a knee or hip fracture.

Whenever applying the traction splint, always be sure to assess distal PMS both before and after applying the splint.

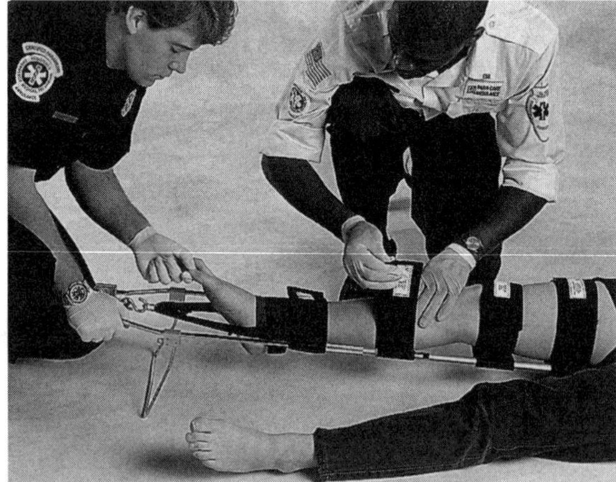

Figure 2-13 The Hare traction splint.

Case Study ANSWERS

Case Study I Full-Thickness Burns

Question 1: Why is this injury considered a significant MOI?

Answer 1: It is a serious burn that involves a large amount of body surface area as well as a potential airway burn.

Question 2: What is the significance of the hoarse and raspy sounding voice?

Answer 2: When the airway is swollen and potentially burned from inhaling super-heated gasses, the patient's voice will sound raspy and hoarse and the tidal volume may be lower than normal.

Question 3: The first drug of choice for this patient was oxygen. Why?

Answer 3: Burn patients go into shock and with the resultant poor perfusion to the tissues they become hypoxic at the cellular level. Early administration of high concentration supplemental oxygen is helpful in improving the oxygenation at the cellular level.

Question 4: Would a medication for pain relief be appropriate to administer?

Answer 4: Patients in severe pain expend too much energy that could be better utilized in their fight to live or compensate for their condition or begin the healing process. It is also inhumane to allow patients to continue to be in extreme pain if the means exist to manage that pain. In the case of a child, it may be prudent to consult with medical control to ensure correct dosing.

Question 5: How might an end-stage COPD patient, who you suspect is on hypoxic drive, alter your oxygen administration?

Answer 5: A COPD patient (eg, emphysema, chronic bronchitis, black lung, or other terminal stage lung disorder) retains CO_2 in their lower airways. The primary impetus for normal patients to breathe is a high CO_2 level in the arterial blood. With chronic CO_2 retention, a secondary mechanism is sometimes employed, called hypoxic drive. This occurs when lowered arterial oxygen levels supply the impetus to breathe. That is why you need to use high concentrations of oxygen with caution in the patient with advanced COPD as they are likely to be on a hypoxic drive and higher concentrations of supplemental oxygen could cause them to have respiratory depression and ultimately stop breathing. The bottom line is that patients who need oxygen should get it. Patients whose respiratory drive is from low oxygen levels (ie, CO_2 retainers) may need ventilatory assistance with provision of supplemental oxygen.

Question 6: If the patient's respiratory effort becomes depressed after the administration of morphine, what action should you take and why?

Answer 6: If the patient who has been given morphine develops respiratory depression, it is best to improve their ventilation by assisting with a bag-mask, providing supplemental oxygen, and on rare occasions, administering naloxone hydrochloride [Narcan]. Remember the naloxone hydrochloride [Narcan] is antagonistic with the morphine sulfate [Astramorph PF] and will reverse the effect of the morphine sulfate. Also remember that if the negative effects of the morphine go away, so do the positive effects and the patient's pain will return. Since the half-life of morphine sulfate is longer than the half-life of the naloxone hydrochloride [Narcan], be aware that the effect of the naloxone hydrochloride [Narcan] could diminish and the patient may need additional doses. If this is the situation, it is not recommended that you intubate the patient right away or else you may end up with a respiratory depressed patient who, after receiving the naloxone hydrochloride [Narcan], suddenly wakes up intubated and fighting!

Question 7: If the patient had a sudden drop in blood pressure, what should you do?

Answer 7: Slow down or stop the morphine sulfate administration, place the patient in the Trendelenburg position, and increase the IV/IO fluid infusion rate.

Question 8: If the patient had rales, rhonchi, or crackles in both lungs (ie, pulmonary edema), what should you consider and are there any medications that may be useful?

Answer 8: Monitor the vital signs, consider administration of naloxone hydrochloride [Narcan], and sit the patient up. It may be necessary to assist ventilations. This child is not generally a patient whose pulmonary edema is improved by a drug such as furosemide [Lasix] since the pulmonary edema is most likely noncardiogenic and due to lower airway burns and resultant edema or narcotic overdose. Some EMS systems might also consider the use of either noninvasive or invasive ventilation (CPAP/BiPAP, ETT placement) in this situation. It is best to consult with medical control in the management of this child should this change occur.

Case Study ANSWERS

Case Study II Epidural Hematoma

Question 1: What is the significance of the location of the injury being on the side of the head?

Answer 1: When a patient is struck on the side of the head, it is likely that the thinnest bone in the skull, the temporal bone, has been injured. This bone contains the middle meningeal artery, which can easily be injured by a fracture or high force injury to the surrounding bone.

Question 2: Why is the assessment of the mental status so important to this patient?

Answer 2: Any patient who has a mechanism of injury that points to a potential traumatic brain injury needs to have frequent reassessments of the mental status since the earliest signs of intracerebral pressure increasing are subtle changes in the patient's mental status.

Question 3: Although Mike has been quiet, had he become suddenly violent and combative, what would be the most likely cause of this change in affect?

Answer 3: The head injury may have affected the frontal lobe as well as the temporal lobe. The patient who has hypoxemia can also become combative.

Question 4: Why is it important to be prepared for vomiting when treating a patient who was struck in the head?

Answer 4: All patients who have central nervous system insults (brain and spinal cord) are likely to vomit. Vomiting results in unacceptable elevations in ICP, and also poses the distinct threat of airway compromise, especially worrisome in a patient who has been immobilized for transport. In some cases, these patients will actually have projectile vomiting. Be prepared!

Question 5: How would you define and manage hypoxia and hypotension in the field?

Answer 5: Frank hypoxia is a pulse oximetry reading of below 90%, whereas relative hypoxia includes oximetry of less than 95% while breathing supplemental oxygen. Hypotension is a systolic blood pressure of below 90 mm Hg in an adult patient. Follow your local protocols in the treatment of fluid therapy as well as high concentration oxygen administration.

Question 6: Can a head-injured patient have hypotension and what would be examples of hypotension for children in the field?

Answer 6: Yes, a head-injured patient can have hypotension. Systemic blood pressure increases as a physiologic response to increased ICP, as the brain attempts to maintain adequate cerebral perfusion pressure in the presence of intracranial injury, so as the pressure in the head goes up so does the BP. When herniation has occurred, it is not uncommon to see hypotension as the brain is no longer able to satisfactorily autoregulate itself via normal hemodynamic mechanisms. However, injuries do not only occur by themselves and it is common for the patient to sustain multiple injuries from a fall, collision, assault, or other mechanism of injury. If the patient sustains an injury to cause severe internal or external bleeding in addition to the head trauma, they may also become hypotensive as shock develops and the body is no longer able to compensate for the blood loss. Hypotension for an adult as well as a child from 13 to 16 years old is <90 mm Hg systolic, for an infant 0 to 1 year of age is <65 mm Hg systolic, for a child between 2 to 5 years old is <75 mm Hg systolic, and for a child between 6 to 12 years old is <80 mm Hg systolic.

Question 7: Why is it so important that the ED be informed as early as possible of your arrival and the patient's condition?

Answer 7: The patient is bleeding from an artery so the hematoma is rapidly developing. This collection of blood shifts the brain downward and may herniate the tentorium or other membranes within the head. You need to give the hospital as much time as possible to muster their resources and staff so they can be ready to manage this patient immediately upon your arrival.

Question 8: What do you expect is likely to be done to treat this patient?

Answer 8: This patient will get further assessment, a CT scan to confirm the epidural hematoma, and then rapid transport to the awaiting neurosurgeon in the OR. The hematoma needs to be evacuated and the bleeding controlled as soon as possible.

Case Study ANSWERS

Case Study III Spinal Cord Injury

Question 1: Why are spinal cord injuries so devastating?

Answer 1: Compressed nerve tissue may recover most of its function. However, severed or degenerated nerves cannot be regenerated and the loss of function is permanent.

Question 2: What single factor in the prehospital setting can make the most difference in the patient's prognosis?

Answer 2: Proper handling of the patient with a suspected or actual SCI can prevent further injury. The highest risk of secondary injury occurs immediately after the primary injury when the patient moves or untrained helpers attempt to move the patient without stabilizing the spine.

Question 3: At what level of the cervical spine do you estimate the primary injury has occurred?

Answer 3: Jim has no sense of touch below the clavicle so you can estimate the injury is between C5 and C6.

Question 4: What is the body's initial response to a spinal cord injury?

Answer 4: Immediately following the primary injury the spinal cord swells to fill the entire cavity of the spinal canal at the level of injury cutting off blood flow, which also cuts off oxygen to the spinal cord tissue.

Question 5: Why is methylprednisolone sodium succinate [Solu-Medrol] not administered in the prehospital setting for the ASCI patient?

Answer 5: High dose corticosteroid therapy is not without risk. There are many problems associated with the use of high dose steroids including: increased incidence of sepsis, pneumonia, hyperglycemia, and gastrointestinal complications. Its potential benefit is so far unproven.

Question 6: What changes in vital signs should you be alert for with severe ASCI?

Answer 6: Injury to the spinal cord at or above C3, C4, and C5 levels, which supply the phrenic nerves leading to the diaphragm, can stop breathing. The patient will need immediate ventilatory support. When injuries are at the C5 level and below, diaphragm function is preserved, but breathing tends to be rapid and shallow and people have trouble coughing and clearing secretions from their lungs because of loss of innervation to the thoracic and intercostal muscles and subsequent weakness of those muscles. Loss of sympathetic nerve tone and thermoregulation can produce massive vasodilation that can lead to shock with bradycardia and skin that is pink, warm, and dry.

Question 7: What two factors may be contributing to the change in lung sounds?

Answer 7: It is highly likely that Jim swallowed or aspirated water in the pool. This could be the cause of the rapid change in lung sounds. Also, patients with injuries at the level of C5 and below tend to have respirations that are rapid and shallow. As this injury progresses, Jim's risk of developing pneumonia will increase. Even though his diaphragm is functioning, he will have problems coughing and clearing secretions from his lungs because of weak thoracic muscles.

Question 8: Why does Jim try to move his head even though it could make the injury worse?

Answer 8: There are a number of reasons why Jim is attempting to move. He is emotionally overwhelmed, distraught, and is experiencing many emotions at the thought of being paralyzed for life. His nervous system is in shock. The only things he has physical control over right now are the ability to speak and move his head.

Case Study ANSWERS

Case Study IV Musculoskeletal Injury

Question 1: What type of joint is the knee?

Answer 1: The knee is a hinge joint like the elbow joint.

Question 2: Why is the knee easily injured when it is forced laterally?

Answer 2: There is only a small amount of range of motion laterally in the knee joint. If overstretched laterally or medially, the joint literally tears apart. The knee is a very important joint that is well supported by a series of ligaments holding bones of the distal femur to the bones of the proximal tibia and fibula. Certain activities, such as sports like skiing, soccer, football, racquetball, or squash can pin the leg while the weight of the body is still moving laterally. This will stretch or tear the ligaments, thus requiring surgical repair.

Question 3: Can a patient with a closed fracture be in shock and likely require fluid resuscitation and analgesia?

Answer 3: Yes, definitely! Some patients can go into shock from the pain of the injury. Bones are living structures with a blood supply and when injured they bleed. In a typical uncomplicated fracture (no artery or vein involvement), it is not uncommon for the following fractures to bleed the following volumes over the first 2 hours:

Fracture	Typical Blood Loss in First 2 hours
Pelvic	1,500 to 3,000 mL
Femur	1,000 to 1,500 mL
Humerus, Tibia, Fibula	250 to 500 mL
Ankle or Elbow Joints	250 to 500 mL
Radius, Ulna	150 to 250 mL

With all this blood loss in mind, it is easy to see that patients who break multiple bones can easily lose a considerable amount of blood and be in either the compensated or the decompensated phases of shock.

Question 4: Which comes first, the pain relief or the splinting of a painful long bone or joint injury?

Answer 4: As is often the case in medicine, there is no clear answer on this! Clearly analgesia, such as morphine sulfate, can be helpful in preparing the patient for the small amount of movement it will take to position them securely in a splint and the often painful bumpy ride to the hospital in the back of an ambulance. On the other hand, an assessment of the patient's clinical condition is important to determine their baseline vital signs and other associated symptoms (ie, nausea) as well as the cardiovascular status. The administration of an analgesic will have an effect on their vitals and in some instances, such as hypotension, will be contraindicated. Therefore, in a patient with stable vital signs it would be reasonable to administer analgesia prior to splinting the injury, otherwise consider the administration of analgesia en route to the ED. Oftentimes, the promise that the ED will medicate the patient turns into a considerable delay in the administration of analgesia since the patient may not be the highest priority when arriving at a busy ED.

Question 5: What other pain medication could be considered if the patient has an allergy to morphine sulfate?

Answer 5: Some EMS systems are using fentanyl citrate [Sublimase] which is a narcotic pain reliever. It can be given IM or slow IV injection. Fentanyl citrate [Sublimase] has a faster onset of effect and time to peak effect than morphine sulfate, making it easier and safer to titrate to effect than morphine sulfate. There is also a shorter duration of effect with fentanyl citrate [Sublimase] than morphine sulfate, as well as less masking of undiagnosed conditions. (for more information see Chapter 10).

Question 6: If the patient starts to complain of nausea, should an antiemetic be considered?

Answer 6: Yes, definitely. Actually a side effect of both morphine sulfate [Astramorph] and fentanyl citrate [Sublimase] is nausea so the antiemetic can be helpful. There are a number of drugs to consider in the management of nausea and vomiting. Commonly used medications include promethazine hydrochloride [Phenergan], metoclopramide hydrochloride [Reglan], prochlorperazine [Compazine], or ondansetron hydrochloride [Zofran].

Question 7: Why is it helpful to have a concerned conversation with the patient?

Answer 7: It calms the patient down, relieves their pain, may provide further insight into the nature of their problem, and shows that you are a caring provider!

Question 8: Will Shelly be back this season and if asked, how should you answer that question?

Answer 8: If she has actually stretched or torn a ligament she may need surgery. Also, there is always the possibility that she may have fractured the bone very close to the joint. Do not make any promises you cannot keep! It is best to tell her more will be known once the physician in the ED examines her and additional ED and outpatient testing (radiographs, MRI, arthroscopy) is performed.

Medication Review

Benzocaine Spray (Hurricane)

Indications Used as a lubricant and topical anesthetic to facilitate passage of diagnostic and treatment devices. Suppresses the pharyngeal and tracheal gag reflex.

Contraindications Patients with a known hypersensitivity to benzocaine.

Dosage and administration Adult: 0.5–1.0-second spray, repeat as needed. Pediatric: 0.25–0.5-second spray, repeat as needed.

Dexamethasone Sodium Phosphate (Decadron, Hexadrol)

Indications Anaphylaxis, asthma, croup.

Contraindications Hypersensitivity to product, systemic sepsis, bacterial infection.

Dosage and administration Adult: 10–100 mg IV (1 mg/kg slow IV bolus) (considerable variance through medical control). Pediatric: 0.25–1.0 mg/kg/dose IV, IO, IM.

Diazepam (Valium)

Indications Acute anxiety states, acute alcohol withdrawal (delirium tremens), muscle relaxant, seizure activity, agitation. Analgesia for medical procedures (fracture reduction, cardioversion).

Contraindications Hypersensitivity, glaucoma, coma, shock, substance abuse, head injury.

Dosage and administration Seizure activity: Adult: 5–10 mg IV every 10–15 minutes as needed (5 mg over 5 min) (maximum dose, 30 mg). Seizure activity: Pediatric: 0.2–0.5 mg slowly every 2–5 minutes up to 5 mg (maximum dose, 10 mg/kg). Rectal diazepam: 0.5 mg/kg via rectal catheter and flush with 2–3 mL air after administration. Sedation for cardioversion: 5–15 mg IV over 5–10 minutes prior to cardioversion.

Flumazenil (Romazicon)

Indications Reversal of respiratory depression and sedative effects from pure benzodiazepine overdose.

Contraindications Hypersensitivity, tricyclic antidepressant overdose, seizure-prone patients, coma of unknown etiology.

Dosage and administration Adult: First dose: 0.2 mg IV/IO over 15 seconds. Second dose: 0.3 mg IV/IO over 30 seconds. If no response, give third dose. Third dose: 0.5 mg IV/IO over 30 seconds. If no response, repeat once every minute until adequate response or a total of 3 mg is given. Pediatric: Not recommended.

Hydrocortisone Sodium Succinate (Solu-Cortef)

Indications Shock due to acute adrenocortical insufficiency.

Contraindications None if given as single dose.

Dosage and administration Adult: 4 mg/kg slow IV bolus. Pediatric: 0.16–1.0 mg/kg slow IV bolus.

Hydroxyzine Hydrochloride (Atarax, Vistaril)

Indications To potentiate the effects of analgesics; to control nausea and vomiting, anxiety reactions, and motion sickness; preoperative and postoperative sedation.

Contraindications Hypersensitivity.

Dosage and administration Adult: 25–100 mg IM. Pediatric: 0.5–1.0 mg/kg/dose IM.

Ketorolac Tromethamine (Toradol IM)

Indications Short-term management of moderate to severe pain.

Contraindications Allergy to salicylates or other NSAIDs; patients with history of asthma; bleeding disorders, especially gastrointestinal (GI) related (peptic ulcer disease); renal failure.

Dosage and administration Adult: 30–60 mg IM. Pediatric: Not recommended.

Medication Review

Lorazepam (Ativan)

Indications Initial control of status epilepticus or severe recurrent seizures, severe anxiety, sedation.

Contraindications Acute narrow-angle glaucoma. Coma, shock, or suspected drug abuse.

Dosage and administration Note: When given IV or IO, must dilute with equal volume of sterile water or sterile saline; When given IM, lorazepam is not to be diluted. Adult: 2–4 mg slow IV at 2 mg/min or IM; may repeat in 15–20 minutes to maximum dose of 8 mg. For sedation: 0.05 mg/kg up to 4 mg IM. Pediatric: 0.05–0.20 mg/kg slow IV, IO slowly over 2 minutes or IM; may repeat in 15–20 minutes to maximum dose of 0.2 mg/kg.

Meperidine Hydrochloride (Demerol)

Indications Analgesia for moderate to severe pain.

Contraindications Hypersensitivity to narcotic agents, diarrhea caused by poisoning, patients taking MAOIs, during labor or delivery of a premature infant, undiagnosed abdominal pain or head injury.

Dosage and administration Adult: 50–100 mg IM, SC or 25–50 mg slow IV. Pediatric: 1–2 mg/kg/dose IV, IO, IM, SC.

Methylprednisolone Sodium Succinate (Solu-Medrol)

Indications Acute spinal cord trauma, anaphylaxis, bronchodilator for unresponsive asthma.

Contraindications Premature infants, systemic fungal infections; use with caution in patients with gastrointestinal bleeding, sepsis, local infection.

Dosage and administration Adult: Acute spinal cord injury: 30 mg/kg IV over 30 minutes followed by infusion: 5.4 mg/kg/h. Asthma, COPD: 1–2 mg/kg IV. Pediatric: Acute spinal cord trauma: 30 mg/kg IV over 30 minutes; Infusion: 5.4 mg/kg/h. Asthma: 1–2 mg/kg/dose IV.

Midazolam (Versed)

Indications Sedation, anxiolytic prior to endotracheal or nasotracheal intubation; administer for conscious sedation.

Contraindications Glaucoma, shock, coma, alcohol intoxication, overdose, depressed vital signs, concomitant use with other CNS depressants, barbiturates, alcohol, narcotics.

Dosage and administration Adult: 2.0–2.5 mg slow IV over 2–3 minutes; may be repeated to total maximum: 0.1 mg/kg. Pediatric: Not recommended.

Morphine Sulfate (Astramorph/PF and others)

Indications Severe CHF, pulmonary edema, chest pain associated with acute MI, analgesia for moderate to severe acute and chronic pain (use with caution).

Contraindications Head injury, exacerbated COPD, depressed respiratory drive, hypotension, undiagnosed abdominal pain, decreased level of consciousness, suspected hypovolemia, patients who have taken MAOIs within the past 14 days.

Dosage and administration Adult: Initial dose: 2–4 mg IV (over 1–5 minutes) every 5–30 minutes. Repeat dose: 2–8 mg at 5- to 15-minute intervals. Pediatric: 0.1–0.2 mg/kg per dose via IV, IO, IM, or SC; maximum dose of 5 mg.

Nalbuphine (Nubain)

Indications Chest pain associated with acute MI; moderate to severe acute pain; pulmonary edema, with or without associated chest pain (morphine remains first line).

Contraindications Head injury or undiagnosed abdominal pain, diarrhea caused by poisoning, hypovolemia, hypotension.

Dosage and administration Adult: 2–5 mg slow IV; may repeat 2-mg doses as needed to maximum dose of 10 mg. Pediatric: Not recommended.

Medication Review

Naloxone Hydrochloride (Narcan)

Indications Opiate overdose, coma; complete or partial reversal of CNS and respiratory depression induced by opioids; decreased level of consciousness; coma of unknown origin; narcotic agonist for the following: morphine, heroin, hydromorphone (Dilaudid), methadone, meperidine (Demerol), paregoric, fentanyl citrate (Sublimase), oxycodone (Percodan), codeine, propoxyphene (Darvon); narcotic agonist and antagonist for the following: Butorphanol (Stadol), pentazocine (Talwin), nalbuphine (Nubain).

Contraindications Use with caution in narcotic-dependent patients; use with caution in neonates of narcotic-addicted mothers.

Dosage and administration Adult: 0.4–2.0 mg IV, IM, SC, or ET (diluted); minimum recommended dose, 0.4 mg; repeat at 5-minute intervals to a maximum dose of 10 mg (medical control may request higher amounts). Infusion: 2 mg in 500 mL of D_5W (4 µg/mL), infuse at 0.4 mg/h (100 mL/h). Pediatric: 0.1 mg/kg/dose IV, IM, SC, ET (diluted); maximum dose of 0.8 mg; if no response in 10 minutes, administer an additional 0.1 mg/kg/dose.

Nitrous Oxide: Oxygen (50:50) (Nitronox)

Indications Moderate to severe pain, anxiety, apprehension.

Contraindications Impaired level of consciousness, head injury, inability to comply with instructions; decompression sickness (nitrogen narcosis, air embolism, air transport); undiagnosed abdominal pain or marked distention, bowel obstruction; hypotension, shock, COPD (with history/suspicion of carbon dioxide retention); cyanosis; chest trauma with pneumothorax.

Dosage and administration Adult: (Note: Invert cylinder several times before use.) Instruct the patient to inhale deeply through demand valve and mask or mouthpiece. Pediatric: Same as adult.

Ondansetron Hydrochloride (Zofran)

Indications For the prevention or control of nausea or vomiting. Also used in the hospital setting for patients undergoing chemotherapy or surgical procedures.

Contraindications Known allergy to this medicine or other 5-HT3 receptor antagonists.

Dosage and administration Adult: 4 mg IV or IM (may repeat in 10 minutes). Pediatric: 0.1 mg/kg IV or IM.

Oxygen

Indications Confirmed or expected hypoxemia, ischemic chest pain, respiratory insufficiency, prophylactically during air transport, confirmed or suspected carbon monoxide poisoning, all other causes of decreased tissue oxygenation, decreased level of consciousness.

Contraindications Certain patients with COPD or emphysema who will not tolerate oxygen concentrations over 35%, hyperventilation. Oxygen should never be withheld from a patient who needs it, however. Be prepared to assist with ventilations in a patient with COPD who requires high concentrations, as apnea may result.

Dosage and administration Adult: Cardiac arrest and carbon monoxide poisoning: 100%. Hypoxemia: 10–15 L/min via nonrebreathing mask. COPD: 1–6 L/min via nasal cannula or 28%–35% Venturi mask. Be prepared to provide ventilatory support if higher concentrations of oxygen needed. Pediatric: Same as for adult with exception of premature infant.

Pancuronium Bromide (Pavulon)

Indications Induction or maintenance of paralysis after intubation to assist ventilations.

Contraindications Hypersensitivity, inability to control airway and support ventilations with oxygen and positive pressure, neuromuscular disease (myasthenia gravis), hepatic or renal failure.

Dosage and administration Adult: 0.1 mg/kg slow IV; repeat every 30–60 minutes as needed. Pediatric: 0.1 mg/kg slow IV, IO.

Medication Review

Phenobarbital (Luminal)

Indications Prevention and treatment of seizure activity; prophylaxis for febrile seizures; anxiety, apprehension; status epilepticus.

Contraindications Patients with porphyria, hypersensitivity, severe liver or respiratory diseases.

Dosage and administration Adult: 100–250 mg slow IV, or IM; may repeat as needed in 20–30 minutes. Pediatric: 10–20 mg/kg IV, IO (less than 1 mg/kg/min) or IM; repeat as needed in 20–30 minutes.

Phenytoin (Dilantin)

Indications Prophylaxis and treatment of major motor seizures, digitalis-induced arrhythmias.

Contraindications Hypersensitivity, bradycardia, second- and third-degree heart block.

Dosage and administration Adult: Seizures: 10–20 mg/kg slow IV, not to exceed 1 g or rate of 50 mg/min). Arrhythmias: 50–100 mg (diluted) slow IV every 5–15 min as needed; maximum, 1 g. Pediatric: Seizures: 10–20 mg/kg slow IV (1–3 mg/kg/min). Arrhythmias: 5 mg/kg slow IV; maximum, 1 g.

Promethazine Hydrochloride (Phenergan)

Indications Nausea, vomiting, motion sickness; sedation for patients in labor; potentiation of analgesic effects of narcotics.

Contraindications Hypersensitivity, coma, CNS-depressed patients from alcohol, barbiturates, narcotics, Reye's syndrome.

Dosage and administration Adult: 12.5–25 mg IV, deep IM, PO, rectally. Pediatric: (greater than 2 years old) 0.25–0.5 mg/kg dose IM.

Succinylcholine Chloride (Anectine, Quelicin)

Indications To facilitate intubation, to terminate laryngospasm, to promote muscle relaxation, to facilitate electroconvulsive shock therapy.

Contraindications Acute narrow angle glaucoma, penetrating eye injuries, inability to control airway or support ventilations with oxygen and positive pressure.

Dosage and administration Adult: 1–2 mg/kg rapid IV; repeat once if needed. Pediatric: 1–1.5 mg/kg dose rapid IV, IO; repeat once if needed.

Tetracaine HCL (ophthalmic) (Pontocaine, Supracaine)

Indications Cataract extraction, tonometry, gonioscopy, removal of foreign objects, corneal suture removal, glaucoma surgery. Also used in conjunction with the Morgan Lens for flushing the eyes.

Contraindications Known allergy to this medicine or hypersensitivity PABA (para-aminobenzoic acid).

Dosage and administration Adult and pediatric: 1 to 2 drops before the procedure.

Vecuronium Bromide (Norcuron)

Indications To facilitate intubation, to terminate laryngospasm, to promote muscle relaxation, to facilitate electroconvulsive shock therapy.

Contraindications Acute narrow angle glaucoma, penetrating eye injuries, inability to control airway or support ventilations with oxygen and positive pressure, newborns, myasthenia gravis, hepatic or renal failure.

Dosage and administration Adult: 0.1 mg/kg IV push; maintenance dose within 25–40 minutes: 0.01–0.05 mg/kg IV push. Pediatric: 0.1 mg/kg IV, IO; maintenance dose within 20–35 minutes: 0.01–0.05 mg/kg IV push.

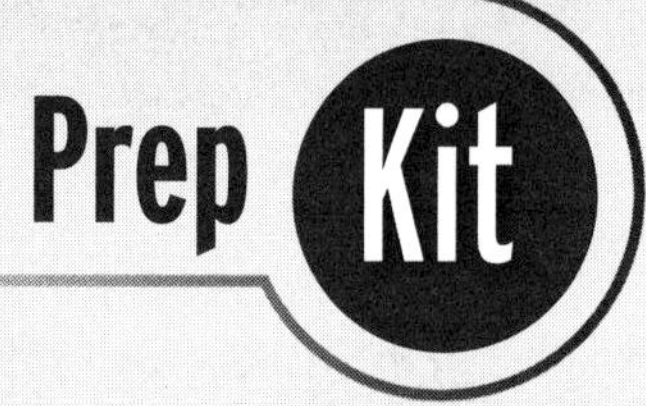

Chapter Summary

- Pharmacologic agents have a limited role for trauma patients.
- Narcotic and nonnarcotic analgesics are the essential component of the appropriate and compassionate treatment of any trauma patient.
- The general management of all critical burns should include the drug oxygen.
- Management for the five categories of burns (thermal, inhalation, chemical, electrical, and radiation) involves care of the airway, ventilation, circulation, pharmacologic and nonpharmacologic strategies, as well as transport, psychological support or communication strategies, and other management such as local protocols.
- Burn victims tend to require an IV for fluid resuscitation and for the administration of an analgesic.
- The prehospital management of the head-injured patient involves assessment and management of the ABCs, cervical spine immobilization, supplemental oxygen, ventilatory assistance, and rapid transport to the trauma center.
- Prehospital treatment of spinal cord injuries includes management of the ABC's, proper immobilization, and immediate transport to an appropriate facility.
- Treating pain is necessary in almost two thirds of patients wth spinal cord injury.
- Prehospital management of musculoskeletal injuries includes management of the ABC's, consideration of an analgesic, and splinting.
- Individuals with age-associated changes in bones are treated with medications specific to their condition (ie, rheumatoid arthritis, gout, or osteoarthritis) which are designed to relieve chronic pain and decrease the inflammation.

Vital Vocabulary

Antiemetic An agent that prevents or arrests vomiting.

Benzodiazepines Any medications of a group of psychotropic agents used as antianxiety, muscle relaxants, sedatives, and hypnotics.

Parkland formula The calculation that is used to determine the fluid volume to be administered to the burn patient in the first day of care. It was developed in the Parkland Burn Center in Dallas, Texas.

Phenothiazines Any of the various phenothiazine derivatives that are used as tranquilizing agents and also used in the treatment of schizophrenia.

Titrate To administer a medication in small doses up to the point where the desired effect occurs (ie, to a normal pulse rate or blood pressure from bradycardia or hypotension).

Traumatic brain injury (TBI) An injury caused by a blow or jolt to the head or penetrating head injury that disrupts the normal function of the brain. The severity of a TBI can range from mild (ie, brief change in mental status) to a severe (ie, extended period of unconsciousness or amnesia post-injury).

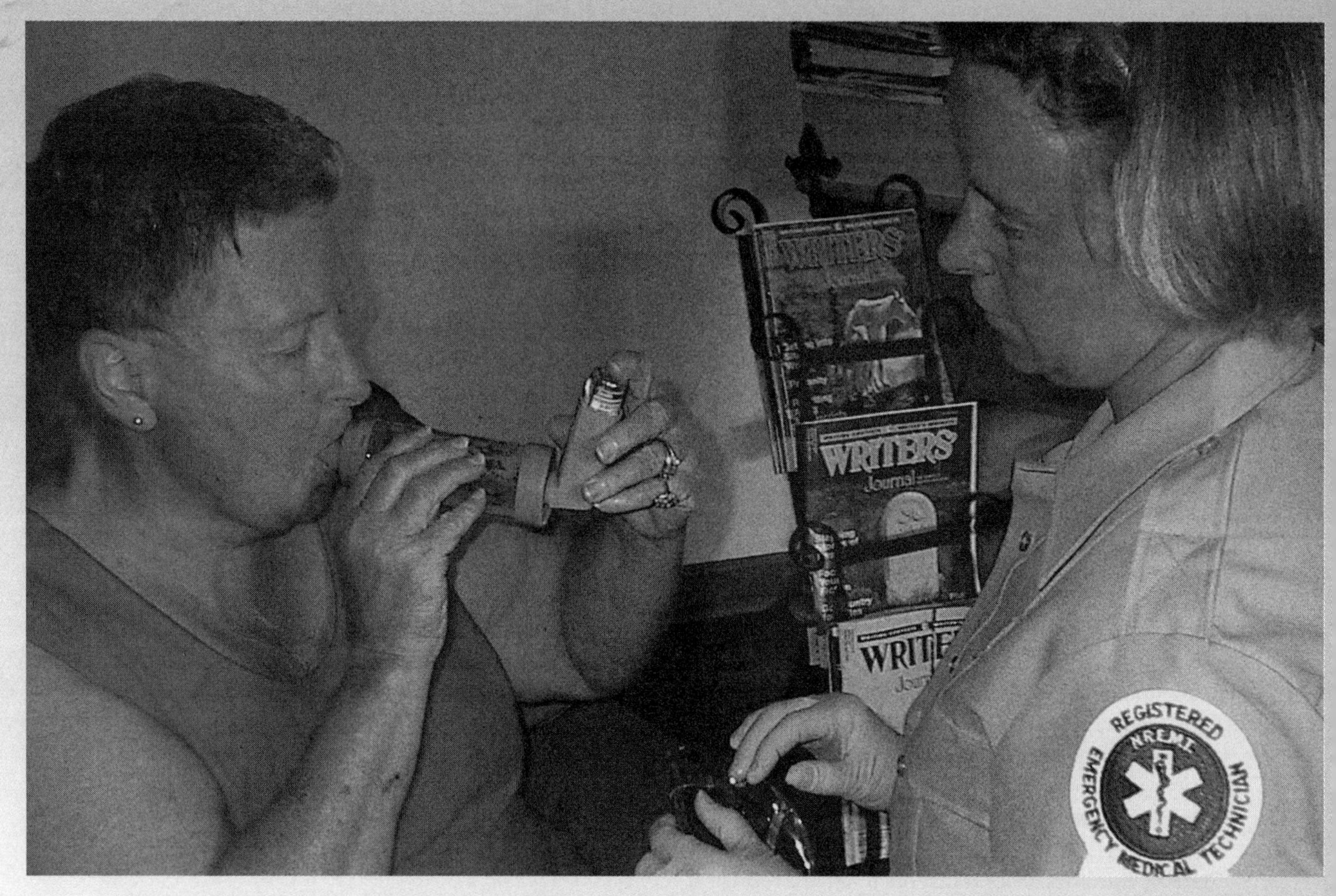
WRITERS
WRITERS
Journal
WRITERS
REGISTERED
NREMT
EMERGENCY MEDICAL TECHNICIAN

Pulmonary and Respiratory Emergencies

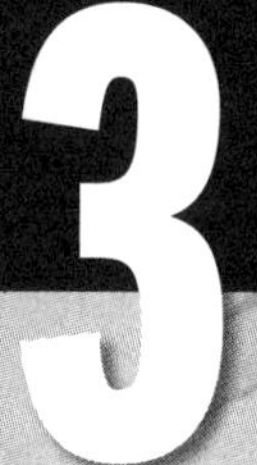

Objectives

Cognitive

5-1.7 Review the pharmacological preparations that paramedics use for management of respiratory diseases and conditions. (pages 82–83)

5-1.8 Review the pharmacological preparations used in managing patients with respiratory diseases that may be prescribed by physicians. (pages 82–83)

Affective

None

Psychomotor

None

Additional Objectives

3-1 Discuss the following medications used in the prehospital setting for respiratory patients: oxygen, albuterol [Proventil, Ventolin], ipratropium bromide [Atrovent], dexamethasone sodium phosphate [Decadron Phosphate], epinephrine hydrochloride [Adrenalin Chloride] 1:1000, morphine sulfate [Astramorph/PF]—for acute pulmonary edema, racemic epinephrine inhalant, [Vaponefrin, Micronefrin], terbutaline sulfate [Brethine, Bricanyl], methylprednisolone sodium succinate [Solu-Medrol], furosemide [Lasix], magnesium sulfate. (pages 82–113)

3-2 Discuss the pathophysiology, assessment findings, and paramedic field management for the following respiratory diseases and conditions:

a. Asthma (pages 84–93)
b. Acute pulmonary edema (pages 98, 100–104)
c. Pulmonary embolism (pages 94–98)

Medications Often Prescribed to Manage Respiratory Conditions

In most EMS systems the complaint of "difficulty breathing" is very common. This is due in part to the increasing age of the population as well as the large number of chronic respiratory conditions and other acute medical problems that primarily present with shortness of breath. Obstruction to the airway is often described as being above the larynx or upper airway or below the larynx or lower airway. Generally, patients who have a partial obstruction of the upper airway describe difficulty in getting air into their lungs. Those with lower airway obstruction describe difficulty getting the air out of their chest. In fact, as thick secretions and inflammation develop in the lungs and smaller airways, accompanied by bronchoconstriction, patients often retain carbon dioxide (CO_2). A patient experiencing bronchoconstriction often describes feeling chest tightness and having to work in order to blow the air out of their lungs. It would be as if you were given a cocktail straw to exhale through, forced to lie on your back, and have a heavy person sit on your chest!

To manage obstructive airway disease or "reactive airways," physicians often prescribe a powerful anti-inflammatory drug to break up the inflammation obstructing the lower airways. A **bronchodilator** works directly on the smooth muscle of the bronchioles to dilate them which in turn decreases airway resistance and makes it easier for the patient to breathe. A **vasodilator** medication acts on the smooth muscles of the arterioles and veins. There are many patients who have grown accustomed to living their life with shortness of breath or **dyspnea**. They usually do not call the ambulance because they have a chronic disease. Their call is often made because they have an acute exacerbation of their disease often brought on by an upper respiratory infection or pneumonia. This new development, on top of their preexisting condition, pushes their respiratory distress over the edge. **Chronic obstructive pulmonary disease (COPD)** can also be exacerbated by stress, exercise, tobacco smoke, allergens, drugs, heart failure, and other occupational hazards.

Special Needs Tip

Changes of bones and teeth in the elderly can alter the shape of the face and mouth, making an airway harder to maintain when attempting to ventilate these patients.

From a pathophysiological perspective, respiratory abnormalities commonly affect ventilation, diffusion, or perfusion (**Table 3-1 ▸**). When ventilation is affected, this impacts the ability to oxygenate and exhale or remove carbon dioxide. When diffusion is affected, the impact is on the movement of oxygen and carbon dioxide across the alveolar membranes in the lungs. Perfusion-related abnormalities impact the pumping of blood from the heart to the body's tissues.

Physicians prescribe a number of medications for the treatment of obstructive or reactive airway conditions. These fall into a number of categories such as: bronchodilators, **sympathomimetics**, **parasympatholytics**, **steroids**, and **leukotriene blockers** (**Table 3-2 ▸**). Sympathomimetics are administered to stimulate the sympathetic nervous system and parasympatholytics work on the parasympathetic division of the autonomic nervous system. Steroids and leukotriene blockers are administered to stop the inflammation process that is obstructing the lower airways. A common leukotriene blocker is montelukast [Singulair] that is taken as a dry powder inhaler by the patient.

Some patients that you manage in the field may be taking **antitussives**, which are medications designed to stop coughing. When taken in excess, the medication can have a sedative effect as well as reduce respiratory effort and cause excessive plugs in the bronchioles. In addition, over-the-counter **expectorants**, or medications that thin out secretions so they can be coughed up, are commonly taken by respiratory patients. These medications can be problematic because they often contain **antihistamines**, which are not always appropriate when the patient has increased secretions. **Methylxanthines**, such as aminophylline or theophylline, were previously the mainstay of prehospital medications for the asthmatic or COPD patient. These medications are rarely used today and have been replaced with more modern preparations that have less adverse cardiac effects on the patient. In addition to fast-acting bronchodilators, some patients may be on a slow-acting bronchodilator for its long-term benefits in improving the quality of their life. Examples would include: salmeterol [Serevent] and cromolyn [Intal, NasalCrom].

Respiratory Conditions Confronted by Paramedics in the Field

There are a number of specific respiratory conditions that you will be confronted with in the field. Some of these are best managed in the field as they can be potentially life-threatening. Your priority in all respiratory emergencies is to size-up the scene for your own safety and to complete an initial assessment of the patient. Respiratory complaints can be associated

Table 3-1 Pathophysiology of Respiratory Abnormalities

Commonly Affecting	Examples
Ventilation	Upper airway obstruction (ie, epiglottitis, foreign body airway obstruction (FBAO), tonsillitis, trauma)
Ventilation	Lower airway obstruction (ie, COPD, mucus accumulation, smooth muscle spasm, bronchospasm, airway edema, trauma)
Ventilation	Impairment of chest wall movement (ie, hemothorax, pneumothorax, pleural inflammation, neuromuscular diseases, multiple sclerosis, muscular dystrophy, trauma)
Ventilation	Problems with neurologic control of the CNS (ie, stroke, CNS depressant drugs)
Ventilation	Problems with neurologic control of the peripheral nervous system (ie, phrenic nerve dysfunction) or spinal nerve dysfunction (ie, trauma or neuromuscular disease)
Diffusion	Inadequate oxygen in the air
Diffusion	Alveolar pathology (ie, inhalation injuries, blebs from COPD, asbestosis)
Diffusion	Primary interstitial space problems (ie, elevations in hydrostatic pressure, pulmonary edema, pulmonary hypertension)
Diffusion	Secondary interstitial space problems (ie, abnormal permeability of pulmonary vessels, acute respiratory distress syndrome (ARDS), submersion, hypoxia, inhalation injuries)
Perfusion	Inadequate blood volume or hemoglobin levels (ie, anemia, hypovolemia)
Perfusion	Impaired circulation blood flow (ie, pneumothorax, pulmonary embolus, cardiac tamponade)
Perfusion	Chest wall injury from trauma

Table 3-2 Medications for Obstructive Lung Diseases

Category of Medication	Examples
Bronchodilators	albuterol [Proventil,Ventolin], terbutaline sulfate [Brethine], epinephrine [Adrenalin], racemic epinephrine [Micronefrin, Vaponefrin], magnesium sulfate, metaproterenol [Alupent], levalbuterol hydrochloride [Xopenex], aminophylline [Phyllocontin, Truphylline], theophylline [Quibron-T], xanthine bronchodilators, oxymetazoline nasal [Afrin, Afrin Nasal Sinus, Allerest 12 Hour Nasal Spray, Duramist Plus, Four-Way Nasal Spray, Genasal, Neo-Synephrine 12 Hour, Nostrilla, Oxyfrin, Oxymeta-12, Sinarest Nasal, Sinex Long-Acting]
Sympathomimetics	salbutamol (albuterol) [Airomir, Asthalin, Asmol, Buventol, Proventil, Salamol, Sultanol, Ventolin, Volmax], terbutaline sulfate [Brethine, Bricanyl], salmeterol xinafoate inhalation powder [Serevent, Diskus], epinephrine [Adrenalin]
Parasympatholytics	ipratropium bromide [Atrovent], tiotropium bromide [Spiriva]
Steroids	prednisone [Prednisone Intensol, Sterapred, Sterapred DS] [Liquid Pred, Deltasone], methylprednisolone sodium succinate [Solu-Medrol]
Leukotriene blockers	montelukast [Singulair], zafirlukast [Accolate], zileuton [Zyflo]

with toxins in the environment, most often high carbon monoxide levels that would be dangerous to you as well as the patient. Be sure that the environment is safe for the rescuer and if not, that appropriately trained personnel wearing proper breathing apparatus quickly move the patient to a safe place to allow assessment and management of their condition.

Conscious patients are often found in the tripod position to help decrease the work of breathing (**Figure 3-1** ▶). Respiratory patients with the most serious, often life-threatening conditions can be found with one or more of the following "respiratory red flags." They may have: an altered mental status, absent breath sounds, an audible stridor, one- or two-word dyspnea, exertional tachycardia (more than 130 beats/min), pallor and diaphoresis, the presence of retractions or use of accessory muscles of respiration, and grunting.

The following list should be a quick review of the commonly found respiratory conditions:

- Asthma—a recurring, *reversible* condition of lower airway airflow obstruction. The patient exhibits constriction of the terminal bronchioles characterized by wheezing, cough, and dyspnea.

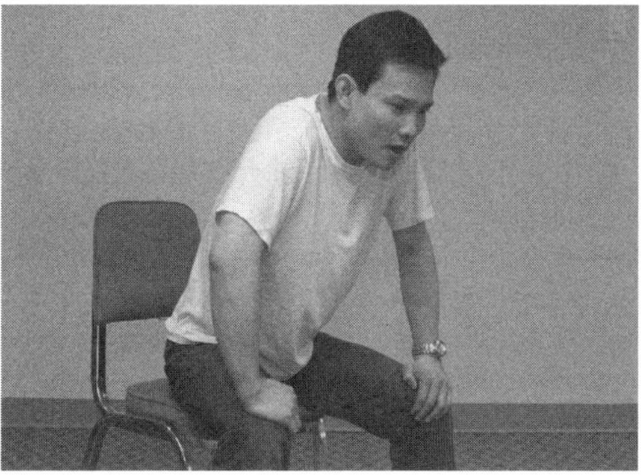

Figure 3-1 The tripod position (elbows out) allows for easier diaphragmatic movement.

Though wheezing is a common sign associated with asthma, it may be found in other respiratory processes as well.

Changes in weather, both temperature and humidity, frequently have an adverse affect on patients with asthma and other pulmonary diseases.

- Chronic Bronchitis—results from an overgrowth of the airway's mucous glands and an excess secretion of mucus causing a partial obstruction to the lower airways. The diagnosis is based on the patient having a productive cough for at least 3 months of the year for 2 or more consecutive years.
- Emphysema—results from a destruction of the alveolar walls leading to a decrease in the elastic recoil on expiration. This results in resistance in expiratory airflow, trapping air in the lungs and leading to poor air exchange.
- Pneumonia—an acute bacterial or viral inflammatory condition of the lungs characterized by dyspnea, cough, pleuritic chest pain, fever, and a variety of focally distributed adventitious breath sounds. Pleuritic chest pain is from the lining of the lungs and hurts more with movement of the chest wall as the patient breathes. Often found in association with COPD and can cause an acute exacerbation of underlying chronic lung disease.
- Pulmonary Edema—refers to the filling of the lungs with fluid. The fluid may be in the alveoli or the interstitial spaces or both, causing the patient to literally drown in his or her own fluids due to a decreasing ability to exchange gases across the alveolar membrane. This condition is not a disease but rather a result of other diseases such as chronic heart failure, a narcotic overdose, acute respiratory distress syndrome (ARDS), or altitude sickness.
- Pulmonary Thromboembolism—a pulmonary embolism (PE) is a blockage of a pulmonary artery by foreign matter such as a blood clot. The term thromboembolism describes the process of a peripheral venous clot formation followed by dislodgement and movement of the clot through the venous circulation, past the right side of the heart and lodging in the lung as an embolus.
- Neoplasms of the Lung—a neoplasm is a new growth, usually a tumor. Tumors are classified as benign or malignant (cancerous). Although these conditions are not managed in the field, their sequelae often are as they present with weakness, nausea, dyspnea, hemoptysis, as well as the debilitating symptoms associated with their therapy.
- Upper Respiratory Infections (URI)—(common cold) an acute, self-limiting infection of any part of the upper respiratory tract. A URI usually involves the patient's mouth, throat, and ears and is not generally managed in the field. Though occasionally caused by bacterial infection, many times URIs are related to a viral source. The presence of a URI often exacerbates underlying COPD or asthma.
- Spontaneous Pneumothorax—a sudden accumulation of air in the pleural space (ie, between the lung and chest wall) causing the lung on the involved side to collapse. May be due to a penetrating or closed injury or a bleb or weak spot on the outside of the lung that bursts (**Figure 3-2 ▸**).
- Hyperventilation Syndrome—an anxiety produced syndrome resulting in tachypnea without associated physiologic demand for the increased oxygen or removal of CO_2. It leads to a respiratory alkalosis by blowing off too much CO_2. Patients may develop symptoms such as paresthesias, carpopedal spasms, cramps, chest tightness, and increased anxiety. Considered a diagnosis of exclusion.

Asthma: A Major Health Problem

In the US, asthma is a disease that affects more than 17 million people, a third of whom are children. Asthma is the most common chronic disease in children accounting for considerable school absences. In 2002, 478,000 hospitalizations and 4,657 deaths were attributed to asthma. Although slightly more common in African Americans, asthma affects people of all races and ages. Costing the US economy nearly $13 billion each year, asthma is one of the most common reasons for ED visits and hospital stays. Approximately 5,000 patients die from asthma yearly.

Always be cautious with patients who have allergies when administering nebulized bronchodilators, a drug that dilates, or expands, the size of the lumina of the air passages of the lungs by relaxing the muscular walls. The chemicals known as "sulfites" are some-

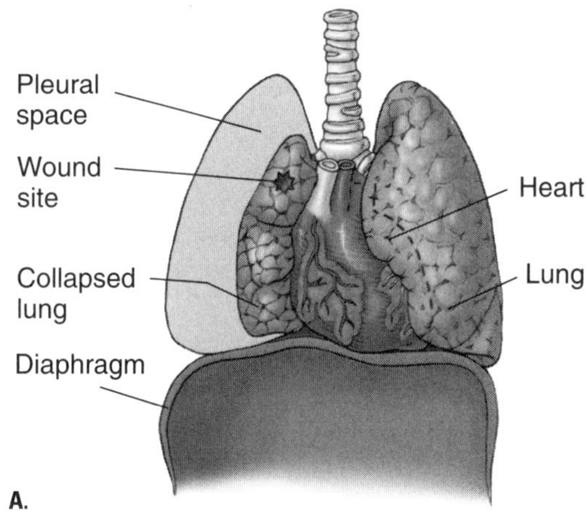

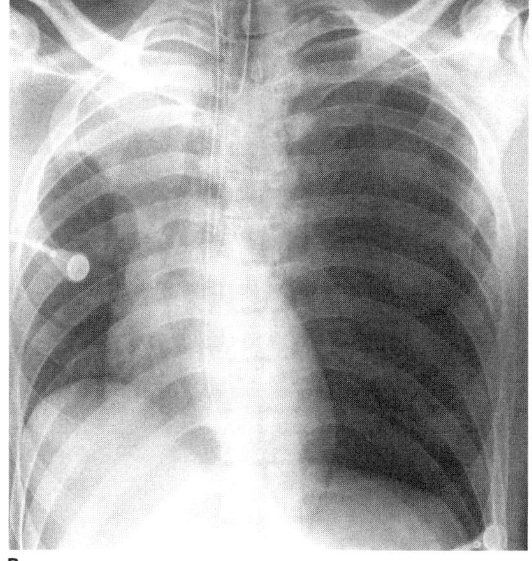

Figure 3-2 A pneumothorax A) illustration and B) radiograph.

times used as a preservative in these medications. If a bronchodilator is given to a sulfite-sensitive patient, the symptoms can quickly worsen. When checking the SAMPLE history, pay close attention for allergies. Inquire if the patient has previously been intubated because this will definitely signal that the patient has had experience with a very serious attack. The patient can also give you some subjective assessment of how today's symptoms compared to that previous event. Other significant historic points specifically related to understanding how severe an asthma attack is and how much therapy early on the patient may require include: last use of steroids to manage an attack, last ED visit for asthma, and last time hospitalized as an in-patient for asthma. Most physicians do not like to prescribe steroids, especially for lengthy periods of time. They are very effective at reducing the inflammation that comes with lower airway diseases. If the patient is on a steroid and has been for quite some time, that is a "red flag" that this patient has a very serious condition and should be handled as such. Remember that patients can and do die from an asthma attack!

In addition to bronchospasm, acute asthma increases mucus production within the lungs. This irritates the airways, clogs the smaller bronchioles, and makes breathing more difficult. The thickness of the secretions makes them difficult to clear with coughing, while the irritation produces swelling and edema that further blocks the flow of air. The inflammatory response is cell proliferation in the airways (only in long-term chronic asthma). These cells secrete substances that worsen muscle spasm and further increase mucus production. Treatment involves reversing bronchoconstriction and muscle spasm by relaxing the smooth muscle and reducing the inflammatory response, resulting in improved airflow and gas exchange and decreased dyspnea (**Figure 3-3 ▸**).

All patients who have a history of obstructive airway disease and are in respiratory distress should be taken very seriously. As an attack worsens, the patient retains CO_2, becomes acidotic, becomes hypoxic, and because of increased insensible water loss, also becomes dehydrated. Patients will complain of lightheadedness or dizziness, with increasing fatigue. The work of breathing consumes all available energy and literally wears out the patient.

A severe and prolonged asthma attack that does not respond to standard medications is called **status asthmaticus**. Its onset is frequently caused by a viral infection and it requires immediate treatment and transport to the ED. These patients are in imminent danger of respiratory failure and often require endotracheal intubation and mechanical ventilation. This is a large problem and a very precarious situation. Intubation should be held off as a last resort, but not too late!

Consideration for Steroid Administration

Dexamethasone sodium phosphate [Decadron phosphate] is a steroid that was used in the earlier prehospital formularies for asthma attacks. Most agencies have switched to methylprednisolone sodium succinate [Solu-Medrol] because there are other popular uses as discussed earlier in this chapter. If your service is still carrying dexamethasone sodium phosphate [Decadron phosphate] instead of methylprednisolone sodium succinate [Solu-Medrol], we would use it in this context, without question. It is really a function of giving some steroid (**glucocorticoid** as opposed to **mineralocorticoid**) to manage the attack, which is a matter of individual system set-up. Dexamethasone sodium phosphate [Decadron phosphate] is appropriate, as are methylprednisolone sodium succinate [Solu-Medrol], hydrocortisone sodium phosphate [Solu-Cortef], methylprednisolone acetate

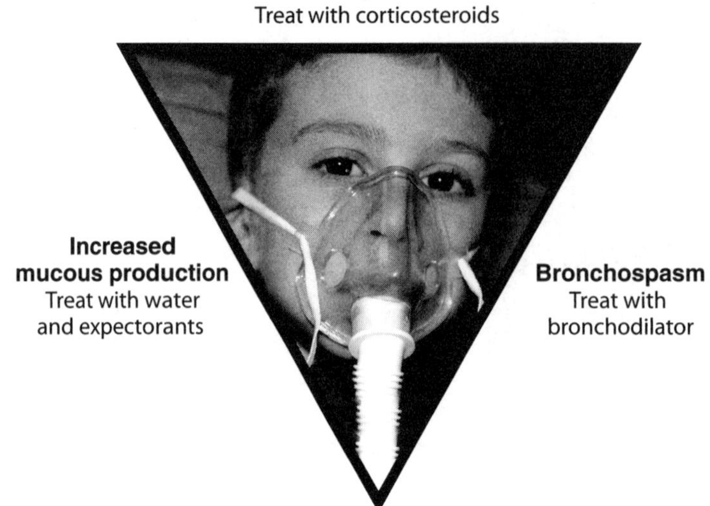

Figure 3-3 The asthma triad demonstrates the three primary components of asthma, and the corresponding treatments for each component.

[Depo-Medrol], and prednisone [Prednisone Intensol, Sterapred, Sterapred DS]. Before methylprednisolone sodium succinate [Solu-Medrol] was available for prehospital care, paramedics were sometimes instructed to administer an augmented dose of whatever prednisone a patient may have had leftover at home.

Therefore, for acute cases giving some steroid is better than no steroid; it does not matter what kind. You should pick one, learn it, and use it. All of these steroids take a fairly long time to take effect (ie, 2 to 24 hours); therefore, giving it sooner (in the prehospital setting) tends to produce better results rather than waiting for the patient's condition to worsen and allowing the inflammation and distress to become overwhelming.

A phrase that you must remember from your paramedic training goes like this: "All that wheezes is not asthma." What does this phrase actually mean? Wheezing is a sign that may be present in a number of respiratory conditions besides asthma. Patients with respiratory conditions such as COPD, heart failure, pulmonary embolism, pneumothorax, near drowning (submersion), toxic inhalation, and foreign body airway obstruction (FBAO) have all been known to wheeze. If the patient is a young child or is elderly, always consider a foreign body in the airway and obtain a complete history before deciding that the patient is suffering from an asthma attack.

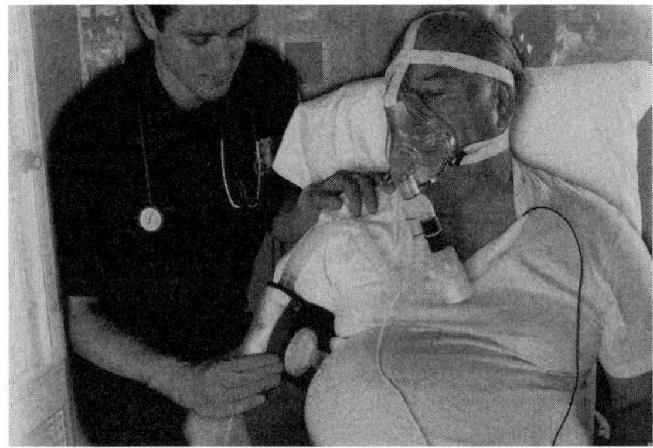

Figure 3-4 The CPAP used in the acute setting is usually administered via a face mask, which must make a tight seal to function properly.

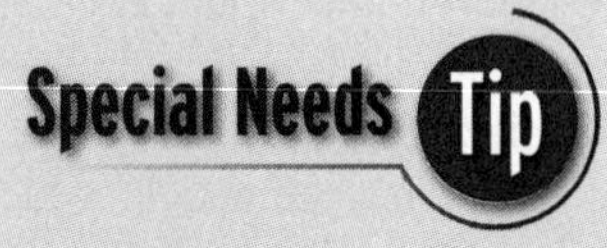

The smooth muscles of the lower airway weaken with age. Strong inhalation can make the walls of the airway collapse inward and cause inspiratory wheezing.

Other Options for Management of Respiratory Conditions

When a patient's breathing becomes ineffective and requires assistance, there are three treatment methods you may consider to assist with the ventilations of the patient: bag-mask device, CPAP, and either oral or nasal endotracheal intubation (**Figure 3-4 ▲**). The patient experiencing a severe asthma attack requires bronchodilator medication to relieve bronchospasm even with ventilatory assistance. These medications can be nebulized through each of the three ventilatory methods. Two oxygen sources are required, one for the nebulizer and one for the ventilation adjunct.

Case Study 1 Asthma Attack

Part 1

You unit has been dispatched to a gas station in town for a patient who is struggling to breathe. The attendant called because a car pulled into the station and almost crashed into the front of the mini-mart. When he ran out to see what was happening, he found the driver in the vehicle struggling to breathe.

Upon your arrival and although the police have just arrived, you make sure that the scene is safe. The patient is a man in his early forties who is sitting in the front seat of the vehicle. The driver's side door is open and he has both of his legs outside the vehicle. You do not need to be right next to the patient to hear he is wheezing or to see he is struggling. You quickly grab your first-in bag and proceed to begin the initial assessment on the patient (see **Table 1**). The police officer says the patient's name is Bill but he is barely able to speak more than a word or two at a time. You note that there are a couple of multiple dose inhalers sitting on the front seat of the vehicle.

Table 1 **Initial Assessment**

Initial Assessment	Recording Time: 1 Minute
General Impression/ Appearance	Middle-aged male, wearing a tee shirt and gym shorts, obviously struggling to breathe
Mental Status	"A" alert (oriented to person, place, and day)
Airway	Open, audible wheezing both inspiratory and expiratory
Breathing	Rapid and shallow, turning pale and blue and only able to speak a word or two at a time
Circulation	Rapid and thready radial pulse, no external bleeding
Priority/Plan	High priority due to severe respiratory distress

As you complete your initial assessment it is clear that this patient is in severe respiratory distress. Apparently he knew it and was attempting to drive himself to the hospital but felt he would not make it so he pulled into the gas station.

Your partner has already placed the patient on a nonrebreathing mask and supplemental oxygen and is getting an albuterol [Proventil, Ventolin] treatment ready. There is also an EMT-B on the scene who you ask to quickly get a set of baseline vital signs and hook up the pulse oximeter. The patient is able to nod his head and blurt out brief answers to your questions although it is clear he is getting very lightheaded and literally wearing himself out.

Question 1: When does a routine asthma attack become a life-threatening asthma attack?

Question 2: Why is this patient so dizzy and appears to be wearing out?

Part 2

A supervisor is now on the scene and has brought the stretcher over to the car where the patient is sitting. You and your partner gently lift the patient over to the stretcher which is now in the semi-Fowler's position. It seems that Bill had tried desperately to use his albuterol [Proventil, Ventolin] many times during his frantic ride in the car. Clearly it has not yet helped. Since Bill is a responsive medical patient, you begin a focused history and physical examination and start by listening to his chest (see **Table 2**). It is difficult to get the OPQRST questions answered because Bill is in so much distress.

You are able to determine that the breathing difficulty began about an hour ago and has gotten progressively worse. He has a history of asthma and a productive cough with green sputum. He thinks all of the coughing today has made him a lot worse.

Bill definitely has that sense of impending doom on his face and only speaks when spoken to. He is concentrating on his breathing, although it is not entirely successful.

Your partner begins getting a quick IV line into Bill as you listen once more to his lungs. He is getting quieter which is not always a good sign. In this

Table 2 **Focused History and Physical Examination**

Baseline Vital Signs	Recording Time: 5 Minutes
Skin CTC (color, temperature, condition)	Pale and cyanotic, warm, clammy
Pulse	Radial pulse of 136 beats/min, regular, and thready
Blood Pressure	146/88 mm Hg
Respirations	32 breaths/min, labored and shallow

Case Study 1 Continued

case it means that Bill is tiring and is unable to move enough air to wheeze. You know he is going to need an advanced airway intervention shortly if he does not start improving.

You ask Bill how this attack compares to his prior experiences and he says it is ". . . definitely . . . the . . . worst . . .!"

Question 3: Why do we sometimes ask the patient if they have ever required a "breathing tube" or to be intubated to treat their asthma?

Question 4: How serious is the asthma problem in the US?

Part 3

From your lung assessment you learned that Bill still has both inspiratory and expiratory wheezes throughout all lung fields but his chest is getting quieter because he seems to be moving less air. If you had a spirometer, you could actually measure the volume of air entering and leaving the lungs, but some might argue the value of measuring something that is obvious. The second albuterol [Proventil, Ventolin] treatment is mixed with ipratropium bromide [Atrovent] by placing 3 mL (2.5 mg) of albuterol [Proventil, Ventolin] premixed solution into 2.5 mL (0.5 mg) of ipratropium bromide [Atrovent]. This mixture is placed into a nebulizer mask and administered to the patient. Bill is still able to hold onto the device and self administer so you do not yet have to consider bagging it in with a bag-mask device.

The ECG monitor has been placed on Bill as you pull away from the scene heading to the nearest hospital. Fortunately the EMT-B on the scene is able to drive your ambulance in so both you and your partner are in the back of the ambulance working on Bill. You obtain a SAMPLE history as your partner is drawing up methylprednisolone sodium succinate [Solu-Medrol] to administer a dose of 1 to 2 mg/kg (usually 125 mg) IV to the patient (see **Table 3**). After this drug goes in, your local protocol is to administer 2 g of magnesium sulfate IV in 100 mL of normal saline over 10 minutes.

Table 3 SAMPLE History

SAMPLE History	Comments
Signs/symptoms	Nausea, chest tightness although no cardiac history and no ST-segment elevation MI (STEMI) on the ECG
Allergies	Most of the "cillin" drugs
Medications	Albuterol metered dose inhaler (MDI) (no spacer), budesonide MDI [Pulmicort Turbuhaler]
Pertinent past medical history	Recent upper respiratory infection, coughing for the past few days, was previously "tubed" in the ED about 6 months ago for a serious asthma attack
Last oral intake	Lunch of chicken soup but ended up only eating a little bit due to a coughing spell
Events leading up to the incident	Prolonged coughing spell, attack began while cleaning up the house

Treatment Plan

This patient will need rapid transport without scaring him with the siren.

1. Maintain the ABCs.
2. Manage his airway using high concentration supplemental oxygen. Evaluate his ability to ventilate as you are likely to need to lay him down and intubate him. While he is still breathing the nasal route may be an option for the tube.
3. The 12-lead ECG should always be checked in cases of severe respiratory distress, as it is possible that myocardial ischemia could have precipitated the current set of symptoms or result from a very severe attack. Obviously, assessing the ECG should not take precedence over evaluating and securing this patient's currently very fragile airway and breathing status.
4. The albuterol [Proventil, Ventolin] by MDI or nebulizer is a good first step but vascular access will be necessary for additional medication administration. Be prepared to administer a mix of albuterol [Proventil, Ventolin] and ipratropium bromide [Atrovent] followed by 1 to 2 mg/kg (approximately 125 mg) of methylpred-

Case Study 1 Continued

nisolone sodium succinate [Solu-Medrol] and 2 g of magnesium sulfate in 100 mL of NS over 10 minutes. This patient will likely also need epinephrine 1:1,000 given subcutaneously.

5. As always with all medications, reevaluate the patient's serial vital signs and lung sounds after each intervention and be prepared to thoroughly document this very challenging case after arriving at the ED.

Medications for Consideration:

There are a number of medications for consideration by the paramedic to begin to manage the asthmatic in distress in the prehospital setting. These drugs include: oxygen, albuterol [Proventil, Ventolin], ipratropium bromide [Atrovent], methylprednisolone sodium succinate [Solu-Medrol], magnesium sulfate [Magnesium], epinephrine [Adrenalin], and levalbuterol hydrochloride [Xopenex] (see **Table 4**, **Table 5**, **Table 6**, **Table 7**, and **Table 8**).

Table 4 Albuterol

Do you know?	Comments
Right drug? Generic name: [**Albuterol**] Trade name: [Proventil, Ventolin]	Used to acutely treat wheezing, cough, and dyspnea from reactive airways. Often patients may have already self administered using a metered-dose inhaler (MDI), most effectively used with a spacer device. This is one of the typical drugs that EMT-Bs are trained to assist the patient with (provided the medication is prescribed to the patient). In some regions, the basic level ambulances actually carry MDIs or nebulizers.
Right patient?	The patient with reactive airway disease who has bronchoconstriction.
Right dose?	A spray from an MDI canister delivers approximately 90 μg per actuation. The dose when using a MDI is 1 to 2 inhalations or 90 to 180 μg. Each canister contains 17 grams and is designed to administer up to 200 doses. When given by paramedics in the field using a nebulizer, the standard dose is 2.5 mg and is typically repeated up to 3 times.
Right route?	Given as an inhaled MDI, as a nebulizer treatment, or may be ventilated into the patient using a bag-mask device.
Right time?	While the patient is still able to breathe and hold the mask for the nebulizer on his/her own.
Right documentation?	Document the administration of the medication as well as the ongoing assessment findings, including lung sounds on the patient care report.
Expected action	Bronchodilation and ease of breathing with less wheezing and improved airflow and gas exchange.
Side effects	The effects are many and may include: tremulousness, nervousness, palpitations, nausea, vomiting, cough, throat irritation, tachycardias, difficulty swallowing, and hoarseness.
Contraindications	None depending upon chosen route of administration.
Precautions	Use with caution in patients with coronary heart disease or in patients with significant cardiac arrhythmias. Use of albuterol [Proventil, Ventolin] together with other stimulant medications is discouraged because of their combined effects on the heart rate, blood pressure, and the potential for causing chest pain in patients with underlying coronary heart disease. Tricyclic antidepressants should not be used together with albuterol [Proventil, Ventolin] because of their combined toxicity to the vascular system.

Table 5 Ipratropium Bromide

Do you know?	Comments
Right drug? Generic name: [**Ipratropium Bromide**] Trade name: [Atrovent]	This drug may be taken alone or as a mixture with albuterol [Proventil, Ventolin] and given by a nebulizer treatment. The retail versions of the combinations are known as Combivent (MDI) and Duo-Neb (nebulizer solution).
Right patient?	Used to prevent or treat wheezing, difficulty breathing, chest tightness, and coughing in patients with asthma or COPD.
Right dose?	The dose given by nebulizer treatment is 0.5 mg in 2.5 mL of solution which is poured into the nebulizer. This dose can be repeated 3 to 4 times a day or combined with albuterol [Proventil, Ventolin]. When using an MDI, the patient should not take more than 12 puffs in a 24-hour period.

continues

Case Study I Continued

Table 5 Ipratropium Bromide (*Continued*)

Do you know?	Comments
Right route?	Comes in a liquid form to be nebulized for inhalation. It also comes in a MDI.
Right time?	Use as prescribed and as a treatment for reactive airway disease in its acute condition.
Right documentation?	Document the administration of the medication as well as the ongoing assessment findings, including lung sounds on the patient care report.
Expected action	As a bronchodilator it works by relaxing smooth muscle and opening the smallest airways.
Side effects	Some of the side effects are minor such as: dizziness, nausea, heartburn, constipation, dry mouth, difficulty or pain when urinating, frequent urination, and back pain. Other side effects can be more serious such as: rash, hives, itching, swelling of the eyes, face, lips, tongue, throat, hands, feet, ankles, or lower legs, difficulty breathing or swallowing, a fast and pounding heartbeat, and chest pain.
Contraindications	None depending upon chosen route of administration.
Precautions	If using an inhaler, be careful not to get the medication in your eyes as it may cause glaucoma or worsen the disease if it is preexisting.

Table 6 Epinephrine Hydrochloride

Do you know?	Comments
Right drug? Generic name: [**Epinephrine Hydrochloride**] Trade name: [Adrenalin Chloride 1:1000]	Sympathomimetic drug which is a direct acting alpha and beta agonist. In asthma, the drug is being given for its beta-2 stimulation. It also has alpha and beta-1 effects which were discussed in Chapter 1.
Right patient?	Used for the patient experiencing a severe allergic reaction or asthma attack. Also used in the cardiac arrest patient and further described in Chapter 4.
Right dose?	In a mild allergic reaction or asthma, the patient is given 0.3–0.5 mg of the 1:1,000 solution. According to the manufacturer, epinephrine dosing is based on body weight. The EpiPen auto-injector (0.3 mg) is for individuals weighing 66 lb or more. The EpiPen Jr auto-injector (0.15 mg) is for individuals weighing between 33 and 66 lb.
Right route?	Given by the SC injection. If the patient is severely ill, it can be given by the IV route but the concentration used is the 1:10,000. For a severe allergic reaction or anaphylaxis, it is given by the IM route with the use of an EpiPen auto-injector. (EpiPens are all 1:1,000 concentration, 0.15 or 0.3 mg, IM auto-injected only)
Right time?	Rarely used in cases of a severe refractory asthma attack.
Right documentation?	Document the administration of the medication as well as the ongoing assessment findings, including vital signs, 12-lead ECG tracings, and lung sounds on the patient care report.
Expected action	Immediate action of bronchial smooth muscle relaxation and dilation of the skeletal vasculature.
Side effects	Hypertension, tachycardias, arrhythmias, anxiety, restlessness, psychomotor agitation, nausea, headache, angina, and myocardial infarction.
Contraindications	Hypertension, hypothermia, pulmonary edema, acute coronary syndrome, and hypovolemic shock.
Precautions	May increase the myocardial oxygen demand. It potentiates other sympathomimetic agents and is deactivated by alkaline solutions.

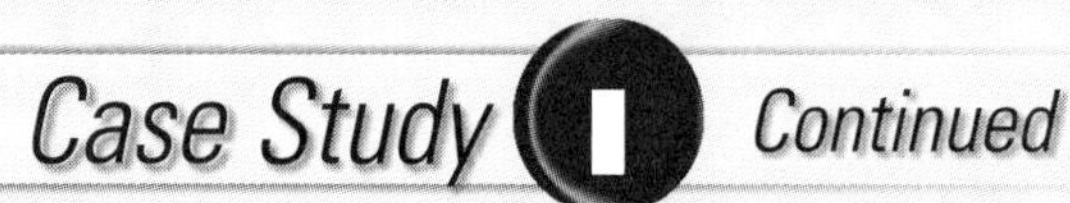

Table 7 Methylprednisolone Sodium Succinate

Do you know?	Comments
Right drug? Generic name: [**Methylprednisolone Sodium Succinate**] Trade name: [Solu-Medrol]	A potent anti-inflammatory glucocorticoid, it is a synthetic corticosteroid that suppresses inflammation. It also potentiates vascular smooth muscle relaxation by beta-adrenergic agonism.
Right patient?	Used with the acute spinal cord trauma patient, anaphylaxis, and as a bronchodilator for unresponsive acute asthmatics.
Right dose?	For asthma or COPD, adults should receive 1–2 mg/kg IV. Some systems simply give 125 mg IV.
Right route?	Given by the IV route.
Right time?	Administered to the asthmatic who is not responsive to other therapy.
Right documentation?	Document the administration of the medication as well as the ongoing assessment findings, including lung sounds on the patient care report.
Expected action	Used as a bronchodilator for asthma. Also can be used for spinal cord injury and anaphylaxis.
Side effects	May cause headache, hypertension, sodium and water retention, CHF, hypokalemia, alkalosis, peptic ulcer disease, nausea, or vomiting.
Contraindications	Systemic fungal infections, use with caution in patients with gastrointestinal bleeding, sepsis, local infection.
Precautions	Use with caution in patients with gastrointestinal bleeding. The drug can interact by blunting the effects of insulin and hypoglycemic agents. Potassium-depleting agents may exacerbate hypokalemic effects.

Table 8 Magnesium Sulfate

Do you know?	Comments
Right drug? Generic name: [**Magnesium Sulfate**] Trade name: [Magnesium]	Not a first-line drug but may be helpful. It is an electrolyte that reduces the striated muscle contractions and blocks peripheral neuromuscular transmission by reducing acetylcholine release at the myoneural junction. It manages seizures in toxemia of pregnancy and causes uterine relaxation in premature labor.
Right patient?	The patient with a severe asthma attack unresponsive to other therapy.
Right dose?	The adult dose for cardiac arrest from torsades de pointes, or hypomagnesemia, or severe asthma is 1–2 g (2–4 mL of a 50% solution) diluted in 100 mL of D_5W/NS IV/IO over 5–20 minutes. If the patient is in torsades with a pulse, the loading dose is 1–2 g mixed in 50–100 mL D5W over 5–60 minutes IV. It should be followed with 0.5–1 g/h IV titrated to control the torsades.
Right route?	IV or IO.
Right time?	In a severe attack while other first-line medications are being administered or have yet to achieve the desired effect.
Right documentation?	Document the administration of the medication as well as the ongoing assessment findings, including lung sounds and vital signs on the patient care report.
Expected action	Given for seizures in eclampsia, torsades de pointes, hypomagnesemia, or refractory pulseless ventricular fibrillation or ventricular tachycardia. Can also be used for bronchodilation after beta-agonists and anticholinergics have been used.
Side effects	May cause CNS depression, facial flushing, diaphoresis, depressed reflexes, circulatory collapse, or hypotension.
Contraindications	Heart blocks and myocardial damage.
Precautions	Use with caution in patients with renal failure. IV calcium chloride or calcium gluconate should be available as an antagonist if needed.

Case Study I Continued

Other considerations for medications would include: epinephrine racemic [Micronefrin, Vaponefrin], promethazine hydrochloride [Phenergan], or ondansetron hydrochloride [Zofran] for the nausea (see **Table 9**). Ondansetron hydrochloride [Zofran] is discussed in more detail in chapter 2. Terbutaline sulfate [Brethine, Bricanyl] should be considered to reverse the bronchospasm (see **Table 10**).

Table 9 Epinephrine Racemic

Do you know?	Comments
Right drug? Generic name: [**Epinephrine Racemic**] Trade name: [Micronefrin, Vaponefrin]	Really no indication for nebulized epinephrine to manage acute lower airway bronchospasm, though it is useful to manage upper airway problems like laryngeal edema and stridor; very effective in cases of laryngotracheobronchitis (croup). Over-the-counter epinephrine inhalers are still sold [Primatene] as an aid to "bronchial asthma" but significant risk associated with overuse both in terms of the direct actions of the medication itself and the fact that overuse tends to be related to severe poorly treated asthma that may rapidly progress and be less responsive to more typical treatments that are considerably safer and more effective (albuterol).
Right patient?	Indicated for patients with bronchial asthma, prevention of bronchospasm, laryngotracheobronchitis (croup), or laryngeal edema.
Right dose?	The MDI dose is 2 to 3 puffs that can be repeated every 5 minutes as needed. In solution dilute 5 mL in 5.0 mL of normal saline and administer over 15 minutes.
Right route?	May be administered by MDI or nebulizer inhalation.
Right time?	During the patient's reactive airway distress.
Right documentation?	Document the administration of the medication as well as the ongoing assessment findings, including lung sounds on the patient care report.
Expected action	A sympathomimetic that stimulates beta-2 receptors in the lungs causing bronchodilation as the bronchial smooth muscles relax. It also inhibits a histamine release.
Side effects	May cause tachycardia and other arrhythmias.
Contraindications	Hypertension, underlying cardiovascular disease, and epiglottitis.
Precautions	Monitor vital signs and watch for bronchospasm caused by excessive use. Note that monoamine oxidase inhibitors (MAOI) may potentiate the effects. Beta-blockers may blunt the effects.

Table 10 Terbutaline Sulfate

Do you know?	Comments
Right drug? Generic name: [**Terbutaline Sulfate**] Trade name: [Brethine, Bricanyl]	A sympathomimetic bronchodilator that works in 15–30 minutes by SC and 5–30 minutes by MDI route.
Right patient?	Bronchial asthma, reversible bronchospasm associated with exercise, and COPD.
Right dose?	Adults are given 0.25 mg SC that may be repeated in 15 to 30 minutes up to a maximum dose of 0.5 mg in 4 hours. Also may be given in 400 μg (two MDI inhalations) every 4–6 hours. Allow 1 to 2 minutes between each inhalation.
Right route?	SC or MDI inhalation.
Right time?	Given in response to bronchospasm associated with an asthma attack or exacerbation of COPD.
Right documentation?	Document the administration of the medication as well as the ongoing assessment findings, including lung sounds on the patient care report.

continues

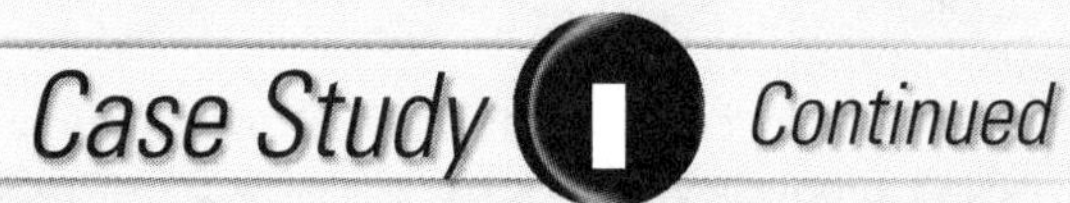

Table 10 Terbutaline Sulfate (*Continued*)

Do you know?	Comments
Expected action	As a selective beta-2 adrenergic receptor site stimulator, this drug causes relaxation of smooth muscle of the bronchial tree and peripheral vasculature. There are minimal cardiac effects of the drug.
Side effects	Usually transient and dose related, restlessness, apprehension, palpitations, tachycardia, chest pain, coughing, bronchospasm, nausea, facial flushing.
Contraindications	Hypersensitivity or tachyarrhythmias.
Precautions	Use with caution in patients with cardiovascular disease or hypertension. The patient should receive oxygen before and after administration of this drug. Be aware that cardiovascular effects may be exacerbated by other sympathomimetics. MAOIs may potentiate arrhythmias. Beta-blockers may antagonize terbutaline sulfate [Brethine, Bricanyl].

Most EMS systems reserve the use of injectable sympathomimetics for the patient whose respiratory efforts are so diminished that the ventilatory volume would not allow nebulized treatments to be effective.

Question 5: What is the significance of the patient being on steroids for his disease?

Question 6: Why are you giving him additional steroids?

Part 4

En route to the ED you reassess the patient as well as call in to let them know Bill's condition (see **Table 11**). After administration of the medications, he is starting to improve. You decide to hold off on the nasal tube as his mental status is improving and he is finally starting to pink up.

You are also beginning to notice that he is using more words in each sentence and he seems less confused about what is going on around him.

Question 7: What is the purpose of administering a steroid in the prehospital setting?

Question 8: If the patient was intubated, how does that affect their hospital care?

Table 11 Reassessment and Ongoing Assessment of the Patient

Serial Vital Signs and Relevant Data	Recording Time: 15 Minutes
Skin CTC	Pale, warm, and dry
Pulse	128 beats/min, weak and regular at radial
Blood Pressure	140/82 mm Hg
Respirations	26 breaths/min, labored, and shallow
Mental Status	"A" Alert (oriented to person, place, and day)
ECG	Sinus tachycardia with no ectopy
SpO_2	90%
Lung Sounds	Expiratory wheezes in both lungs
Other (ie, glucose, core temperature)	Warm body temperature but not hot enough to do a rectal temperature

Part 5

Bill is very lucky to make it to the ED with some clear signs that all of those drugs have helped to improve his condition. Asthma and reactive airway disease are very common and very dangerous. Always pay close attention to the asthmatic who does not respond to his own prescribed medications. The ED staff will reevaluate Bill and determine if he should be intubated. They will also administer additional medication treatments and continuously monitor his color, vitals, lung sounds, and mental status to see how he is doing after each intervention. Next time you have an asthmatic patient in trouble, think of Bill.

Pulmonary Embolism

When a pulmonary artery becomes blocked by an embolus such as a blood clot, fat particle, air, gas, amniotic fluid, or tumor tissue, the lung tissue distal to the occlusion becomes ischemic from decreased blood flow and can die (infarct). The insult causes a response that includes release of vasoactive substances (ie, histamine) from white blood cells which cause bronchospasm and may produce wheezing. The risk factors for a pulmonary embolism (PE) are many (**Table 3-3▼**).

Signs and Symptoms of Pulmonary Embolism

The signs and symptoms of a pulmonary embolism, though occasionally classic, are often vague, develop suddenly, and vary in intensity depending on the amount of area affected. Smaller emboli can present with sudden pleuritic chest pain, anxiety, dyspnea, wheezing, or hemoptysis. When the PE is massive, the signs and symptoms may appear the same as those of a spontaneous pneumothorax, an acute myocardial infarction (AMI) with right heart failure, cardiac tamponade, or septic shock. The patient can collapse with syncope and go into cardiac arrest.

Signs of Pulmonary Embolism

- Dyspnea
- Coughing
- Pale skin or cyanosis may develop
- Diaphoresis
- Jugular vein distention
- Elevated blood pressure (hypotensive with saddle embolus)
- Pulmonary edema
- Blood-tinged sputum obtained by coughing (hemoptysis)
- Anxiety or confusion
- Sudden onset of chest pain
- Tachycardia

The typical development of a pulmonary embolism involves a number of stages. The blood flow is altered in the peripheral vein from an injury to the vein's wall, decreased movement of the patient from a period of immobilization, or an increase in the coagulability of the blood. The altered blood flow leads to platelet aggregation and activation of the coagulation system. A clot or thrombosis forms in the deep vein and pieces dislodge into the venous circulation, returning to the heart as emboli. The emboli pass through the right side of the heart to the pulmonary circulation. As the clot passes into smaller and smaller pulmonary circulation, it becomes lodged and blocks the vessel. This causes the lung tissue supplied by the vessel to become ischemic and ultimately infarcts the delicate lung tissue if not reperfused.

The pathophysiologic changes that result from a PE include impaired gas exchange and defects in pulmonary mechanics and hemodynamics. The changes are proportional to the area affected by the obstruction and can produce pulmonary hypertension with right heart failure, shock, and cardiac arrest. When lung tissue infarcts, pleuritic chest pain may be present or the pain may be anginal when right ventricular ischemia develops from pulmonary hypertension. See Case Study II for the management of PE.

Table 3-3 Risk Factors for Pulmonary Embolism

Risk Factor	Problem
Obesity	Effects on the coagulation system as well as decreased movement.
Infection	In sepsis, abnormal activation of the coagulation system can cause thrombus formation and subsequent embolization.
Cancer	Kidney and lung tumors in particular can produce substances that increase the propensity of blood to clot.
Oral contraceptives	Affect the woman's level of natural anticoagulants resulting in an increased coagulability state (particularly in the context of associated cigarette smoking).
Sedentary lifestyle	Prolonged inactivity or being bedridden decreases the normal muscular contractions involved in venous return of blood to the heart. As venous flow is slowed, the blood clotting system is activated causing clots to form and thrombi to break off and travel through the vessels into the lungs.
Long bone fracture	Fat and other marrow contents travel through the bloodstream in the form of emboli and lodge in the pulmonary circulation.
Pregnancy	Amniotic fluid embolism may occur during delivery, hypercoagulability and increased venous stasis in the legs and pelvis tends to occur during the third trimester.
Recent surgery	Blood clots can form in the pelvis and legs during surgical procedures.
Blood diseases	Rare conditions can make the patient's blood more likely to clot (Factor V leiden, protein C and S deficiencies).
Autoimmune disease (ie, systemic lupus)	Conditions that may produce a hypercoagulable state in the blood.

Case Study II Pulmonary Embolism

Part 1

Your unit has been dispatched to a local bike path where a cyclist found a runner in distress. There was very little information provided and it takes a while to find the nearest entrance to the bike path. You park the ambulance and you and your partner grab some portable equipment and begin your trek down the path in search of the patient. An in-line skater stops to tell you that the patient is just around the bend about 50 yards away.

As you come around the bend you can see the patient sitting on a tree stump at the side of the path. Several people have stopped to offer help. It is clear that the scene is safe. You also hear over the radio that a backup unit was dispatched to the next entryway and will probably arrive at the patient's side a few minutes after you. You can advise them to bring in additional equipment, if needed.

Table 1 Initial Assessment

Initial Assessment	Recording Time: 1 Minute
General Impression/ Appearance	In tripod position, female in her 30's
Mental Status	"A" alert (oriented to person, place, and day)
Airway	Open and clear
Breathing	Rapid and shallow
Circulation	Weak radial, regular at 130 beats/min
Priority/Plan	High due to respiratory complaint

You see a thin woman in her late 30's who appears to be healthy looking; however, it is clear she is having trouble breathing. You begin to conduct your initial assessment by first introducing yourself and evaluating her mental status (see **Table 1**).

Due to the medical nature of the complaint and the fact that there is no obvious trauma involved, you decide you will do a focused history and physical examination of the patient. As you continue to question the patient, your partner starts oxygen with a nonrebreathing mask. The chief complaint of difficulty breathing came on suddenly during exercise. She states that her name is Ginny and that she is trying to get back in shape as she has not been running for the past 8 weeks. Of course, all of her statements are a few words at a time. She does not have any history of asthma, COPD, or reactive airway disease. She states she feels sharp pain like someone has stabbed her in the chest. Your partner gets a set of baseline vital signs while you listen to Ginny's breath sounds.

Question 1: This patient is in good physical shape. From your EMT-B and paramedic training, what are three examples of respiratory conditions that could be occurring to Ginny?

Question 2: What is the significance of the patient saying she does not have any history of asthma?

Part 2

Ginny is anxious and appears breathless. You administer high-flow oxygen by nonrebreathing mask and coach her to breathe slower. You ask the bystanders if they saw or know anything about Ginny that may be helpful. Someone saw her jogging and then stop and drop to her knees. No loss of consciousness was confirmed by the same witness. Ginny is able to tell you that she was well earlier today. She had been jogging for 20 minutes when the chest pain and shortness of breath began. Even though she stopped jogging 15 minutes ago, the breathing is not getting any easier. Ginny is a nonsmoker, she takes fexofenadine hydrochloride [Allegra] for seasonal allergies and uses a topical patch for birth control. Your partner has the vital signs: skin is flushed, warm, and moist, distal pulse is 134 beats/min, strong and regular, respirations are 34 breaths/min and shallow, and blood pressure is 160/110 mm Hg. You perform a focused history and physical examination of her cardiopulmonary and vascular systems (see **Table 2**). Lung sounds are diminished with no adventitious sounds, chest pain increases with deep breaths, there are no bruising marks or scars on the chest or back, and there is no pain on palpation of the thorax. ECG is sinus tachycardia, 12-lead shows a right bundle branch block, and SpO_2 is 92% on the oxygen. Ginny's pain is severe at 8 on a scale from 1 to 10.

Case Study II Continued

Table 2 Focused History and Physical Examination

Baseline Vital Signs	Recording Time: 5 Minutes
Skin CTC (color, temperature, condition)	Flushed, warm, and moist
Pulse	134 beats/min with tachycardia, regular and thready
Blood Pressure	160/110 mm Hg
Respirations	34 breaths/min, tachypneic and shallow (SpO_2 is low 90's).

Question 3: Does Ginny have any risk factors for pulmonary embolism?

Question 4: Which of Ginny's vital signs is of most concern?

Part 3

The backup crew has brought the stretcher and now it is time to move Ginny to the ambulance. Once inside, transport begins and you reassess vital signs. You start an IV and obtain blood samples. Oxygen has done little to improve her condition. She remains anxious and restless, and she is hyperventilating, tachycardic, and a little hypertensive. When you reassess her lungs, there are fine crackles in the bases. She coughs and spits up into a tissue. You note the pink-tinged sputum in the tissue. The pain in her chest increases when she coughs and is now radiating up to the left shoulder. It is time to call medical control to give them an early notification for a possible PE and request an order for analgesia for the pain. You complete a SAMPLE history (see **Table 3**).

Table 3 SAMPLE History

SAMPLE History	Comments
Signs/symptoms	Anxiety, breathless, pleuritic chest pain
Allergies	Seasonal
Medications	fexofenadine hydrochloride [Allegra], norelgestromin/ethinyl estradiol transderm system [Ortho Evra]
Pertinent past medical history	Healthy with no significant past medical history
Last oral intake	Breakfast
Events leading up to the incident	Moderate outdoor aerobic exercise

Treatment Plan

1. For this patient, you will need to focus on maintaining the ABCs and manage her airway with high concentration supplemental oxygen.
2. The position of comfort is most likely to be on her side; this will help the PE migrate into the smallest of the pulmonary circulation vessels.
3. A 12-lead ECG was done given her markedly abnormal vital signs and presenting complaints (just in case this is actually a case of pulmonary edema with **ST-Segment Elevation Myocardial Infarction (STEMI)** as the proximate cause).
4. You would not be wrong to try an albuterol nebulizer treatment here. You may even want to consult with medical control for furosemide [Lasix] and a possible dose of morphine sulfate [Astramorph/PF] (in judicious amounts) (see **Table 4**). Even a single dose of a steroid is not going to harm this patient and could potentially help given the history and the fact that the saturation on the nonrebreathing mask is only 92%.
5. The key is to recognize the need for prompt transport, high flow oxygen, ventilation assistance/CPAP, expectant management (endotracheal intubation as needed), and early notification to the ED. Pain management, as with any patient, is important for Ginny. Additional medications that are typically administered to the asthmatic are not likely to help much in Ginny's situation. Rapid transport is likely to be your best bet in her case.
6. As with all medications, reevaluate the patient's serial vital signs and lung sounds after each intervention and be prepared to properly document this potentially difficult call when you arrive at the ED.

Case Study II Continued

Table 4 **Morphine Sulfate**

Do you know?	Comments
Right drug? Generic name: [**Morphine Sulfate**] Trade name: [Astramorph/PF]	Opiate analgesic for relief of moderate to severe pain, relief of anxiety, reduces left ventricular work by reducing preload pressure, pulmonary edema, and sedative effects.
Right patient?	Analgesic for chest pain and to reduce apprehension.
Right dose?	2-4 mg IV (over 1–5 minutes) every 5–30 minutes. Repeat 2–8 mg at 5- to 15-minute intervals.
Right route?	IV or IM.
Right time?	After physical examination and vital signs are obtained and contraindications have been considered.
Right documentation?	Document the administration of the medication as well as the ongoing assessment findings, including lung sounds on the patient care report.
Expected action	Pain relief and reduced anxiety.
Side effects	Respiratory depression, hypotension, decreased level of consciousness, nausea, vomiting (consider antiemetic), bradycardia, tachycardia, syncope, facial flushing, euphoria, bronchospasm, dry mouth.
Contraindications	Known allergy, hypotension.
Precautions	Respiratory depression, hypotension.

Question 5: What other conditions can the signs and symptoms of a pulmonary embolism mimic?

Question 6: What is the significance of blood in Ginny's sputum?

Part 4

After speaking with medical control, you prepare to administer morphine sulfate to help reduce Ginny's chest pain. The hospital is 10–15 minutes away depending on traffic. Serial vital signs and focused physical examinations of her cardiothoracic systems will be completed in the time remaining during transport. In the prehospital setting there is no pharmacological treatment for PE. Treatment is supportive for the patient's signs and symptoms. The morphine you are using for pain relief has side effects that can produce respiratory depression and a drop in blood pressure so you will watch for these.

The ongoing assessment of the patient is performed (see **Table 5**).

Question 7: Based on what information you have obtained thus far, would you consider Ginny's chest pain to be cardiac or pleuritic in nature?

Question 8: In addition to pain relief, how can morphine sulfate help Ginny?

Table 5 **Reassessment and Ongoing Assessment of the Patient**

Serial Vital Signs and Relevant Data	Recording Time: 10 Minutes
Skin CTC	Warm, moist, and pale
Pulse	118 beats/min, strong and regular
Blood Pressure	150/100 mm Hg
Respirations	30 breaths/min and shallow
Mental Status	Alert, less anxious
ECG	12-lead—sinus tachycardia with no ST-segment elevation
SpO_2	95% on high flow oxygen
Lung Sounds	Crackles that clear with coughing
Other (ie, glucose, core body temperature)	Chest pain with radiation up to the shoulder. Pain is an 8 on a scale of 1 to 10, core body temperature unremarkable.

Case Study II Continued

Part 5

En route to the hospital you notice that the morphine sulfate you administered via IV has reduced Ginny's pain and anxiety. You reassure Ginny and continue to explain what you suspect is happening to her and what she can expect when you arrive at the ED. If the hospital confirms that Ginny does have a PE, the treatments may include:

- Analgesia.
- Short-term anticoagulation therapy (heparin, low-molecular weight heparin) followed by long-term anticoagulation (warfarin [Coumadin]).
- Thrombolytic therapy (tPA) for cases of saddle emboli and associated hemodynamic instability.
- Pulmonary embolectomy (very risky and rarely done today).
- Partial interruption of the inferior vena cava by a filter for recurrent deep venous thrombosis or pulmonary emboli.

Pulmonary emboli and deep venous thrombosis (venous thromboembolism) represent an abnormality with the body's usual balance between making and dissolving blood clots, a process that normally occurs continuously within the body. In the case of venous thromboembolism, the balance is tipped more in the direction of clot formation. Most often these clots develop in the large veins of the legs and pelvis. When one of these clots forms, all or a portion of it can break free and flow via the right side of the heart through the pulmonary artery to the lungs where it lodges and causes the embolism. The severity of a pulmonary embolism varies depending on the size of the embolism and the location it gets lodged. The classic presentation of a PE is sudden severe chest pain, often pleuritic in nature, with shortness of breath or coughing that progressively intensifies. Getting a good history from the patient will often reveal one or more risk factors for developing a PE and can help to make a better differential diagnosis. Prehospital treatment is supportive for the signs and symptoms. Analgesia may be a pharmacological option for pain and anxiety.

Pulmonary Edema

Pulmonary edema is a condition in which excessive fluid accumulates in the interstitial spaces and the alveoli. Pulmonary edema is not a disease but is a condition associated with various diseases and causes. This condition causes problems with the exchange of oxygen and carbon dioxide across the alveolar membrane. Pulmonary edema occurs in two ways and can be classified as "high pressure" or "high permeability."

High pressure pulmonary edema occurs when the hydrostatic pressure (water pressure) in the pulmonary capillaries increases. Causes include:

- Acute MI with left ventricular failure
- Chronic heart failure
- Renal insufficiency
- Diving accidents (overpressurization and rapid ascent)
- Brain injury
- Scorpion bites
- Opiate overdose

In high permeability pulmonary edema, the alveolar-capillary membrane is disrupted, causing fluid to leak into the interstitial space. High permeability pulmonary edema is less common than high pressure pulmonary edema. Causes include:

- High altitude
- Inhalation of toxins
- Septic shock
- Acute respiratory distress syndrome (ARDS)
- Severe hypotension
- Severe hypoxemia (post-cardiac arrest, prolonged seizure, prolonged hypoventilation, post-submersion)

Signs and Symptoms of Pulmonary Edema

Whatever the cause of pulmonary edema, the classic symptom is acute onset of shortness of breath. As fluid leaks into the lungs, the patient's dyspnea increases, he or she becomes more hypoxic and can drown in his or her own fluids. See Case Study III for management of acute pulmonary edema.

Congestive Heart Failure (CHF)

Heart failure can be primarily right sided or left sided and may develop slowly (chronically) or acutely (as with acute pulmonary embolism). It is a progressive disorder that many patients chronically live with, punctuated by occasional episodes of decompensation. Heart failure has no cure but can be treated successfully. Treatment includes lifestyle changes such as regular exercise, weight loss, drinking less alcohol, smoking cessation, and healthy diets low in sodium and saturated fats, and pharmacologic treatment. Medications may include several classes of drugs, such as diuretics, ACE inhibitors, digitalis, nitrates, and beta-blockers. Many patients are treated with at least two of these classes:

- **Diuretics**—help reduce blood pressure and water retention. Potential side effects include hypotension, hypokalemia, and hyponatremia.
- **ACE inhibitors**—relax blood vessels and may slow or prevent the loss of heart pumping activity. Many potential side effects include: chronic dry cough, fluid retention, hyperkalemia, renal problems, and skin rashes.
- **Digitalis**—improves circulation by increasing the force of the heart's contraction. Many potential side effects including toxicity.
- **Nitrates**—relaxes blood vessels and improves circulation. May be used by patients who cannot take ACE inhibitors and angiotensin II receptor blockers.
- **Beta-blockers**—reduce the heart rate and blood pressure. Not typically recommended for severe heart failure.

One of the treatment aspects of CHF that is often overlooked and undermanaged is sodium restriction. Neglecting this aspect is a frequent cause of refractory exacerbations. For many, just avoiding salted foods and eliminating table salt to maintain a 2- to 4-gram restriction is adequate. Severe cases require restriction below 2 grams daily. Advanced CHF may require more severe restrictions of sodium to 0.5–1.5 grams and the use of potent diuretics.

Diuretics are used to lower blood pressure and help the body eliminate excess water and sodium. There are three types of diuretics you may find prescribed to patients:

- **Loop diuretics**—furosemide, ethacrynate sodium, bumetanide, torsemide
- **Thiazides**—hydrochlorothiazide,indopamide, metalozone, chlorothiazide, trichlomethiazide
- **Potassium "K" sparing drugs**—triamterene, spironolactone, eplerenone, amiloride

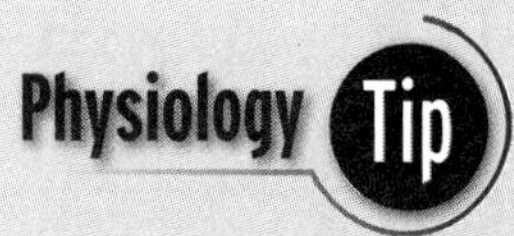

Many diuretics cause the patient to lose not only fluid but also potassium. Patients who do not take their potassium may have low potassium levels, and a subsequent predisposition to cardiac arrhythmias and chronic muscle cramping.

Loop diuretics are usually preferred because of their rapid effectiveness given IV or PO. The disadvantage of loop diuretics is their potency, which when given in overdose can cause hypovolemia, hyponatremia, and hypokalemia. They are also potentially nephrotoxic, and can result in renal insufficiency and failure. Thiazides are helpful in cases of mild CHF. Low dosages are effective and increasing the dosage does not significantly increase its effect. The disadvantage is supplemental potassium chloride is commonly needed to avoid hypokalemic alkalosis. When the body eliminates excessive amounts of water, it also loses potassium and this can cause potassium levels to become too low (hypokalemia). Potassium-sparing diuretics are useful in cases of mild CHF and often are used in combination with other diuretics and antihypertensives such as ACE inhibitors. ACE inhibitors lower blood pressure by helping to relax blood vessels. They also increase potassium levels.

Treatment of hypokalemia may include increasing potassium in the diet. This is most commonly achieved with the use of potassium supplements as well as changing to a potassium-sparing diuretic if indicated.

Case Study III Acute Pulmonary Edema

Part 1

Your unit is dispatched to a private residence in a suburban area of your district. You note that it is 3:00 am. The call is for a patient with difficulty breathing. It is easy to find the address since the house is the only one with the outside lights on. The scene appears to be safe so you and your partner grab the equipment needed to perform an initial assessment, the ECG monitor, and the drug box. Just before ringing the doorbell the patient's wife opens the door and tells you to come quickly. She states that her husband is upstairs in the bedroom.

Table 1 Initial Assessment

Initial Assessment	Recording Time: 1 Minute
General Impression/ Appearance	Obvious distress, male in his early 60's
Mental Status	"A" alert (oriented to person, place, and day)
Airway	Open
Breathing	Distressed, rapid, and noisy (heard from the stairs)
Circulation	Rapid, weak, and irregular radial pulse
Priority/Plan	High due to respiratory distress

As you walk up the stairs to the second floor, you can already hear the patient breathing. It sounds like he is bubbling as he takes a breath. You introduce yourself and he greets you. It is obvious that he is in distress. You perform the initial assessment (see **Table 1**).

Based on the chief complaint of difficulty breathing and given a lack of a trauma history, you note that you will need to perform a focused history and physical examination for a medical patient who is responsive. The patient's wife tells you his name is Bill and he is 64 years old. She says she has never seen him so bad despite his two previous heart attacks. He is extremely pale and diaphoretic. Your partner offers him supplemental oxygen by nonrebreathing mask. Bill grabs the mask, a clear sign he is starving for oxygen. Your partner begins to gather a set of baseline vital signs, apply ECG electrodes, and attach the pulse oximeter to the patient's fingertip. Getting the ECG electrodes to stick is a chore in itself because Bill is diaphoretic and sweating profusely. You proceed to ask a few essential questions and begin your examination.

Question 1: Would you expect to find pedal edema in this patient and what would be its significance?

Question 2: Why does the patient literally grab the nonrebreathing mask from your partner?

Part 2

You learn from Bill's wife that the onset was slow during the night. Bill usually sleeps with three pillows since he often gets **proxsysmal nocturnal dyspnea (PND)**. Tonight he woke up around 2:30 am very short of breath and in a cold sweat. He feels very weak and exhausted. He describes a crushing sensation in the center of his chest which changes as he breathes. He describes this shortness of breath as worse than previous incidents in which he was admitted to the ED.

Table 2 Focused History and Physical Examination

Baseline Vital Signs	Recording Time: 6 Minutes
Skin CTC (color, temperature, condition)	Pale, warm, and diaphoretic
Pulse	120 beats/min, weak, rapid, and irregular
Blood Pressure	148/98 mm Hg
Respirations	24 breaths/min and labored

The discomfort is focused on the front center area of the chest and he feels like he is suffocating for air. Although the onset has been in the middle of the night, approximately 30 minutes has gone by since the symptoms got so bad Bill was willing to have the call made to EMS. He admits that he has been tired the last couple of days. You prepare for the focused history and physical examination (see **Table 2**).

Your focused medical examination will involve a cardiopulmonary examination and include assessment of the lung sounds, neck veins, ankles, and belly. Meanwhile, your partner has attached the electrodes and you review a quick strip which shows rapid atrial fibrillation. Bill states that he has had an irregular heartbeat for the past few years.

Question 3: What significant medical problems can be caused by atrial fibrillation in a patient who has respiratory distress?

Question 4: What type of adventitious breath sounds would you expect to hear on this patient?

Part 3

After determining that Bill has some distant crackles and wheezes in the upper lung fields, frothy red sputum, distended neck veins, and both ascites and pitting pedal edema, you decide to insert an IV and get ready to transport him. Since he is likely to run out of "steam" or energy for his breathing effort, you and your partner decide that Bill would be a good candidate for the CPAP device that your service recently acquired.

You take a look at the SAMPLE history obtained primarily from the patient's spouse (see **Table 3**).

Treatment Plan

1. The focus on Bill will be to maintain the ABCs and manage his airway with high concentration supplemental oxygen.
2. The position for transport will be the high Fowler's position as long as he is still alert.
3. You will need to obtain vascular access and draw blood as well as obtain a 12-lead ECG.
4. If CPAP is available, it can be helpful so the patient does not need to be intubated.

Table 3 SAMPLE History

SAMPLE History	Comments
Signs/symptoms	Weak, exhausted, and short of breath
Allergies	Codeine, novacaine
Medications	Hydrochlorothiazide, furosemide [Lasix], potassium chloride [Slow-K]
Pertinent past medical history	2 past acute myocardial infarctions (AMIs) (3 years apart), coronary artery bypass graft (CABG) 4 years ago
Last oral intake	Tomato juice before going to bed
Events leading up to the incident	Poor general health, less and less energy over the past few days

5. Administer chewable aspirin 160- to 325-mg tablets for their antiplatelet effects and not as an analgesic. Intravenous furosemide [Lasix] dosed at twice the patient's usual oral dose over 1 to 2 minutes would also be appropriate (see **Table 4**). Administer nitroglycerin tablets 0.3 to 0.4 mg sublingual every 3 to 5 minutes (maximum of 3 doses as long as the blood pressure is stable) (see **Table 5**). If there is any concern about this patient's mental status and the potential need for mechanical ventilation and/or endotracheal intubation, it would be prudent to defer any medication administration by mouth. Similarly, if using a bag-mask device for noninvasive ventilation, repeatedly breaking the mask seal to administer sublingual nitroglycerin may be counterproductive; in that case transdermal nitroglycerin application may be a better choice.
6. Medical control should be contacted as they are likely to order additional furosemide [Lasix] and morphine sulfate [Astramorph/PF] (see **Table 6**). Transport Bill to the ED after ensuring that he is kept covered and as warm as possible, preferably seated in an upright position. Patients often get better with this treatment plan in the prehospital setting.
7. As always with all medications, reevaluate the patient's serial vital signs and lung sounds after each intervention and be prepared to properly document this call when you arrive at the ED.

Medications for Consideration:

Oxygen, nitroglycerin, and aspirin were all covered previously in this book.

Table 4 Furosemide

Do you know?	Comments
Right drug? Generic name: [**Furosemide**] Trade name: [Lasix]	A loop diuretic used for the treatment of hypertension and/or fluid retention, to reduce the volume of total body water.
Right patient?	Suspected acute pulmonary edema.
Right dose?	40 to 80 mg slow IV (usually 0.5 to 1 mg/kg). Inject over 1 to 2 minutes.
Right route?	IV, IM.
Right time?	After assessment including vital signs.

continues

Case Study III Continued

Table 4 Furosemide (*Continued*)

Do you know?	Comments
Right documentation?	Document the administration of the medication as well as the ongoing assessment findings, including lung sounds on the patient care report.
Expected action	Relief of pulmonary edema via diuresis and initial preload reduction.
Side effects	Potent diuretic that may cause profound diuresis with hypovolemia, hypokalemia, and hyponatremia; possible allergic reaction.
Contraindications	Do not use with ethacrynate sodium (another loop diuretic).
Precautions	Use lower doses with geriatric patients and children (usual dose via mg/kg).
Pharmacokinetics	Onset 5 minutes through IV; peak effects in 20–60 minutes; duration 4–6 hours; metabolized in the liver and excreted through urine.

Table 5 Nitroglycerin

Do you know?	Comments
Right drug? Generic name: [**Nitroglycerin**] Trade name: [Nitrostat, NitroTab, NitroQuick, Nitro-Bid, Nitrol, ImDur, Isosorbide, Tridil]	This drug is a coronary vasodilator and peripheral venodilator that comes in several forms: lingual spray, sublingual tablets, topical ointment, oral tablets, transdermal patches, intravenous drip.
Right patient?	This drug may be used to manage pain associated with acute coronary syndrome (ACS), angina prophylaxis, and to vasodilate blood vessels in acute pulmonary edema.
Right dose?	0.3 to 0.4 mg SL. May be repeated in 3 to 5 minutes to a maximum of 3 doses (provided the blood pressure remains adequate).
Right route?	Can be administered by lingual, sublingual, oral tablets, or topical routes but in this specific case sublingual would be our choice.
Right time?	After cardiothoracic assessment, vital signs, and history.
Right documentation?	Document the administration of the medication as well as the ongoing assessment findings, including lung sounds, on the patient care report.
Expected action	Relief of chest pain, dyspnea, and pulmonary edema, and reduced blood pressure.
Side effects	Hypotension, increased chest pain, cardiac arrhythmias, potential allergic reaction.
Contraindications	Hypotension.
Precautions	Monitor respiratory effort and blood pressure.
Pharmacokinetics	Onset for sublingual route: 1–3 minutes and then peaks in 1–4 minutes. The drug is metabolized in the liver and excreted in urine.

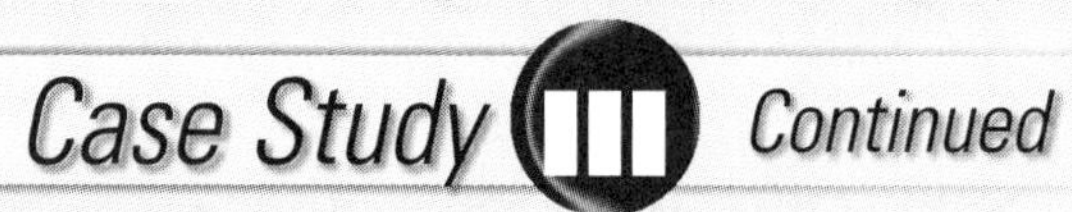

Table 6 **Morphine Sulfate**

Do you know?	Comments
Right drug? Generic name: [**Morphine Sulfate**] Trade name: [Astramorph/PF]	This is a narcotic analgesic. It can be used for pain relief, sedation, reduce left ventricular work by reducing afterload pressure, treat dyspnea associated with acute pulmonary edema and acute left ventricular failure.
Right patient?	In this situation the medication is being administered to relieve dyspnea and also reduce the workload on the heart by afterload reduction.
Right dose?	0.05 mg/kg IV (generally 2 to 4 mg IV first dose and 2 to 8 mg for the second dose).
Right route?	IV, IM, SC, PR.
Right time?	After assessment including vital signs.
Right documentation?	Document the administration of the medication as well as the ongoing assessment findings, including lung sounds on the patient care report.
Expected action	Relief of pulmonary edema, decreased cardiac workload, and anxiety.
Side effects	Hypoventilation, hypovolemia, possible allergic reaction.
Contraindications	Known allergy, mental status changes, hypotension.
Precautions	Monitor respiratory effort and blood pressure, narcotic may depress respirations.
Pharmacokinetics	Onset is 0 to 15 minutes via IV, 10–30 minutes IM/SC/PR; peak 10–15 minutes; duration 2–7 hours IM/SC; metabolized in the liver and excreted in urine.

Questions 5: What specific precautions should you take when administering morphine sulfate [Astramorph/PF] to this patient?

Question 6: Why is aspirin given to this patient?

Part 4

After administering the aspirin and nitroglycerin spray, you recheck the CPAP and it seems to be working properly. As your partner pulls away from the scene heading for the ED, you administer the furosemide [Lasix] and contact medical control for the orders for the morphine sulfate. After presenting the case to the physician on the radio you receive an order for the narcotic and then administer the dose with your Tubex syringe.

Bill's 12-lead ECG has just been obtained and you begin to reassess and obtain some serial vital signs (see **Table 7**).

Bill's wife is riding in the front of the ambulance. She is very nervous and your partner is trying to comfort her by having a conversation as he navigates the ambulance to the ED. It is clear from the conversation that his wife has been taking care of him for many years.

Question 7: Is it possible for a patient to go into acute pulmonary edema with his first MI?

Table 7 **Reassessment and Ongoing Assessment of the Patient**

Serial Vital Signs and Relevant Data	Recording Time: 10 Minutes
Skin CTC	Pale, warm, clammy
Pulse	120 beats/min, rapid and irregular
Blood Pressure	140 palpation mm Hg
Respirations	22 breaths/min and less labored
Mental Status	"A" alert (oriented to person, place, and day)
ECG	Atrial fibrillation (possible MI unconfirmed)
SpO_2	95% on CPAP
Lung Sounds	Considerably louder crackles throughout the lung fields
Other (ie, glucose, core temperature)	n/a

Question 8: Will this patient be admitted to the hospital based on the information presented in this case?

Case Study III Continued

Part 5

As you arrive at the ED you review the prehospital management with the receiving nurse and physician. You are impressed by how much better Bill looks. He is still clammy but not as pale and certainly not as diaphoretic as he was when you arrived at his home. He still has some rhonchi but you need your stethoscope to hear the adventitious sounds up close rather than from the doorway as you did when you arrived in his home. The CPAP has helped improve his condition and he seems to be a little more talkative at this point. That is always a good sign of improvement in a patient with respiratory distress!

You know Bill will have at least a couple of days of intense observation and management in the hospital. He will be back on his no-salt diet and will certainly not be having any late night glasses of tomato juice! You complete your patient care report and greet the patient's son as he arrives from out of town.

Case Study ANSWERS

Case Study I Asthma Attack

Question 1: When does a routine asthma attack become a life-threatening asthma attack?

Answer 1: When it cannot be broken with simple bronchodilators and continues to exist causing the patient to become hypercarbic and/or hypoxic. The term "status asthmaticus" has been used in the past to refer to a life-threatening asthma attack.

Question 2: Why is this patient so dizzy and appears to be wearing out?

Answer 2: As the attack worsens the patient retains CO_2, becomes acidotic and hypoxic, and because of increased insensible water loss also becomes dehydrated. The patient will complain of lightheadedness or dizziness, with increasing fatigue. The work of breathing consumes all available energy and literally wears out the patient.

Question 3: Why do we sometimes ask the patient if they have ever required a "breathing tube" or to be intubated to treat their asthma?

Answer 3: If a patient has previously been intubated, that was definitely a significant and serious attack and the patient will remember the incident. They can also give you some subjective assessment of how today's symptoms compare to that prior event. Other significant historic points specifically related to understanding how severe an asthma attack is and how much therapy early on the patient may require include their last use of steroids to manage an attack, last ED visit for asthma, and last time hospitalized for asthma.

Question 4: How serious is the asthma problem in the US?

Answer 4: In the US, asthma is a disease that affects more than 17 million people, a third of whom are children. Asthma is the most common chronic disease in children, accounting for considerable school absences. Approximately 5,000 patients die from asthma yearly.

Question 5: What is the significance of the patient being on steroids for his disease?

Answer 5: Most physicians do not like to prescribe steroids, especially for lengthy periods of time. They are very effective at reducing the inflammation that comes with lower airway diseases. If the patient is on a steroid and has been for quite some time, that is a "red flag" that this patient has a very serious condition and should be handled as such. Remember, patients can and do die from asthma attacks!

Question 6: Why are you giving him additional steroids?

Answer 6: Because they are effective in fighting the inflammation and secretions that are clogging up his lower airways. Regardless of route of administration, they take time to work (anywhere from 2 to 24 hours), so starting to administer in the prehospital setting is an important part of this patient's care.

Question 7: What is the purpose of administering a steroid in the prehospital setting?

Answer 7: It is important to administer a steroid (glucocorticoid as opposed to mineralocorticoid) to deal with the attack. All steroids take some time to work so they should be started in the prehospital setting to get them "on-board." It really does not matter which specific steroid is used by your EMS system (ie, dexamethasone sodium phosphate [Decadron], methylprednisolone sodium succinate [Solu-Medrol], hydrocortisone sodium phosphate [Solu-Cortef], methylprednisolone acetate [Depo-Medrol], or prednisone [Prednisone Intensol, Sterapred, Sterapred DS]).

Question 8: If the patient was intubated, how does that affect their hospital care?

Answer 8: Asthmatics receiving mechanical ventilation are at serious risk of developing barotrauma. They tend to be very hyperinflated because of expiratory bronchiole collapse, and require careful attention to furnishing adequate expiratory time during the breathing cycle to allow for as complete an exhalation as possible. Failure to do so results in a phenomenon called "breath stacking" also known as "auto-peep." This puts the patient at exceptional risk of developing a pneumothorax, which would progress rapidly into tension given that the patient is also receiving positive-pressure ventilation. Respiratory patients who are serious enough to require prehospital intubation will need to be weaned off the respirator. This could take days to a week and there is always the possibility of pneumonia developing in the intubated patient.

Case Study ANSWERS

Case Study II Pulmonary Embolism

Question 1: This patient is in good physical shape. From your EMT-B and paramedic training, what are three examples of respiratory conditions that could be occurring to Ginny?

Answer 1: Exercise-induced asthma, spontaneous pneumothorax, and pulmonary embolism.

Question 2: What is the significance of the patient saying she does not have any history of asthma?

Answer 2: It explains why she is not taking her own MDI and could help to narrow down the cause of the problem.

Question 3: Does Ginny have any risk factors for pulmonary embolism?

Answer 3: The use of birth control medications is a risk factor because these medications affect levels of natural anticoagulants resulting in a hypercoagulable state. Many PEs occur without any apparent cause.

Question 4: Which of Ginny's vital signs is of most concern?

Answer 4: Ginny's respiratory rate and effort are of most concern. Even after resting her rate remains fast. She has no history of respiratory problems or medical conditions that cause persistent tachypnea.

Question 5: What other conditions can the signs and symptoms of a pulmonary embolism mimic?

Answer 5: The signs and symptoms of a PE are similar to those of an AMI with right heart failure, spontaneous pneumothorax, cardiac tamponade, and shock.

Question 6: What is the significance of blood in Ginny's sputum?

Answer 6: When attempting to make a differential diagnosis, this finding may be helpful. Hemoptysis is not a common finding associated with spontaneous pneumothorax, cardiac tamponade, or shock. Hemoptysis is associated with PE, pneumonia, bronchitis, excessive anticoagulation, heart failure, trauma, tumors in the upper and lower airways, exacerbations of respiratory diseases, and clotting defects.

Question 7: Based on what information you have obtained thus far, would you consider Ginny's chest pain to be cardiac or pleuritic in nature?

Answer 7: Ginny's chest pain is constant and increases with movement, coughing, and radiates up to the shoulder. Her pain is pleuritic when you consider that it increases with movement, coughing, and taking a deep breath, but it could also be cardiac in nature as angina is constant and radiates up to the neck, face, back, and arm.

Question 8: In addition to pain relief, how can morphine sulfate help Ginny?

Answer 8: Morphine sulfate is an opiate analgesic with sedative effects. This drug also helps to relieve anxiety and pulmonary edema, and it reduces left ventricular work by reducing preload pressure. Morphine sulfate can lower blood pressure and cause respiratory depression; therefore, the effects must be monitored closely to avoid an excess in either one of these effects.

Case Study III Acute Pulmonary Edema

Question 1: Would you expect to find pedal edema in this patient and what would be its significance?

Answer 1: Finding pedal edema in this patient would not be a surprise. Usually patients with swollen ankles are having difficulty moving fluids in their body. It could be the result of a cardiac problem, such as chronic heart failure, or a problem of the kidney not removing sufficient fluids from the body. The fluid collects in the dependant areas. If the patient was bedridden, you would expect to see the fluid collected in the sacral area of the spine.

Question 2: Why does the patient literally grab the nonrebreathing mask from your partner?

Answer 2: The patient is so hypoxic and anxious that he grabs the mask to place it on his own face. Sometimes we find these patients up in the middle of the night with their head sticking out of the window trying to get some air.

Case Study ANSWERS

Question 3: What significant medical problems can be caused by atrial fibrillation in a patient who has respiratory distress?

Answer 3: Atrial fibrillation decreases cardiac output because of the loss of atrial kick when the atria do not fill adequately. When a patient is in distress for whatever reason, the normal response is an increased heart rate. With atrial fibrillation, an increased heart rate further decreases cardiac output and the patient gets worse.

Question 4: What type of adventitious breath sounds would you expect to hear on this patient?

Answer 4: This patient would likely have wheezes and crackles (rales). The sounds do not clear with coughing.

Question 5: What specific precautions should you take when administering morphine sulfate [Astramorph/PF] to this patient?

Answer 5: Monitor the respirations closely as the narcotic may depress the patient's respirations.

Question 6: Why is aspirin given to this patient?

Answer 6: The patient may have had another MI exacerbating his underlying heart failure. The aspirin is given for its antiplatelet effects and not as an analgesic.

Question 7: Is it possible for a patient to go into acute pulmonary edema with his first MI?

Answer 7: Yes but it is unlikely. Usually patients who go into acute pulmonary edema do so from heart failure because the mass of damaged myocardial tissue has significantly reduced pumping capacity. Oftentimes patients will present with acute pulmonary edema and CHF several days after an MI because the heart is unable to adequately maintain cardiac output. Occasionally a patient will have CHF as a presenting problem with active MI when the infarct is very large and involves the left ventricle, or if the inferior wall of the heart is involved and results in papillary muscle rupture and associated valve incompetence. As they say, the pump won't work because the vandals took the handles!

Question 8: Will this patient be admitted to the hospital based on the information presented in this case?

Answer 8: Our patient will be admitted to the hospital and may be there for a few days to weeks depending on how quickly he recovers. The patient will likely have bladder catheterization to precisely measure urine output, and will be continued on diuretic and nitrate therapy. Oral and IV input versus output measurements and patient weights will be carefully kept. Oxygen supplementation and positive-pressure ventilation will be continued as a function of patient comfort and arterial blood gas measurement. He will be carefully monitored for persistent or worsening of symptoms, probably in the coronary care unit to begin with. Depending on the source of his problem, the patient could require treatment from the cardiology, renal, pulmonary, and infectious disease services while staying in the hospital.

Medication Review

Albuterol (Proventil, Ventolin)

Indications Treatment of bronchospasm in patients with reversible obstructive airway disease (COPD/asthma). Prevention of exercise-induced bronchospasm.

Contraindications Known prior hypersensitivity reactions to albuterol. Tachycardia arrhythmias, especially those caused by digitalis. Synergistic with other sympathomimetics.

Dosage and administration Adult: Administer 2.5 mg (0.5 mL of the 0.5% solution) added to 2 mL of normal saline for inhalation by nebulizer treatment and administer over 10–15 minutes. May repeat every 20 minutes up to three times. MDI: 1–2 inhalations (90–180 µg). Five minutes between inhalations. Pediatric (between the ages of 2 and 12): administer 2.5 mg (0.5 mL of the 0.083% solution) added to 2 mL of normal saline for inhalation by nebulizer treatment and administer over 10–15 minutes. May repeat every 20 minutes up to three times.

Benzocaine Spray (Hurricane)

Indications Used as a lubricant and topical anesthetic to facilitate passage of diagnostic and treatment devices. Suppresses the pharyngeal and tracheal gag reflex.

Contraindications Patients with a known hypersensitivity to benzocaine.

Dosage and administration Adult: 0.5–1.0 second spray, repeat as needed. Pediatric: 0.25–0.5 second spray, repeat as needed.

Dexamethasone Sodium Phosphate (Decadron, Hexadrol)

Indications Anaphylaxis, asthma, croup.

Contraindications Hypersensitivity to product, systemic sepsis, bacterial infection.

Dosage and administration Adult: 10–100 mg IV (1 mg/kg slow IV bolus) (considerable variance through medical control). Pediatric: 0.25–1.0 mg/kg/dose IV, IO, IM.

Diazepam (Valium)

Indications Acute anxiety states, acute alcohol withdrawal (delirium tremens), muscle relaxant, seizure activity, agitation. Analgesia for medical procedures (fracture reduction, cardioversion).

Contraindications Hypersensitivity, glaucoma, coma, shock, substance abuse, head injury.

Dosage and administration Seizure activity: Adult: 5–10 mg IV every 10–15 minutes as needed (5 mg over 5 min) (maximum dose, 30 mg). Seizure activity: Pediatric: 0.2–0.5 mg slowly every 2–5 minutes up to 5 mg (maximum dose, 10 mg/kg). Rectal diazepam: 0.5 mg/kg via rectal catheter and flush with 2–3 mL air after administration. Sedation for cardioversion: 5–15 mg IV over 5–10 minutes prior to cardioversion.

Medication Review

Epinephrine (Adrenalin)

Indications Cardiac arrest (V-fib/pulseless V-tach, asystole, PEA), symptomatic bradycardia as an alternative infusion to dopamine, severe hypotension secondary to bradycardia when atropine and transcutaneous pacing are unsuccessful, allergic reactions, anaphylaxis, asthma.

Contraindications Hypertension, hypothermia, pulmonary edema, myocardial ischemia, hypovolemic shock.

Dosage and administration Adult: Mild allergic reactions and asthma: 0.3–0.5 mg (0.3–0.5 mL of 1:1,000) SC. Anaphylaxis: 0.1 mg (1 mL of 1:10,000) IV/IO over 5 minutes. Cardiac arrest: IV/IO dose: 1 mg (10 mL of 1:10,000 solution) every 3–5 minutes during resuscitation. Follow each dose with 20 mL flush and elevate arm for 10 to 20 seconds after dose. Higher dose: Higher doses (up to 0.2 mg/kg) may be used for specific indications (beta-blocker or calcium channel blocker overdose). Continuous infusion: Add 1 mg (1 mL of 1:1,000 solution) to 500 mL normal saline or D_5W. Initial infusion rate of 1 μg/min titrated to effect (typical dose: 2–10 μg/min). Endotracheal (ET) dose: 2–2.5 mg diluted in 10 mL normal saline. Profound bradycardia or hypotension: 2–10 μg/min; titrate to patient response. Pediatric: Mild allergic reactions and asthma: 0.01 mg/kg (0.01 mL/kg) of 1:1,000 solution SC (maximum of 0.3 mL). Cardiac arrest: IV/IO dose: 0.01 mg/kg (0.1 mL/kg) of 1:10,000 solution every 3–5 minutes during arrest. All endotracheal (ET) doses: 0.1 mg/kg (0.1 mL/kg) of 1:1,000 solution. Symptomatic bradycardia: IV/IO dose: 0.01 mg/kg (0.1 mL/kg) of 1:10,000 solution. Continuous IV/IO infusion: Begin with rapid infusion, then titrate to response. Typical initial infusion: 0.1–1 μg/min. Higher doses may be effective.

Epinephrine Racemic (Micronefrin, Vaponefrin)

Indications Bronchial asthma, prevention of bronchospasm. Croup, laryngotracheobronchitis, laryngeal edema.

Contraindications Hypertension, underlying cardiovascular disease, epiglottitis.

Dosage and administration Adult: MDI: 2–3 inhalations, repeated every 5 minutes as needed. Solution: dilute 5 mL (1%) in 5.0 mL NS, administer over 15 minutes. Pediatric: Solution: dilute 0.25 mL (0.1%) in 2.5 mL NS (if less than 20 kg); dilute 0.5 mL in 2.5 mL NS (if 20–40 kg); dilute 0.75 mL in 2.5 mL NS (if greater than 40 kg). Administer by aerosolization.

Furosemide (Lasix)

Indications CHF, pulmonary edema, hypertensive crisis.

Contraindications Hypovolemia, anuria, hypotension (relative contraindication); hypersensitivity, hepatic coma.

Dosage and administration Adult: 0.5–1.0 mg/kg injected IV over 1 to 2 minutes. If no response, double the dose to 2 mg/kg over 1 to 2 minutes. Pediatric: 1 mg/kg/dose IV, IO.

Hydrocortisone Sodium Succinate (Solu-Cortef)

Indications Shock due to acute adrenocortical insufficiency.

Contraindications None if given as single dose.

Dosage and administration Adult: 4 mg/kg slow IV bolus. Pediatric: 0.16–1.0 mg/kg slow IV bolus.

Medication Review

Ipratropium Bromide (Atrovent)

Indications Maintenance treatment of bronchospasm in patients with reversible obstructive airway disease (COPD/asthma). Can be used alone or in combination with other bronchodilators (especially beta-adrenergics).

Contraindications Known prior hypersensitivity reactions to ipratropium bromide. Hypersensitivity to atropine or any anticholinergic derivatives or to soya lecithin or related food products.

Dosage and administration Adult: Administer 500 μg (1 Unit-Dose vial) administered three to four times a day by oral nebulization, with doses 6 to 8 hours apart. Ipratropium Bromide Inhalation Solution Unit-Dose vials contain 500 μg Ipratropium bromide anhydrous in 2.5 mL normal saline. Ipratropium Bromide Inhalation Solution can be mixed in the nebulizer with albuterol or metaproterenol if used within 1 hour. Pediatric: Safety and effectiveness in the pediatric population younger than age 12 years have not been established.

Isoetharine (Bronchosol, Bronkometer)

Indications Acute bronchial asthma, bronchospasm (especially in COPD patient).

Contraindications Use with caution in patients with diabetes, hyperthyroidism, cardiovascular and cerebrovascular disease.

Dosage and administration Adult: 1–2 inhalations with MDI. COPD: 2.5–5.0 mg (0.25 mL–0.5 mL) diluted in 3 mL normal saline (NS) and nebulized. Pediatric: 0.01 mL/kg; maximum dose: 0.5 mL diluted in 3 mL NS and nebulized.

Metaproterenol 5% (Alupent)

Indications Bronchial asthma, reversible bronchospasm secondary to bronchitis, COPD.

Contraindications Tachyarrhythmias, hypersensitivity, tachycardias due to digitalis toxicity.

Dosage and administration Adult: MDI: 2–3 inhalations every 3–4 hours (2 minutes between inhalations). Inhalation solution 5%: via hand-held nebulizer 0.2–0.3 mL diluted in 2.5 mL saline. Inhalation solution unit-dose 0.4% or 0.6% vials: intermittent positive-pressure breathing device only: one vial/treatment. Pediatric: MDI: not recommended. Inhalation solution 5%: age 6–12 years: 0.1–0.2 mL diluted in 3 mL saline.

Methylprednisolone Sodium Succinate (Solu-Medrol)

Indications Acute spinal cord trauma, anaphylaxis, bronchodilator for unresponsive asthma.

Contraindications Premature infants, systemic fungal infections; use with caution in patients with gastrointestinal bleeding.

Dosage and administration Adult: Acute spinal cord injury: 30 mg/kg IV over 30 minutes followed by infusion: 5.4 mg/kg/h. Asthma, COPD: 1–2 mg/kg IV. Pediatric: Acute spinal cord trauma: 30 mg/kg IV over 30 minutes; infusion: 5.4 mg/kg/h. Asthma: 1–2 mg/kg/dose IV.

Midazolam (Versed)

Indications Sedation, anxiolytic prior to endotracheal or nasotracheal intubation; administer for conscious sedation.

Contraindications Glaucoma, shock, coma, alcohol intoxication, overdose, depressed vital signs, concomitant use with other CNS depressants, barbiturates, alcohol, narcotics.

Dosage and administration Adult: 2.0–2.5 mg slow IV over 2–3 minutes; may be repeated to total maximum: 0.1 mg/kg. Pediatric: Not recommended.

Medication Review

Morphine Sulfate (Astramorph/PF and others)

Indications Severe CHF, pulmonary edema, chest pain associated with acute MI, analgesia for moderate to severe acute and chronic pain (use with caution).

Contraindications Head injury, exacerbated COPD, depressed respiratory drive, hypotension, undiagnosed abdominal pain, decreased level of consciousness, suspected hypovolemia, patients who have taken MAOIs within the past 14 days.

Dosage and administration Adult: Initial dose: 2–4 mg IV (over 1–5 minutes) every 5–30 minutes. Repeat dose: 2–8 mg at 5- to 15-minute intervals. Pediatric: 0.1–0.2 mg/kg per dose via IV, IO, IM, or SC; maximum dose of 5 mg.

Nalbuphine (Nubain)

Indications Chest pain associated with acute MI; moderate to severe acute pain; pulmonary edema, with or without associated chest pain (morphine remains first line).

Contraindications Head injury or undiagnosed abdominal pain, diarrhea caused by poisoning, hypovolemia, hypotension.

Dosage and administration Adult: 2–5 mg slowly IV; may repeat 2-mg doses as needed to maximum dose of 10 mg. Pediatric: Not recommended.

Naloxone Hydrochloride (Narcan)

Indications Opiate overdose, coma; complete or partial reversal of CNS and respiratory depression induced by opioids; decreased level of consciousness; coma of unknown origin; narcotic agonist for the following: morphine sulfate, heroin, hydromorphone (Dilaudid), methadone, meperidine (Demerol), paregoric, fentanyl citrate (Sublimase), oxycodone (Percodan), codeine, propoxyphene (Darvon); narcotic agonist and antagonist for the following: butorphanol (Stadol), pentazocine (Talwin), nalbuphine (Nubain).

Contraindications Use with caution in narcotic-dependent patients; use with caution in neonates of narcotic-addicted mothers.

Dosage and administration Adult: 0.4–2.0 mg IV, IM, SC, or ET (diluted); minimum recommended dose, 0.4 mg; repeat at 5-minute intervals to a maximum dose of 10 mg (medical control may request higher amounts). Infusion: 2 mg in 500 mL of D_5W (4 µg/mL), infuse at 0.4 mg/h (100 mL/h). Pediatric: 0.1 mg/kg/dose IV, IM, SC, ET (diluted); maximum dose of 0.8 mg; if no response in 10 minutes, administer an additional 0.1 mg/kg/dose.

Nifedipine (Procardia)

Indications Hypertensive crisis, angina pectoris, pulmonary edema (investigational).

Contraindications Compensatory hypertension, hypotension, hypersensitivity.

Dosage and administration Adult: 10 mg SL or buccal (puncture end of capsule with needle and squeeze; may administer SL or buccally or may have patient bite and swallow); may repeat in 30 minutes. Pediatric: Not recommended.

Nitroglycerin (Nitrostat, Tridil, and others)

Indications Acute angina pectoris, ischemic chest pain, hypertension, CHF, pulmonary edema.

Contraindications Hypotension, hypovolemia; intracranial bleeding or head injury; previous administration of Viagra, Revatio, Levitra, Cialis, or similar agents within past 24 hours.

Dosage and administration Adult: Tablets: 0.3–0.4 mg SL; may repeat in 3–5 minutes to maximum of 3 doses. Nitroglycerin (NTG) spray: 0.4 mg under the tongue; 1–2 sprays. NTG IV infusion: begin at 10 to 20 µg/min; increase by 5–10 µg/min every 5 minutes until desired effect. Pediatric: Not recommended.

Medication Review

Nitropaste (Nitro-Bid Ointment)

Indications Angina pectoris and chest pain associated with acute MI.

Contraindications Same as NTG.

Dosage and administration Adult: Paste: Apply ½ to ¾ (1–2 cm), 15–30 mg, cover with wrap and secure with tape; maximum, 5 (75 mg) per application. Transdermal: Apply unit to intact skin (usually chest wall) in varying doses. Pediatric: Not recommended.

Ondansetron Hydrochloride (Zofran)

Indications For the prevention or control of nausea or vomiting. Also used in the hospital setting for patients undergoing chemotherapy or surgical procedures.

Contraindications Known allergy to this medicine or other 5-HT3 receptor antagonists.

Dosage and administration Adult: 4 mg IV or IM (may repeat in 10 minutes). Pediatric: 0.1 mg/kg IV or IM.

Oxygen

Indications Confirmed or expected hypoxemia, ischemic chest pain, respiratory insufficiency, prophylactically during air transport, confirmed or suspected carbon monoxide poisoning, all other causes of decreased tissue oxygenation, decreased level of consciousness.

Contraindications Certain patients with COPD or emphysema who will not tolerate oxygen concentrations over 35%, hyperventilation. Oxygen should never be withheld from a patient who needs it, however. Be prepared to assist with ventilations in a patient with COPD who requires high concentrations, as apnea may result.

Dosage and administration Adult: Cardiac arrest and carbon monoxide poisoning: 100%. Hypoxemia: 10–15 L/min via nonrebreathing mask. COPD: 1–6 L/min via nasal cannula or 28%–35% Venturi mask. Be prepared to provide ventilatory support if higher concentrations of oxygen needed. Pediatric: Same as for adult with exception of premature infant.

Pancuronium Bromide (Pavulon)

Indications Induction or maintenance of paralysis after intubation to assist ventilations.

Contraindications Hypersensitivity, inability to control airway and support ventilations with oxygen and positive pressure, neuromuscular disease (myasthenia gravis), hepatic or renal failure.

Dosage and administration Adult: 0.1 mg/kg slow IV; repeat every 30–60 minutes as needed. Pediatric: 0.1 mg/kg slow IV, IO.

Promethazine Hydrochloride (Phenergan)

Indications Nausea, vomiting, motion sickness; sedation for patients in labor; potentiation of analgesic effects of narcotics.

Contraindications Hypersensitivity, coma, CNS-depressed patients from alcohol, barbiturates, narcotics, Reye's syndrome.

Dosage and administration Adult: 12.5–25 mg IV, deep IM, PO, rectally. Pediatric: (older than 2 years old) 0.25–0.5 mg/kg dose IM.

Succinylcholine Chloride (Anectine, Quelicin)

Indications To facilitate intubation, to terminate laryngospasm, to promote muscle relaxation, to facilitate electroconvulsive shock therapy.

Contraindications Acute narrow angle glaucoma, penetrating eye injuries, inability to control airway or support ventilations with oxygen and positive pressure.

Dosage and administration Adult: 1–2 mg/kg rapid IV; repeat once if needed. Pediatric: 1–1.5 mg/kg dose rapid IV, IO; repeat once if needed.

Medication Review

Terbutaline Sulfate (Brethine, Bricanyl)

Indications Bronchial asthma, reversible bronchospasm associated with exercise, chronic bronchitis, and emphysema.

Contraindications Hypersensitivity, tachyarrhythmias.

Dosage and administration Adult: 0.25 mg SC; may repeat in 15–30 minutes to maximum dose of 0.5 mg in 4-hour period. 400 µg (two inhalations by MDI) every 4–6 hours; allow 1–2 minutes between inhalations. Pediatric: Not recommended for children younger than 12 years of age; 0.01 mg/kg/dose SC every 15–20 minutes as needed to maximum 0.25 mg dose. 0.03–0.05 mg/kg in 1.25 mL saline for aerosolization every 4 hours.

Vecuronium Bromide (Norcuron)

Indications To facilitate intubation, to terminate laryngospasm, to promote muscle relaxation, to facilitate electroconvulsive shock therapy.

Contraindications Acute narrow angle glaucoma, penetrating eye injuries, inability to control airway or support ventilations with oxygen and positive pressure, newborns, myasthenia gravis, hepatic or renal failure.

Dosage and administration Adult: 0.1 mg/kg IV push; maintenance dose within 25–40 minutes: 0.01–0.05 mg/kg IV push. Pediatric: 0.1 mg/kg IV, IO; maintenance dose within 20–35 minutes: 0.01–0.05 mg/kg IV push.

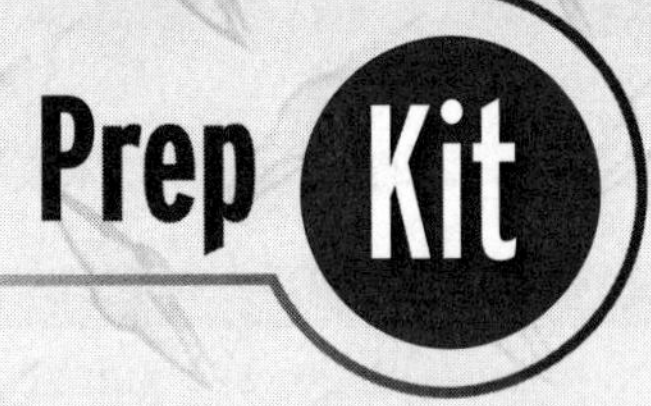

Chapter Summary

- Patients who have a partial obstruction of the upper airway describe difficulty getting air into their lungs. Those with lower airway obstruction describe difficulty getting the air out of their chest.
- Physicians prescribe a number of medications for the treatment of obstructive or reactive airway conditions. These medications fall into a number of categories such as: bronchodilators, sympathomimetics, parasympatholytics, steroids, and leukotriene blockers.
- Common respiratory conditions include asthma, chronic bronchitis, emphysema, pneumonia, pulmonary edema, pulmonary embolism, neoplasms of the lung, upper respiratory infections, spontaneous pneumothorax, and hyperventilation syndrome.
- Providing steroids in the prehospital setting tends to produce better results than waiting for the patient's condition to worsen in the hospital setting.
- When a patient's breathing becomes ineffective and requires assistance, there are three treatment options the paramedic may use to ventilate the patient: bag-mask device, CPAP, and oral or nasal endotracheal intubation.
- Heart failure medications may include several classes of drugs: diuretics, ACE inhibitors, digitalis, nitrates, and beta-blockers.
- Diuretics are used to lower blood pressure and help the body eliminate excess water and sodium. There are three types of diuretics you may find prescribed to patients: loop diuretics, thiazides, and Potassium "K" sparing drugs.

Vital Vocabulary

ACE inhibitors Relax blood vessels and may slow or prevent the loss of heart pumping activity.

Antihistamine A drug that counteracts the release of histamine such as occurs in allergic reactions.

Antitussives Medications designed to stop coughing.

Beta-blockers Reduce the heart rate and blood pressure.

Bronchodilators Medications that are designed to dilate the smooth muscle of the bronchioles which in turn decreases airway resistance and often eliminates wheezing from obstructed or reactive lower airways.

Chronic obstructive pulmonary disease (COPD) A general category of airway diseases involving long-term obstruction. This includes conditions such as emphysema, chronic bronchitis, asbestosis, and black lung disease.

Digitalis Improves circulation by increasing the force of the heart's contraction.

Diuretics Help reduce blood pressure and water retention.

Dyspnea The sensation of shortness of breath.

Expectorants Medications that thin out secretions so they can be coughed up.

Glucocorticoid Any group of anti-inflammatory steroidlike compounds, such as hydrocortisone, that are produced by the adrenal cortex, are involved in carbohydrate, protein, and fat metabolism, and are used as anti-inflammatory agents.

Leukotriene blockers Medications that have been designed to inhibit the release of leukotrines which are 1,000 times more potent than histamine in producing inflammation in the asthmatic patient.

Loop diuretics Powerful diuretic medication used in the management of heart failure (ie, furosemide [Lasix]). The drug acts on the loop of Henlé, a structure of the kidney involved in reabsorbing water.

Methylxanthines Previously the mainstay of prehospital medications for the asthmatic or COPD patient.

Mineralocorticoid Any of a group of steroid hormones that are secreted by the adrenal cortex and regulate the balance of water and electrolytes in the body.

Nitrates Relax the blood vessels to improve circulation.

Parasympatholytics An anticholinergic drug producing effects resembling those of interruption of the parasympathetic nerve supply to block the transmission of impulses.

Potassium "K" sparing drugs Diuretics that do not promote the secretion of potassium into the urine.

Proxsysmal nocturnal dyspnea (PND) The sensation of difficulty in breathing that comes on in the middle of the night, usually after the patient has been sleeping in a supine position.

ST-segment elevation myocardial infarction (STEMI) A heart attack, or MI, that is caused by a prolonged period of blocked blood supply. It affects a large area of the heart muscle, and so causes changes on the ECG involving elevation of the ST segments in two or more leads, as well as changes in blood levels of key chemical markers.

Status asthmaticus Severe and prolonged asthma attack that does not respond to standard medications.

Steroids There are three types of steroids: corticosteroids, estrogens and progesterones, and androgens. The corticosteroids are related to the hormones in the body associated with the adrenal cortex (ie, OTC creams for rashes). The estrogens and progesterones are steroids associated with the female sex hormones (ie, in prescription birth control). The androgens are the most controversial as they are related to the male sex hormone testosterone and have been used to build up muscle mass.

Sympathomimetics Drugs that mimic the effects of the sympathetic nervous system on the body.

Thiazides A type of diuretic drug derived from benzothiadiazine. They inhibit Na^+Cl^- reabsorption from the distal convoluted tubules in the kidneys by blocking the thiazide-sensitive Na^+Cl^- symporter. Thiazides also cause loss of potassium and an increase in serum uric acid.

Vasodilator Medication that acts on the smooth muscles of the arterioles and veins.

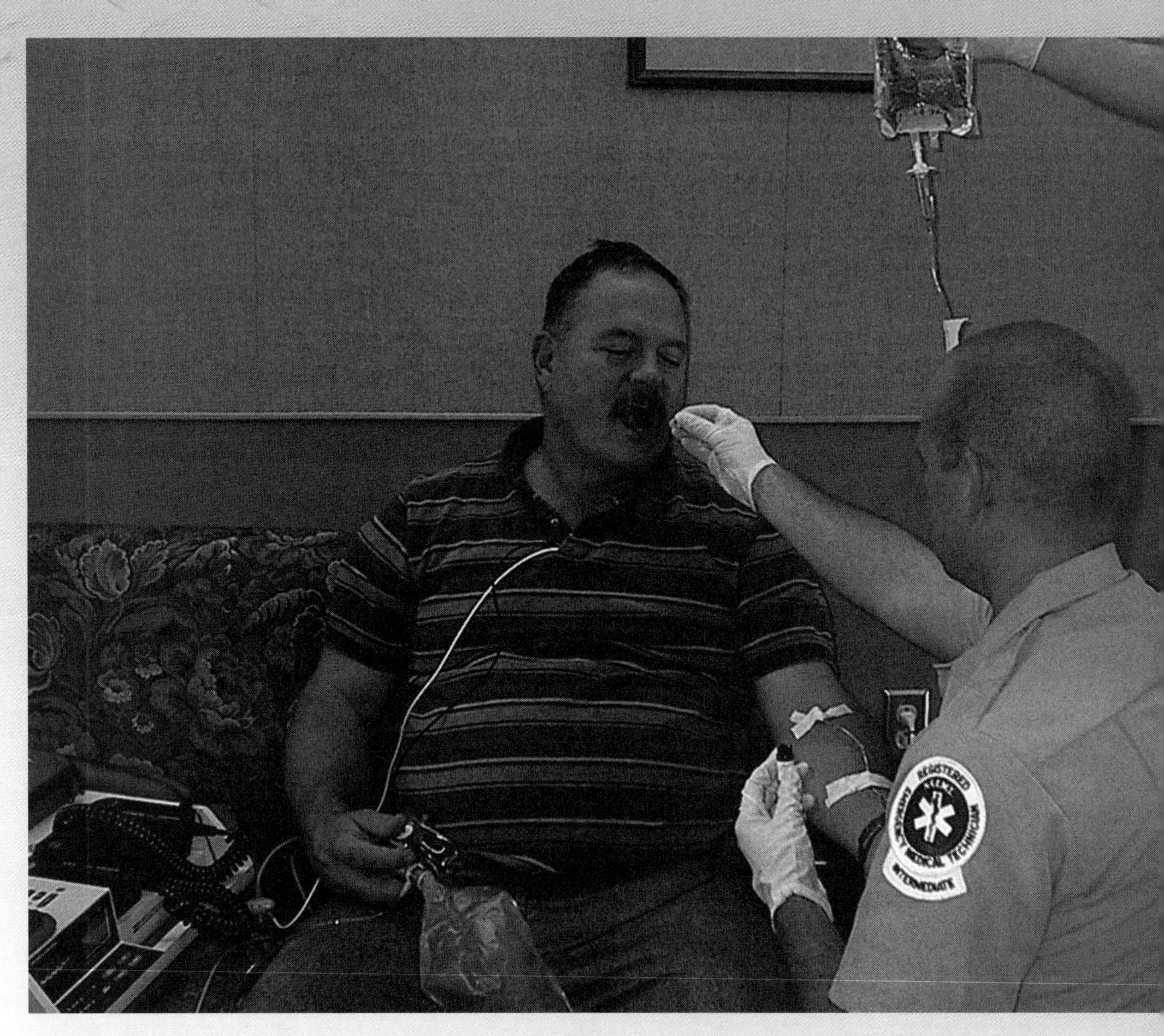
REGISTERED

Cardiovascular Emergencies 4

Objectives

Cognitive

5-2.51 Identify the major therapeutic objectives in the treatment of the patient with any arrhythmia. (pages 126–134)

5-2.52 Identify the major mechanical, pharmacological and electrical therapeutic interventions. (pages 126–136)

5-2.84 Describe the most commonly used cardiac drugs in terms of therapeutic effect and dosages, routes of administration, side effects and toxic effects. (pages 118–185)

5-2.95 Describe the most commonly used pharmacological agents in the management of congestive heart failure in terms of therapeutic effect, dosages, routes of administration, side effects and toxic effects. (pages 162–167)

5-2.110 Identify the drugs of choice for hypertensive emergencies, rational for use, clinical precautions and disadvantages of selected antihypertensive agents. (pages 162–172)

5-2.118 Describe the most commonly used pharmacological agents in the management of cardiogenic shock in terms of therapeutic effects, dosages, routes of administration, side effects and toxic effects. (pages 162–167)

5-2.129 Describe the most commonly used pharmacological agents in the management of cardiac arrest in terms of therapeutic effects. (pages 126–134)

Affective

None

Psychomotor

None

Additional Objectives

4-1 Discuss the following medications used in the prehospital and/or in-hospital setting for patients with acute pulmonary edema or acute coronary syndrome: acetylsalicylic acid [Aspirin], adenosine [Adenocard], amiodarone [Cordarone], atropine sulfate [Atropine], ß-Adrenergic receptor blockers (beta-blockers), calcium chloride, clopidogrel [Plavix], diltiazem hydrochloride [Cardizem], dopamine [Intropin], dobutamine [Dobutrex], epinephrine [Adrenalin], furosemide [Lasix], Glycoprotein IIb/IIIa inhibitor (eptifi batide [Integrelin]), isoproterenol hydrochloride [Isuprel], heparin (unfractioned and low-molecular weight [Lovenox]), labetalol [Normodyne], lidocaine hydrochloride [Xylocaine], magnesium sulfate [Magnesium], metoprolol tartrate/metoprolol succinate [Lopressor], morphine sulfate [Astramorph/PF], nitroglycerin [Nitrostat] tablet, paste, spray, nitroglycerin infusion [Tridil], norepinephrine bitartrate [Levophed], ondansetron hydrochloride [Zofran], oxygen, procainamide hydrochloride [Procanbid, Pronestyl], sodium bicarbonate [Citrocarbonate], tissue plasminogen activator [t-PA, Alteplase], vasopressin [Pitressin], ACE inhibitors/angiotensin receptor blocker (ARB). (pages 118–185)

4-2 Discuss the following medications used in the prehospital setting and/or in-hospital setting for the patient with hypotension of a cardiac origin, and/or cardiogenic shock: oxygen, epinephrine [Adrenalin], dopamine [Intropin], dobutamine [Dobutrex]. (pages 162–167)

4-3 Discuss the following medications used in the prehospital and/or in-hospital setting for a hypertensive emergency: nicardipine [Cardene], sodium nitroprusside [Nitropress], nitroglycerin infusion [Tridil], labetalol [Normodyne]. (pages 167–172)

4-4 List the following medications that may be used in the prehospital and/or in-hospital setting for patients with symptomatic arrhythmias and/or cardiac arrest: amiodarone [Cordarone], diltiazem hydrochloride [Cardizem], epinephrine, lidocaine hydrochloride [Xylocaine], vasopressin, verapamil [Isoptin, Calan], atropine sulfate [Atropine], adenosine [Adenocard], ibutilide fumarate [Corvert], milrinone lactate [Primacor], atenolol [Tenormin], propranolol hydrochloride [Inderal], esmolol [Brevibloc], calcium chloride, digoxin [Digitek], isoproterenol hydrochloride [Isuprel], procainamide hydrochloride [Pronestyl, Procanbid], sodium bicarbonate [Citrocarbonate], magnesium sulfate [for torsades de pointes and cross reference to preeclampsia]. (pages 126–161)

Acute Coronary Syndrome (ACS)

Rather than specifically discussing the **acute myocardial infarction (AMI)**, current educational materials and research all refer to a broader category of cardiovascular disorders associated with coronary **atherosclerosis**. These disorders may be associated with a spectrum of clinical syndromes that represent varying degrees of coronary occlusion. The general heading for the syndromes (ie, unstable angina, non-Q wave MI, Q wave MI, and sudden cardiac death) is acute coronary syndrome or ACS.

The Value of Aspirin in ACS

Prostaglandins are one of a number of hormone-like substances that participate in a wide range of body functions (ie, contraction/relaxation of smooth muscle, dilation/constriction of blood vessels, control of blood pressure, and modulation of inflammation). These substances, derived from arachidonic acid, are found in tissues throughout the body, but are especially associated with being found in places where there is pain and inflammation, as they are key in the activation of inflammatory responses both locally and systemically. They are derived from fatty acids. Some types of prostaglandins cause platelets in blood to stick together to form a blood clot. This is good when you want to stop a nosebleed or bleeding from a laceration, but this is bad when a blood clot is causing a heart attack. Aspirin has the property of inhibiting prostaglandin production. For this reason, many adults take a low dose (81–325 mg/day) to help prevent heart attacks and it is why aspirin is administered when a person is suspected of having ACS.

Case Study 1 A Potential Candidate for Fibrinolysis

Part 1

It is mid-afternoon when a call for chest pain comes in. The address is in the high finance business area and the location is on the third floor. Security is there to meet you and direct you to an executive suite. The scene is safe so you and your partner proceed with your full equipment piled on the stretcher. When you enter the office there is an overweight male in his 50s who is pale/gray and diaphoretic. He is sitting on a couch clutching his chest in the typical "Levine's sign" fashion. You recall from your paramedic training that when you see a patient who has their fist pressed to their sternum and is expressing pain (Levine's sign), this is often a typical presentation in a coronary event. He does not look good so you and your partner waste no time. The first priority is to alleviate the patient's physical and emotional distress and then proceed with obtaining a history and a set of baseline vital signs as part of the initial assessment (see **Table 1**).

Table 1 Initial Assessment

Initial Assessment	Recording Time: 1 Minute
General Impression/ Appearance	Sick, pale/gray, diaphoretic
Mental Status	Alert and distressed
Airway	Open
Breathing	Short of breath
Circulation	Poor color and weak distal pulse
Priority/Plan	High

Case Study 1 Continued

The patient is Rob Jenson and he works here in this office as an attorney. Today he received news regarding a huge loss in the stock market. Soon after, he developed 8/10 substernal chest pain with radiation to the neck and left arm. He also became sweaty and is having difficulty breathing. He tells you that the pain has increased to a 10 since the onset. Mr. Jenson tells you that he feels like a horse is sitting on his chest. Vital signs are taken and reveal a weak and slightly irregular distal pulse. High flow oxygen is applied right away and his blood pressure is obtained. His lung sounds will need to be assessed, and because he is extremely diaphoretic it will be difficult to get the cardiac electrodes to stick.

Since there is no apparent trauma and the patient is responsive, you will need to conduct a focused history and physical examination for a responsive medical patient with a chief complaint of chest pain. The OPQRST questions will be used to elaborate on the chief complaint while you begin to conduct your focused history and physical examination. You recall your medical director saying, "once you have some baseline vitals get MONA in place for the ACS patient!" MONA is an acronym that stands for morphine, oxygen, nitrates (nitro), and aspirin. It is not given in that order but MONA is easier to remember than AONM or OANM, depending on your local protocols.

Question 1: Do all patients who may be experiencing a heart attack have crushing chest pain?

Question 2: If the patient has his fist on his chest, what is that sign called and what is its relevance?

Part 2

Mr. Jenson's pain began 20 minutes ago while on the phone. The heaviness in the chest and shortness of breath is like nothing he has experienced before and he says he knows he is having a heart attack. He is scared and wants to know if he is going to die. You reassure him that he is in good hands and that you will get him to the hospital right away. Mr. Jenson takes atorvastatin calcium [Lipitor], labetalol [Normodyne], and aspirin daily and he has no allergies to medications. Your partner has finished taking vital signs and respirations are 26 breaths/min, pulse rate is 88 beats/min weak and slightly irregular, and blood pressure is 118/64 mm Hg (see **Table 2**). The neck veins are flat, abdomen is obese, soft, and non-tender, and he has no peripheral

Table 2 Focused History and Physical Examination

Baseline Vital Signs	Recording Time: 5 Minutes
Skin CTC (color, temperature, condition)	Pale/gray, diaphoretic
Pulse	88 beats/min weak, slightly irregular
Blood Pressure	118/64 mm Hg
Respirations	26 breaths/min with clear lung sounds

Case Study 1 Continued

(pedal) edema. The three-lead ECG is abnormal with **ST segment** elevation in lead I, and depression in II and III with occasional premature ventricular contractions (PVCs). You administer nitroglycerin sublingual (SL) and aspirin with instructions to chew first and then swallow. You then obtain a 12-lead ECG while getting ready to start the IV. You remember that the administration of nitroglycerin is not only a treatment but also a diagnostic indicator. The failure of the nitroglycerin to relieve the chest pain could be an indication of AMI instead of simply angina. Of course as you have always been reminded by your instructors, "the true diagnosis of AMI is made based on a good history as well as the findings of the 12-lead ECG and serial cardiac enzymes." In this instance, the 12-lead ECG is also abnormal with significant ST segment elevation in aVL, V3-6 and depression in II, III, and aVF which, in concert with the clinical picture, you interpret as representative of an anterolateral wall **ST segment elevation myocardial infarction (STEMI)**. The left anterior descending artery and circumflex artery and its branches are most likely affected. Mr. Jenson is experiencing the classic signs of a heart attack or AMI with chest pain, dyspnea, diaphoresis, neck and arm pain, and an abnormal ECG.

Question 3: If the patient does not have relief after taking two sprays of nitroglycerin, what may this indicate?

Question 4: What is the significance of a patient taking an aspirin every day?

Part 3

Once the IV is established, another blood pressure reading is obtained. Mr. Jenson's pain is 9 of 10 and his blood pressure is holding at 118/64 mm Hg. Another dose of nitroglycerin is administered as you move him to the ambulance. Once settled in the ambulance you will reassess the patient and give early notification to the ED of the interpretation of the 12-lead ECG in this suspected ACS patient. This will reduce the door-to-catheterization or door-to-fibrinolytics time and that is why it has been written into your regional ALS protocols for the suspected ACS patient. You judge that this patient needs to go to the interventional cardiac catheterization laboratory as soon as possible. In the elevator the remaining SAMPLE history is obtained (see **Table 3**). Mr. Jenson takes medication for hypertension and is compliant with all his medications. He is a smoker and is trying to lose weight. For lunch he had a low sodium vegetable dish with white rice. He feels nauseous now and is going to vomit. Your partner is quick to remove the oxygen mask and hand him an emesis basin. He will get a dose of antiemetic in the ambulance.

Table 3 SAMPLE History

SAMPLE History	Comments
Signs/symptoms	Chest pain described as heaviness, dyspnea, diaphoretic, poor signs of circulation
Allergies	No known drug allergies (NKDA)
Medications	atorvastatin calcium [Lipitor], labetalol [Normodyne], acetylsalicylic acid [aspirin].
Pertinent past medical history	Hypertension, stress, overweight, smoker
Last oral intake	Low sodium vegetable dish with white rice for lunch
Events leading up to the incident	Shockingly bad news

Treatment Plan

1. Administer supplemental oxygen.
2. Administer acetylsalicylic acid [Aspirin] (see **Table 4**).
3. Administer nitroglycerin [Nitrostat] (see **Table 5**).
4. Relieve the stress on the heart.
5. Obtain a 12-lead ECG.
6. Administer morphine sulfate [Astramorph PF] (see **Table 6**) and consider ondansetron hydrochloride [Zofran] (see **Table 7**).
7. Consider metoprolol tartrate [Lopressor] (see **Table 8**).
8. Move the patient to a facility where they can provide thrombolytic therapy (fibrinolysis) or coronary catheterization because "time is muscle!"

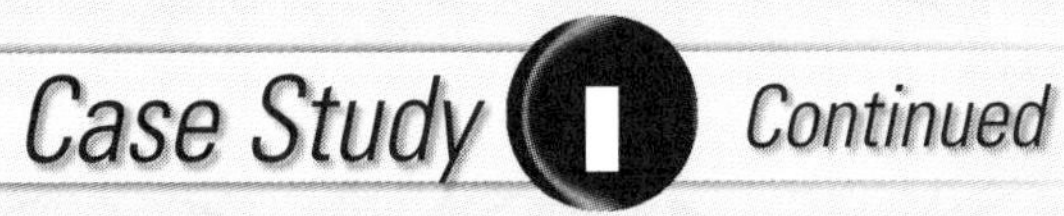

Table 4 Acetylsalicylic Acid

Do you know?	Comments
Right Drug? Generic name: [**Acetylsalicylic Acid**] Trade name: [Aspirin, ASA, Empirin, Genprin, Genuine Bayer Aspirin, Norwich Extra Strength, Bayer Children's Aspirin, St. Joseph Adult Chewable Aspirin, Ecotrin, Halfprin 81, Heartline, Zorprin, Easprin, Asaphen, Entrophen, Novasen]	This drug is a nonsteroidal anti-inflammatory with analgesic and antipyretic effects. Its ability to stop prostaglandin production and inhibit platelet aggregation is why it is used for cardiovascular reasons.
Right patient?	Suspected ACS.
Right dose?	81- to 325-mg tablets—follow local protocol.
Right route?	Chewed and swallowed.
Right time?	As soon as possible after developing signs and symptoms of a suspected ACS.
Right documentation?	Document the administration of the medication as well as the ongoing assessment findings, including lung sounds on the patient care report.
Expected action	Inhibiting clot formation.
Side effects	Stomach irritation, increased bleeding, allergic reaction.
Contraindications	Known hypersensitivity to salicylates, severe bleeding, or anemia. Relative contraindication to patients with active ulcer disease or asthma.
Precautions	Generally not recommended for children. Should definitely not be used in children or teenagers with flu symptoms or chickenpox due to the possibility of Reye's syndrome.
Pharmacokinetics	Rapidly absorbed in the GI tract; peak is variable depending on dose; excreted in urine.

Table 5 Nitroglycerin

Do you know?	Comments
Right drug? Generic name: [**Nitroglycerin**] Trade name: [Nitrostat, NitroTab, NitroQuick, NitroBid, Nitrol]	This drug is a coronary vasodilator.
Right patient?	This drug may be used to manage pain associated with ACS, angina pectoris (chronic, stable, and unstable) and to relax blood vessels in acute pulmonary edema (APE).
Right dose?	0.4 mg (1/150 grain) SL pill, or 0.4 mg spray SL. May be repeated up to 3 doses with an adequate blood pressure.
Right route?	Lingual, sublingual, topical, IV, PO.
Right time?	After placing the patient at rest, administering oxygen and aspirin, obtaining baseline vital signs as well as a cardiothoracic assessment and history.
Right documentation?	Document the administration of the medication as well as the ongoing assessment findings, including lung sounds on the patient care report.
Expected action	Relief of chest pain, pulmonary edema, and reduced blood pressure.
Side effects	Hypotension, increased chest pain, cardiac arrhythmias, potential allergic reaction.
Contraindications	Known sensitivity, hypotension.
Precautions	Monitor respiratory effort and blood pressure.
Pharmacokinetics	Onset 1–3 minutes SL, peak effect 5–10 minutes; duration 20–30 minutes or so if IV (1–10 minutes after discontinuation of use); metabolized in the liver and excreted in urine.

Case Study I Continued

Table 6 Morphine Sulfate

Do you know?	Comments
Right drug? Generic name: [**Morphine Sulfate**] Trade name: [Astramorph PF, Kadian, MS Contin, MSIR, Oramorph SR, Rescudose, Roxanol]	This drug is an opiate analgesic for relief of moderate to severe pain, relief of anxiety, pulmonary edema; it reduces left ventricular work by reducing preload pressure and has sedative effects.
Right patient?	For ACS as an adjunct following treatment with acetylsalicylic acid [Aspirin] and nitrates for the relief of chest pain, to reduce anxiety and decrease left ventricular work.
Right dose?	2–4 mg.
Right route?	IV.
Right time?	After physical examination and baseline vital signs are obtained; oxygen, aspirin, and nitrates have been considered.
Right documentation?	Document the administration of the medication as well as the ongoing assessment findings, including lung sounds on the patient care report.
Expected action	Pain relief and reduced anxiety, decreased myocardial workload.
Side effects	Respiratory depression and hypotension.
Contraindications	Known allergy, hypotension.
Precautions	Respiratory depression, hypotension.
Pharmacokinetics	Onset immediate IV; duration 2–7 hours; metabolized in the liver, excreted in urine.

Table 7 Ondansetron Hydrochloride

Do you know?	Comments
Right drug? Generic name: [**Ondansetron Hydrochloride**] Trade name: [Zofran]	This drug is an antiemetic. It is used to relieve or prevent nausea and vomiting in a variety of situations.
Right patient?	Nauseous with suspected ACS and ST Segment Elevation Myocardial Infarction (STEMI).
Right dose?	4 mg initial dose; may be repeated in 10 minutes. Follow your local protocol.
Right route?	IV or IM.
Right time?	Adjunct treatment in suspected ACS after treating with acetylsalicylic acid [Aspirin], nitrates, and/or morphine sulfate [Astramorph/PF].
Right documentation?	Document the administration of the medication as well as the ongoing assessment findings, including lung sounds on the patient care report.
Expected action	Relief of nausea.
Side effects	Typically chest pain, wheezing, or hives/skin rash may occur. Other side effects can include: seizures, tachycardia, bradycardia, heart attack, sedation, blurred vision, hypokalemia, and fever. Acute dystonic reactions, involving painful muscular twisting and twitching, may also occur.
Contraindications	Known sensitivity.
Precautions	May worsen preexisting symptoms.
Pharmacokinetics	Onset: 30 minutes. Peak effect: 2 hours. Duration: 3–6 hours; metabolized in the liver, excreted in urine.

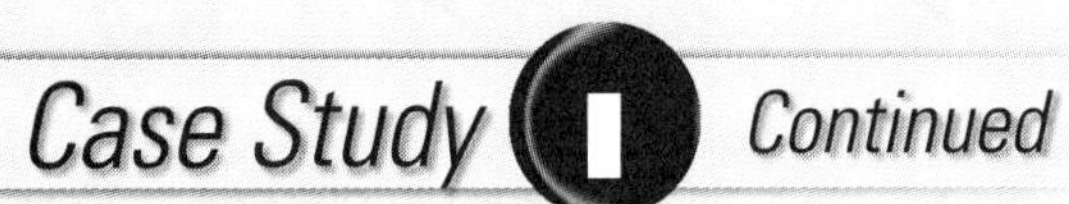

Table 8 Metoprolol Tartrate

Do you know?	Comments
Right drug? Generic name: [**Metoprolol Tartrate, Metoprolol Succinate**] Trade name: [Lopressor, Toprol]	This drug is a **beta-adrenergic blocking agent** that can be used alone or with other drugs to control hypertension, chronic angina pectoris, and heart failure. Metoprolol tartrate is also used to treat migraines and ventricular arrhythmias.
Right patient?	Suspected ACS with STEMI.
Right dose?	5 mg initial dose; may be repeated up to 3 doses—follow local protocol.
Right route?	IV.
Right time?	Adjunct treatment to suspected ACS after treating with acetylsalicylic acid [aspirin] and nitrates.
Right documentation?	Document the administration of the medication as well as the ongoing assessment findings, including lung sounds on the patient care report.
Expected action	Decreases workload of the heart, slows heart rate, and lowers blood pressure.
Side effects	Bradycardia and hypotension.
Contraindications	Known hypersensitivity, bradycardia, and hypotension.
Precautions	Use with caution in patients with impaired hepatic function.
Pharmacokinetics	Onset 1–5 minutes; peak 90 minutes; metabolized in liver, excreted in urine.

Question 5: What is meant by the phrase, "Time is muscle?"

Question 6: What is the value of communicating directly with the ED as soon as possible about the 12-lead ECG findings in the suspected ACS patient?

Part 4

Medical control has been advised of the patient and is notifying the "cath lab." You have received and confirmed orders to continue nitroglycerin, administer 4 mg morphine sulfate [Astramorph/PF], and 5 mg metoprolol tartrate [Lopressor] IV bolus. Once these medications are administered, an ongoing assessment reveals that Mr. Jenson's pain is now at 6 of 10 (see **Table 9**). He is still pale and diaphoretic and has the following vital signs: respirations are 20 breaths/min with clear lung sounds, pulse rate is 78 beats/min and regular, blood pressure is 116/58 mm Hg, and SpO_2 is 98%. The ECG shows further increasing ST segment elevations and depressions in reciprocal leads leading you to believe he is definitely experiencing an AMI.

You are almost to the ED, but you are still very busy completing the regional fibrinolytic checklist that is based on the AHA criteria. This information

Table 9 Reassessment and Ongoing Assessment of the Patient

Serial Vital Signs and Relevant Data	Recording Time: 10 Minutes
Skin CTC	Pale and diaphoretic
Pulse	78 beats/min and regular
Blood Pressure	116/58 mm Hg
Respirations	20 breaths/min
Mental Status	Alert/less anxious
ECG	ST elevations in anterolateral leads and depression in reciprocal leads
SpO_2	98%
Lung Sounds	Clear
Other (ie, glucose, core temperature)	None

Case Study I Continued

helps to determine if the patient is likely to go directly to the catheterization lab or receive fibrinolytics in the ED, or if he needs additional testing and evaluation in the ED upon your arrival. Your Medical Director's policy is that when there are choices of hospitals, to take the patient to the hospital that has a cardiac catheterization lab if there are significant findings on the 12-lead ECG or they have evidence of STEMI.

Question 7: What does the acronym "MONA" stand for in the care of the ACS patient?

Question 8: Why is it important to do a fibrinolytic checklist on the suspected ACS patient?

Part 5

Upon arrival at the ED, the staff is waiting for you and your patient. The physician looks at your 12-lead ECG and agrees with your interpretation and the actions you have taken so far. A member of the catheterization lab is also there and ready to take the patient upstairs. Because of your rapid assessment skills, thorough history taking, accurate ECG interpretation, and aggressive treatment, including bringing your patient to a facility with reperfusion capabilities, Mr. Jenson's window of opportunity for surviving this heart attack is significant.

In some cases an emergency cardiac catheterization or percutaneous coronary intervention (PCI) would be the most appropriate course of action for the patient. A **cardiac catheterization** or percutaneous coronary intervention (PCI) is the insertion of a catheter through the femoral artery in the groin, through the femoral and iliac arteries into the aorta, and finally into the heart's coronary arteries. By entering the coronary arteries the physician can inject radiopaque dye so an X-ray can be taken of the heart and its vessels. This process of injecting dye into the catheter is called angiography and it allows a view of the flow, or lack of flow, of blood through all of the arteries in the heart. The movement of the walls of the heart and the regurgitation of blood, due to problems with heart valves flowing backwards into the wrong chamber, can also be seen on angiography.

Not all hospitals have a specialized catheterization lab so this will definitely factor into the transportation decision for the patient. Of course, all therapies are most successful if done within the first hour or two from the onset of the ischemia as determined by the onset of pain, so time clearly is a factor. Most EDs and catheterization labs track the door-to-catheterization time because focusing on this time period helps them to make appropriate administrative decisions to remove the obstacles or lengthy steps that might otherwise delay the catheterization procedure.

Why Is It Necessary to Get a Good History?

Even in the hospital, diagnosing an AMI or heart attack is difficult in many cases based on any one component of an examination or diagnostic test. Three primary components are used for diagnosing an AMI or ruling out an ACS; the subjective and objective assessments, an abnormal ECG or ECG with changes, and an analysis of the patient's cardiac enzymes done in serial blood tests in the hospital setting.

Not everyone who experiences an ACS will have the classic signs and symptoms or an abnormal ECG. For many people, especially women, the elderly, and diabetics, the severity or absence of pain is often unrelated to the life-threatening potential of the coronary event they are experiencing. These patients sometimes present with only one or more of the following atypical signs:

- Fatigue
- Weakness
- Dyspnea
- Confusion
- Syncope
- New onset of congestive heart failure (CHF)

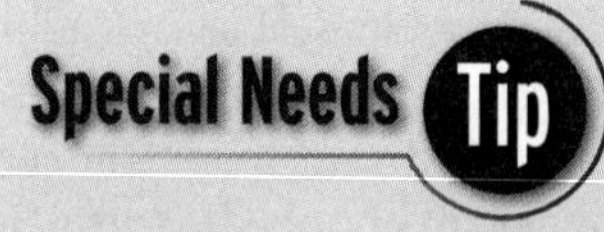

Elderly patients, women, and diabetics commonly have "silent MIs" that do not present with the classic crushing chest pain.

Obtaining a history is especially important for the patient with atypical signs and symptoms and is considered significant to making a diagnosis to include or exclude an acute coronary syndrome (ACS) or the presence of an AMI. For the paramedic, it involves fully investigating the answers to the questions using OPQRST and SAMPLE.

Other Acute Coronary Syndrome Issues

Over the past 20 years or so, several other medications, focused at in-hospital care, have been developed to help manage the patient with ST segment elevation myocardial infarction (STEMI) and ACS. Though there are several different physiologic pathways involved, they all share the common goal of either intra-arterial clot thrombolysis, platelet aggregation inhibition (which therefore limits infarct extension), or preventing reocclusion of a previously reopened coronary artery. These medicines may include tissue plasminogen activator (TPA) [Alteplase], clopidogrel [Plavix], various types of heparins (unfractionated and low-molecular weight [Lovenox]), and glycoprotein IIb/IIa inhibitors (eptifibatide [Integrelin]). Most of these medications come in a least one parenteral form, and it would not be unreasonable to expect that you would be called upon to supervise an infusion of these products while providing interfacility transport, or perhaps even initiate care with one or more of these agents while on-scene with an unstable patient.

Other medications that may be used during the in-hospital phase of either the acute or continuing management of ACS patients include β-adrenergic blockers (metoprolol tartrate [Lopressor]), ACE (angiotensin converting enzyme—captopril [Capoten]) inhibitors and ARBs (angiotensin receptor blockers—irbesartan [Avapro]), and HMG Co-A reductase inhibitors (atorvastatin [Lipitor]). These medications are used to better manage provocative coronary heart disease risk factors, and help to limit the occurrence of secondary cardiovascular events.

The 12-Lead ECG

A 12-lead ECG is used to localize the site of injury to heart muscle and it allows the heart to be looked at from several angles. As soon as possible a 12-lead ECG should be applied and obtained on any patient suspected of having an ACS. When correctly placed on the chest, the leads form a triangle around the heart, called the Einthoven triangle (**Figure 4-1**▲).

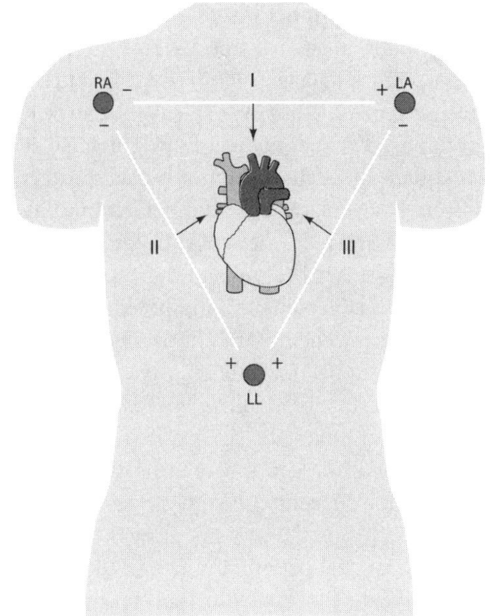

Figure 4-1 The Einthoven triangle.

Knowing the size and location of injury helps you to anticipate common complications associated with the area affected and thus helps you better prepare and treat the patient. For example, one of the more common areas to infarct, or die, is the inferior wall for which treatment includes nitrates. A less common area to infarct is the right ventricle (RV). RV infarcts are sensitive to drugs to reduce **preloads** (ie, nitrate). Giving nitrates to a patient who is having a RV infarct may cause the blood pressure to fall precipitously, thereby reducing blood flow to the lungs and brain and eventually worsening the AMI. The specific ECG changes typically found with infarction to different locations in the heart are shown in **Table 4-1**▼.

Table 4-1 Acute Coronary Syndrome

Location	Leads showing direct ECG changes	Leads showing reciprocal ECG changes
Inferior wall (RCA, LCx)	II, III, aVF	I, aVL
Anteroseptal (LAD)	V_1, V_2, V_3, V_4	
Anterolateral (LAD, LCx)	V_3, V_4, V_5, V_6	
Lateral (LCx)	V_5, V_6	
High lateral (LAD, LCx)	I, aVL	II, III, aVF
Right ventricular (RCA, LCx)	V_4R, V_5R, V_6R	
*Posterior (RCA, LCx)	V_7, V_8, V_9	V_1, V_2 (can extend to V_3–V_5)

*Note: Posterior wall MI is initially diagnosed using the reciprocal leads. Additional leads are then made to confirm the diagnosis.
RCA = right circumflex artery
LCx = left circumflex artery
LAD = left anterior descending artery.

The Window of Opportunity

Taking the patient with a suspected AMI to the appropriate hospital can make a significant difference in the patient's outcome and quality of life. When an ischemic part of the heart tissue (myocardium) infarcts because of inadequate blood flow from a blocked artery, the area affected can enlarge even more if left untreated or if treatment is delayed. After an AMI, the myocardium that infarcts first is the "core" and the tissue surrounding the core remains ischemic and potentially salvageable if reperfusion therapy (ie, fibrinolytics, coronary artery bypass, or balloon angioplasty) can be started right away to restore blood flow. The time when injury is developing and has not yet resulted in permanent damage is called "the window of opportunity." Taking a patient with a suspected AMI to a facility that does not offer reperfusion therapy can close the window of opportunity for that patient and can result in death.

If significant blockages in the coronary arteries are uncovered while the patient is undergoing angiography, the cardiologist will make a decision as to the best course of treatment. In some cases, a procedure called angioplasty is used whereby a small balloon-tipped catheter is inserted and inflated to open up the blocked vessel. In other cases, the cardiologist injects a tiny amount of clot busting drug directly on the site of the clot to help dissolve it. Oftentimes following angioplasty a stent will be placed into the affected portion of the coronary artery. The stent is like a tiny spring mesh tube that adheres to the walls of the vessel. It is used to help keep a previously opened vessel patent and clear of blockage. There has been considerable controversy on the effectiveness of stents but this procedure is still commonly done today. Another option the cardiologist may consider is replacement of the arteries when they are simply too blocked. In this case, the procedure involves a coronary artery bypass graft or CABG surgery. Depending on the arteries that are involved, this can involve a small incision and microsurgery techniques or a major open chest procedure. Either way, both procedures are invasive, have considerable risks, and yet are life-saving. When a patient has a "bypass," a small segment of a blood vessel, often a vein from the leg, is removed and used as a replacement for the diseased segment of the coronary artery. Some patients may require multiple bypasses, involving replacement of two, three, or even four small segments of a blocked artery. This procedure is commonly performed every day in cardiac centers with the general public becoming more aware of bypass surgery from celebrities like David Letterman and President Bill Clinton.

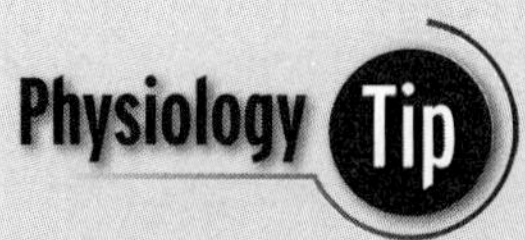

Of the nearly 5,000 acute care hospitals in the United States, about 1,200 have heart catheterization laboratories capable of performing PCI. Each EMS system should have a plan in place to ensure that the patient identified in the field with STEMI will be taken to the most appropriate facility based on the resources in the region.

Patients with Symptomatic Arrhythmias and Cardiac Arrest

Each year there are 1.2 million Americans who have a new heart attack. Close to 452,000 of these patients will die, making heart disease a leading cause of death. It is estimated that 7.9 million adult Americans have survived a myocardial infarction and about 8.9 million have **angina pectoris** (angina). Sudden cardiac arrest (SCA) accounts for some 325,000 deaths occurring in the ED or prehospital setting each year.

The precipitating factors to sudden cardiac arrest (SCA) include:

- coronary artery disease
- valvular disease
- congenital heart disease
- long QT syndrome
- Wolff-Parkinson-White (WPW) syndrome
- previous cardiac arrest or heart attack
- drug abuse
- hyperthyroidism
- considerable electrolyte changes
- a low (< 35%) ejection fraction (blood pumped out of the heart).

Case Study II Ventricular Fibrillation/ Ventricular Tachycardia

Part 1

Your unit has been dispatched to the county airport for a patient who collapsed in the security check-in area. There are airport fire department first responders on the scene and the report is they have initiated CPR on a middle-aged male patient. Fortunately you and your partner were just coming back from another call so you are already on the road and it is a quick response to the airport. The airport fire department, ticket counter personnel, and flight attendants have all been trained in CPR.

As your partner is negotiating the traffic on the perimeter road leading to the airport, you review in your mind the ACLS algorithm for pulseless arrest. "Well, it's a good thing they put up all of those automated external defibrillators (AED) last winter at the terminal," says your partner. You know that defibrillation will stun the heart muscle momentarily and allow the patient's normal conduction system to regain control. You also know the rule of thumb for placement of AEDs is clearly marked locations in a place of public occupancy that are within 1 minute's brisk walk from all locations in a building.

As you pull up in front of the terminal building there are two police officers clearing traffic and directing you to the entrance. You and your partner load up all of the necessary equipment on the stretcher and head inside. Your supervisor is also en route and she is supposed to bring the Thumper CPR System with her on any confirmed arrest call. The Thumper CPR System is an adjunct to CPR that provides both continuous chest compressions (100/min) and ventilations. It can be used with a pocket mask or an advanced airway.

As you approach the area where the patient is located you can see there are two firefighters and a bystander doing CPR on the patient. They have performed their initial assessment (see **Table 1**). You learn the patient's name is Dan Wilde. The AED is open at his side and has just been brought there by a Transportation Security Administration (TSA) employee moments before your arrival. The AED will analyze Mr. Wilde's ECG rhythm and determine whether or not a defibrillating shock is needed. The scene is safe and it appears that the patient never actually made it through the airport screening. You have just finished going over the ACLS algorithm for pulseless arrest in your head when the firefighter looks to you and says, "we have completed 2 minutes of CPR and analyzed. The AED says to shock, is that okay?" You quickly respond, "yes, by all means clear all personnel and proceed with the defibrillation!"

As the shock is administered Mr. Wilde's body jumps a bit but he does not wake up. Chest compressions are started again immediately. Your partner switches the bag-mask device to a manual transport ventilator with an **impedance threshold device (ITD)** on it. Since the ventilations are effective at this time, your partner will have ample time to prepare to insert an advanced airway.

The remainder of the initial assessment reveals additional information.

It appears that Mr. Wilde did not experience any obvious trauma. His wife was with him and stated he was all worked up about the long line and he had thought they might miss the flight. She said he got edgy and short-tempered with all of the waiting around. He became sweaty, clutched his chest, and collapsed. She explains that she does not understand what is happening but she can see he is very sick. She says that Mr. Wilde is healthy overall, 53 years old, and exercises every day. You note that he looks about 30 lb overweight. You call for the AED and recall that the rhythms that an AED prompts the rescuer to shock include **ventricular fibrillation (V-fib)** and **ventricular tachycardia**

Table 1 **Initial Assessment**

Initial Assessment	Recording Time: 1 Minute
General Impression/ Appearance	Poor impression (just does not look well), middle-aged male in arrest
Mental Status	"U" unresponsive
Airway	Open and clear at this time
Breathing	Being ventilated with a bag-mask device
Circulation	None aside from the 100 compressions/min from CPR
Priority/Plan	High due to recent arrest with short downtime

Case Study II Continued

(V-tach) (usually over 180 beats/min). Since the AED does not actually take the patient's pulse there is a slim chance it could suggest shocking V-tach in a patient who still has a pulse. This is why the AED should not be applied to a conscious patient. Always follow the protocol in your EMS system for the proper application and use of the AED on unconscious patients.

Question 1: If the patient is being shocked with a defibrillator, the patient is most likely experiencing what cardiac arrhythmia?

Question 2: What is a good "rule of thumb" for the placement of AEDs in busy public places such as an airport, music hall, or sports arena?

Part 2

After 2 more minutes of CPR you have switched over the AED to your monitor and are getting ready to reanalyze the patient's rhythm. For your bag-mask ventilations you incorporate the use of an ITD since this is standard procedure for all resuscitations in your agency. You recall learning that the ITD helps to improve the venous return to the heart by maintaining negative pressure during the filling phase or diastole. This in turn improves the coronary perfusion. The heart needs to work like a straw, drawing blood from the venous system during the recoil phase of your CPR compressions. Thus it is important to allow for complete chest recoil and avoid any pressure on the patient's chest between compressions. The ITD enhances this effect by capping the ET tube at the right moment to allow the heart to work as the piston it was intended to work as, constantly filling and emptying with each stroke.

Your partner has inserted an advanced airway and confirmed placement with capnography while you were able to start an IV and start a normal saline drip. The first dose of epinephrine [Adrenalin] 1 mg of 1:10,000 will be delivered by an IV bolus. Epinephrine is a **vasopressor**. Since the rhythm is still ventricular fibrillation (V-fib), you clear the patient and deliver another shock. The patient does not wake up. CPR is immediately resumed with compressions. Since an advanced airway is now in place, the ventilations and compressions can be asynchronous with the ventilator at 8–10 breaths/min and the compressions at a rate of 100/min. Of course this will result in the compressor tiring faster so you will need to switch compressors every 2 minutes.

With a chief complaint of sudden cardiac arrest (SCA) you have an initial assessment problem that needs immediate resuscitation, leaving little time for the focused history and physical examination of the patient (see **Table 2**). The EMS supervisor is just arriving on the scene so you know the Thumper will be coming in with her.

Question 3: What are the risk factors for SCA?

Question 4: How does an impedance threshold device (ITD) work to improve the quality of the CPR?

Table 2 Focused History and Physical Examination

Baseline Vital Signs	Recording Time: 5 Minutes
Skin CTC (color, temperature, condition)	Pale, cool, and clammy
Pulse	None; being compressed at 100/min
Blood Pressure	None
Respirations	None; being ventilated

Part 3

As the EMS supervisor and the "on-deck" compressor work to set up the Thumper without interrupting the CPR, you note that it is time for administration of the next vasopressor. A vasopressor is an agent that constricts the blood vessels, thus causing the blood pressure to rise. In this instance, and 3 to 5 minutes after the initial dose, you decide to administer additional epinephrine [Adrenalin] 1 mg of 1:10,000. You realize that you could just as easily have administered one 40-unit dose of vasopressin [Pitressin synthetic]. The rhythm is reanalyzed and the patient is still in V-fib so another shock is administered. This time there is a brief run of pulseless electrical activity (PEA) and then the patient reverts back to V-fib. Seeing no change in mental status, CPR compressions are restarted without delay.

Case Study II Continued

Your partner is able to take a moment to talk with the patient's wife and gather some information for the SAMPLE history (see **Table 3**). She says that he is a type II diabetic on oral medications and diet control. He has had a lot of stress due to a very busy workload and is looking forward to this vacation in California.

As you approach the next 2-minute point, the Thumper is working properly, freeing up a rescuer to begin preparing for transport. You draw up the first dose of antiarrhythmic which is amiodarone [Cordarone] 300 mg.

In summarizing your treatment plan for the adult cardiac arrest patient who is in a shockable rhythm, you will be taking these actions:

Table 3 SAMPLE History

SAMPLE History	Comments
Signs/symptoms	Diaphoresis and a witnessed sudden cardiac arrest (SCA)
Allergies	Novacaine
Medications	Glyburide [Diabeta], folic acid, and atorvastatin calcium [Lipitor]
Pertinent past medical history	Type II diabetes, eye surgery 6 months ago
Last oral intake	Breakfast 2 hours ago
Events leading up to the incident	Stress and anxiety

1. Provide CPR using proper hand position (push hard, fast and allow full chest recoil).
2. Administer supplemental oxygen as available.
3. Give one shock, then immediately resume CPR.
4. After 2 minutes (5 cycles of CPR), reassess the patient.
5. If patient is still in a shockable rhythm, you will give one shock, then immediately resume CPR.
6. Next start an IV/IO and administer a vasopressor (ie, epinephrine [Adrenalin]) 1 mg every 3 to 5 minutes of the arrest or a single dose of vasopressin [Pitressin] 40 unit dose can be substituted for the first or second epinephrine [Adrenalin] dose, but not both (see **Table 4** and **Table 5**).
7. After 2 additional minutes (5 cycles of CPR), reassess the patient.
8. If still in a shockable rhythm, you will give one shock, then immediately resume CPR.
9. Next action will be to administer an antiarrhythmic (ie, amiodarone [Cordarone] or lidocaine hydrochloride [Xylocaine] or magnesium sulfate if the rhythm is torsade de pointes) (see **Table 6** and **Table 7**).
10. Then you will reassess the patient to decide what would be the next most appropriate action (per your local protocols).

Table 4 Epinephrine

Do you know?	Comments
Right drug? Generic name: [**Epinephrine**] Trade name: [Adrenalin]	This drug is a **sympathomimetic**. It has the property (vasopressor) to cause contraction of smooth muscle of arteries and arterioles, thereby increasing cardiac afterload and coronary perfusion pressure. In a cardiac arrest, a vasopressor is administered every 3–5 minutes. Epinephrine is the drug of choice in cardiac arrest as well as severe allergic reaction and asthma. It can also be effective in symptomatic bradycardia as an alternative to dopamine [Intropin], severe hypotension that is secondary to bradycardia and not responsive to atropine sulfate or transcutaneous pacing.
Right patient?	The vasopressor of choice for the pulseless arrest patient.
Right dose?	1 mg is administered every 3–5 minutes for the duration of the arrest.
Right route?	The 1:10,000 concentration of epinephrine is administered by the IV or IO route. It is possible to administer by the ET route but its effectiveness is believed to be questionable at best.
Right time?	Every 3-5 minutes of the cardiac arrest.
Right documentation?	Dose, route, time administered, and reassessment should be clearly documented on your patient care report.
Expected action	This drug is a direct acting alpha- and beta-agonist. The alpha effect is vasoconstriction and Beta-1 has positive inotropic, chronotropic, and dromotropic effects. The Beta-2 effects, which are not immediately relevant to the cardiac arrest patient, are bronchial smooth muscle relaxation and dilation of the skeletal vasculature.

continues

Case Study II Continued

Table 4 Epinephrine (*Continued*)

Do you know?	Comments
Side effects	Can cause hypertension, tachycardia, arrhythmias, pulmonary edema, anxiety, restlessness, agitation, nausea, headache, and angina, also local tissue necrosis if extravasated at IV site, or limb ischemia/necrosis if given intra-arterially.
Contraindications	Hypertension, hypothermia, pulmonary edema, myocardial ischemia, and hypovolemic shock.
Precautions	Epinephrine can potentiate other sympathomimetics. It can be deactivated by alkaline solutions (ie, sodium bicarbonate). Use of monamine oxidase inhibitors (MAOIs) may potentiate effects and beta-blockers may blunt its effects.
Pharmacokinetics	Onset: immediate IV, 5–10 minutes SC/IM; metabolism takes place in both the liver and other tissues by monoamine oxidase (MAO) and catechol-O-methyltransferase (COMT) to inactive metabolites. Peak effect: minutes. Duration: several minutes.

Table 5 Vasopressin

Do you know?	Comments
Right drug? Generic name: [**Vasopressin**] Trade name: [Pitressin synthetic]	This drug is a pituitary antidiuretic hormone that stimulates smooth muscle receptors. It is also a potent vasoconstrictor when given in high doses.
Right patient?	The patient in cardiac arrest.
Right dose?	40-unit one-time dose.
Right route?	Given by the IV or IO route.
Right time?	Vasopressin [Pitressin synthetic] can be given as a single dose as a substitute for the first or second (but not both) dose of epinephrine [Adrenalin].
Right documentation?	Dose, route, time administered, and reassessment should be clearly documented on the patient care report.
Expected action	An alternative vasopressor to the first or second dose of epinephrine [Adrenalin] (but not both) during a cardiac arrest.
Side effects	May cause bronchospasm, ischemic chest pain, nausea and vomiting, and abdominal pain.
Contraindications	Responsive patients with coronary artery disease. (FYI—we do use it in the ICU setting for management of severely septic patients).
Precautions	No reported drug interactions.
Pharmacokinetics	Onset: immediate IV/IO; duration of action: variable; metabolized rapidly in the liver and kidneys.

Table 6 Amiodarone

Do you know?	Comments
Right drug? Generic name: [**Amiodarone**] Trade name: [Cordarone or Pacerone]	This drug is an antiarrhythmic medication given in cardiac arrest with an ECG of V-fib/pulseless V-tach. It is also used for recurrent life-threatening tachycardia arrhythmias (ie, ventricular tachycardia) and may also be used for atrial fibrillation.
Right patient?	Primarily given to the cardiac arrest patient in V-fib/V-tach/pulseless V-tach. Also SVTs unresponsive to other treatment.

continues

Case Study II Continued

Table 6 Amiodarone (*Continued*)

Do you know?	Comments
Right dose?	For cardiac arrest administer 300 mg IV/IO (recommended dilution in 20–30 mL D_5W). Initial dose can be followed in 3–5 minutes by a one-time bolus of 150 mg. For recurrent life-threatening ventricular arrhythmia the maximum cumulative dose is 2.2 g per 24 hours administered as follows: rapid infusion 150 mg IV/IO over 10 minutes (15 mg/min). May repeat the infusion (150 mg IV/IO) every 10 minutes as needed. Slow infusion of 360 mg IV/IO over 6 hours (1 mg/min). Maintenance infusion of 540 mg IV/IO over 18 hours (0.5 mg/min).
Right route?	IV or IO for the bolus or IV or IO drip for the infusion. There are no recommendations on administering this medication down the ET tube.
Right time?	For the patient in cardiac arrest after high quality CPR, defibrillation, and vasopressors have been administered without return of spontaneous circulation. Can be used to prevent the patient from deteriorating back to V-fib following a successful conversion.
Right documentation?	Dose, route, time administered, and reassessment should be clearly documented on the patient care report.
Expected action	Blocks sodium channels and myocardial potassium channels, as well as alpha- and beta-adrenergic blockade.
Side effects	Hypotension (usually related to rate of infusion), bradycardia, prolongation of the **P-R interval**, **QRS complex/interval**, and **Q-T interval**.
Contraindications	Known hypersensitivity, cardiogenic shock, sinus bradycardia, and high level (second or third degree) atrioventricular (AV) block.
Precautions	Use with digoxin can cause digitalis toxicity. Antiarrhythmics have been known to cause increased serum levels. In addition, beta-blockers and calcium channel blockers may potentiate bradycardia, sinus arrest, and AV heart blocks. Draw up the medicine slowly from the ampule or else it will bubble up like soap. This drug has a slow absorption rate and accumulates in the liver, lungs, spleen, and adipose tissue and the effects may persist for weeks and months after therapy is ended.
Pharmacokinetics	An iodine-containing compound, it is highly lipid soluble and is stored in high concentrations in fat, muscle, the liver, lungs, and skin. The drug's bioavailability is approximately 40% and excretion is minimal through the hepatic route. The minimal effective serum concentration has not been established with certainty, and the unique pharmacokinetics of this agent has made it difficult to perform dose-response studies. Onset: immediate with peak effect in 10–15 minutes. Duration of action: 30–45 minutes.

Table 7 Lidocaine Hydrochloride

Do you know?	Comments
Right drug? Generic name: [**Lidocaine Hydrochloride**] Trade name: [Xylocaine]	This drug is an antiarrhythmic and for many years was the first-line ventricular antiarrhythmic medication. It is also commonly used as a local anesthetic agent. Currently an alternative to the first-line antiarrhythmic medication amiodarone [Cordarone]. The prophylactic use of lidocaine [Xylocaine] is no longer recommended in the presence of ACS. Lidocaine [Xylocaine] is a potent left-ventricular end-diastolic depressant. Experts note that a patient in arrest has an already markedly compromised cardiac output, and administering a medication as such will likely result in a poorer response to other aspects of the resuscitation.
Right patient?	The cardiac arrest patient in V-fib/pulseless V-tach or for stable V-tach, wide-complex tachycardia of uncertain type, or significant ectopy.
Right dose?	For cardiac arrest the patient should receive an initial dose of 1–1.5 mg/kg IV/IO. The dose can be repeated at 0.5 to 0.75 mg/kg in 5 to 10 minutes to a maximum dose of 3 mg/kg. The dose for stable V-tach, wide complex tachycardia of uncertain type or significant ectopy is 0.5 to 0.75 mg/kg and up to 1 to 1.5 mg/kg. Repeat the dose at 0.5 to 0.75 mg/kg every 5 to 10 minutes. The maximum total dose is 3 mg/kg. A maintenance infusion of 1 to 4 mg/min can be administered with the lidocaine [Xylocaine] diluted in D_5W or normal saline.

continues

Case Study II Continued

Table 7 Lidocaine Hydrochloride (*Continued*)

Do you know?	Comments
Right route?	Given in IV or IO bolus. If given by the ET route (cardiac arrest only), twice the dose should be administered although its effectiveness is questionable. The maintenance dose is often given by an IV drip. Some EMS systems that have short transport times have chosen to simply rebolus the patient instead of setting up an IV drip.
Right time?	For the patient in cardiac arrest after high quality CPR, defibrillation, and vasopressors have been administered without return of spontaneous circulation. Can be used to prevent the patient from converting back to V-fib following successful resuscitation.
Right documentation?	Dose, route, time administered, and reassessment should be clearly documented on the patient care report.
Expected action	It decreases automaticity by slowing the rate of phase 4 depolarization.
Side effects	Slurred speech, seizures (with high doses), altered mental status, confusion, lightheadedness, blurred vision, and bradycardia.
Contraindications	Hypersensitivity, second-degree AV block, or third-degree AV blocks in the absence of an artificial pacemaker, Stokes-Adams syndrome, wide-complex ventricular escape beats in a patient with bradycardia. Should not be used in patients allergic to other "caine" drugs.
Precautions	Be extremely careful not to administer the 2-gram concentrated dose that is intended to be used only to prepare a drip, directly into the IV/IO site as the patient is likely to have a seizure and die. Apnea induced with succinylcholine chloride [Anectine, Quelicin] may be prolonged with high doses of lidocaine [Xylocaine]. Cardiac depression may occur with IV phenytoin [Dilantin]. Procainamide hydrochloride [Pronestyl, Procanbid] may exacerbate CNS effects. Elimination of the drug is decreased with patients who have liver disease or are on beta-blockers.
Pharmacokinetics	Onset 1–3 minutes IV and 5–15 minutes IM; peak effect is 5–10 minutes, duration is variable 15 minutes–2 hours; Metabolized in the liver.

Question 5: Once an antiarrhythmic is chosen for this patient, why is lidocaine hydrochloride [Xylocaine] not routinely recommended?

Question 6: What are the key issues in the management of an adult patient in pulseless arrest with an ECG of V-fib or pulseless V-tach?

Part 4

Once you have administered amiodarone [Cordarone], you prepare for a third shock. After the third shock the patient starts to move and opens his eyes. You continue to assist ventilations and your partner gets a quick set of vital signs as part of the reassessment (see **Table 8**). A drip of amiodarone [Cordarone] is started and you switch over to a nonrebreathing mask. Your partner has the suction ready as he considers extubating the patient who at this point is biting the tube. It does not help the patient to allow him to continue to gag. Gagging stimulates the vagus nerve and will slow down the heart rate. You will need to assess the patient for clinical stability and consider a sedative medication should you decide that it is necessary to maintain the mechanical ventilation.

Next you get a full set of vital signs and begin transport of the patient to the ED. The ED staff will

Table 8 Reassessment and Ongoing Assessment of the Patient

Serial Vital Signs and Relevant Data	Recording Time: 8 Minutes
Skin CTC	Pale, warm, dry
Pulse	108 beats/min and irregular
Blood Pressure	130/68 mm Hg
Respirations	18 breaths/min on his own now
Mental Status	"V" verbal
ECG	Sinus tachycardia with occasional premature ventricular contractions (PVC)
SpO_2	95%
Lung Sounds	Some basilar rales
Other (ie glucose, core temperature)	Blood glucose is 150 g/dL

Case Study II Continued

be happy to hear the radio report on this patient and will be looking to quickly move him through the ED and possibly up to the coronary catheterization lab. In preparation for arrival at the ED and once everything calms down a bit, you decide to run a 12-lead ECG on the patient.

Question 7: Why might it be advantageous for ED staff to remove the advanced airway upon the patient's arrival?

Question 8: How is an amiodarone [Cordarone] drip prepared?

Part 5

This patient was extremely fortunate that he had his cardiac arrest in a public place where a considerable amount of preparation had occurred involving CPR training and placement of AEDs. Actually some of the safest places in the United States are in airports like Chicago's O'Hare where they have trained many of the airport personnel as well as placed AEDs every minute or so around the terminal buildings.

Since the bystanders were first to begin CPR and the fire department quickly responded to the call for help, the patient received plenty of qualified help, and quickly. In addition, because there were a number of trained helpers the paramedic who took over the role of the code team leader was able to frequently rotate the compressors before the Thumper arrived on the scene. Research has shown that each of the links in the chain of survival is important but the quality of the early CPR is essential to the success of the code. If this patient had arrested in a private residence (more than 75% do), and unless his family members had found him right away and were trained in CPR, the story may have had a very different ending.

The arriving EMS providers continued the CPR and the defibrillation, timing the code around cycles of 2 minutes. The airway was managed first with basic life support techniques and then with an advanced airway. The patient's venous system was accessed with a peripheral IV and vasopressors were administered followed by antiarrhythmic medications. Upon reanalyzing and determining that the patient remained in ventricular fibrillation, additional defibrillations ultimately caused the patient's heart rhythm to convert to a tachycardia with palpable pulses. The patient also began breathing on his own and woke up.

On arrival at the ED the patient's serial vital signs were within normal range and he was actually awake and alert. The ED arranged for the patient to go right up to the catheterization lab where a catheterization revealed a serious blockage in his left anterior descending artery. Another part of the story that his wife told your partner en route to the hospital was that the patient's father had died from heart disease in his 40's.

You have a busy day but return to the hospital that evening to check on the patient. He is resting in the coronary care unit after having a stent put in his artery.

Sudden Cardiac Arrest Risk Factors

The risk factors for sudden cardiac arrest (SCA) are the same as those for diseases of the heart in general and include a family history of heart disease, smoking, high blood pressure (hypertension), high cholesterol, obesity, diabetes, or a sedentary lifestyle.

On a personal level you can stop using tobacco, be physically active, eat healthy food, watch your weight, avoid excessive alcohol, control your cholesterol, watch your blood pressure, take medication to control hypertension as directed by your physician, and keep your diabetes in check. The risks you cannot control are your age, gender, and heredity.

To improve cardiac arrest survival on a community level, it is essential to train the lay public and all levels of responders in CPR and public access defibrillation. The relative value of early defibrillation to reduce the interval from arrest to the first defibrillation by 1 to 2 minutes does more to improve the probability of survival for a patient than all of the medications you are likely to administer, airway interventions, and newly designed defibrillators combined. Since between 75% to 80% of the cardiac arrests occur in the home, it is also very important that your family be trained to recognize, access, and begin CPR so when the professional rescuers arrive they have a much better chance of successfully resuscitating the patient. Studies have shown that high quality CPR applied quickly after the patient's collapse can double if not triple the chance of survival.

Simply requiring CPR training in high school health class would result in a far greater number of bystanders who are able to serve as potential rescuers each year. Public training in CPR is now simpler with the advent of streamlined focused training programs that use watch-and-do DVDs to make learning easier and fun. In fact with the advent of the CPR Anytime product, it is now possible for citizens to learn CPR on their own in approximately 30 minutes. The kit comes with a DVD as well as an inflatable manikin that can be reused from time to time to refresh the skills of CPR.

Research has shown that CPR can double and in some cases triple the rate of survival of cardiac arrest. The CPR must be of high quality, consisting of fast compressions at a rate of 100/min, hard compressions producing a depth of 1½″ to 2″ on an adult and one third the anterior-posterior (AP) diameter on an infant or child, and full chest recoil after each compression. Further research on rescuer fatigue has shown that there is a delay between the point when the compressor is actually tired and the point where they perceive they are tired. This "delay" leads to a period of poor quality compressions that can reduce coronary perfusion dramatically. Remember that the entire resuscitation centers around perfusion. If the patient's perfusion diminishes due to poor quality compressions or lengthy interruptions in the compressions, the patient is likely to not survive. We suggest that compressors be rotated every 2 minutes and that if there are sufficient rescuers, the "on-deck" compressor kneel at the side of the patient ready to begin. In this way the switch will not drop any beats. Remember to review the ACLS Pulseless Arrest Algorithm regularly (**Figure 4-2 ▸**).

Some EMS systems have recognized that bystanders are often reluctant to do CPR for fear of hurting the patient, for fear of obtaining an infectious disease, or for fear of not remembering the right steps of CPR. In a number of these systems, the public are taught compression-only CPR with the theory that most arrests in adults are primary V-fib and not a primary respiratory event. Thus the blood is potentially still oxygenated so immediate perfusion is essential. Although the Guidelines 2000 and 2005 both discussed "compression-only" CPR for dispatcher assisted (telephone instruction) or those cases where the public is reluctant to do ventilations, this is not the conventional method taught in CPR courses at this time. After careful consideration of the available scientific research, in April 2008, the American Heart Association released a Science Advisory recognizing hands-only CPR as an effective alternative for the training of bystanders to manage the adult witnessed cardiac arrest. The conventional method includes the ventilation component and is still required for an infant, child, and adult cardiac arrest incident that is not witnessed.

What better advice should paramedics follow than to be role models for the public, demonstrating fitness, nutrition, weight control, wearing seat belts, and not smoking!

The success of cardiac arrest resuscitation is built on early action for each of the links in the chain of survival. This means there must be early access, early CPR, early defibrillation, and early advanced care. In turn, this means the bystanders should be trained to recognize an unresponsive patient, access the EMS System (call 911), begin CPR, and send someone for the AED. The professional rescuers should continue the resuscitation with a strong emphasis on the layers in the resuscitation pyramid (**Figure 4-3 ▸**). The pyramid is built on a base of high-quality chest compressions (fast, deep, full recoil). Defibrillation, as needed, comes next and then is followed by quality BLS ventilations. The advanced airway placement (ie, ET tube, LMA, or Combitube) is considered next and then medications, or drugs. The space in the pyramid focused on medications is smallest because resuscitation studies have shown that few medications contribute to the long-term success of the code as opposed to all the research supporting the tremendous value of chest compressions and defibrillation.

Adjuncts to Assist in CPR

Three devices are being closely studied since they seem to be improving the quality and consistency of CPR compressions (rate, depth, and chest recoil) as well as improving blood flow: the impedance threshold device (ITD) (**Figure 4-4 ▸**), the AutoPulse (**Figure 4-5 ▸**), and the Thumper (**Figure 4-6 ▸**).

The ITD is marketed as the ResQPOD® and has been shown to enhance the vacuum in the chest during the recoil phase of the compression. This device helps to create the natural negative pressure in the lungs. Just like a bellows fanning a fire, when the bellows opens it sucks air in and when the bellows is closed it forces the air out. In the same manner, the air is sucked into the lungs and blood sucked into the heart during the recoil phase of the compression.

An ITD limits the air being drawn into the lungs and enhances the effect of the blood from the venous system being sucked into the heart during the recoil

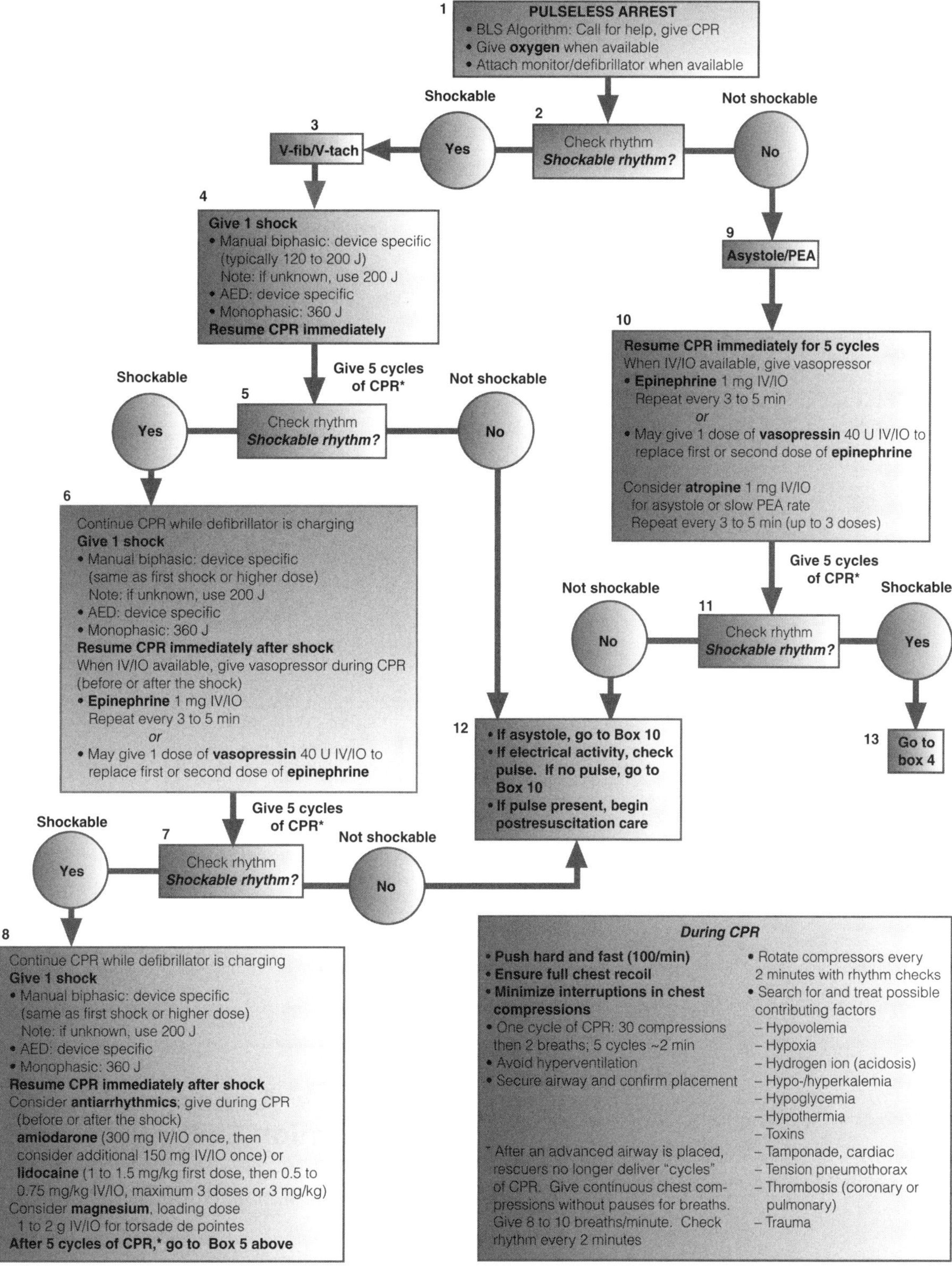

Figure 4-2 The ACLS algorithm for pulseless arrest.

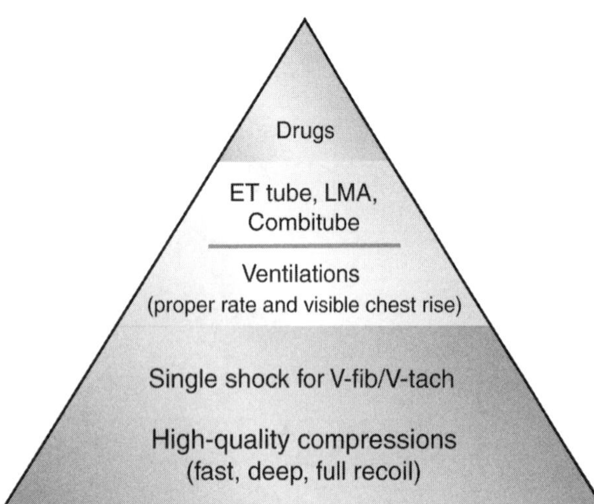

Figure 4-3 The resuscitation pyramid. The success of a code relies on high-quality CPR.

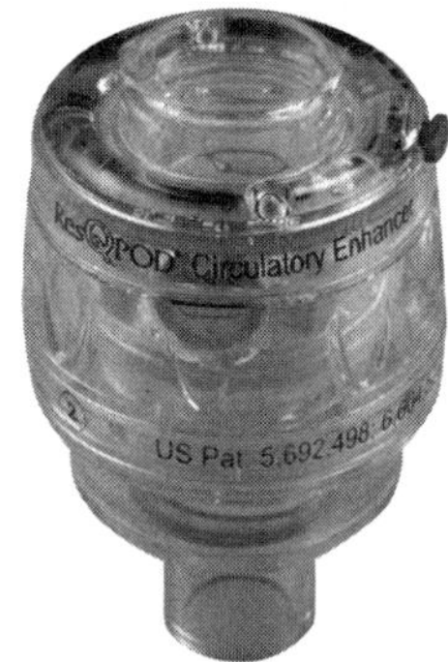

Figure 4-4 The ResQPOD®, an impedance threshold device, improves perfusion during CPR.

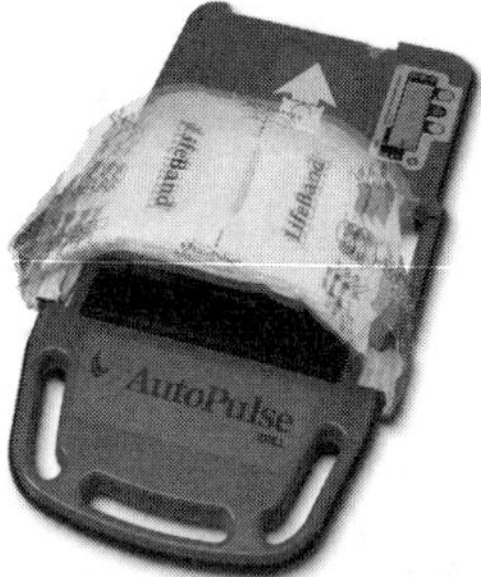

Figure 4-5 The AutoPulse® noninvasive cardiac support pump.

phase (diastole). Studies have shown that excessive ventilation rates or volumes are detrimental on cardiac perfusion. With the proper ventilation rate and with an ITD in use during cardiac arrest, the blood flow is enhanced through the heart as the proper amount of ventilation is allowed to enter the chest at the right time. It even has a series of colored lights that prompt the ventilator when to ventilate so as not to overventilate inadvertently.

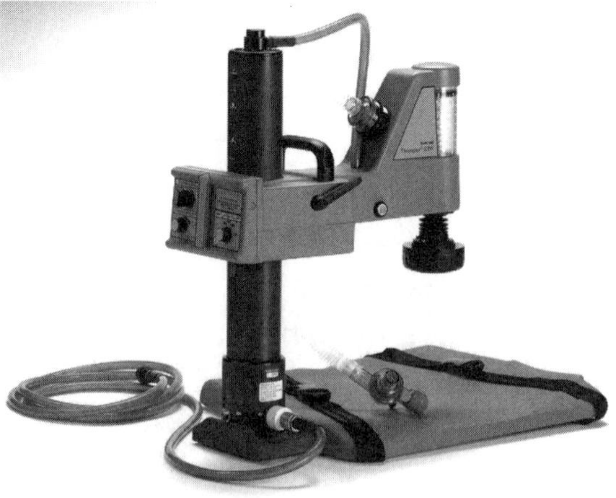

Figure 4-6 The Thumper CPR System.

The AutoPulse® is a load-distributing band CPR device designed to deliver compressions in a consistent and uninterrupted manner. The Thumper has a piston designed to provide both consistent high-quality compressions and ventilations.

Use of these devices should improve the hemodynamics during chest compressions provided to the pulseless arrest patient. Both devices can help to free up rescuers to focus on other lifesaving interventions and eliminate rescuer fatigue. In the past these devices were often reserved for the transport to the hospital. Since the Guidelines 2005 (*2005 American Heart Association Guidelines for Cardiopulmonary Resuscitation and Emergency Cardiovascular Care, Circulation: Journal of the American Heart Association (Volume 112, Number 24), December 13, 2005*) for CPR were so clear in emphasizing that the success of the code is based on the quality of the compressions and not the medications, the current philosophy is to get the mechanical adjuncts on as soon as possible! With improved circulation and quality of CPR there may be a greater likelihood that the vasopressors and antiarrythmics can be effective.

Teamwork: An Essential Resuscitation Skill

Teamwork is a very important part of preparing to be successful in managing cardiac arrest. During a resuscitation or "code" there are many tasks that need to be performed. Teamwork divides the tasks while multiplying the chances of success in the code. There is a role for each EMS provider who is committed to fulfilling his or her part. Experience tells us that teams who practice together regularly are more successful in their resuscitation attempts. Code team members (meaning you and your crew), need to be rested, fit, and well nourished. They need to bring a positive attitude to their work, practice their skills, know the "plays," and work together as a team to be able to achieve success. The best teams know how important it is to take the following key steps of preparation:

- Knows the plays expertly and automatically. This takes a lot of practice.
- Listen to your "coaches." They have the best interests of the patients in mind and yours too.
- Recognize the value of "practice." Pull out the manikins and run mock codes frequently. Collect data on the cumulative time of interruptions of compressions so that the team has feedback and can work to improve its performance.
- Remember that success equals practice, practice plus a positive mental attitude, well-designed plays (ie, algorithms), and excellent coaching.
- Recognize that the effectiveness of the team is not about you. It is about succeeding as a group. Patients are counting on you to get this right!

The stress level of the paramedic can be reduced by practicing codes and following a plan with clearly defined roles as we described here using the team member and team leader concept.

The Role of Code Team Members

The code team members often have different experiences and levels of training. It is the part of the code team leader's responsibility to use each member of the team to enhance their strengths, which in turn improves the effectiveness of the entire team effort. Code team members in the prehospital setting may be called on to perform a number of skills at a resuscitation including:

- As the ventilator managing the airway:
  - Suctioning the patient.
  - Applying cricoid pressure.
  - Ventilating the patient with a bag-mask device or ATV.
  - Inserting an advanced airway device (ie, LMA, ET tube, or Combitube).
  - Maintaining manual in-line immobilization of the head/neck.
- As the active compressor providing chest compressions. There are NO other "jobs" assigned to this team member other than to compress for 2 minutes and be the on-deck compressor for 2 minutes.
- As the on-deck compressor there is a limited amount of time to do other functions, but at the 2-minute point the team member needs to be ready to relieve the compressor without any interruption in compressions. Other functions may include:
  - Assisting with application of a mechanical CPR adjunct device (ie, Thumper, AutoPulse, etc.) if one is used.
  - Checking on vital signs.
  - Preparing the patient for transport.
- As other support personnel:
  - Analyzing the ECG and delivering shocks.
  - Gaining venous (IV or IO) access.
  - Providing documentation for the patient care report.
  - Supporting family members.

If it is not your responsibility to "run" the resuscitation as a code team leader, then it is understandable that you may not have mastered all the specific tasks (eg, medications and interpretation of ECGs, as well as decision-making), but it is expected that you will have mastered your own responsibilities and be firmly committed to the success of the attempt.

The Role of The Code Team Leader

Every resuscitation team needs a leader to organize the efforts of the group. The code team leader must know all the skills and know how to perform each skill. This is necessary because occasionally the code team leader will serve as the backup for a team member who may be having a tough time inserting a tube or gaining IV access. The code team leader is often responsible for making sure everything gets done at the right time in the right way.

Examples of the roles of the code team leader include:

- Taking the patient's history and performing the physical examination.
- Interpreting the ECG.
- Keeping track of the time.
- Making a medication decision following the ACLS pulseless arrest algorithm.
- Delegating tasks to code team members.
- Completing documentation after the resuscitation attempt.
- Talking with medical control.
- Controlling the resuscitation scene.

Code team leaders also have the important role of modeling excellent behavior and leadership skills for their team and all others who may be involved in the resuscitation. The code team leader should serve as a coach to help train future team leaders and seek to improve the effectiveness of the entire team through continuous quality improvement and practice after the resuscitation to help prepare for the next code.

Defibrillation or Compressions: Which Comes First?

Early defibrillation has been well proven to be an intervention that saves lives. Actually, the defibrillator is one of the few pieces of equipment carried on an ambulance that studies confirm makes a difference. We like to think all the rest of the gear we lug into people's homes is useful. However, most of our gear has either not been studied or the evidence of its effectiveness is based on low-level rational conjecture (common sense), common practices, or was accepted before evidence-based guidelines were put into place. The Guidelines 2005 (*2005 American Heart Association Guidelines for Cardiopulmonary Resuscitation and Emergency Cardiovascular Care, Circulation: Journal of the American Heart Association (Volume 112, Number 24), December 13, 2005*) emphasize the need for timely defibrillation in public places, in the homes of high-risk patients, and in commercial aircraft, airports, hospitals, doctor's offices, and outpatient clinics.

Here is the real question: In a recognized unresponsive patient, should the patient be shocked first or should the compressions be provided first? At the point where the heart goes into ventricular fibrillation (V-fib) and the patient becomes pulseless, they are very receptive to treatment with a dose of electricity (200 joules is the default dose for an adult). As time passes, the probability of a successful conversion to an acceptable rhythm, involving return of spontaneous circulation, declines. Therefore, the policy should be that if the EMS provider witnesses the arrest and has immediate access to a defibrillator (in hand or within reach), the electrodes should be applied and if the patient is in V-fib/pulseless V-tach, defibrillation should be provided right away. However, if the arrest is not actually witnessed, a period of five cycles of CPR (approximately 2 minutes) is the most appropriate management prior to checking the ECG and attempting defibrillation if the patient is in V-fib/pulseless V-tach. The research seems to indicate that the perfusion will improve the success of the defibrillation attempt.

To implement this policy, most EMS medical directors have stated that if you arrive on the scene and CPR is in progress by a bystander or family member, the quality of the compressions should be assessed. If the patient has been receiving high-quality compressions (pushing hard, pushing fast (100/min), and allowing full chest recoil), then their CPR would be considered the 2-minute trial. However, if you assess that the compressions were not of high quality, you then need to institute a full 2 minutes of high-quality compressions to improve myocardial perfusion prior to administering a dose of electricity.

Case Study III Asystole/Pulseless Electrical Activity

Part 1

Your unit has been dispatched to the local shopping mall where a day shift security guard found one of the midnight shift guards, Joey, slumped over in a chair in a remote storage area. Apparently the rest of the day shift have been wondering where he was because he has not been answering the radio for the last hour. You and your partner load up all of the equipment and head into a storage area behind one of the stores. You were told that there is another security guard doing CPR on Joey. As you approach, you can tell by the compressions and lack of ventilations that it has been a long time since he has performed CPR! Fortunately, you know your medical director has been working to ensure that all the security personnel refresh their CPR skills and that AEDs be placed throughout the mall.

On the radio you hear that your supervisor is also en route. He is supposed to bring the mechanical compression device with him on any confirmed arrest calls. As you approach the patient you review the ACLS adult pulseless arrest algorithm in your mind and prepare to perform the initial assessment (see **Table 1**).

Table 1 Initial Assessment

Initial Assessment	Recording Time: 2 Minutes
General Impression/ Appearance	Pale and cyanotic, poor general impression
Mental Status	Unresponsive, CPR compressions in progress
Airway	No ventilations, appears to be some vomitus near patient
Breathing	None
Circulation	Poor quality compressions
Priority/Plan	High

The first priority will be to relieve the security guard doing compressions since he is obviously tiring already. Your partner will set up the ventilator and begin ventilations while you do 2 minutes of compressions. Since this is a medical patient and there is no reason to consider trauma, he will need the assessment of a medical patient who is not responsive. However, there is a lot to do before you get to that point! Compressions are difficult because Joey is obese. Another security guard shows up and he is able to do compressions to relieve you. You get the electrodes attached and quickly determine the patient's ECG rhythm. Joey does not have a shockable rhythm. He is in asystole. You check another lead to confirm the strip and they agree. You ask the security guard who began the compressions to make sure someone meets the supervisor to lead him in with the AutoPulse. You then ask, "how long had you been calling Joey on the radio before you found him like this?" You realize that this situation is going to be emotionally charged because the patient is a co-worker, but it is important to determine the "downtime" because the patient may have been in arrest for most of the shift.

Question 1: What is the significance of establishing the potential downtime in this patient?

Question 2: If the security guard who started the compressions skipped ventilations because the patient had vomited and the compressions were too slow, not deep enough, and there was poor chest recoil, is it likely that the CPR has been helpful?

Part 2

Now that the patient is in confirmed asystole, CPR is immediately resumed and the priorities are attended to. This will include better airway management since the patient is likely to vomit again; continuing to rotate the compressor every 2 minutes; starting an IO to administer a vasopressor agent (1-mg epinephrine [Adrenalin] in this case); and considering the "Hs and Ts" as you learned in the ACLS course: hypovolemia, hypoxia or ventilation problems, hydrogen ion (acidosis), hypo-/hyperkalemia, hypoglycemia, hypothermia, toxins, tamponade (cardiac), tension pneumothorax, thrombosis (coronary or pulmonary), and trauma (ie, hypovolemia, increased ICP). You will use the "Hs and Ts" to consider the possible cause of adult pulseless arrest.

Considering the "Hs and Ts" as well as this patient's history, the probable cause could include hypoxia, thrombosis (coronary or pulmonary), and hydrogen ion (acidosis) possibly from the liquid diet the patient was on. Another security guard has arrived on the scene and he states that they have contacted Joey's wife and she is upset, but not entirely surprised because Joey has been complaining of chest pain all week. She says he was on a liquid-only diet as well as trying to quit smoking. She said he has done

Case Study III Continued

this before and was probably cheating by smoking cigarettes. He has a history of hypertension and high cholesterol and is taking medications to control both. She said she would get right into her car and be there in a few minutes. You begin the focused history and physical examination (see **Table 2**).

Question 3: What is the memory jogger "Hs and Ts" used for?

Question 4: With the information about the patient from his wife, what is the probable cause of the arrest?

Table 2 Focused History and Physical Examination

Baseline Vital Signs	Recording Time: 5 Minutes
Skin CTC (color, temperature, condition)	Pale and cyanotic
Pulse	None, CPR is in progress
Blood Pressure	None
Respirations	None, being ventilated at 6–8 breaths/min

Part 3

There is some difficulty obtaining IO access since the patient is obese and his veins are hard to find. Your partner tries the new IO bone drill and is successful. You administer the first round of epinephrine [Adrenalin] and perform 2 more minutes of CPR. Because the ECG has an occasional beat or complex (but they come very slowly—about 5/min), you decide to administer a 1-mg dose of atropine sulfate [Atropine]. This may be repeated every 3 to 5 minutes for a maximum of 0.4 mg/kg of atropine sulfate (Atropine).

Your supervisor arrives on scene with the AutoPulse as does Joey's wife. As the adjunct to compressions is applied to the patient, you are able to obtain some additional information from Joey's wife (see **Table 3**).

Table 3 SAMPLE History

SAMPLE History	Comments
Signs/symptoms	Chest pain and nausea for the last week. He refused to get it checked out.
Allergies	Sulfa drugs and many antibiotics
Medications	Atorvastatin calcium [Lipitor] and hydrochlothiazide, and nitroglycerin spray
Pertinent past medical history	Recent dieting, high levels of stress, angina, smoker
Last oral intake	A number of glasses of water before reporting to work at midnight
Events leading up to the incident	Dieting, limited sleep, and chest pains other days this week

Treatment Plan

You review in your mind the treatment that has taken place so far:

1. High-quality CPR is started.
2. Supplemental oxygen is administered.
3. The AED/monitor is attached and reveals asystole, which is not a shockable rhythm.
4. The reassessment and focus of this resuscitation is to immediately resume CPR.
5. An attempt is made at venous access. An IV is not successful but IO access is obtained.
6. Next the vasopressor epinephrine [Adrenalin] 1 mg is administered.
7. While CPR continues, the first dose of atropine sulfate [Atropine] 1 mg (see **Table 4**) is administered IO.

Basically the next actions in this case will involve continuing high-quality CPR and ensuring that the compressors are being rotated so no one is getting tired. The patient will receive up to two more doses of atropine sulfate [Atropine] at 1 mg each (the maximum dose is 0.4 mg/kg.) The epinephrine [Adrenalin] will be continued every 3 minutes of the arrest at 1-mg doses all focused around 2-minute cycles of high-quality CPR. There will come a time, after considering the "Hs and Ts" where consultation with medical control is the likely course of action to consider termination of the resuscitative efforts. Of course, this consideration assumes that there is no change of ECG rhythm or return of spontaneous circulation which research has shown is unlikely.

Sodium bicarbonate could be considered if there is a lengthy downtime and acidosis is not likely to be

Case Study III Continued

resolved with ventilation (see **Table 5**). In previous years, most of the drug box was filled with sodium bicarbonate prefilled syringes. Research has shown that parenteral bicarbonate may influence serum acidosis but does little to help out with intracellular pH problems. Overall it is believed that acidosis initially can be better managed with proper ventilation of the patient.

Table 4 **Atropine Sulfate**

Do you know?	Comments
Right drug? Generic name: [**Atropine Sulfate**] Trade name: [Atropine]	This drug is an anticholinergic agent. It is used to increase and restore the cardiac rate. It is also used as an antidote for toxicity due to organophosphate nerve agents and cholinergic drugs.
Right patient?	In this case it will be used for a patient with a hemodynamically unstable bradycardia, asystole, bradycardic (< 60 beats/minute) PEA.
Right dose?	For asystole or PEA: 1 mg IV/IO push. May repeat every 3–5 minutes to a maximum of 0.04 mg/kg.
Right route?	IV/IO. ET involves 2–3 mg diluted in 10 mL of normal saline or water.
Right time?	After the patient has received high-quality CPR for two cycles and the vasopressor has yet to work.
Right documentation?	Dose, route, time administered, and reassessment should be clearly documented on the patient care report.
Expected action	Parasympatholytic reaction that inhibits the action of acetylcholine at the postganglionic parasympathetic neuroeffector sites. It should increase the heart rate in life-threatening bradyarrhythmias.
Side effects	Headache, dizziness, palpitations, nausea and vomiting, tachycardia, arrhythmias, anticholinergic effects (blurred vision, dry mouth, urinary retention), paradoxical bradycardia when pushed slowly or at low doses, flushed, hot, dry skin.
Contraindications	Tachycardia, hypertension, unstable cardiovascular status in acute hemorrhage and myocardial ischemia, narrow-angle glaucoma. It is not appropriate in second-degree AV block and third-degree AV block.
Precautions	Potential adverse effects when administered with digoxin, cholinergics, physostigmine. Effects enhanced by antihistamines, procainamide hydrochloride, quinidine, antipsychotics, benzodiazepines, and antidepressants.
Pharmacokinetics	Onset immediate; peak effect rapid 1–2 minutes; metabolized by the liver, excreted through urine unchanged. About 30% to 50% is excreted unchanged in urine and the rest as metabolites; half life 4 hours.

Table 5 **Sodium Bicarbonate**

Do you know?	Comments
Right drug? Generic name: [**Sodium Bicarbonate**] Trade name: [Citrocarbonate, Neut]	This drug is an alkalinizing agent, antacid, and electrolyte. It is used to treat acute metabolic acidosis caused by shock, severe dehydration, anoxia, uncontrolled diabetes, renal disease, cardiac arrest, and severe lactic acidosis. It is also used to treat hyperacidity, and prophylaxis for renal calculi.
Right patient?	In this case it can be used for prolonged downtime in cardiac arrest.
Right dose?	1 mEq/kg.
Right route?	IV bolus in a secondary line.
Right time?	After vasopressors, antiarrythmics, and any other drugs. It is typically used as a last option drug in cardiac arrest.

continues

Case Study III Continued

Table 5 Sodium Bicarbonate (*Continued*)

Do you know?	Comments
Right documentation?	Dose, route, time administered, and reassessment should be clearly documented on the patient care report.
Expected action	Relief of metabolic acidosis.
Side effects	Hypernatremia, alkalosis, tetany, and fluid overload.
Contraindications	Metabolic and respiratory alkalosis, hypertension, convulsions, and CHF.
Precautions	Used with caution in patients with impaired renal and hepatic function, and cardiovascular insufficiency with or without CHF.
Pharmacokinetics	Rapidly metabolized to carbonic acid which rapidly dissociates into water and carbon dioxide. The carbon dioxide is excreted via the lungs.

Question 5: What are the key issues in the management of an adult in pulseless arrest who has an ECG of either PEA or asystole?

Question 6: How often is the patient reassessed?

Part 4

An advanced airway was placed and the primary route of medications is the IO route. Your Medical Director shows up on the scene and after a brief report of lack of progress and the fact that there has been no return of spontaneous circulation, he feels that termination of the code is the most appropriate course of action (see **Table 6**). It was agreed that the downtime was probably a considerable amount of time, even before the radio calls were first placed for the patient.

You now turn your attention to the patient's wife, trying to comfort her and offering to call a family member as well as a clergy member. The other security guards are arranging for a police report and a local funeral director to come and pick up Joey's body per the orders of the Medical Director.

Table 6 Reassessment and Ongoing Assessment of the Patient

Serial Vital Signs and Relevant Data	Recording Time: 10 Minutes
Skin CTC	Pale and less cyanotic than before
Pulse	No pulse
Blood Pressure	None
Respirations	None
Mental Status	Unresponsive
ECG	Asystole
SpO_2	In the 60s
Lung Sounds	Clear and the tube is in the correct location
Other (ie, glucose, core body temperature (CBT))	$EtCO_2$ is about 40, CBT is normal

Question 7: If the patient was in a cold part of the warehouse and his body temperature was low, would this change your management of this patient?

Question 8: What do the CPR Guidelines say about lengthy resuscitative efforts and the transportation of cardiac arrest patients?

Part 5

The response to this cardiac arrest was appropriate, but like many cardiac arrests it did not have a successful outcome. Certainly it was an eye-opening experience for the other members of security at the mall. After the funeral has passed, it will be appropriate for your Medical Director to make one more attempt to convince the security guards that it is important for them to learn CPR and how to use AEDs. It would also be appropriate to find the money to install AEDs throughout the mall so that the next cardiac arrest can be rapidly managed. It may also be a good window of opportunity to discuss the need for the guards to exercise on a regular basis, alter poor eating habits, and control their cholesterol and blood pressure. Sometimes it takes a life to pass to wake up those left behind.

Chest Compressions: Do Not Disturb!

Studies have shown that interruption of chest compressions is associated with reduced coronary perfusion pressure and the more frequent or prolonged the interruption, the lower the mean coronary perfusion pressure. Think of the resuscitation as a rock song where the bass guitar and the drums create the underlying beat. The other instruments (ie, keyboard, lead guitar) and the vocals are layered on top of the underlying rhythm. The same holds true for a resuscitation where the compressions create the beat or perfusion and all other interventions are layered on top of the chest compressions (ie, defibrillation, drugs, airway management). When the drums stop so does the song . . . when the compressions stop so does the resuscitation, so do not disturb!

Expansion of the Use of Intraosseous Access

Intraosseous (IO) access has been around for a long time but in the past it was commonly practiced in pediatric patients younger than the age of 6 years. The Guidelines 2005 (*2005 American Heart Association Guidelines for Cardiopulmonary Resuscitation and Emergency Cardiovascular Care, Circulation: Journal of the American Heart Association (Volume 112, Number 24), December 13, 2005*) expanded the use of IO access to all ages of patients in extremis where a peripheral line was not immediately available. The algorithm for the adult pulseless arrest patient clearly states that IO is an acceptable type of access to the patient's circulation. Due to the hollow nature of the patient's long bones, the infused fluids make it to the central circulation as fast as an injection into a central venous line (ie, internal jugular or subclavian vein). With the introduction of modern IO placement devices, such as the F.A.S.T.1 (First Access for Shock and Trauma) for the sternum site, the EZ-IO bone drill for the tibia or more recently the humerus site, and the Bone Injection Gun (BIG) for the tibia site, this technique has become much easier to perform (these devices are shown in Chapter One).

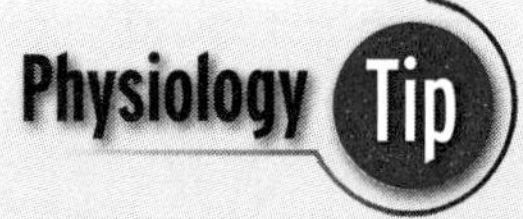

Medications administered into the long bone of the tibia access the central circulation as fast as a central line. This is especially helpful when compared to other slower routes such as SC or IM to administer a medication to the patient.

Termination in the Field

There are very few instances that require transporting a cardiac arrest patient who has failed a successfully executed prehospital ACLS resuscitation effort to an ED to continue the resuscitation attempt. In the absence of mitigating factors, prolonged resuscitative efforts are unlikely to be successful. If return of spontaneous circulation (ROSC) of any duration occurs, however, it may be appropriate to consider extending the resuscitative effort. Rare exceptions may include severe prehospital hypothermia (eg, submersion in icy water), and drug overdose. A successfully executed prehospital resuscitation includes an "adequate trial" of BLS and ALS.

Transporting a deceased patient refractory to proper BLS/ACLS is considered unethical (and unsafe). If the efforts have failed in the prehospital setting, how could the same treatment succeed in the ED? It is well known that any lights and siren transport to the ED increases the risk of a collision and death or injury to the EMS providers. Protocols for pronouncement of death and appropriate transport of the body by non-EMS vehicles should be established in every region. For more information on this topic you should consult with your service medical director. Instead of focusing on the deceased patient, The International Liaison Committee of Resuscitation (ILCOR) recommends that paramedics should be trained to focus on dealing sensitively with family.

Defibrillation and the Hypothermic Patient

When a patient is unresponsive and thought to be potentially hypothermic, you should extend the time to assess the pulse from 5 to 10 seconds to 30 to 45 seconds. The hypothermic patient is likely to be in profound bradycardia, experiencing a heart rate of less than 60 beats/min. If the patient is not breathing, rescue breaths should be started immediately. If the patient is pulseless, chest compressions should be started immediately. Do not wait for the patient to be rewarmed until you begin CPR! Wet clothing should be removed to prevent further heat loss. Insulate the patient from the wind and cold and if possible ventilate with warmed humidified oxygen. Avoid rough movement and transport the patient to the ED as soon as possible. If the patient is in V-fib/pulseless V-tach, a single shock should be attempted. If the shock is not effective in converting the patient, the algorithm suggests two additional shocks separated by 2 minutes (5 cycles) of CPR. After three shocks have been unsuccessful, simply transport the patient. The medications typically administered to the patient in pulseless arrest are not given when the patient is in hypothermia. They are not designed to be effective with the colder body temperature and will simply accumulate in the body and may "kick in" all at once when the core body temperature is raised.

Successful Implementation of Public Access Defibrillation

Research has shown that public access defibrillation and first responder AED programs may increase the number of sudden cardiac arrest victims who receive bystander CPR and early defibrillation, improving survival from prehospital sudden cardiac arrest. The most effective programs have an organized and practiced response with rescuers trained and equipped to implement the chain of survival (ie, early access, early CPR, early defibrillation, and early advanced care) including the AED. There have been reports of lay rescuer AED programs that include the placement as well as the training of employees (ie, airports, on airplanes, casinos) and first responder programs with police officers achieving survival rates of as high as 49% to 74% from prehospital witnessed V-fib sudden cardiac arrest. In these cases there was a system in place for initiation of immediate bystander CPR and defibrillation within 3 to 5 minutes of collapse.

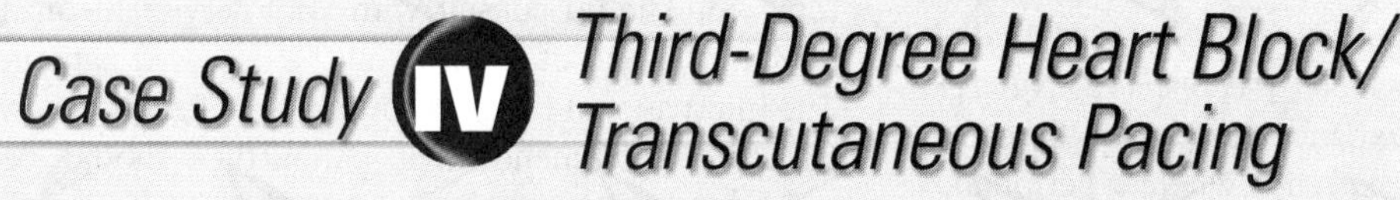

Part 1

Your unit has been dispatched to a supermarket where a woman in her 50s collapsed at the checkout line. The police are on the scene and state that she is awake at this time and resting in a chair. As you pull up in front of the store, you think about all of the typical reasons that people pass out or experience syncope in public places. You and your partner load up the stretcher and are lead into the store by an employee. As you approach the patient you can see she is sitting back in one of those inexpensive plastic yard chairs the store sells. She looks very pale and clammy.

The scene is safe and the officer is questioning the patient. Apparently her daughter works nearby and has already been called. The cashier states that Mrs. Greene must have passed out from the heat. She was unconscious for less than a minute and when she woke up they had put her in the chair. She also adds that the patient did not strike her head when she passed out.

You introduce yourself to the patient and begin doing your initial assessment to see if there are any life-threats that need to be immediately managed (see **Table 1**).

Table 1 Initial Assessment

Initial Assessment	Recording Time: 2 Minutes
General Impression/ Appearance	Pasty looking, very sweaty
Mental Status	"V" verbal (knows name, where she is but is confused about the day)
Airway	Open and clear
Breathing	24 breaths/min and shallow
Circulation	Very slow heart rate
Priority/Plan	High, as general impression is poor

Case Study IV Continued

Since the patient did not experience any trauma and did not fall and injure herself, you decide that the assessment will need to follow the pathway of that for a responsive medical patient. You will also need to elaborate on the chief complaint of an altered mental status and fainting spell. You know there are many potential causes of fainting, a syncope episode, or sudden transient loss of consciousness, so this should not be underplayed. First and foremost is to determine if true syncope occurred. In many instances, near-syncope is truly what happened, and prognostically that is an entirely different matter. Additionally, separating cardiogenic (Stokes-Adams) syncope from other forms of syncope can be challenging. Other differentials that may present need to be considered (seizure, migraine, vertigo). Generally speaking, the causes of syncope can be divided up into three general categories: cardiac causes, non-cardiac causes, and medication induced (see **Table 2**).

If a patient takes beta-blocker medications, he or she could be bleeding internally and the typical sign of tachycardia would be prevented by the medication. Watch out for patients who may have accidentally overdosed on multiple medications. If the patient is overmedicated with the beta-blocker itself or in combination with another medication, that could prove problematic. Always be aware of polypharmacy when obtaining a history. Lastly, we must consider the overall patient situation when dealing with syncope. Syncope in a diabetic 80-year-old individual with prior CAD is different than syncope in an otherwise healthy 22-year-old individual.

Table 2 Causes of Syncope

Cardiac Causes	Heart blocks and bradycardias Arrhythmias (ie, supraventricular tachycardia, Stokes-Adams syndrome, sick sinus syndrome) Aortic stenosis AMI Angina
Non-Cardiac Causes	Neurologic Hemorrhagic Vasovagal Micturition (urination) Dehydration Respiratory Pharmacologic Emotional (ie, stress, anxiety, fright)
Medications that can cause syncope	Beta-blockers Diuretics Antihypertensives Narcotic analgesics Antiarrhythmics Nitrates Digitalis ACE inhibitors Psychiatric medications (ie, tricyclics)

Question 1: What are some of the causes of a patient passing out?

Question 2: What is the significance of a very slow heart rate?

Part 2

Mrs. Greene says that this is not the first time she has felt dizzy and almost like she was going to pass out this month. She also says she has been getting hot flashes and figured it was all due to her going through her "change of life." She is otherwise healthy looking but when you ask if she normally works out she said she does not know where the gym is in this town. Your OPQRST elaboration on the chief complaint reveals that she did feel dizzy, hot, and sweaty just prior to waking up on the floor with the store's employees putting a cool towel on her forehead. She denies any pain in her head or chest but does say she feels rather nauseous and weak sitting in the chair. You and your partner decide to lift her over to your stretcher and place her in the Trendelenburg position. Your partner is also getting a nonrebreathing mask ready to place supplemental oxygen on her. After asking a few key questions you decide to do a focused history and physical examination including lung

Case Study IV Continued

sounds, and a quick neurologic examination to verify there is no trauma (see **Table 3**).

Question 3: Why would it be helpful to ask when she last had something to eat or drink?

Question 4: During your questioning, why would it be helpful to find out if the patient takes any specific medications?

Table 3 Focused History and Physical Examination

Baseline Vital Signs	Recording Time: 5 Minutes
Skin CTC (color, temperature, condition)	Pale, cool, and clammy
Pulse	48 beats/min and regular
Blood Pressure	90/68 mm Hg
Respirations	24 breaths/min and shallow

Part 3

As you continue to acquire a SAMPLE history from Mrs. Greene, your partner obtains an IV and the ECG electrodes are applied (see **Table 4**). She is very dizzy, diaphoretic, and her mental status is confused. She states she feels like she is fading in and out. Her daughter arrives on the scene and explains that her mother has been having dizzy spells for the past few months. The family physician referred her to a cardiologist because she has an abnormal cardiogram but she has yet to see the specialist. Apparently she canceled the last appointment because she was too busy and the next appointment is next week.

When you examine the ECG it looks like she will be seeing that cardiologist sooner than next week. You recall from your paramedic course that a normal heartbeat is generated by the **SA node**, travels through the **internodal pathways** to the **AV node**, through the **Bundle of His**, and then down into the right and left bundle branches and Purkinje fibers of the ventricles (**Figure 1**). The P-R interval is a measurement of the time an impulse takes to get through the atrium and into the ventricles where it produces the QRS complexes/intervals (**Figure 2**). A high-degree block is one where the ventricle is basically cut off from the impulses of the atrium's SA node. The inherent rate of the ventricles (20–40) kicks in when this happens. This can produce very poor perfusion and is likely to allow lethal ventricular rhythms to

Table 4 SAMPLE History

SAMPLE History	Comments
Signs/symptoms	Dizziness, nausea, weakness, fainting
Allergies	None
Medications	Folic acid, multivitamin, aspirin
Pertinent past medical history	Fainting spells, hysterectomy 4 years ago, gall bladder removed 10 years ago
Last oral intake	Tea and toast about 2 hours ago
Events leading up to the incident	Busy day, feeling dizzy and passed out in store

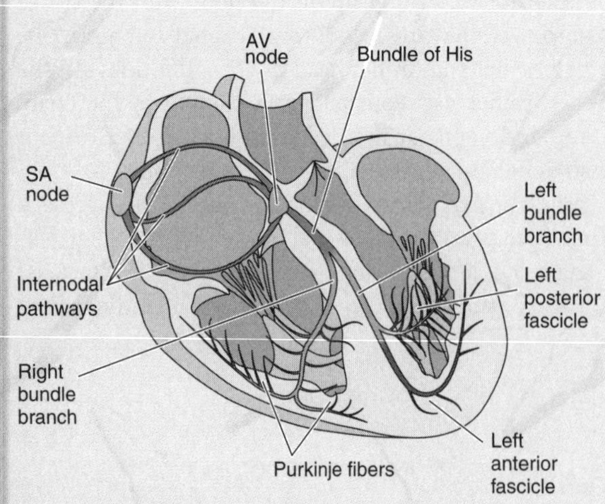

Figure 1 The heart's conduction system.

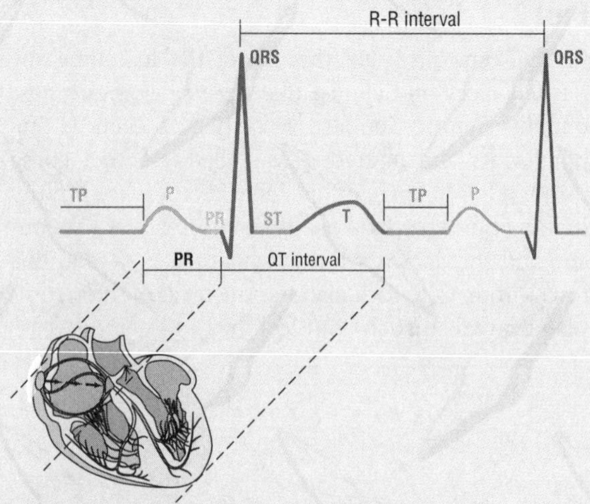

Figure 2 The ECG and cardiac events.

Case Study IV Continued

intercede. The high-degree blocks are second-degree type II and third-degree or complete heart block.

The patient's ECG is very slow and she has a third-degree AV block. You will need to prepare for transcutaneous pacing (TCP). Atropine sulfate [Atropine] would be useful in a first- or second-degree type I block (**Figure 3**), but it is generally not the first approach in this type of symptomatic bradycardia (ie, second-degree type II or third-degree AV block (**Figure 4**). Generally, the approach with high-level blocks is to use electricity rather than medications. The drugs we give help to increase the transmission of impulses from the AV node. In a high-degree block, very few, if any, of the impulses from the atria make it through to the ventricles; therefore, treating with a medication, such as atropine sulfate [Atropine] is generally not effective in improving the rate of the ventricles. At this point the highest priority is to apply the external pacemaker and begin TCP on the patient. Because an IV is already in place you quickly contact medical control for approval to give the patient 5 mg diazepam [Valium] as an IV push. Some EMS systems still make it a practice to administer the atropine sulfate [Atropine] as they are preparing to pace the patient but the drug is usually not the solution.

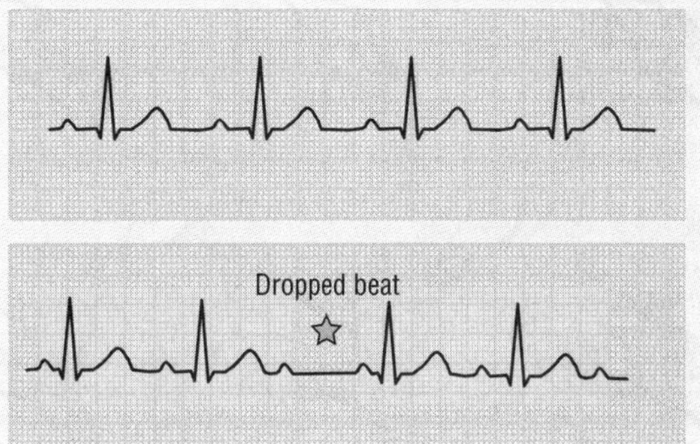

Figure 3 First-degree heart block and second-degree heart block (Wenckebach).

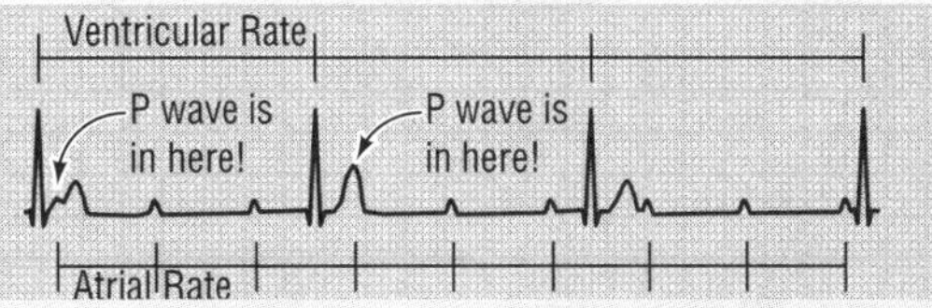

Figure 4 Third-degree heart block.

Treatment Plan

This patient needs a fast track approach involving management of the ABCs including:

1. Administer supplemental oxygen.
2. Obtain a complete set of baseline vital signs and assess the ECG.
3. Start an IV for a keep vein open line of normal saline.
4. Determine your course of action: drug, electricity, or both as defined by your local protocols and ACLS.

Many paramedic units would then administer 0.5 mg atropine sulfate (Atropine) as an IV bolus as they were setting up for transcutaneous pacing (TCP) although it is generally not effective for the high-degree blocks (see **Table 5**). Depending on your regional protocols, you may need to make quick contact with medical control for a diazepam [Valium], etomidate [Amidate], or midazolam [Versed] order to make the discomfort of the pacing more tolerable for the patient (realize that all of the specified medications are sedatives and not analgesics; therefore, they should not actually reduce the pain of pacing). Do not delay TCP because it is likely to keep this patient from going into cardiac arrest. Other medications for consideration if the pacer is ineffective include

Table 5 Atropine Sulfate

Do you know?	Comments
Right drug? Generic name: [**Atropine Sulfate**] Trade name: [Atropine]	This drug is an anticholinergic agent. It is used to restore cardiac rate and arterial pressure. It is also used as an antidote for toxicity due to organophosphate nerve agents, cholinergic drugs, pilocarpine, physostigmine, or isoflurophate.
Right patient?	In this case it will be used for a patient with a hemodynamically unstable bradycardia (< 60 beats per minute).
Right dose?	For asystole or PEA: 1 mg IV/IO push. May repeat every 3–5 minutes to a maximum of 0.04 mg/kg.

continues

Case Study IV Continued

Table 5 **Atropine Sulfate (*Continued*)**

Do you know?	Comments
Right route?	IV/IO. If the patient had an ET tube and there was no other access you could administer the drug in that way. ET involves 2–3 mg diluted in 10 mL of saline and has questionable effectiveness.
Right time?	After the patient has received high-quality CPR for two cycles and the vasopressor has yet to work.
Right documentation?	Dose, route, time administered, and reassessment should be clearly documented on the patient care report.
Expected action	Parasympatholytic reaction that inhibits the action of acetylcholine at the postganglionic parasympathetic neuroeffector sites. It should increase the heart rate in life-threatening bradyarrhythmias.
Side effects	Headache, dizziness, palpitations, nausea and vomiting, tachycardia, arrhythmias, anticholinergic effects (blurred vision, dry mouth, urinary retention), paradoxical bradycardia when pushed slowly or at low doses, flushed, hot, dry skin.
Contraindications	Tachycardia, hypertension, unstable cardiovascular status in acute hemorrhage and myocardial ischemia, narrow-angle glaucoma.
Precautions	Potential adverse effects when administered with digoxin, cholinergics, physostigmine. Effects enhanced by antihistamines, procainamide hydrochloride, quinidine, antipsychotics, benzodiazepines, and antidepressants.
Pharmacokinetics	Onset immediate; peak 1–2 min; metabolized by the liver, excreted through urine unchanged. About 30% to 50% is excreted unchanged in urine and the rest as metabolites; half life 4 hours.

epinephrine [Adrenalin] infusion at 2 to 10 µg/min or dopamine [Intropin] infusion of 2 to 10 µg/min drip. Mrs. Greene should be transported quickly and your ongoing assessment should include repeating the serial vital signs as well as the cardiopulmonary examination.

Once at the hospital, the staff will review the patient's current and recent past medical situation. Should it be revealed that she uses any medications that may predispose to bradycardia, they would be discontinued. If by chance she happens to have a case of tertiary Lyme disease, she would be treated with appropriate antibiotics. If she remained critically ill with bradycardia despite EMS interventions, she would be taken to the electrophysiology laboratory to have a more permanent indwelling pacemaker installed. If there were any concern about myocardial ischemia or acute coronary syndrome, she would also be taken to the catheterization laboratory to undergo an appropriate intervention. She will then be admitted to either a telemetry or coronary care unit for further monitoring and for continued work-up of the cause of the arrhythmia.

Question 5: What is a high-degree block?

Question 6: Why is TCP the appropriate treatment for this type of block?

Part 4

As you are loading the patient into the ambulance, you observe that the pacemaker seems to have improved her mental status. She is alert and able to answer all of your questions. She also has a number of questions to ask you about this electrical device you are placing on her chest. You tell her she is slightly medicated with the diazepam [Valium] and that she should let you know if the pain starts to return and you will attempt to help her. She also confirms that she does not have a history of diabetes or stroke. Now that she is able to give you additional history you can explore other potential causes of the syncope during a reassessment (see **Table 6**).

You remember your medical director telling the group at a recent class, "Basically if the cause of the bradycardia is a medication overdose, then you should attempt to manage it. If the patient fell and

has a hip fracture, always remember to monitor the patient and do a complete work-up because syncope may have been the cause of the fall. If the cause is cardiac, such as a decaying conduction system, that too should be managed. Symptomatic bradycardias can be very complicated and often require expert consultation from the cardiologist once the patient gets to the hospital. Your job, as the paramedics in the field, is to follow the ACLS algorithm to the letter and get the patient to the experts as soon as possible!"

Question 7: If the TCP is ineffective, are there any other options in the prehospital setting?

Question 8: The algorithm says to treat the contributing causes and consider expert consultation. What does that mean?

Table 6 Reassessment and Ongoing Assessment of the Patient

Serial Vital Signs and Relevant Data	Recording Time: 10 Minutes
Skin CTC	Pale and less clammy
Pulse	70 beats/min with the TCP
Blood Pressure	110/72 mm Hg with pacing
Respirations	24 breaths/min and normal
Mental Status	"A" alert since TCP began
ECG	Paced ECG at 70 beats/min
SpO_2	98% on nonrebreathing mask
Lung Sounds	Clear bilaterally
Other (ie, glucose, core temperature)	Normal body temperature

Part 5

Fortunately for Mrs. Greene she was in a very public place when she passed out. Had this occurred in her home when she was fixing dinner on the stove, the situation could have been disastrous. She was given some warnings in the prior weeks as to something not being quite right with her health but she had put off following up with the cardiologist as her family physician had urged her to do.

The next day when you are taking another patient into the ED you happen to run into Mrs. Greene's daughter. She is very thankful and invites you to come up to the critical care unit to visit her mother. Maybe she will even show you the photos of the new pacemaker she had installed late last night!

Dangerously Slow Heart Rate

Heart disease, arrhythmias, heart attack, medications, and vasovagal stimuli are just a few possible reasons that can cause the heart rate to become too slow. When the heart rate becomes slow enough for the patient to experience symptoms, this usually results in a call to 9-1-1. Prescription medications used to treat heart disease, arrhythmias, hypertension, and other chronic conditions sometimes produce serious side effects or become toxic due to overdosing or liver and renal failure and can lead to cardiac arrest. In those rare instances when the cause of a cardiac arrest is known, such as a new onset of complete heart block or a look at the patient's medication list gives a clue to a possible cause (ie, an overdose of verapamil [Calan, Isoptin] which is a calcium channel blocker), the patient should be treated with additional medications that are tailored to the cause. Calcium chloride is an electrolyte that can be used in either cardiac arrest or patients with known toxicity or overdose of calcium channel blockers and magnesium sulfate (**Table 4-2**▼). Isoproterenol hydrochloride [Isuprel]

Table 4-2 Calcium Chloride

Right drug? Generic name: **[Calcium Chloride]** Trade name: [Calcium Chloride]	This drug is an electrolyte. It is used as an adjunct to manage severe hyperkalemia, hypocalcemia, hypermagnesemia, and calcium channel blocker or magnesium sulfate toxicity/overdose.
Right patient?	For use in post-cardiac arrest if known hyperkalemia, hypocalcemia, hypermagnesemia, and calcium channel blocker or magnesium sulfate toxicity/overdose.

continues

Table 4-2 Calcium Chloride (*Continued*)

Right dose?	0.5 to 1 gram.
Right route?	IV.
Right time?	After assessment and recognition of one of the indications for its use.
Right documentation?	Dose, route, time administered, and reassessment should be clearly documented on the patient care report.
Expected action	It increases cardiac contractility and automaticity. It reverses the symptoms of calcium channel blocker or magnesium sulfate overdose.
Side effects	Rapid administration may cause hypotension and cardiac syncope.
Contraindications	V-fib, hypercalcemia, and hypocalcemia of renal insufficiency.
Precautions	Used with caution in patients taking digitalis.
Pharmacokinetics	Onset 3–5 minutes; peak 5–15 minutes; 80% excreted in feces as insoluble salts and 20% in urine.

Table 4-3 Isoproterenol Hydrochloride

Right drug? Generic name: [**Isoproterenol Hydrochloride**] Trade name: [Isuprel]	This drug is a sympathomimetic. It is used to treat mild or transient heart block that does not require electric shock or pacemaker therapy and for cardiac arrest until electric shock or pacemaker therapy is available. It is also used as an adjunct to fluid and electrolyte replacement therapy to treat hypovolemic and septic shock, low cardiac output states, CHF, and cardiogenic shock.
Right patient?	At this point this medication is only used in the hospital setting and is not considered a first-line drug.
Right dose?	IV injection dilute 1 mL of the 1:5,000 (2 mg) to 10 mL with NS or D_5W. Initial dose is typically 1–3 mL (0.02–0.06 mg) of diluted solution. For drip dilute 5 mL of the 1:5,000 (1 mg) in 250 mL of D_5W or NS (1.25 mcg/min) deliver 5 μg/min.
Right route?	IV injection or drip.
Right time?	After assessment and recognition of one of the indications for its use.
Right documentation?	Dose, route, time administered, and reassessment should be clearly documented on the patient care report.
Expected action	Speeds up the heart, often at the expense of enlarging the infarcted tissue in the heart.
Side effects	Cardiac arrest, Adams-Stokes attack, hypotension, chest pain, and dyspnea.
Contraindications	Tachycardia, tachyarrhythmias, or heart block caused by digitalis toxicity.
Precautions	Has negative interactions with many other drugs (ie, tricyclic antidepressants).
Pharmacokinetics	Onset immediate; duration < hour; partially metabolized, excreted in urine.

is a sympathomimetic only used in the hospital setting to treat mild or transient heart block that does not require electric shock or pacemaker therapy and for cardiac arrest until electric shock or pacemaker therapy is available (**Table 4-3**▲). Its use has been significantly downplayed in the past few years due to its potential for increasing the size of an MI in the context of ACS. Procainamide hydrochloride [Procanbid (old name was Pronestyl)] is an antiarrhythmic used in the hospital setting to treat ventricular tachycardia and persistent V-fib/V-tach arrest (**Table 4-4**▶). It is also used to treat atrial fibrillation, a rhythm in which the atria no longer contract, but rather fibrillate or quiver without any organized contraction (**Figure 4-7**▶).

For many years procainamide hydrochloride [Procanbid] was listed as the last drug or near last drug of choice in the persistent V-fib/V-tach arrest algorithm, but was discontinued because of the risks associated with its use and the lack of evidence to show its effectiveness.

Nausea and Vomiting

With the symptom of nausea being so common, it is helpful to review what causes nausea and vomiting. Vomiting is often, but not always, preceded by nausea. The vomiting reflex is located in the vomiting center in the medulla. The reflex can be stimulated by several mechanisms (**Table 4-5**▶).

Table 4-4 Procainamide Hydrochloride

Right drug? Generic name: [**Procainamide Hydrochloride**] Trade name: [Pronestyl, Procanbid]	This drug is an antiarrhythmic. It is used to treat ventricular tachycardia, atrial fibrillation and flutter. It has some anticholinergic and local anesthetic effects.
Right patient?	In life-threatening indications where the benefits of treatment outweigh risks.
Right dose?	For recurrent VF/VT administer 20 mg/min IV infusion (maximum dose 17 mg/kg). In urgent situations, up to 50 mg/min may be administered. For other indications: administer 20 mg/min until one of the following occurs: arrhythmia suppression, hypotension, QRS widens by > 50% or total dose of 17 mg/kg is given.
Right route?	IV drip.
Right time?	After assessment and recognition of one of the indications for its use.
Right documentation?	Dose, route, time administered, and reassessment should be clearly documented on the patient care report.
Expected action	Prolongs the refractory period of the atria and to a lesser extent the Bundle of His-Purkinje system and ventricles.
Side effects	May cause AV block or complete heart block, V-fib or asystole, hypotension, GI symptoms, dizziness, weakness, thrombocytopenia, hives, and rash.
Contraindications	Known sensitivity, complete heart block, lupus, torsades de pointes, and asymptomatic PVCs.
Precautions	Should only be used with life-threatening ventricular arrhythmias. For Wolff-Parkinson-White (WPW) syndrome, use beta-blocker first.
Pharmacokinetics	Onset 10–30 minutes; peak variable; duration 3–6 hours; metabolized/eliminated 50% renal and 50% hepatic.

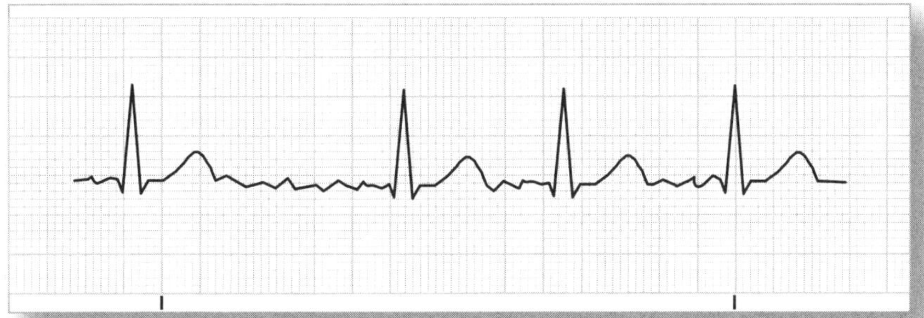

Figure 4-7 Atrial fibrillation.

Table 4-5 Stimulating the Vomiting Reflex

Sensory receptors in the stomach and intestines may stimulate the reflux due to infection, gastric irritation, or injury.
Chemoreceptor trigger zones in the vestibular system are stimulated by: 1. Inner ear disorders (ie, dizziness, vertigo, motion sickness). 2. Various drugs (ie, morphine, digitalis, and various anesthetics). 3. Endogenous toxins.
Increased intracranial pressure can stimulate the reflex as seen with brain disorders (ie, TBI, infections, tumors, migraine).
Stimulation of the cerebral cortex and limbic system by noxious stimuli or stress.
Voluntary stimulation of the gag reflex.

Alpha and Beta Receptors

Many of the medications used in cardiovascular emergencies are designed to have an effect on the nervous system's adrenergic receptors, particularly those found in the heart, lungs, and vessels of the body. The adrenergic receptors have been subdivided into: alpha 1, alpha 2, beta 1, beta 2, beta 3, and beta 4 receptors. In this text we will be focusing on how medications work with these receptors to either stimulate (agonist) or block (antagonist) the sympathetic response. Beta 3 receptors may affect how the body metabolizes fatty acids and could be the site of antiobesity drugs in the future. The purpose of beta 4 receptors has yet to be discovered. Certain drugs can affect only one receptor (selective), whereas others affect all receptors (nonselective). Some drugs can stimulate one receptor at low doses and other receptors at higher doses.

Alpha 1 receptors cause contraction (vasoconstriction) of smooth muscle, blood vessels to the skin, GI system, kidney, and brain. The **alpha 2 receptors** are inhibitory and stop the release of norepinephrine, inhibit insulin release in the pancreas, contract the sphincters of the GI tract, and induce glucagons release from the pancreas. **Beta 1 receptors**, when stimulated, are responsible for increasing the cardiac output and increasing the rate and force of myocardial contraction. **Beta 2 receptors**, when stimulated, relax the smooth muscles (ie, bronchi), dilate the skeletal muscles, relax the urinary sphincter, and contract the sphincters of the GI tract. Beta antagonists block the sympathetic nervous system from increasing the rate and force of myocardial contraction. Beta 1 receptors also regulate the release of renin from the kidney; this reduces the formation and activity of angiotensin II which affects blood pressure. Beta 1 antagonists decrease blood pressure. Beta-blockers are also used to treat ischemic heart disease and prevent reinfarction following an MI because they decrease myocardial oxygen consumption by decreasing the rate and force of myocardial contraction. Some beta-blockers are used to treat supraventricular tachycardia that is caused by excess stimulation of beta 1 receptors. Other beta-blockers are used to treat CHF. Beta-blockers are also used to treat conditions unrelated to cardiovascular problems.

Some patients who have a history of angina take beta-blockers. Excessive use of beta-blockers can lead to a symptomatic bradycardia (discussed in Case Study IV). There are many commonly prescribed beta-blockers you may come across in the field (**Table 4-6 ▸**).

Table 4-6 Commonly Prescribed Beta-Blockers

Generic name	Trade name
Acebutolol	Sectral
Atenolol	Tenormin
Betaxolol	Kerlone
Bisoprolol	Zebeta
Cartelol	Cartrol
Carvedilol	Coreg
Esmolol	Brevibloc
Labetalol (mixed alpha- and beta-blockade)	Normodyne, Trandate
Metoprolol	Lopressor, Toprol-XL
Nadolol	Corgard, Corzide
Penbutolol	Levatol
Pindolol	Visken
Propranolol hydrochloride	Inderal, Inderal-LA
Sotalol	Betapace
Timolol	Biocadren, Timolide

Common sense safety practices should always be first priority to avoid rescuer or patient harm. For example if you only administer part of a syringe of medication you had to draw up from a multi-dose vial to the patient, always label the syringe so it is clear what is left in that syringe. It will not serve the patient well for the paramedic to administer a dose of atropine sulfate [Atropine] instead of diazepam [Valium]. In addition, even though the dose of electricity administered by an automatic implantable cardioverter defibrillator (AICD) is considerably less than the dose you administer with your external defibrillator or AED, it is still strongly suggested that you do not come in contact with the patient as the device is firing.

Pacemakers

Pacemakers come in three types: external or noninvasive transcutaneous pacer (TCP), transvenous temporary wires, and internal or invasive (surgically implanted). TCPs are now routinely found as a component in cardiac monitor/defibrillators, or they can be freestanding and are battery or wall current powered. They have adjustable control settings for heart rate and amplitude. The device comes with two large external pacer pads that adhere to the chest wall similar to the pads of an AED. TCPs are used as a temporary treatment until an invasive pacer can be placed in the patient. In some instances a TCP may be used as a temporary measure because the battery in a patient's artificial internal pacemaker is failing and there is no capture. Transvenous pacemakers are installed in emergency situations where the bradycardia is insensitive to the TCP and a patient is not ready to have an implanted pacer placed. A central vein is accessed percutaneously with a large bore introducer and the transvenous wire is placed using a blind approach. If the patient has cardiac output, a balloon-tipped pacing wire is used to help direct the wire tip into the right ventricle. If there is no appreciable cardiac output, a semirigid device is employed and blindly steered into the ventricle. Implanted pacers come with various features depending on patient requirements. These devices are placed under the skin, commonly in the left or right upper chest wall. Electrode catheters are attached to the pacer at one end, with the other end inserted into the heart through the subclavian vein. Battery-operated invasive pacers have the feature of being on all the time (non-demand) or on only when needed (demand). Another important feature of invasive pacers is how they stimulate the heart to contract. They are typically categorized as either single chamber or dual chamber. Some pacers stimulate the atria (atrial pacers) which in turn produce atrial contraction followed by ventricular contraction. Others stimulate only the ventricles (ventricular pacer). This is the feature of the TCP. The third type of invasive pacer stimulates both the atria and ventricles (AV sequential). Additionally, some patients require placement of a biventricular pacer.

One other device that may be implanted in the patient is an automatic implantable cardioverter defibrillator (AICD). This device is placed under the skin in the abdomen. It has two sensors that are placed on the left ventricle and monitor the cardiac rhythm, as well as two defibrillation patches that are placed on the outside of the heart (epicardium). The AICD is battery powered and can be activated or deactivated with a magnet. If the device senses a rapid ventricular rate (ie, V-fib/V-tach), it delivers a shock of approximately 30 joules.

There are many medications available to control rapid heart rates. Some of these drugs are prescribed for daily use, some are for emergency use, and some are used both ways. These drugs come in various classifications and work in different ways to slow or control heart rates alone or in combination with other drugs. Some are beta-blockers, either beta selective or nonselective or are calcium channel blockers; others are inotropic, or occur naturally in the cells like adenosine [Adenocard] or a cardiac glycoside like digoxin [Digitek]. **Table 4-7** ▾ lists some of these medications with its classification and a brief description of its use.

Table 4-7 Medications Available to Control Rapid Heart Rates

Atenolol [Tenormin]	This drug is a beta blocker. It is predominately beta 1, and beta 2 in higher doses.	Used to treat hypertension, control heart rate, angina, and acute myocardial infarction (AMI).
Esmolol [Brevibloc]	This drug is a beta-blocker.—Beta-1 selective.	Used to treat supraventricular tachycardia (SVT) without atrial fibrillation or atrial flutter. Also used to treat rapid atrial fibrillation, atrial flutter, tachycardia, and hypertension during intubation and surgery.
Propranolol hydrochloride [Inderal]	This drug is a beta-blocker. Nonselective, both beta 1 and 2 blocker.	Used to treat hypertension, AMI, SVT, ventricular, and tachyarrhythmias of digitalis intoxication.
Digoxin [Digitek, Lanoxin]	This drug is a cardiac glycoside.	Used to control rapid a-fib/flutter and treat CHF.
Diltiazem [Cardizem]	This drug is a calcium channel blocker.	Used both daily and for rapid conversion of rapid A-fib/flutter.
Verapamil [Calan, Isoptin]	This drug is a calcium channel blocker.	Used both daily and for rapid conversion of rapid A-fib/flutter.
Milrinone lactate [Primacor]	This is an inotropic drug.	It is used IV short-term for treatment of CHF, usually in patients taking digoxin and diuretics, typically administered in a critical care unit setting.
Inamrinone lactate	This is an inotropic drug.	Used in short term therapy for patients in CHF who are taking digitalis, or who are unresponsive to digitalis, diuretics, and/or vasodilators.
Ibutilide fumarate [Corvert]	Sodium channel inhibitor.	Used for rapid conversion of atrial fibrillation and atrial flutter.
Adenosine [Adenocard]	Endogenous nucleotide formed from the breakdown of ATP.	Used for rapid conversion of SVT that is not atrial fibrillation and atrial flutter.
Amiodarone hydrochloride [Cordarone]	Sodium channel blocker, as well as alpha and beta adrenergic blockade.	Initial treatment and prophylaxis of frequently occurring tachyarrhythmias, both SVT and V-tach/V-fib.

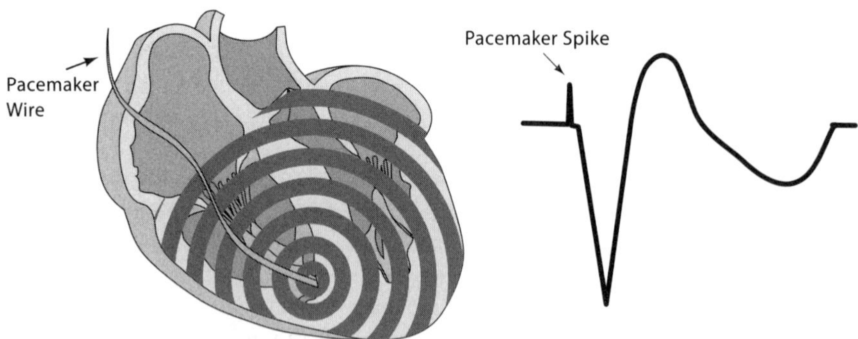

Figure 4-8 Pacemaker spike followed by QRS complex.

Using a Pacer in the Field

All paramedics should be well versed in operating their external pacemaker as it can be a life-saving tool.

Follow these steps to initiate TCP:

1. Apply pacing electrodes (similar location to defibrillation electrodes). Alternate position is anterior left lower sternum and posterior below the left scapula.
2. Switch the pacer power on.
3. Set the pacing rate at 70 bpm.
4. Start increasing current by 10 to 20 milliamps every few seconds.
5. Check for electrical capture—QRS following each pacemaker spike (**Figure 4-8**▲).
6. Check for mechanical capture—palpable radial pulse.
7. Lower the current to the lowest setting achieving mechanical and electrical capture.
8. Transport the patient monitoring the ECG and serial vital signs.

Rapid Heart Rate: Too Much Coffee or a Life-Threat?

There are many reasons why our patients have a rapid heart beat. Ask a person who is not in good physical shape to climb a couple of flights of stairs and their heart will be chugging along at a rapid rate. If a patient sustains blood loss or is dehydrated, their body's normal compensatory mechanisms send a message to the adrenal glands to "dump epinephrine and norepinephrine" into the bloodstream so they can increase the force and rate of the heart beat as well as vasoconstrict the periphery. When a patient is in pain or sick, they often have an increased heart rate. Then there are those patients who tell us "my heart is racing and I can feel it." It is acceptable for your heart rate to rise for a brief period of time but when it involves lengthy periods of time or very high rates, a rapid heart rate can produce dangerous symptoms. When referring to a patient as tachycardic, this means a heart rate of over 100 beats/min. When you look to treat the patient who is symptomatic and tachycardic you always must try to answer the question, "Why is this patient tachycardic?" As you consider the possible answers, you should be reviewing the patient's ECG and providing supplemental oxygen. Some of the conditions that can cause a tachycardia are shock, heat, anxiety, pain, fever, cardiac arrhythmia, dehydration, and drugs (ie, atropine, epinephrine, amphetamines, cocaine, caffeine, nicotine, and alcohol).

When a patient has a very rapid heart rate, the heart may not be filling adequately with blood. As blood flow becomes inadequate, so does oxygenation. The patient may experience shortness of breath because he or she is becoming hypoxic.

In the past, the ACLS algorithm for the treatment of the patient with a tachycardia was the most complex algorithm issued. With the 2005 Guidelines (*2005 American Heart Association Guidelines for Cardiopulmonary Resuscitation and Emergency Cardiovascular Care, Circulation: Journal of the American Heart Association (Volume 112, Number 24), December 13, 2005*) the algorithm got much simpler by recognizing that expert consultation is often the best course of action (**Figure 4-9**▸). Basically, you need to break down the potential pathways to follow based on the following: the presence of symptoms, whether the patient is stable or unstable, if the QRS complex is wide or narrow, and if the rhythm is regular or irregular.

Let's take a look at four fast ECGs: sinus tachycardia, atrial flutter, supraventricular tachycardia (SVT), and ventricular tachycardia (these are just a sampling as there are many more). They are all fast heart rates. Sinus tachycardia is fast but usually not a life-threat although the reason it has developed might be the life-threat (ie, a ruptured spleen in a car crash) (**Figure 4-10**▸).

Atrial flutter is an ECG that is easy to visualize when you think of the teeth of a saw. The rate is very fast and often there are two or more atrial beats to each ventricular beat (**Figure 4-11**▸). When the heart beat gets this fast the ventricles do not completely fill

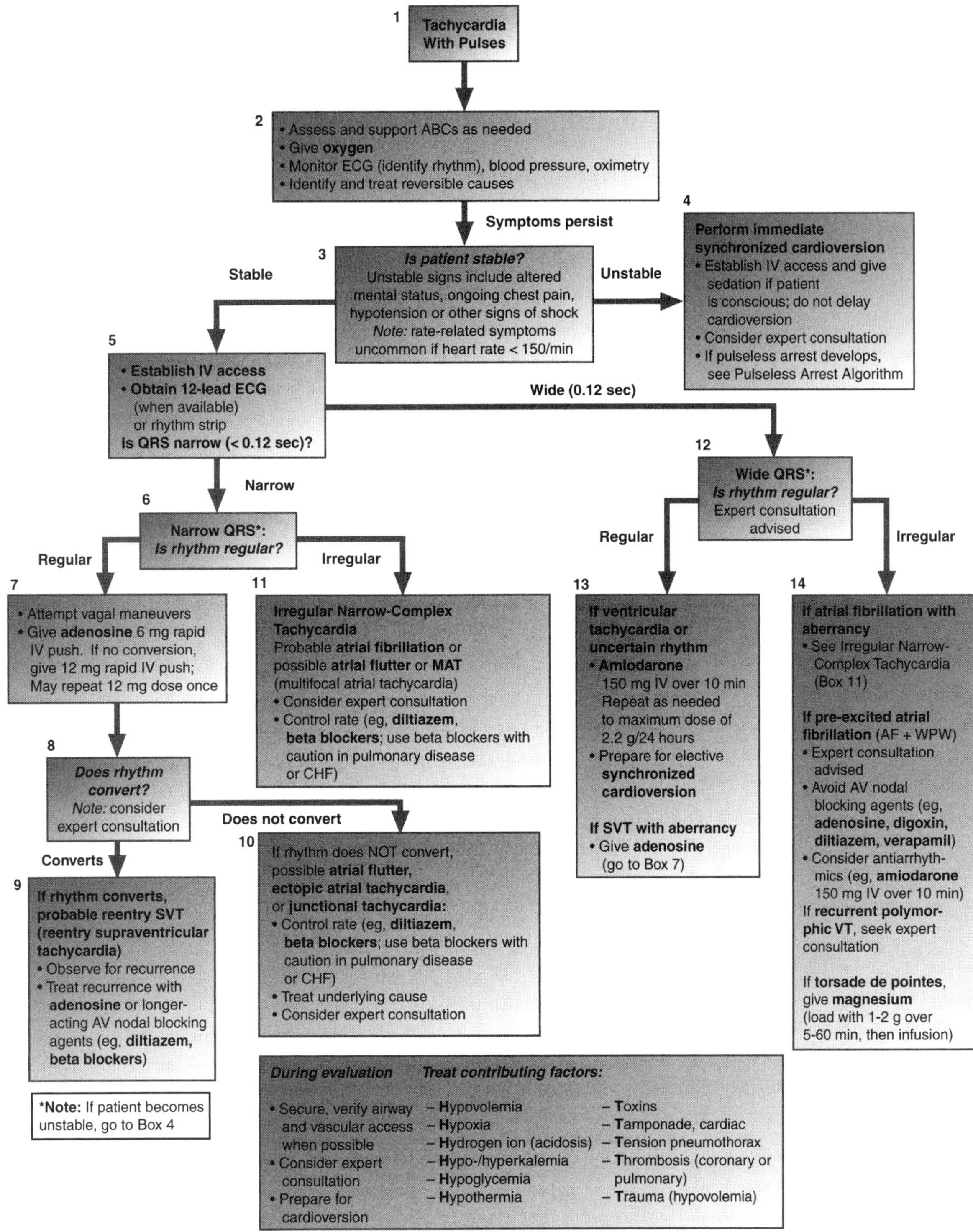

Reprinted with permission, *2005 American Heart Asssociation Guidelines for Cardiopulmonary Resuscitation and Emergency Cardiovascular Care, Part 4: Adult Basic Life Support. Circulation. 2005; 112(suppl IV): IV-1-IV-111* © 2005, American Heart Association, Inc.

Figure 4-9 Algorithm for tachycardia.

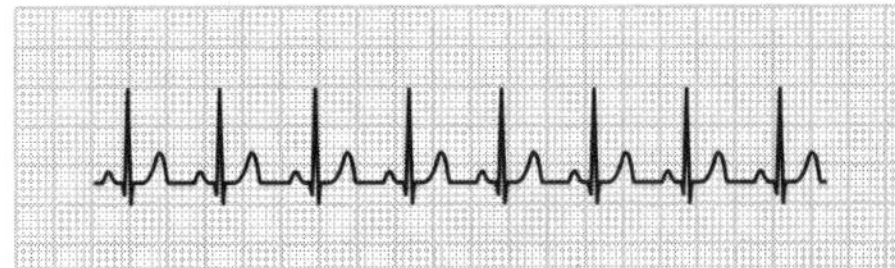

Figure 4-10 Sinus tachycardia.

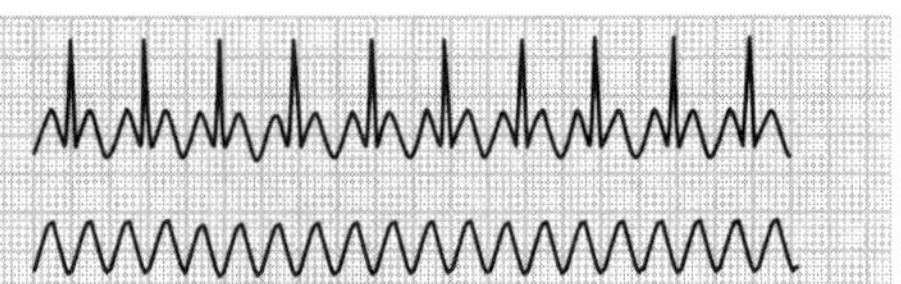

Figure 4-11 Atrial flutter.

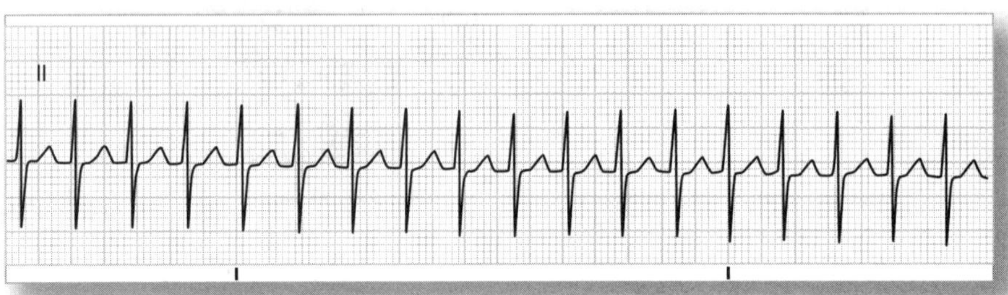

Figure 4-12 Supraventricular tachycardia.

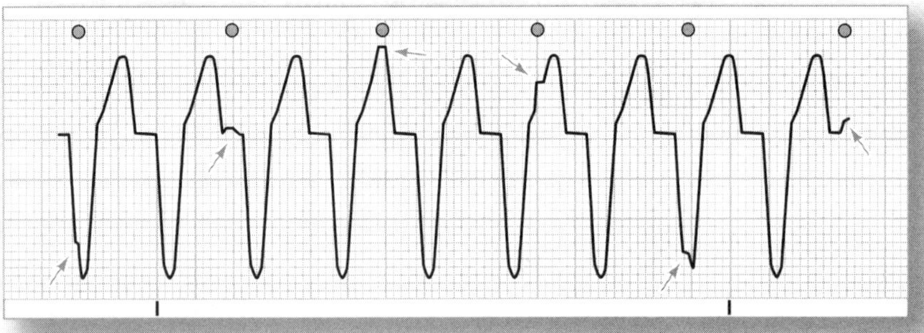

Figure 4-13 Monomorphic ventricular tachycardia: similar in shape, most likely originating from the same site.

and do not completely empty, thus diminishing the stroke volume and cardiac output.

When a tachycardia is so fast it may be difficult to tell if it is **sinus tachycardia**, **atrial tachycardia**, or **junctional tachycardia** but you can be sure it was generated in the atria by the narrow QRS complex. This is preceded by **P waves**; the general term that is used is supraventricular tachycardia (SVT) (**Figure 4-12▲**). If you actually see this rhythm develop in front of you, it is a paroxysmal (suddenly appeared) SVT. The other term that is commonly used for SVT is a reentry SVT. When you encounter this, you try various maneuvers to get the patient out of the rhythm (ie, drugs, vagal maneuvers, and electricity) if the patient is symptomatic.

The last of our four fast rhythms originates in the ventricles. Ventricular tachycardia (VT), when a pulse is associated, is a precursor for pulseless VT and a cardiac arrest requiring defibrillation and high quality CPR (**Figure 4-13▲**). Patients cannot stay in VT for a long period of time so they must be quickly and aggressively managed or else you will be performing compressions on their chest.

This rhythm occurs in a very sick or hypoxic heart. Certainly an extra couple of cups of coffee (caffeine) can cause some extra beats but it does not cause VT!

Case Study V Atrial Fibrillation

Part 1

Your unit has been dispatched to a video store where a man in his 50's is sitting on a chair after getting very dizzy. The fire department first responders are on the scene and report on the radio that the patient is conscious and complaining that his heart is racing. They are obtaining a set of vital signs at this point, just as you pull into the parking lot in front of the store. You and your partner unload the stretcher and are led into the store by a firefighter who was standing next to the engine waiting for your arrival. As you approach the patient you can see he is sitting on a stool and looks very pale, clammy, and scared.

The scene is safe and the firefighters are already questioning the patient. The video store employee states the man was wandering around the store for about 15 minutes before he asked for help. He said he was very dizzy. She said she does not know how to handle medical emergencies so she just called for help right away.

You introduce yourself to the patient and begin doing your initial assessment to see if there are any life-threats that need to be immediately managed (see **Table 1**).

The patient did not experience any trauma so you decide to proceed with the focused history of a responsive medical patient. The patient states that this has happened to him before and usually goes away after a few minutes. This time it seems worse and has not gone away.

Question 1: What is a tachycardia?

Question 2: What are some examples of conditions that can cause a tachycardia?

Table 1 Initial Assessment

Initial Assessment	Recording Time: 1 Minute
General Impression/ Appearance	Poor impression, fails the look test (the patient does not look right)
Mental Status	Alert but very anxious
Airway	Open and clear
Breathing	Rapid but regular
Circulation	Very fast radial pulse rate
Priority/Plan	High at this point

Part 2

The firefighters have the baseline vital signs and part of the focused history and physical examination (see **Table 2**). They have placed a nonrebreathing mask on the patient and are calling his wife. The patient is alert, pale, cool, and diaphoretic. The respirations are 28 breaths/min, distal pulse is weak, rapid, and irregular at 120 beats/min, and the blood pressure is 154/86 mm Hg. A firefighter introduces you and your partner to the patient, William Bently, and you begin a rapid medical examination of his cardiothoracic systems. William smells of cigarettes, his lung sounds are clear bilaterally, his neck veins are flat, there are no scars on his chest or abdomen, and he has no signs of peripheral edema or clubbing of the finger tips. He is however, obese. You confirm that is not the first time something like this has happened. Last year William went to the hospital for a rapid heart rate that was converted with adenosine [Adenocard]. Since then, the palpitations have occurred twice but resolved in a short time with no specific intervention. He has not seen a cardiologist since the hospital visit. William tells you he still feels dizzy and is a little short of breath despite the oxygen. Your partner is attaching the leads, pulse oximeter, and obtaining the blood pressure while you continue obtaining a history.

Table 2 Focused History and Physical Examination

Baseline Vital Signs	Recording Time: 10 Minutes
Skin CTC (color, temperature, condition)	Pale, cool, and diaphoretic
Pulse	120 beats/min rapid, weak, irregular distal pulse
Blood Pressure	154/86 mm Hg
Respirations	28 breaths/min and complains of feeling short of breath

Question 3: Why is a rapid heart rate often associated with shortness of breath or dyspnea?

Question 4: What are some of the possible cardiac rhythms you might expect to see once an ECG is obtained?

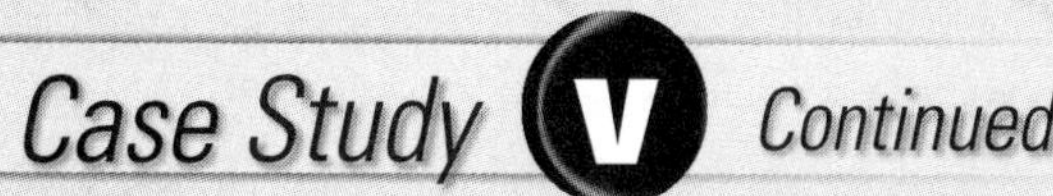

Part 3

The initial ECG is a rapid narrow QRS complex around 210 beats/min. At this fast rate it is difficult to tell if the rhythm is atrial fibrillation. You start an IV and your partner obtains a 12-lead ECG. You could give William a dose of adenosine [Adenocard] for SVT, but if the rhythm is atrial fibrillation or atrial flutter, diltiazem hydrochloride [Cardizem] will be more effective. You will wait for the 12-lead results and get more of the SAMPLE history (see **Table 3**). William has a history of anxiety, hypertension, and hypothyroidism. He takes medications regularly for his conditions. He is allergic to promethazine hydrochloride [Phenergan] and enalapril maleate [Vasotec]. Last oral intake was salad and pasta for lunch a few hours ago. The blood pressure is 150/90 mm Hg, the SpO_2 is 100% with the oxygen, and the 12-lead shows atrial fibrillation with a rapid ventricular response of 208 beats/min. As you watch the monitor you can see the rate change between 190 and 210 which is indicative of atrial fibrillation (atrial flutter and SVT typically remain more constant). You recall that a baseline pulse is 120 beats/min; however, the ECG is much faster. You also recall that when the palpated distal pulse is less than the apical pulse and the rate on the ECG, this is called a pulse deficit. You know this is typically present with very rapid heart rates and is a condition associated with irregular filling of the ventricles which causes inconsistent cardiac output.

Table 3 SAMPLE History

SAMPLE History	Comments
Signs/symptoms	Palpitations, anxious, dizzy, short of breath, and diaphoretic
Allergies	Promethazine hydrochloride [Phenergan] and enalapril maleate [Vasotec]
Medications	Atenolol [Tenormin], fluoxetine hydrochloride [Prozac], and levothyroxine sodium [Levothroid]
Pertinent past medical history	Hypertension, anxiety, and hypothyroidism
Last oral intake	Salad and pasta for lunch 2 hours ago
Events leading up to the incident	Walking around in the video store

Treatment Plan

William is stable for the moment so the treatment plan is to:

1. Encourage and instruct the patient to try a vagal maneuver (bear down).
2. Draw up a dose of diltiazem hydrochloride [Cardizem] in the event the vagal maneuver does not work (see **Table 4**).
3. If the patient's condition persists, consider a second dose of diltiazem hydrochloride [Cardizem].

Diltiazem hydrochloride [Cardizem] is a calcium channel blocker used to slow atrial fibrillation and atrial flutter with a rapid ventricular response. Calcium channel blockers work by decreasing SA and AV conduction which slows the ventricular rate. They also decrease myocardial contractility and peripheral vascular resistance. William has no contraindications so the first dose will be 0.25 mg/kg slow IV. The first dose often slows the rate for a short time and then it speeds up again (refractory) so a second dose of 0.35 mg/kg may be required 15 minutes later.

Table 4 Diltiazem Hydrochloride

Do you know?	Comments
Right drug? Generic name: [**Diltiazem Hydrochloride**] Trade name: [Cardizem]	This drug is a calcium channel blocker. It is used as a rapid and temporary relief for uncontrolled atrial fibrillation or flutter. It works by decreasing SA and AV conduction. This will most likely slow the ventricular rate rather than convert the rhythm. It also decreases myocardial contractility and peripheral vascular resistance.
Right patient?	Symptomatic rapid atrial fibrillation or flutter.
Right dose?	0.25 mg/kg initial dose over 2 minutes, after 15 minutes may repeat with 0.35 mg/kg for a second dose.
Right route?	IV (also frequently given as a slow drip).
Right time?	After assessment and recognition of one of the indications for its use.
Right documentation?	Dose, route, time administered, and reassessment should be clearly documented on the patient care report.

continues

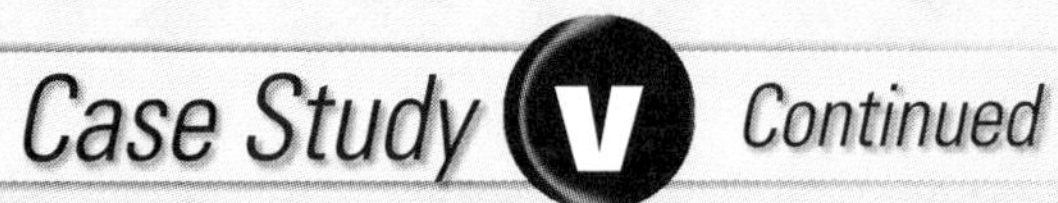

Table 4 Diltiazem Hydrochloride (*Continued*)

Do you know?	Comments
Expected action	Slowed ventricular response and relief of symptoms.
Side effects	Hypotension, syncope, tachycardia, bradycardia, AV block, bundle branch block (BBB), CHF, angina, weakness, headache, and nausea.
Contraindications	Hypotension, cardiogenic shock, high-degree AV block, sick sinus syndrome, V-tach, WPW, AMI, and APE.
Precautions	Use with caution in patients with hepatic failure and CHF.
Pharmacokinetics	Onset 2–5 minutes; Peak effect: variable. Duration: 1–3 hours excreted through both bile and urine.

Adenosine [Adenocard] is a naturally occurring hormone found in the cells and is used as an antiarrhythmic to convert SVT to a normal sinus rhythm (see **Table 5**). Adenosine does not slow atrial fibrillation or atrial flutter with a rapid ventricular response and should not be used when these rhythms are present. Amiodarone [Cordarone] is another antiarrhythmic option. Amiodarone [Cordarone] is discussed in Case Study II.

The current ILCOR guidelines state that using one antiarrhythmic works better than multiple drugs and recommend correctly identifying the arrhythmia prior to administering any antiarrhythmic. When the patient's condition is unstable, the guidelines recommend the use of electricity. The use of a beta-blocker as an adjunct to electricity may be effective to avoid postconversion arrhythmias.

Question 5: What is a pulse deficit?

Question 6: What is a vagal maneuver?

Table 5 Adenosine

Do you know?	Comments
Right drug? Generic name: [**Adenosine**] Trade name: [Adenocard]	This drug is an antiarrhythmic. It is an endogenous nucleotide formed from the breakdown of adenosine triphosphate (ATP). It is used for rapid conversion of reentry SVT that is not atrial fibrillation or flutter.
Right patient?	Symptomatic reentry supraventricular tachycardia (SVT) or paroxysmal supraventricular tachycardia (PSVT) that is not atrial fibrillation or flutter.
Right dose?	6 mg over 1–3 seconds, followed by a 20-mL saline flush. If no response, may administer 12 mg after 1–2 minutes over 1–3 seconds. If no response, repeat 12 mg again. Maximum dose of 30 mg.
Right route?	Rapid IV bolus.
Right time?	After assessment and recognition of SVT.
Right documentation?	Dose, route, time administered, and reassessment should be clearly documented on the patient care report.
Expected action	Conversion of reentry SVT to normal sinus rhythm.
Side effects	Short-lasting first-, second-, or third-degree heart block, prolonged asystole, V-fib, or cardiac arrest.
Contraindications	Second- or third-degree heart block, sick sinus syndrome, atrial fibrillation or flutter, V-tach, history of MI or cerebral hemorrhage.
Precautions	Facial flushing, shortness of breath, chest pain, headache, paresthesia, diaphoresis, palpitations, hypotension, nausea, metallic taste.
Pharmacokinetics	Onset and peak in seconds; duration 12 seconds; metabolized to inosine and adenosine monophosphate (AMP).

Part 4

William gave a good effort with the vagal maneuver (and he did not stroke out) but it did not work so you administered diltiazem and loaded him on the stretcher and into the ambulance. En route to the hospital you reassess him and obtain the following serial vital signs and diagnostics: skin CTC is a better color, warmer, and dryer; breathing feels easier; distal pulse is stronger and slower at 106 to 114 beats/min; blood pressure is 144/76 mm Hg; ECG is still atrial fibrillation but with a much slower ventricular response that matches the distal pulse; and he seems less anxious (see **Table 6**).

Question 7: Why didn't the vagal maneuver work?

Question 8: Why didn't the diltiazem convert the rapid atrial fibrillation to a normal sinus rhythm?

Table 6 **Reassessment and Ongoing Assessment of the Patient**

Serial Vital Signs and Relevant Data	Recording Time: 15 Minutes
Skin CTC	Pink, warm, and dryer
Pulse	106 beats/min strong and irregular
Blood Pressure	144/76 mm Hg
Respirations	20 breaths/min
Mental Status	More relaxed
ECG	Atrial fibrillation with a ventricular response of 106 to 114 beats/min
SpO_2	100%
Lung Sounds	Clear bilaterally
Other (ie, glucose, core temperature)	Not obtained

Part 5

The transport to the hospital is short and William's rate did increase between 20–30 beats/min by the time you arrived. It appears as if William has a new onset of atrial fibrillation and may now need new daily medication for rate control and anticoagulation. The goal is to keep the ventricular response "controlled," below 100. Keeping atrial fibrillation controlled helps to reduce the risk for developing a systemic emboli that can cause a stroke or other peripheral vascular ischemic complications. As stated earlier, there are many causes for rapid heart rates. Some of the possible causes for atrial fibrillation include coronary artery disease, hypertension, rheumatic heart disease, hyperthyroidism, sepsis, and heavy alcohol intake. Atrial fibrillation is often a sign of another problem, and may spontaneously revert to normal sinus rhythm once that problem is corrected. Atrial fibrillation that persists for longer than 48 to 72 hours markedly increases the risk of atrial thrombus formation and subsequent embolization. This is dealt with via anticoagulation and elective cardioversion.

Treatment of symptomatic atrial fibrillation in the prehospital setting includes the use of vagal maneuvers, diltiazem or amiodarone for stable patients, and synchronized cardioversion for unstable patients. The use of a beta-blocker as an adjunct to electricity may be effective to avoid postconversion arrhythmias.

Vagus Nerve Stimulation

The vagus nerve is the 10th of 12 cranial pairs of nerves and the only cranial nerve that extends out of the skull into the body. The vagus lies beside the carotid arteries and extends down to the atria of the heart and into the GI tract. When stimulated, the vagus slows the heart rate. A vagal maneuver can occur in many ways: touching the back of the throat (ie, intubating or suctioning), vomiting, rubbing the carotid artery, applying pressure on the eyeball, changes in intrathoracic pressure (ie, bearing down for a bowel movement), or placing the face in ice water. For most individuals, vagal stimulation is not dangerous, but for the patient who has an arrhythmia or is having an MI or a serious medical condition, the effects can be very serious. In some cases vagal stimuli can cause cardiac arrest. However, when indicated, vagal stimuli can be used as a treatment option to slow SVT. When used to treat atrial fibrillation or atrial flutter, it may make the flutter or fibrillation waves more apparent, making the ECG diagnosis easier to identify.

Special Needs Tip

When considering the methods of vagal stimulation, administered either purposely or by accident, remember that children are especially sensitive to vagal stimuli when the back of the throat or gag reflex is stimulated. If you are suctioning a child, keep this in mind and be aware that lengthy suctioning of the throat could cause the heart rate to drop rapidly.

When a reentry SVT is rapid enough to produce symptoms that cause the patient's condition to deteriorate to unstable, electricity is the recommended emergency therapy. The rationale is to quickly deliver electricity to the heart, causing it to stop and reset the sinoatrial (SA) pacemaker (originating in the SA node), thus allowing the heart to return to a normal sinus rhythm. Synchronized cardioversion is a calculated and timed shock of electricity designed to be delivered after the peak of the **R wave** of the cardiac cycle so as to avoid the vulnerable relative refractory phase. Also called countershock, cardioversion is unlike defibrillation which is a higher dose of electricity delivered with no particular point as to when in the cardiac cycle the shock is delivered.

Cardioversion Technique

All paramedics should be well versed in operating a defibrillator in the synchronized cardioversion mode. Cardioversion involves using the defibrillator to terminate arrhythmias other than ventricular fibrillation (V-fib).

Follow these steps to initiate cardioversion:

1. Turn on the main power and then turn the synchronize switch to the "on" position.
2. Prepare and apply the pads or paddles similar to defibrillation.
3. Set the energy level to the appropriate dose: 100 J, 200 J, 300 J, then 360 J (monophasic energy levels) for V-tach and atrial fibrillation. Rentry SVT and atrial flutter should start with 50 J. The biphasic energy dose depends on the manufacturer of the device.
4. Charge the paddles.
5. Clear the area, "I'm clear, you're clear, we are all clear."

Always check to see if the cardioverter is showing a marking of the "R" waves. In some cases this may require turning up the height of the QRS complex so the unit recognizes the R wave. The unit should mark the R wave by showing a light at the top of the wave, or some other technique specific to the device you are using. After cardioversion has been administered, some units will default to the defibrillation setting. This may mean that if you wish to deliver another dose of electricity by cardioversion you must reset the unit or else it will not mark the R wave and automatically defibrillate the patient.

6. Depress the shock buttons until the cardioverter discharges (which could take a few seconds).
7. Reassess the patient's condition (ECG rhythm and pulse).
8. Repeat the shock at a higher dose as necessary making sure the cardioversion setting is turned on.
9. If a cardioversion shock produces a V-fib, immediately:
   - Recharge the defibrillator to the setting for defibrillation.
   - Turn the synchronizer circuit to the "off" position if it has not defaulted to that position.
   - Deliver the defibrillation.

Wolff-Parkinson-White (WPW) Syndrome

Wolff-Parkinson-White syndrome, or WPW, is an abnormal rhythm that presents as SVT. In WPW an accessory pathway links the atria and ventricles bypassing the atrioventricular (AV) node, a specialized structure located in the AV junction that slows conduction through the AV junction. The ECG has a short P-R interval (< 0.12) and slurred QRS called a delta wave which widens the complex. Treatment is the same as with stable SVT. A danger exists when WPW is associated with atrial fibrillation. The drugs (calcium channel blockers) used to treat stable atrial fibrillation actually enhance the ventricular rate and may lead to V-fib. Therefore, the treatment of choice is synchronized cardioversion for both stable and unstable patients with WPW-associated atrial fibrillation.

Acute Pulmonary Edema: Not Just a Cardiac Condition

In most instances where you encounter acute pulmonary edema (APE) in the field, it will be in the context of a cardiac patient. That is not to say that heart failure is the only reason a patient goes into APE. For this reason, we have chosen to deal with this important topic in the respiratory chapter of this book. Patients in acute pulmonary edema should be assessed and managed based on the circumstances of their disease and presentation. For example, it would not be appropriate to automatically give the patient a round of furosemide [Lasix] when the patient has altitude sickness or a narcotic overdose that has caused APE. Conversely, this may be a very appropriate drug to consider in the cardiac patient with a good BP and pedal edema.

Hypotension or Cardiogenic Shock

Living with heart failure often includes being on many medications. You will see patients with medication lists that include: antianginal agents (ie, nitrates), beta-blockers, calcium channel blockers, antihypertensives, anticoagulants, ACE inhibitors, antiarrhythmics (ie, digitalis), and diuretics. This may be in addition to medications they may be taking for other underlying conditions such as diabetes, thyroid, anemia, COPD, etc. Some of these drugs have the potential to cause serious complications because they may have a narrow therapeutic window. Patients can become toxic or have serious complications because of either too much or too little available drug (ie, digitalis, beta-blocker, warfarin).

For a patient who has signs of both acute and chronic heart failure (ie, severe dyspnea, orthopnea, wheezes, crackles, distended neck veins, pedal or presacral edema), the emergency treatment is going to be focused on improving oxygenation and ventilation. High flow oxygen and positioning is important in this case. The patient needs to be sitting in a semi-upright position to help venous pooling and prevent pulmonary edema, which is the accumulation of fluid in the lungs. Ventilations may need to be assisted using a bag-mask device or continuous positive airway pressure (CPAP), or the patient may need an advanced airway, especially if he or she becomes comatose. Consider a diuretic such as furosemide [Lasix] administered by IV or an angiotensin converting enzyme inhibitor such as captopril [Capoten], provided the patient is not hypotensive. Captopril [Capoten] is not generally carried on the paramedic unit and therefore not listed in the formulary but has been shown to be effective in combination with diuretics and digitalis to treat CHF. It has also proven to be effective in improving survival following AMI in clinically stable patients with left ventricular dysfunction by reducing the incidence of heart failure and subsequent trips back to the hospital.

If the patient is normotensive or hypertensive, nitrates and morphine have been the traditional treatment and are thought to decrease the myocardial oxygen demand and preload. Use of morphine has some controversy associated with it due to the potential increase in mortality. If the patient has severe hypotension, an inotropic agent such as dopamine [Intropin] (**Table 4-8** ▾) or dobutamine [Dobutrex] (**Table 4-9** ▸) may be helpful as well.

Table 4-8 Dopamine

Right drug? Generic name: [**Dopamine**] Trade name: [Intropin]	This drug is a sympathomimetic that is chemically related to epinephrine and norepinephrine. Variable doses stimulate alpha 1 and beta 1 receptors. Though it has a substantial side effect profile, it may be useful in the treatment of cardiogenic shock.
Right patient?	Hypotension due to cardiac problems.
Right dose?	400 mg diluted in 500 mL NS continuous IV infusion; 2 to 4 μg/kg/min for low dose, 4 to 10 μg/kg/min for mid-dose and 10 to 20 μg/kg/min for high dose. Usually titrated to effect when administered IV drip in the field. The actions are dose specific with dopaminergic response at low doses (dilates vessels in the kidneys and increases urine output), beta-adrenergic in mid doses (positive chronotropic and iontropic adrenergic response), and primarily alpha stimulation (vasoconstriction) at the high doses.
Right route?	IV drip.
Right time?	After assessment and recognition of one of the indications for its use.
Right documentation?	Dose, route, time administered, and reassessment should be clearly documented on the patient care report.
Expected action	Improved blood pressure and tissue perfusion.

continues

Table 4-8 Dopamine (*Continued*)

Side effects	Increased myocardial oxygen demand, tachycardia, bradycardia, ectopy, arrhythmias, hypertension, angina, dyspnea, and headache.
Contraindications	Known sensitivity, uncorrected tachycardia, V-fib, cardiac arrest.
Precautions	Works best when used with volume correction.
Pharmacokinetics	Onset 1–4 minutes; Peak effect 5–10 minutes; duration: effects cease immediately after infusion is stopped. Metabolized in the liver, excreted in urine.

Table 4-9 Dobutamine

Right drug? Generic name: [**Dobutamine**] Trade name: [Dobutrex]	This drug is a sympathomimetic. Stimulates alpha, beta 1 and beta 2 receptors. It increases the force of myocardial contraction and has little effect on heart rate at therapeutic doses.
Right patient?	Used to treat CHF when an increased heart rate is not desired.
Right dose?	Mix 250 mg into 250 mL NS and run a continuous IV infusion at 2 to 20 μg/kg/min titrated to desired effect.
Right route?	IV drip.
Right time?	After assessment and recognition of one of the indications for its use.
Right documentation?	Dose, route, time administered, and reassessment should be clearly documented on the patient care report.
Expected action	Increased blood pressure.
Side effects	Ventricular ectopy, marked increase in heart rate, blood pressure, angina, palpitations, heart attack, and nausea. Can cause a decrease in blood pressure.
Contraindications	Hypertrophic subaortic stenosis.
Precautions	May not be safe to use after AMI.
Pharmacokinetics	Onset 2 minutes; peak 10 minutes; duration: 1–2 minutes after infusion discontinued; metabolized in liver and excreted in urine.

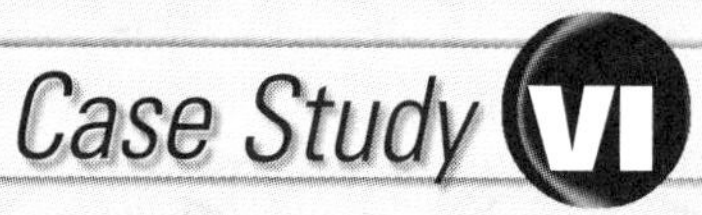

Cardiogenic Shock/Hypotension

Part 1

You receive a call to one of the local nursing homes and the dispatch information reports a patient experiencing difficulty breathing and chest pain. The patient is on the fifth floor at the end of the hall. One nurse just ran by you to the nurse's station and said that she will be right back with the patient's paperwork. As you and your partner enter the room you see and hear a very sick elderly woman lying flat on her back gurgling. There is an aide in the room who can only tell you that the patient was okay about an hour ago and then suddenly complained of chest pain and difficulty breathing. The name plate over the bed reads Emma Wilson. Emma looks cyanotic and is responsive to verbal stimuli as you call her name. With the help of your partner, you sit her up. Your partner quickly suctions Emma's airway and replaces the nasal cannula with a nonrebreathing mask. You begin an initial assessment of the patient (see **Table 1**). She is tachypneic and when you listen to lung sounds they are better than you thought. She has rales in the bases and the apices are clear; however, you do hear an abnormal heart sound called a gallop (rarely heard) that is sometimes associated with heart failure and cardiogenic shock. Emma has signs of acute and chronic heart failure: jugular vein distention two thirds of the way up the

Table 1 Initial Assessment

Initial Assessment	Recording Time: 2 Minutes
General Impression/ Appearance	Looks sick and in respiratory distress
Mental Status	Alert to voice
Airway	Open with gurgling
Breathing	Difficulty breathing
Circulation	Cyanotic, cool, moist, no distal pulse
Priority/Plan	High priority

Case Study VI Continued

neck, +4 pitting edema in all extremities, and fluid in the lungs. There is no distal pulse so you elevate her legs and place her in semi-Fowler's position in order to avoid flooding the lungs. Your partner is attempting to get a blood pressure.

Emma is unstable right now and that makes her a high priority patient. However, a rapid medical examination will be completed, vitals signs and diagnostics obtained, and treatment started before you leave the floor.

Question 1: What is the first treatment priority for Emma?

Question 2: Do you believe that Emma is in respiratory failure or is she having an AMI?

Part 2

The nurse is back with the paperwork. She tells you that Emma is 81 years old, has a history of three MIs, CHF, hypertension, angina, diabetes, and recently a urinary tract infection (UTI). Normally she is alert with mild dementia. She has a do not resuscitate order. As you begin the focused history and physical examination, Emma tells you she has chest pain (see **Table 2**). The blood pressure was difficult to obtain and is 64/20 mm Hg (hypotensive), and the pulse is 52 beats/min (bradycardia) and irregular. She needs IV fluids so you prepare to start an IV while your partner gets an ECG and SpO_2 reading. Emma may be having another MI which is causing a decreased cardiac output. She has an old midline scar on her chest presumably from cardiac surgery. There is a nitroglycerin patch on her chest that you remove because she is hypotensive. When Emma first complained of chest pain she was given 324 mg of aspirin and a nitroglycerin tablet as these are the orders in her chart. Usually this relieves her angina, but today it got worse. You ask the nurse to read the medications listed in her chart because many drugs can cause bradycardia and a slow heart rate. Nitroglycerin does drop the blood pressure by dilating the arteries. However, Emma takes nitroglycerin on a regular basis for angina with no significant drop in blood pressure. Today Emma may be having an MI which is causing the decreased cardiac output and the nitroglycerin may have contributed to the significant state of hypotension.

Table 2 Focused History and Physical Examination

Baseline Vital Signs	Recording Time: 5 Minutes
Skin CTC (color, temperature, condition)	Cyanotic, cool, dry, +4 pitting edema in all extremities
Pulse	52 beats/min and irregular
Blood Pressure	64/20 mm Hg
Respirations	34 breaths/min and labored

Question 3: What drugs might Emma be taking that could cause hypotension and bradycardia?

Question 4: Could the nitroglycerin have caused Emma's hypotension?

Part 3

The IV of normal saline is started and running open for now, the 12-lead ECG shows that Emma has ST segment elevation in V3 and V4, and there is a bundle branch block and occasional PVCs. The SpO_2 is 88%. While starting the IV you obtained a glucose reading of 112 mg/dL. With repositioning and high flow oxygen the cyanosis is improving, but Emma is still breathing fast and shallow. You obtain a quick SAMPLE history from the patient and bystanders as best you can considering how serious her condition is at this point (see **Table 3**). You will put her on CPAP and consider a dose (40 mg) of furosemide [Lasix]. However since the patient's blood pressure is a bit low it would be smart to withhold the furosemide [Lasix] for the moment and consult medical direction before administering that medication. Your partner obtains another blood pressure reading which is 70/30 mm Hg so you will definitely not be giving the furosemide [Lasix]. Emma may need to be taken to the catheterization lab again (provided she is an acceptable candidate). En route to the hospital you will start a second IV and hang a dopamine [Intropin] drip. She will need the alpha effects (peripheral vasoconstriction and the release of norepinephrine) from dopamine [Intropin].

Case Study VI Continued

Table 3 SAMPLE History

SAMPLE History	Comments
Signs/symptoms	Altered mental status, difficulty breathing, chest pain
Allergies	None
Medications	Furosemide [Lasix], potassium [Klor-Con], nitroglycerin patch (which you are planning to remove), metoprolol [Lopressor], glipizide, metformin hydrochloride [Glucophage], digoxin [Digitek, Lanoxin], warfarin [Coumadin]
Pertinent past medical history	Heart failure, 3 MIs, hypertension, diabetes, A-fib
Last oral intake	Nothing today
Events leading up to the incident	Sudden onset of chest pain which was treated with acetylsalicylic acid [Aspirin] and nitroglycerin

Treatment Plan

Emma has a history of previous MIs, heart failure, diabetes type II, and mild dementia. The treatment plan will include:

1. Monitor and manage the ABCs.
2. Administer supplemental oxygen.
3. Improve ventilation and oxygenation with CPAP.
4. Improve cardiac output with judicious use of intravenous fluids.
5. Consult with medical control for administration of dopamine [Intropin] or dobutamine [Dobutrex] while you quickly get her to definitive care.

Another thought to consider would be the possibility of exacerbated heart failure provoking the myocardial ischemia, and the blood pressure might actually come back up once you remove the nitroglycerin patch. Based on the complete assessment findings, the former is more likely than the latter theory.

Question 5: What do the early signs and symptoms of cardiogenic shock look like?

Question 6: Why is cardiogenic shock associated with high mortality?

Part 4

Emma is on the stretcher, the CPAP is on, and now it is time to get down to the ambulance. Once in the ambulance it takes a few minutes to get settled before you begin the reassessment and ongoing assessment of the patient (see **Table 4**). You can see the SpO_2 reading is up to 92% and she is now pale instead of cyanotic. Now more alert, Emma complains of chest pain when asked. Lung sounds are clear in the apices and rales in the bases, but not as much as when you first listened. A repeat ECG shows continued ST segment elevation in leads V3–4; the rate is 58 beats/min with some multifocal PVCs. Blood pressure is dropping again 62/30 mm Hg. After you start the dopamine [Intropin] drip you will call the hospital to give a report on Emma's critical status.

Question 7: Epinephrine is a vasopressor. Why is this not the preferred drug in Emma's case?

Question 8: Would dobutamine [Dobutrex] be a good choice as a vasopressor for Emma?

Table 4 Reassessment and Ongoing Assessment of the Patient

Serial Vital Signs and Relevant Data	Recording Time: 10 Minutes
Skin CTC	Pale, dry, and cool
Pulse	58 beats/min slightly irregular
Blood Pressure	62/30 mm Hg
Respirations	Rapid, assisted with CPAP
Mental Status	More alert
ECG	Abnormal with ST segment elevation V3–4
SpO_2	Improved to 92%
Lung Sounds	Improved with fewer rales
Other (ie, glucose, core temperature)	Glucose 112 mg/dL

Case Study VI Continued

Part 5

Just before arriving at the hospital Emma's blood pressure starts to rise. With the 12-lead ECG in hand you are ready to head into the ED and provide a report. En route you were able to get the dopamine [Intropin] drip started as well as provide an early report to the ED.

Emma is a very sick lady with a significant cardiac history. Today she developed chest pain and difficulty breathing. Initially she appeared to be in respiratory failure and was hypotensive. A rapid assessment showed that she is most likely having another MI which likely exacerbated her heart failure and dropped her blood pressure. This is the picture of cardiogenic shock. The goal of treatment is to improve oxygenation, ventilation, and cardiac output. The treatment plan is to improve ventilation with CPAP and diuretics, and improve cardiac output with fluids and dopamine [Intropin] while you quickly get her to a catheterization lab before her pressure drops any further. Even with all your aggressive and appropriate actions she is not likely to survive this event because cardiogenic shock is associated with a high mortality rate.

Dopamine [Intropin]

Dopamine [Intropin] can be used to treat congestive heart failure and cardiogenic shock. In congestive heart failure, the heart is not able to eject blood efficiently. As a result there is a decrease in cardiac output that triggers a series of compensatory actions. These actions include fluid retention, vasoconstriction, an increase in peripheral vascular resistance, an increase in the levels of circulating catecholamines (chemical compounds such as **epinephrine** (adrenaline), norepinephrine bitartrate (noradrenaline) and dopamine) and tissue hypoxia. Dopamine [Intropin] is used because it has the potential to improve these negative circulatory events. For example, by inducing renal vasodilation (via DA_1 receptors), theoretically blood flow to the kidney should be improved and urine output should increase. By increasing the force of myocardial contraction the cardiac output is increased. Dopamine is used on an outpatient basis via infusion centers to improve chronic congestive heart failure.

Similar to epinephrine [Adrenalin] and norepinephrine bitartrate [Levophed], dopamine [Intropin] has a short plasma half life. It can only be used intravenously in constant or intermittent infusions. Dopamine [Intropin] has a complex pharmacology. It can activate at least four different receptors: the $beta_1$, $dopamine_1$ (DA_1), $alpha_1$, and $alpha_2$. DA_1 receptors exist in the renal vascular bed. Activation of these receptors produces a decrease in renal vascular resistance and an increase in renal blood flow. Activation of the $beta_1$ receptor increases the force of myocardial contraction. Dopamine [Intropin] has a very unusual action on the heart in that it selectively increases the force of myocardial contraction without too significant an effect on heart rate. However, high doses of dopamine [Intropin] can induce rhythm disturbances.

Cardiogenic Shock

Cardiogenic shock is the most serious form of heart failure, resulting in insufficient cardiac output due to left ventricular malfunction. When the heart cannot effectively pump blood through the body, organ tissues deteriorate rapidly and death follows. There are several mechanisms that can produce cardiogenic shock: drugs, acute MI or ischemia, myocarditis, pulmonary embolism, tension pneumothorax, cardiac tamponade, tachycardia, bradycardia, acute mitral or aortic regurgitation, and ruptured interventricular septum.

The first signs and symptoms of cardiogenic shock are the same as an AMI: dyspnea, chest pain, nausea, cyanosis, pallor, diaphoresis, normotension, and hypotension. As compensatory mechanisms fail, severe hypotension develops and organ tissues die. Once shock and hypotension develop, there is a high mortality rate.

Treatment of cardiogenic shock begins with improving oxygenation and peripheral perfusion without adding work to the heart and correcting any arrhythmias. Arrhythmias may bring about hypotension by causing severe disturbances in CO, thus, until major arrhythmias are corrected, you cannot be certain that the patient's hypotension is caused by cardiogenic shock. Depending on the circumstances, you may be asked to administer a vasopressor drug, such as dopamine [Intropin], norephinephrine [Levophed], or epinephrine [Adrenalin] (**Table 4-10** ▼ and **Table 4-11** ▶). The definitive treatment for a patient in cardiogenic shock may include fibrinolytics, cardiac catheterization, balloon angioplasty, stents, or coronary artery bypass graft (CABG). All of these are in-hospital treatments that are usually offered in cardiac specialty centers.

Cardiology: Hypertension (not eligible for fibrinolytic therapy)

Some patients present with cardiovascular-related symptoms (ie, altered mental status, headache and dizziness, and/or difficulty breathing) as well as hypertension, and yet their history is not typical ACS that would make them a candidate for fibrinolytic therapy. As you have learned in your EMT and paramedic education, there are many causes of altered mental status (ie, epilepsy, infection, overdose, uremia, hypoglycemia, head trauma, hypoxia, hypertension, heat stroke, dementia, etc.). Cardiac irregularities such as arrhythmias, poor perfusion states, and irregular heart rates each can affect the patient's mental status and leave them anywhere from dizzy to unresponsive.

When a patient has an elevated blood pressure there can be an increased risk of aneurysm, TIA, or stroke, all which can lead to a cardiovascular catastrophe for the patient. Sometimes the patient may simply have a bounding pulse that seems to bounce your finger off the pulse site because it is so forceful. This may be your first indication that the patient has hypertension, only to be confirmed when you actually take the blood pressure. Sometimes a patient with hypertension presents with a red face although this can also be an indication of alcohol intoxication, fever, CO poisoning, or a sunburn. Pay attention to the visible signs of hypertension and always consider all the potential causes in your differential diagnosis of the patient.

Hypertensive crisis is a broad term associated with significantly elevated blood pressure, occurring along with a variety of serious symptoms or problems. Typically a hypertensive crisis is classified as either a hypertensive emergency (HE) or a hypertensive urgency (HU). HE involves marked elevations in blood pressure linked to some degree of end-organ dysfunction. HU involves elevation in the blood pressure without end-organ dysfunction. Treatment of a hypertensive crisis involves blood pressure reduction, though typically not immediately to so-called normal levels as that might be a bit extreme in the

Table 4-10 Norepinephrine Bitartrate

Right drug? Generic name: [**Norepinephrine Bitartrate**] Trade name: [Levophed]	Stimulates mostly alpha and some beta 1 receptors. It increases peripheral vascular resistance and myocardial contractility. Used with great caution to treat hypotension due to MI and cardiogenic shock, also neurogenic and septic shock.
Right patient?	Hypotension caused by cardiogenic shock without hypovolemia.
Right dose?	4 mg diluted in 250 mL NS continuous IV infusion at 0.5 to 1.0 μg/min, titrated to improve the blood pressure (up to 30 μg/min).
Right route?	IV drip.
Right time?	After assessment and recognition of one of the indications for its use.
Right documentation?	Dose, route, time administered, and reassessment should be clearly documented on the patient care report.
Expected action	Increased systemic blood pressure.
Side effects	Tachycardia, bradycardia, arrhythmias, hypertension, angina, and headache.
Contraindications	Hypotension with hypovolemia.
Precautions	Must correct hypovolemia prior to using. Constricts renal and mesenteric blood vessels.
Pharmacokinetics	Onset immediate; duration 1–2 minutes; metabolized in liver, excreted in urine.

Table 4-11 Epinephrine

Right drug? Generic name: [**Epinephrine**] Trade name: [Adrenalin]	Stimulates alpha and beta 1 and beta 2 receptors. It is used as a vasopressor in shock.
Right patient?	States of reduced cardiac output.
Right dose?	1 mg diluted in 250 mL NS administer over 15 minutes titrated to effect.
Right route?	IV drip.
Right time?	After assessment and recognition of one of the indications for its use.
Right documentation?	Dose, route, time administered, and reassessment should be clearly documented on the patient care report.
Expected action	Improved cardiac output. This drug is a direct acting alpha and beta agonist. The alpha effect is vasoconstriction and beta-1 is positive inotropic, chronotropic, and dromotropic effects.
Side effects	Can cause hypertension, tachycardia, arrhythmias, pulmonary edema, anxiety, restlessness, agitation, nausea, headache and angina, V-fib, cerebral or subarachnoid hemorrhage, and has many negative interactions with other drugs.
Contraindications	Known sensitivity, narrow angle glaucoma, hypertension, hypothermia, pulmonary edema, myocardial ischemia, and hypovolemic shock. May worsen developing MIs.
Precautions	Use with caution in cases of peripheral vascular disease. Epinephrine can potentiate other sympathomimetics. It can be deactivated by alkaline solutions (ie, sodium bicarbonate). Use of MAOIs may potentiate effects and beta-blockers may blunt its effects.
Pharmacokinetics	Onset immediate; metabolism takes place in both the liver and other tissues by monoamine oxidase (MAO) and catechol-O-methyltransferase (COMT) to inactive metabolites.

short term for the patient. Common problems that occur with HE include hypertensive encephalopathy, intracranial hemorrhage, acute coronary syndrome, acute CHF with pulmonary edema, aortic aneurysm or dissection, and eclampsia. Though blood pressure numbers in general can be quite high in HE (systolic blood pressure > 220 mm Hg and/or a diastolic blood pressure > 120 mm Hg are not uncommon), it is the patient's clinical status that determines the degree of intervention required to manage the problem and therefore how it is classified.

If the patient is pregnant in her third trimester or postpartum, you should consider preeclampsia as a potential cause of the hypertension. It is important for you to resist the temptation to merely treat the blood pressure as an abnormal number. Certainly it is reasonable to react to an abnormal vital sign by reevaluating it and establishing any significant trends, plus assessing for significant associated problems that may help distinguish HE from HU. Providing expectant management with appropriate monitoring, vascular access, and oxygenation is a very reasonable first-line approach for EMS to employ. Simply noting that a patient with an elevated blood pressure detected on vital signs assessment is due their regularly scheduled antihypertensive medications is important. It is certainly possible that the patient failed to take his/her medications due to the fall and fractured ankle for which EMS was called to their home. The blood pressure will likely improve with conservative treatments (ie, ice, elevation, and splinting of the painful ankle) and with the regular oral medications given in the hospital setting at a later point.

Some paramedic protocols may incorporate medications such as a nitroglycerin drip [Nitro-Bid or Tridil] or labetalol [Normodyne or Transdate] which are typically an in-hospital option. Most paramedic protocols stick to the more traditional medications, typically carried on the paramedic unit that may be useful with guidance from medical direction (ie, furosemide [Lasix], diazepam [Valium], nitroglycerin paste, metoprolol tartrate [Lopressor], diltiazem hydrochloride [Cardizem], and magnesium sulfate). In the in-hospital setting, medications such as nicardipine [Cardene] or sodium nitroprusside [Nitropress] may be used, and if the paramedic unit is to provide an interhospital transfer of a patient with either of these medications running, it will be necessary to receive some inservice as well as guidance from medical control if in fact either of these medications are authorized in your system.

Lastly, realize that when it comes to medicating hypertensive patients, the adage that "the enemy of good is better" certainly applies. Occasionally an elevated blood pressure may be more of a help to the critically ill patient, and failing to realize this by rapidly or transiently lowering it to so-called "normal" levels may provoke more harm than good.

Case Study VII Hypertension

Part 1

Your unit has been dispatched to a local church where the Sunday morning services have just completed. You are met by two women who lead you into a sitting room in the back of the church. You find a middle-aged woman who is conscious and sitting in a chair. The scene is safe and quiet as most of the crowd is exiting the church from a different location. You quickly grab your first-in bag and proceed to talk to the patient as you begin the initial assessment (see **Table 1**). The woman's daughter and husband are nearby and are very helpful to you.

After completing the intial assessment and ensuring there are no immediate life-threats, you decide to apply supplemental oxygen and begin the focused history and physical examination for a medical patient who is responsive. At this point your partner is present and gets a set of baseline vital signs as you begin to interview your patient and the bystanders to try to figure out this puzzle.

Question 1: What are some of the causes of an altered mental status?

Question 2: What is a "bounding" pulse and what is its most likely cause?

Table 1 **Initial Assessment**

Initial Assessment	Recording Time: 1 Minute
General Impression/ Appearance	Female in late 50's, conscious but disoriented and in obvious pain
Mental Status	"V" verbal (oriented to person, confused about day and place)
Airway	Open and clear
Breathing	Normal rate and quality
Circulation	Normal radial pulse, strong and bounding
Priority/Plan	High due to the pain and altered mental status

Part 2

Because the patient is a responsive medical patient you begin with exploring and elaborating on the chief complaint. In this case the patient has head pain and an altered mental status and your partner informs you that her blood pressure is 228/124 mm Hg. Your partner states he has checked that blood pressure on both arms and gets the same reading. This case will involve the OPQRST, obtaining baseline vital signs, and a focused history and physical examination (see **Table 2**).

Table 2 **Focused History and Physical Examination**

Baseline Vital Signs	Recording Time: 5 Minutes
Skin CTC (color, temperature, condition)	Red face, warm and dry
Pulse	66 beats/min and strong
Blood Pressure	228/124 mm Hg
Respirations	20 breaths/min and regular

With a chief complaint of head pain, altered mental status, and hypertension, the OPQRST questions asked of the patient reveal the following information (see **Table 3**):

Table 3 **OPQRST Questions**

Chief Complaint	Head Pain and AMS
Onset	After very stressful news of the health of a very close friend she received in a conversation at the end of today's service. It started to get worse and worse over time.
Provocation	Probably bad news on top of an extremely busy schedule
Quality	Throbbing pain
Region/radiation/ referral	Top of the head and throbbing
Severity	Patient states she has had headaches but this is one of the worst yet
Time	Approximately 45 minutes so far

Question 3: What is the relevance of the blood pressure reading?

Question 4: What could the red face indicate?

Case Study VII Continued

Part 3

From the SAMPLE history you have learned that the patient received some bad news that may have been the cause of her rapidly rising blood pressure (see **Table 4**). Apparently this is not the first time she has had a transient rise in her blood pressure and she also has a history of hypertension. She is a large woman who is probably over 250 pounds. You proceed with the SAMPLE history while your partner places her on the ECG monitor and then prepares to start an IV of normal saline.

Your physical examination includes the neuro examination and she has equal strength in all extremities as well as no positive Cincinnatti Stroke Score findings. Her lungs are clear bilaterally, she has no jugular vein distention or pedal edema. The ECG is normal sinus rhythm with no ectopy and her glucose is normal.

Table 4 SAMPLE History

SAMPLE History	Comments
Signs/symptoms	Nausea, throbbing headache
Allergies	Penicillin
Medications	Hydrochlorothiazide, potassium chloride [K-Dur]
Pertinent past medical history	Hypertension for the past 5 years and a hysterectomy about 6 months ago
Last oral intake	Ate a light breakfast (juice and coffee) about 2 hours ago
Events leading up to the incident	Headache all morning, severe pain getting worse after hearing bad news

Treatment Plan

This patient needs a fast track approach involving:

1. Monitor and manage the ABCs.
2. Administer supplemental oxygen therapy.
3. Obtain a complete set of baseline vital signs and assess the ECG.
4. Start an IV for a keep vein open line of normal saline.
5. Most paramedic units would then contact medical control to consider medication options for blood pressure control while transporting the patient to the ED. There are some EMS systems that have standing orders for this situation.

The nature of the problem associated with the hypertension will dictate the specific medication used to control it. Anginal chest pain will respond well to sublingual or transdermal nitrates and beta-blockade. It is reasonable to manage hypertension and pulmonary edema with diuretics and nitrates. Agitated delirium and hypertension should be managed with benzodiazepines like diazepam [Valium] and phenothiazines like haloperidol [Haldol]. Hypertension and mental status changes or seizures in the third trimester of pregnancy must include magnesium sulfate in its management (see **Table 5**). Commonly used prehospital medications such as labetalol [Normodyne,Trandate] (see **Table 6**) and diltiazem can also be very useful during emergency blood pressure control, as would IV metoprolol tartrate [Lopressor] during treatment of suspected aortic pathology and hypertension. Obtaining a history of preexisting hypertension and the routine medications prescribed to the patient will often help guide ongoing therapy. This patient should be transported quickly without agitation, and your ongoing assessment should include repeating the serial vital signs as well as the neuro examination.

Once at the hospital the patient may receive escalating doses of labetalol (40 or 80 mg to a total dose of 300 mg). The hospital also has more options to control the patient's blood pressure such as a nitroglycerin drip (see **Table 7**).

Table 5 Magnesium Sulfate

Do you know?	Comments
Right drug? Generic name: [**Magnesium Sulfate**] Trade name: [Magnesium]	Used as an anticonvulsant for seizures associated with eclampsia.
Right patient?	Pregnant patient in third trimester who has preeclampsia history. Preeclampsia is usually defined as a blood pressure > 140/90 mm Hg in a pregnant patient or one who has recently given birth, with severe headache, confusion and/or hyperreflexia.
Right dose?	1 to 4 g slow IV over 3 minutes.
Right route?	IV.

continues

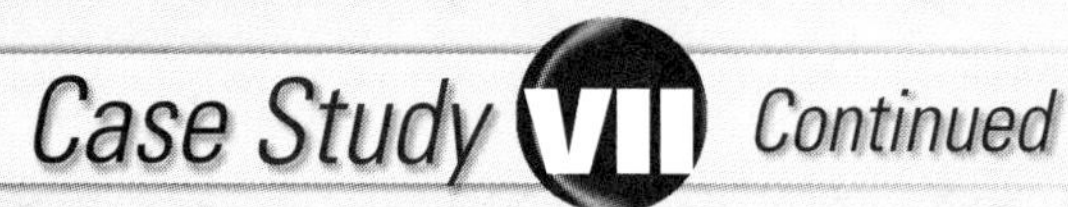

Table 5 Magnesium Sulfate (*Continued*)

Do you know?	Comments
Right time?	If the patient had a witnessed seizure, consult with medical control.
Right documentation?	Dose, route, time administered, and reassessment should be documented on the patient care report.
Expected action	Magnesium sulfate is an essential element for muscle contraction, certain enzyme systems, and nerve transmission. Prevention or control of the seizure by blocking neuromuscular transmission and decreasing the amount of acetylcholine liberated at the end plate by the motor nerve impulse. Magnesium works without producing deleterious CNS depression in the mother or infant.
Side effects	CNS: depression, Cardiovascular: flushing, hypotension, circulatory collapse, depression of the myocardium.
Contraindications	Not to be given in toxemia of pregnancy during the 2 hours prior to delivery. Should not be given to patients with heart blocks or AMI.
Precautions	Drop in blood pressure with rapid administration. Use with caution if renal failure is present because the drug is removed from the body solely by the kidneys.
Pharmacokinetics	Onset is immediate and duration is 30 minutes; excreted in urine.

Table 6 Labetalol

Do you know?	Comments
Right drug? Generic name: [**Labetalol**] Trade name: [Normodyne or Trandate]	This drug is an alpha-beta blocker and is designed to block the adrenergic nervous system receptors that are stimulated by the body's norepinephrine. It relaxes the smooth muscle in the linings of the arterioles which allows them to dilate and in turn decreases the patient's blood pressure.
Right patient?	Used for the patient with a hypertensive emergency.
Right dose?	20 mg IV over 2 minutes (repeated in 10 minutes at double the dose).
Right route?	IV infusion (there is an oral medication form but that is not used in an emergency situation).
Right time?	As soon as possible after obtaining two sets of vital signs to trend the BP.
Right documentation?	Dose, route, time administered, and reassessment.
Expected action	Controlled lowering of the blood pressure.
Side effects	Fainting, leg pain, increased sweating, increased urination, and thirst.
Contraindications	COPD, asthma, severe heart blocks, or severe bradycardia.
Precautions	History of liver or heart problems, diabetes, or allergies.
Pharmacokinetics	Onset 5 minutes IV; duration 5.5 hours; metabolized in the liver, excreted in urine.

Table 7 Nitroglycerin Infusion

Do you know?	Comments
Right drug? Generic name: [**Nitroglycerin Infusion**] Trade name: [Tridil] or [Nitro-Bid]	This drug can be used to control blood pressure, and is especially useful for that purpose in the setting of ischemic chest pain or congestive heart failure and pulmonary edema. It is commonly employed in the in-hospital setting, though some aeromedical units will use it as well. The nitro infusion is given to dilate the vessels which in turn reduces the workload (**preload**) on the heart.
Right patient?	Used for the patient with a hypertensive emergency where stroke is not suspected.

continues

Case Study VII Continued

Table 7 **Nitroglycerin Infusion (*Continued*)**

Do you know?	Comments
Right dose?	5 to 20 μg/min.
Right route?	IV infusion.
Right time?	As soon as possible after obtaining two sets of vital signs to trend the blood pressure.
Right documentation?	Dose, route, time administered, and reassessment should be documented on the patient care report.
Expected action	Controlled lowering of the blood pressure. Note that the body may develop a tolerance to the drug and require higher doses over time.
Side effects	Headache is expected and shows the medication is actually working (dilating vessels). The patient may complain of dizziness, weakness, nausea, vomiting and sweating. More severe side effects may include syncope, incontinence, vision problems, and tachy/bradycardia.
Contraindications	Hypotension is a contraindication. Do not administer within 24 hours of sildenafil and vardenafil or within 48 hours of tadalafil administration (erectile dysfunction medications).
Precautions	Use with caution when the patient is already taking heparin, ACE inhibitors for hypertension (eg, fosinopril or lisinopril), alpha blockers (eg, doxazosin or prazosin), beta-blockers (eg, propranolol), antipsychotics (eg, haloperidol or chlorpromazine), and other medications (eg, isosorbide or bromocriptine or cabergoline.
Pharmacokinetics	Onset 1–2 minutes; duration 3–5 minutes.

Question 5: If your paramedic unit does not carry medications such as a nitroglycerin drip [Nitro-Bid or Tridil] or labetalol [Normodyne or Trandate], what may be another option?

Question 6: If in response to a nitrate your patient gets very dizzy and feels like she may pass out, what should you do?

Part 4

After administration of medication en route to the hospital, you perform a reassessment and ongoing assessment of the patient (see **Table 8**).

Question 7: The patient is still very nauseated. Is there anything you can do about this?

Question 8: You have noted she is now alert. Is this a positive finding?

Part 5

The patient is doing better as she arrives at the emergency department. The treatment has been effective in bringing her hypertension under immediate control. She will be admitted to the hospital and watched closely. Now comes the hard part which involves reevaluating her physiology, medications, and lifestyle to determine why her blood pressure went dangerously high.

Table 8 **Reassessment and Ongoing Assessment of the Patient**

Serial Vital Signs and Relevant Data	Recording Time: 20 Minutes
Skin CTC	Pale, warm, and clammy
Pulse	60 beats/min strong and regular
Blood Pressure	198/106 mm Hg
Respirations	20 breaths/min and regular
Mental Status	Alert
ECG	Normal sinus rhythm with no ectopy
SpO_2	98% on supplemental oxygen
Lung Sounds	Clear bilaterally
Other (ie, glucose, core temperature)	Glucose is normal, temperature is 98.6° F

Case Study ANSWERS

Case Study I A Potential Candidate for Fibrinolysis

Question 1: Do all patients who may be experiencing a heart attack have crushing chest pain?

Answer 1: No. Not everyone who experiences an ACS will have the classic signs and symptoms or an abnormal ECG. For many people, especially women, the elderly, and diabetics, pain perception may be altered and the severity or absence of pain is often unrelated to its life-threatening potential. These patients often present with only one or more of the following atypical signs: fatigue, weakness, dyspnea, confusion, syncope, or new-onset of CHF. Getting a good history is especially important for the patient with atypical signs and symptoms and is significant to making a diagnosis to include or exclude an MI.

Question 2: If the patient has his fist on his chest, what is that sign called and what is its relevance?

Answer 2: A sick looking patient holding his hand or fist on his chest or rubbing his chest is in significant distress. This presentation is known as Levine's sign and is commonly associated with ischemic chest pain.

Question 3: If the patient does not have relief after taking two sprays of nitroglycerin, what may this indicate?

Answer 3: It could lead you to believe that the patient's problem is not angina and might be an AMI. Of course, the true diagnosis of AMI is made based on a good history as well as the results of the 12-lead ECG and serial cardiac enzymes.

Question 4: What is the significance of a patient taking an aspirin every day?

Answer 4: In most cases it could mean that the patient's physician suggested doing so because it has been shown to be helpful in keeping the platelets from sticking to each other and less viscous, which in turn helps prevent clots from occurring. Of course some patients do not take aspirin because of allergy or stomach ulcers.

Question 5: What is meant by the phrase, "Time is muscle?"

Answer 5: The transition from ischemic myocardial tissue to necrotic or dead myocardial tissue is an ongoing process during an evolving MI. This is why as the ischemic ring is ever enlarging and the volume of dead tissue is increasing, you must rapidly administer supplemental oxygen, relieve the stress on the heart, administer an aspirin, and move the patient to a facility that can provide thrombolytic therapy (fibrinolysis) or coronary catheterization.

Question 6: What is the value of communicating directly with the ED as soon as possible about the 12-lead ECG findings in the suspected ACS patient?

Answer 6: Studies have shown that the door-to-fibrinolytics and/or door-to-catheterization lab time is reduced when the hospital has advanced notice of your clinical impression as well as interpretation of the 12-lead ECG in the suspected ACS patient.

Question 7: What does the acronym "MONA" stand for in the care of the ACS patient?

Answer 7: "MONA" is an acronym for the essential drugs to treat the suspected ACS patient, provided they meet the indications and are not contraindicated based on the patient's vital signs. It stands for Morphine, Oxygen, Nitroglycerin, and Aspirin. They are all usually given but not in that order.

Question 8: Why is it important to do a fibrinolytic checklist on the suspected ACS patient?

Answer 8: Running through the same criteria that the ED will be using will help speed the door-to-fibrinolytics or door-to-catheterization lab decision and in some cases may just require the physician in the ED to verify some history before making the decision to provide significant interventions. In many cases, if you have run the checklist and communicated that to the ED they will alert cardiology sooner so they are prepared for the patient's arrival.

Case Study II Ventricular Fibrillation/ Ventricular Tachycardia

Question 1: If the patient is being shocked with a defibrillator, the patient is most likely experiencing what cardiac arrhythmia?

Answer 1: The rhythms that an AED prompts the rescuer to shock include ventricular fibrillation (V-fib) and ventricular tachycardia (V-tach) (usually over 180 beats/min). The AED does not take the patient's pulse so it is not appropriate to attach the AED to a conscious patient.

Question 2: What is a good "rule of thumb" for the placement of AEDs in busy public places such as an airport, music hall, or sports arena?

Case Study ANSWERS

Answer 2: The rule of thumb for placement of AEDs is: in clearly marked locations, in a place of public occupancy, such as an airport, casino, or sports arena, within 1 minute's brisk walk from all locations in the building.

Question 3: What are the risk factors for SCA?

Answer 3: Risk factors for SCA are the same as those for heart disease and include: family history of heart disease, smoking, high blood pressure, high cholesterol, obesity, diabetes, or a sedentary lifestyle.

Question 4: How does an impedance threshold device (ITD) work to improve the quality of the CPR?

Answer 4: The impedance threshold device (ITD) helps to improve the venous return to the heart by maintaining negative pressure during the filling phase or diastole. This in turn improves the coronary perfusion. The heart needs to work like a straw drawing the blood from the venous system during the recoil phase of your CPR compressions. Thus it is important to allow complete chest recoil and not maintain any pressure while your hands are on the patient's chest. The ITD enhances this effect by capping the ET tube at the right moment to allow the heart to work as the piston it was intended to work as, constantly filling and emptying with each stroke.

Question 5: Once an antiarrhythmic is chosen for this patient, why is lidocaine hydrochloride [Xylocaine] not routinely recommended?

Answer 5: Lidocaine hydrochloride [Xylocaine] is a potent left-ventricular end-diastolic depressant. A patient in arrest has an already markedly compromised cardiac output, and administering a medication as such will likely result in a poorer response to other aspects of the resuscitation. There may also be a potential for allergy to the "caine" drugs. Although there is an occasional resuscitation where multiple antiarrhythmics may be tried, it is the normal acceptable practice to stay with the first antiarrhythmic chosen and max out its dose as necessary.

Question 6: What are the key issues in the management of an adult patient in pulseless arrest with an ECG of V-fib or pulseless V-tach?

Answer 6: After ensuring that high-quality CPR has been started and supplemental oxygen is being administered, the monitor should be attached. Once determining the patient has a "shockable rhythm," the provider should proceed with one shock followed immediately by 2 minutes of CPR. If after 2 minutes of CPR the patient is still in V-fib or pulseless V-tach, continue CPR while the defibrillator is charging and then administer the second shock. Immediately resume CPR while another provider attempts to gain IV or IO access so that a vasopressor (either epinephrine [Adrenalin] 1 mg or vasopressin [Pitressin] 40 U) can be administered. After 2 more minutes of CPR, once again continue CPR while the defibrillator is charging and then administer the third shock. Resume CPR and consider an antiarrhythmic (amiodarone [Cordarone] 300 mg is the first choice). After 2 more minutes of CPR, consider another shock. During the arrest and as help is available, an advanced airway can be inserted and once in place, the compression:ventilation ratio can switch to continuous compressions at 100/min and 8 to 10 ventilations per minute. Basically once administration of the vasopressor has begun, it is appropriate to repeat every 3 to 5 minutes for the duration of the arrest. Vasopressin [Pitressin] 40 U can be substituted for the first or second epinephrine dose, but not both.

Question 7: Why might it be advantageous for ED staff to remove the advanced airway upon the patient's arrival?

Answer 7: The patient will chew on the airway and gag. Gagging stimulates the vagus nerve and will slow down the heart rate. Consider assessing the patient for clinical stability, then use sedative medications if necessary to maintain mechanical ventilation if indicated.

Question 8: How is an amiodarone [Cordarone] drip prepared?

Answer 8: Add 3 mL amiodarone [Cordarone] IV (150 mg) to 100 mL of D_5W or normal saline for a concentration of 1.5 mg/mL; infuse at a rate of 100 mL/10 minutes.

Case Study III Asystole/Pulseless Electrical Activity

Question 1: What is the significance of establishing the potential downtime in this patient?

Answer 1: The patient was one of the security guards' co-workers. A resuscitation on this patient is likely to be a very emotional event because he is a co-worker.

Case Study ANSWERS

If you can establish that he was down for a long time, they are more likely to understand why he was in asystole and why the CPR was not effective in reversing his condition (regardless of the quality of the CPR).

Question 2: If the security guard who started the compressions skipped ventilations because the patient had vomited and the compressions were too slow, not deep enough, and there was poor chest recoil, is it likely that the CPR has been helpful?

Answer 2: Any CPR is probably better than no CPR for the first couple of moments but clearly the better the quality of the CPR including ventilations, the more likely it is to be effective. Studies have actually shown that high-quality CPR can double if not triple the chance of survival. However, these findings all presume that there was a very short "downtime," and in this instance the downtime is in question because the patient was not answering his radio for a long time.

Question 3: What is the memory jogger "Hs and Ts" used for?

Answer 3: When searching to treat the possible causes of an adult pulseless arrest with an ECG of asystole or PEA, the "Hs and Ts" is a memory jogger to remind you to consider: hypovolemia, hypoxia or ventilation problems, hydrogen ion (acidosis), hypo-/hyperkalemia, hypoglycemia, hypothermia, toxins, tamponade (cardiac), tension pneumothorax, thrombosis (coronary or pulmonary), and trauma (ie, hypovolemia, increased ICP).

Question 4: With the information about the patient from his wife, what is the probable cause of the arrest?

Answer 4: Considering the Hs and Ts, as well as this patient's history, the probable cause could include: hypoxia, thrombosis (coronary or pulmonary), and hydrogen ion (acidosis) from the liquid diet.

Question 5: What are the key issues in the management of an adult in pulseless arrest who has an ECG of either PEA or asystole?

Answer 5: After ensuring high-quality CPR has been started and supplemental oxygen is being administered, the monitor should be attached. After determining the patient has a "not shockable rhythm," you should immediately resume CPR while another provider attempts to gain IV or IO access so that a vasopressor (either epinephrine [Adrenalin] 1 mg or vasopressin [Pitresson] 40 U) can be administered. Next, while CPR continues, consider atropine sulfate [Atropine] 1 mg if the patient has asystole or a slow PEA rate (may be repeated every 3 to 5 minutes for a maximum of 0.4 mg/kg.) After two more minutes of CPR, recheck the rhythm. If the patient is in a shockable rhythm, follow the treatment for V-fib/V-tach. If the patient is not in a shockable rhythm and asystole, consider termination or another round of atropine sulfate [Atropine] or epinephrine [Adrenalin]. If the patient is still in PEA, consider the Hs and Ts to search for the cause of the arrest.

Question 6: How often is the patient reassessed?

Answer 6: The rhythm should be reassessed at 2-minute intervals. If there is no change in the rhythm, it is not necessary to actually delay CPR compressions for a pulse check.

Question 7: If the patient was in a cold part of the warehouse and his body temperature was low, would this change your management of this patient?

Answer 7: The Medical Director may not be willing to terminate the arrest until the patient is warmed up and still dead. The medications usually do not work when a patient is hypothermic.

Question 8: What do the CPR Guidelines say about lengthy resuscitative efforts and transporting cardiac arrest patients?

Answer 8: There are very few instances that require transporting a cardiac arrest patient who has failed a successfully executed prehospital ACLS resuscitation effort to an ED to continue the resuscitation attempt. In the absence of mitigating factors, prolonged resuscitative efforts are unlikely to be successful. If return of spontaneous circulation (ROSC) of any duration occurs, however, it may be appropriate to consider extending the resuscitative effort. Rare exceptions may include severe prehospital hypothermia (eg, submersion in icy water), and drug overdose. A successfully executed prehospital resuscitation includes an "adequate trial" of BLS and ALS. Transporting a deceased patient refractory to proper BLS/ACLS is dangerous and unethical. If the efforts have failed in the prehospital setting, then how could the same treatment succeed in the ED? Protocols for pronouncement of death and appropriate transport of the body by non-EMS vehicles should be established. Paramedics should be trained to focus on dealing sensitively with the family.

Case Study ANSWERS

Case Study IV Third-Degree Heart Block/Transcutaneous Pacing

Question 1: What are some of the causes of a patient passing out?

Answer 1: There are many and syncope, sudden transient loss of consciousness, should not be underplayed. First and foremost is to determine if true syncope occurred. In many instances, near-syncope is truly what happened, and prognostically that is an entirely different matter. Additionally, separating cardiogenic (Stokes-Adams) syncope from other forms of syncope can be challenging. Other differentials that may present need to be considered (seizure, migraine, vertigo). Generally speaking, we can divide the causes of syncope up into three general categories: cardiac causes (ie, heart blocks, bradycardias, arrhythmias, etc.), non-cardiac causes (ie, neurologic, hemorrhagic, vasovagal, etc.), and medication induced (ie, beta-blockers, narcotics, nitrates, etc.).

Question 2: What is the significance of a very slow heart rate?

Answer 2: There are many causes of syncope but severe bradycardia is certainly related. The only time that bradycardia is normal is if the patient is not symptomatic and has a history of aerobic exercise more than three times a week for more than 20 minutes a day for the last few months or more. This type of exercise ultimately improves the cardiac stroke volume, making the heart a more efficient pump. Athletes have been known to have a resting heart rate in the forties but you can be sure they have developed a stroke volume that is significantly larger than most others at rest. Next time you feel a very slow heart rate in a healthy looking patient who is not in distress, be sure to ask them what their normal heart rate is. If they are an athlete they should know what is normal for them!

Question 3: Why would it be helpful to ask when she had something to eat or drink?

Answer 3: One of the causes of syncope could be related to dehydration and it was a hot day out there. Another reason is hypoglycemia.

Question 4: During your questioning why would it be helpful to find out if the patient takes any specific medications?

Answer 4: By reviewing the list of causes of syncope in Table 2, it should be clear that a number of medications can cause syncope. If the patient takes beta-blockers, she could be bleeding internally and the typical tachycardia would be prevented by the medication. Or, the patient is overmedicated with the beta-blocker itself or in combination with another medication—always beware of polypharmacy.

Question 5: What is a high-degree block?

Answer 5: A normal heartbeat is generated by the sinoatrial (SA) node, travels through the internodal pathways to the atrioventricular (AV) node, through the Bundle of His and then down into the right and left bundle branches and Purkinje fibers of the ventricles. The P-R interval is our measurement of the time an impulse takes to get through the atrium and into the ventricles where it produces the QRS complexes. A high-degree block is one where the ventricle is basically cut off from the impulses of the atrium's SA node. The inherent rate of the ventricles (20–40) kicks in when this happens. This can produce very poor perfusion and is likely to allow lethal ventricular rhythms to intercede. The high-degree blocks are second-degree type II and third-degree or complete heart block.

Question 6: Why is TCP the appropriate treatment for this type of block?

Answer 6: The drugs you give help to increase the transmission of impulses from the AV node. In a high-degree block very few, if any, of the impulses from the atria make it through to the ventricles; therefore, it is not effective in improving the rate of the ventricles. At this point the highest priority is to apply the external pacemaker and begin TCP on the patient.

Question 7: If the TCP is ineffective, are there any other options in the prehospital setting?

Answer 7: Fortunately for Mrs. Greene, the TCP was very effective. Had it not been effective in improving her symptoms, you could have administered either an epinephrine [Adrenalin] or dopamine [Intropin] infusion. Both run at 2 to 10 µg/min.

Question 8: The algorithm says to treat the contributing causes and consider expert consultation. What does that mean?

Answer 8: Basically if the cause of the bradycardia is a medication overdose, it should be managed. If the cause is cardiac, such as a decaying conduction

Case Study ANSWERS

system, it too should be managed. Symptomatic bradycardias can be very complicated and often require expert consultation once the patient gets to the ED. Your job, as the paramedic in the field, is to follow the ACLS algorithm to the letter and get the patient to the experts as soon as possible!

Case Study V Atrial Fibrillation

Question 1: What is a tachycardia?

Answer 1: In an adult, a heart rate over 100 beats/min is considered a tachycardia.

Question 2: What are some examples of conditions that can cause a tachycardia?

Answer 2: Shock, heat, anxiety, pain, fever, cardiac arrhythmia, and dehydration are a few examples of conditions that can cause a tachycardia.

Question 3: Why is a rapid heart rate often associated with shortness of breath or dyspnea?

Answer 3: Rapid heart rates do not allow the heart to fill adequately. When blood flow becomes inadequate, so does oxygenation and the patient feels short of breath because he or she is becoming hypoxic.

Question 4: What are some of the possible cardiac rhythms you might expect to see once an ECG is obtained?

Answer 4: You might expect to see SVT including: sinus tachycardia, atrial tachycardia, rapid A-fib/flutter, and V-tach.

Question 5: What is a pulse deficit?

Answer 5: A pulse deficit is a condition associated with irregular filling of the ventricles causing inconsistent cardiac output. Typically present with rapid heart rates, pulse deficit is present when the palpated distal pulse is less than the apical pulse and the rate on the ECG.

Question 6: What is a vagal maneuver?

Answer 6: Vagal stimuli (carotid sinus massage, valsalva maneuvers) can be used as a treatment option to slow SVT. When stimulated, the vagus nerve will slow the heart rate.

Question 7: Why didn't the vagal maneuver work?

Answer 7: When vagal maneuvers do work, they work better on SVTs that are not A-fib or flutter. When used in A-fib/flutter, it may make the flutter or fibrillation waves more apparent, thus making the ECG diagnosis easier to identify. Sometimes a solitary dose of adenosine can be similarly useful in distinguishing cases of poorly defined rapid atrial fibrillation from SVT.

Question 8: Why didn't the diltiazem convert the rapid atrial fibrillation to a normal sinus rhythm?

Answer 8: Diltiazem is a calcium channel blocker and works by slowing the SA and AV conduction. This will most often slow the ventricular rate rather than convert the rhythm. In some cases the patient will convert to normal sinus rhythym when the rapid reentry circuit is slowed.

Case Study VI Cardiogenic Shock/ Hypotension

Question 1: What is the first treatment priority for Emma?

Answer 1: Airway and breathing is the first treatment priority. Simple BLS steps such as sitting her up a little helps to optimize oxygenation and ventilation by allowing pulmonary edema to move dependently in the lungs. Positive-pressure ventilation and suctioning will be enormously helpful to this patient.

Question 2: Do you believe that Emma is in respiratory failure or is she having an AMI?

Answer 2: She could be experiencing one or both. She has a significant cardiac history and could be having another MI right now which is causing her to be in respiratory failure (CHF).

Question 3: What drugs might Emma be taking that could cause hypotension and bradycardia?

Answer 3: Beta-blockers, digitalis, calcium channel blockers, antiarrhythmics, and digoxin all can precipitate negative inotropic responses and are known to drop blood pressure.

Question 4: Could the nitroglycerin have caused Emma's hypotension?

Answer 4: Nitroglycerin does drop the blood pressure by dilating the arteries. However, Emma takes

Case Study ANSWERS

nitroglycerin on a regular basis for angina with no significant drop in blood pressure. Today Emma may be having an MI which is causing the decreased cardiac output and the nitroglycerin may have contributed to the significant state of hypotension.

Question 5: What do the early signs and symptoms of cardiogenic shock look like?

Answer 5: The early signs and symptoms of cardiogenic shock are the same as an acute MI; dyspnea, chest pain, nausea, cyanosis, pallor, diaphoresis, normotension, or hypotension.

Question 6: Why is cardiogenic shock associated with high mortality?

Answer 6: Cardiogenic shock is the most severe form of heart failure, resulting in insufficient cardiac output due to left ventricular malfunction. When the heart cannot effectively pump blood through the body, organ tissues deteriorate rapidly and death follows.

Question 7: Epinephrine is a vasopressor. Why is this not the preferred drug in Emma's case?

Answer 7: Epinephrine [Adrenalin] is a very potent drug with alpha and beta effects that could increase myocardial workload and worsen the developing MI. Epinephrine can produce a rapid and large increase in the blood pressure that could cause aortic rupture or cerebral hemorrhage.

Question 8: Would dobutamine [Dobutrex] be a good choice as a vasopressor for Emma?

Answer 8: Dobutamine [Dobutrex] is another vasopressor with direct acting effects on beta 1 receptors. It increases cardiac stroke volume and cardiac output with little effect on the heart rate when used in therapeutic doses. However, it can produce a precipitous drop in blood pressure, which makes this drug a better choice for patients who are not as hypotensive as Emma.

Case Study VII Hypertension

Question 1: What are some of the causes of an altered mental status?

Answer 1: Altered mental status can be caused by many things, such as epilepsy, infection, overdose, uremia, hyperglycemia, hypoglycemia, head trauma, hypoxia, hyperthermia, heat stroke, and dementia to name a few.

Question 2: What is a "bounding" pulse and what is its most likely cause?

Answer 2: A bounding pulse is a pulse that is so strong that it feels like your finger is bounced right off the spot where you are taking it. It is often caused by conditions that cause hypertension.

Question 3: What is the relevance of the blood pressure reading?

Answer 3: It is an extremely high blood pressure in the range of a hypertensive emergency by most system's protocols.

Question 4: What could the red face indicate?

Answer 4: Red skin on the face could indicate alcohol intoxication, hypertension, fever, CO poisoning, or sunburn.

Question 5: If your paramedic unit does not carry medications such as a nitroglycerin drip [Nitro-Bid or Tridil] or labetalol [Normodyne or Trandate], what may be another option?

Answer 5: Depending on the patient's underlying problem, many medicines can be useful. These include furosemide (Lasix), diazepam (Valium), nitroglycerin paste, metoprolol tartrate (Lopressor), diltiazem hydrochloride (Cardizem), and magnesium sulfate, to name a few.

Question 6: If in response to a nitrate your patient gets very dizzy and feels like she may pass out, what should you do?

Answer 6: Lay the patient down in the supine position and raise the legs about 12" to 18". Consider running a little fluid in if the patient has experienced a precipitous drop in blood pressure and check the ECG monitor.

Question 7: The patient is still very nauseated. Is there anything you can do about this?

Answer 7: Consider giving the patient an antiemetic drug. Vomiting will only result in further exacerbation of the underlying problem and elevated blood pressure.

Question 8: You have noted she is now alert. Is this a positive finding?

Answer 8: Yes, increased alertness is definitely considered an improvement and should be noted.

Medication Review

Adenosine (Adenocard)

Indications Conversion of paroxysmal supraventricular tachycardia to sinus rhythm. May convert re-entry SVT due to Wolff-Parkinson-White syndrome. Not effective in converting atrial fibrillation/flutter or V-tach.

Contraindications Second- or third-degree block or sick sinus syndrome, atrial flutter/atrial fibrillation, ventricular tachycardia, hypersensitivity to adenosine, poison-induced tachycardia.

Dosage and administration Adult: 6 mg over 1–3 seconds, followed by a 20 mL saline flush and elevate extremity; if no response after 1–2 minutes, administer 12 mg over 1–3 seconds, if no response repeat 12 mg again. Maximum total dose, 30 mg; Pediatric: 0.1–0.2 mg/kg rapid IV; maximum single dose, 12 mg.

Amiodarone (Cordarone, Pacerone)

Indications V-fib/pulseless V-tach and unstable V-tach in patients refractory to other therapy. Also persistent SVTs unresponsive to other treatment.

Contraindications Known hypersensitivity, cardiogenic shock, sinus bradycardia, and second- or third-degree AV block (unless a functional pacemaker is available).

Dosage and administration Adult: V-fib/pulseless V-tach unresponsive to CPR, defibrillation, and vasopressors: 300 mg IV/IO push (recommend dilution in 20–30 mL D_5W). Initial dose can be followed one time in 3–5 minutes at 150 mg IV/IO push. Recurrent life-threatening ventricular arrhythmias: Maximum cumulative dose is 2.2 g/24 hours, administered as follows: Rapid infusion: 150 mg IV/IO over 10 minutes (15 mg/min). May repeat rapid infusion (150 mg IV/IO) every 10 minutes as needed. Slow infusion: 360 mg IV/IO over 6 hours (1 mg/min). Maintenance infusion: 540 mg IV/IO over 18 hours (0.5 mg/min). Pediatric: Refractory V-fib/pulseless V-tach: 5 mg/kg IV/IO bolus. Can repeat the 5 mg/kg IV/IO bolus up to a total dose of 15 mg/kg per 24 hours. Maximum single dose is 300 mg. Perfusing supraventricular and ventricular tachycardias: Loading dose of 5 mg/kg IV/IO over 20–60 minutes (maximum single dose of 300 mg). Can repeat to maximum of 15 mg/kg per day.

Aspirin

Indications New onset chest pain suggestive of acute myocardial infarction. Signs and symptoms suggestive of recent cerebrovascular accident.

Contraindications Hypersensitivity. Relatively contraindicated in patients with active ulcer disease or asthma.

Dosage and administration 160 mg to 325 mg PO (chewed if possible).

Atropine Sulfate

Indications Hemodynamically unstable bradycardia, asystole, bradycardic (< 60 beats/min) pulseless electrical activity (PEA), organophosphate poisoning, bronchospastic pulmonary disorders.

Contraindications Tachycardia, hypersensitivity, unstable cardiovascular status in acute hemorrhage and myocardial ischemia, narrow-angle glaucoma.

Dosage and administration Adult: Asystole or bradycardic PEA: 1 mg IV/IO push. May repeat every 3–5 minutes (if asystole or PEA persists) to a maximum of 0.04 mg/kg. Endotracheal administration: 2–3 mg diluted in 10 mL of water or normal saline. Unstable bradycardia: 0.5 mg IV/IO every 3–5 minutes as needed, not to exceed total dose of 0.04 mg/kg. Use shorter dosing interval (3 minutes) and higher doses in severe clinical conditions. Organophosphate poisoning: Extremely large doses (2–4 mg or higher) may be needed. Pediatric: 0.02 mg/kg via IV/IO push; may double this dose for second IV/IO dose. Minimum single dose: 0.1 mg. Maximum doses: child single dose: 0.5 mg, child total dose: 1 mg, adolescent single dose: 1 mg, adolescent total dose: 2 mg. Endotracheal administration: 0.03 mg/kg (absorption may be unreliable).

Medication Review

Calcium Chloride

Indications Hypocalcemia, hyperkalemia, magnesium sulfate overdose, calcium channel blocker overdose, adjunctive therapy in treatment of insect bites and stings.

Contraindications Hypercalcemia, V-fib, digitalis toxicity.

Dosage and administration Adult: 500 mg to 1,000 mg (5–10 mL of a 10% solution) IV/IO push for hyperkalemia and calcium channel blocker overdose. May be repeated as needed. Pediatric: 20 mg/kg (0.2 mL/kg) slow IV/IO push. Maximum 1 g dose; may repeat in 10 minutes.

Diazepam (Valium)

Indications Acute anxiety states, acute alcohol withdrawal (delirium tremens), muscle relaxant, seizure activity, agitation. Analgesia for medical procedures (fracture reduction, cardioversion).

Contraindications Hypersensitivity, glaucoma, coma, shock, substance abuse, head injury.

Dosage and administration Seizure activity: Adult: 5–10 mg IV every 10–15 minutes as needed (5 mg over 5 min) (maximum dose, 30 mg). Seizure activity: Pediatric: 0.2–0.5 mg slowly every 2–5 minutes up to 5 mg (maximum dose, 10 mg/kg). Rectal diazepam: 0.5 mg/kg via rectal catheter and flush with 2–3 mL air after administration. Sedation for cardioversion: 5–15 mg IV over 5–10 minutes prior to cardioversion.

Digoxin (Lanoxin)

Indications Congestive heart failure, re-entry SVT, especially atrial flutter and atrial fibrillation.

Contraindications Ventricular fibrillation, ventricular tachycardia, digitalis toxicity, hypersensitivity to digoxin.

Dosage and administration Adult: Loading dose of 10 to 15 µg/kg. Pediatric: not recommended in the prehospital setting.

Diltiazem Hydrochloride (Cardizem, Lyo-Ject)

Indications Control of rapid ventricular rates due to atrial flutter, atrial fibrillation, and re-entry SVT; Angina pectoris.

Contraindications Hypotension, sick sinus syndrome, second- or third-degree AV block, cardiogenic shock, wide-complex tachycardias, poison/drug-induced tachycardia.

Dosage and administration Adult: Initial bolus: 0.25 mg/kg (average dose 15–20 mg) IV over 2 minutes. If inadequate response, may re-bolus in 15 minutes: 0.35 mg/kg (average dose 20–25 mg) IV over 2 minutes. Maintenance infusion of 5–15 mg/h. Pediatric: Not recommended.

Dobutamine (Dobutrex)

Indications Cardiogenic shock, CHF, left ventricular dysfunction. Often used in conjunction with other drugs.

Contraindications Tachyarrhythmias, idiopathic hypertrophic subaortic stenosis, severe hypotension.

Dosage and administration Adult: IV infusion at 2–20 µg/kg/min titrated to desired effect. Pediatric: 2–20 µg/kg/min titrated to desired effect.

Dopamine (Intropin)

Indications Cardiogenic, septic or spinal shock, hypotension with low cardiac output states, distributive shock.

Contraindications Hypovolemic shock, pheochromocytoma, tachyarrhythmias, V-fib.

Dosage and administration Adult: 2–20 µg/kg/min titrated to patient response; Pediatric: 2–20 µg/kg/min titrated to patient response.

Medication Review

Epinephrine (Adrenalin)

Indications Cardiac arrest (V-fib/pulseless V-tach, asystole, PEA), symptomatic bradycardia as an alternative infusion to dopamine, severe hypotension secondary to bradycardia when atropine and transcutaneous pacing are unsuccessful, allergic reactions, anaphylaxis, asthma.

Contraindications Hypertension, hypothermia, pulmonary edema, myocardial ischemia, hypovolemic shock.

Dosage and administration Adult: Mild allergic reactions and asthma: 0.3–0.5 mg (0.3–0.5 mL of 1:1,000) SC. Anaphylaxis: 0.1 mg (1 mL of 1:10,000) IV/IO over 5 minutes. Cardiac arrest: IV/IO dose: 1 mg (10 mL of 1:10,000 solution) every 3–5 minutes during resuscitation. Follow each dose with 20 mL flush and elevate arm for 10 to 20 seconds after dose. Higher dose: Higher doses (up to 0.2 mg/kg) may be used for specific indications (beta-blocker or calcium channel blocker overdose). Continuous infusion: Add 1 mg (1 mL of 1:1,000 solution) to 500 mL normal saline or D_5W. Initial infusion rate of 1 µg/min titrated to effect (typical dose: 2–10 µg/min). Endotracheal (ET) dose: 2–2.5 mg diluted in 10 mL normal saline. Profound bradycardia or hypotension: 2–10 µg/min; titrate to patient response. Pediatric: Mild allergic reactions and asthma: 0.01 mg/kg (0.01 mL/kg) of 1:1,000 solution SC (maximum of 0.3 mL). Cardiac arrest: IV/IO dose: 0.01 mg/kg (0.1 mL/kg) of 1:10,000 solution every 3–5 minutes during arrest. All endotracheal (ET) doses: 0.1 mg/kg (0.1 mL/kg) of 1:1,000 solution. Symptomatic bradycardia: IV/IO dose: 0.01 mg/kg (0.1 mL/kg) of 1:10,000 solution. All endotracheal (ET) doses: 0.1 mg/kg (0.1 mL/kg) of 1:1,000 solution. Continuous IV/IO infusion: Begin with rapid infusion, then titrate to response. Typical initial infusion: 0.1–1 µg/min. Higher doses may be effective.

Furosemide (Lasix)

Indications CHF, pulmonary edema, hypertensive crisis.

Contraindications Hypovolemia, anuria, hypotension (relative contraindication); hypersensitivity, hepatic coma.

Dosage and administration Adult: 0.5–1.0 mg/kg injected IV over 1 to 2 minutes. If no response, double the dose to 2 mg/kg over 1 to 2 minutes. Pediatric: 1 mg/kg/dose IV, IO.

Labetalol (Normodyne, Trandate)

Indications Moderate to severe hypertension.

Contraindications Bronchial asthma, CHF, cardiogenic shock, second- and third-degree heart block, bradycardia.

Dosage and administration Adult: 5–20 mg slow IV over 2 minutes (additional injections of 10–40 mg can be given at 10-minute intervals). Infusion: 2 mg/min titrated to acceptable supine blood pressure. Pediatric: safety not established.

Lidocaine Hydrochloride (Xylocaine)

Indications Alternative to amiodarone in cardiac arrest from V-fib/pulseless V-tach, stable monomorphic V-tach, stable polymorphic V-tach with normal baseline QT interval.

Contraindications Hypersensitivity, second- and third-degree AV blocks in the absence of artificial pacemaker, Stokes-Adams syndrome, prophylactic use in AMI, wide-complex ventricular escape beats with bradycardia.

Dosage and administration Adult: Cardiac arrest from V-fib/pulseless V-tach: Initial dose: 1–1.5 mg/kg IV/IO. Repeat dose: 0.5–0.75 mg/kg, repeated in 5–10 minutes to maximum dose of 3 mg/kg. Endotracheal (ET) dose: 2–4 mg/kg. Stable V-tach, wide-complex tachycardia of uncertain type, significant ectopy: Doses ranging from 0.5–0.75 mg/kg and up to 1–1.5 mg/kg may be used. Repeat 0.5–0.75 mg/kg every 5–10 minutes. Maximum total dose is 3 mg/kg. Maintenance infusion: 1–4 mg/min (30–50 µg/kg/min); can dilute in D_5W or normal saline. Pediatric: IV/IO dose: 1 mg/kg rapid IV/IO push. Maximum dose: 100 mg. Continuous IV/IO infusion: 20–50 µg/kg/min. Administer bolus dose (1 mg/kg) when infusion is initiated if bolus has not been given within previous 15 minutes. Endotracheal (ET) dose: 2–3 mg/kg.

Medication Review

Magnesium Sulfate

Indications Seizures of eclampsia (toxemia of pregnancy), torsade de pointes, hypomagnesemia, Class IIa agent for V-fib/pulseless V-tach that is refractory to lidocaine.

Contraindications Heart blocks, myocardial damage.

Dosage and administration Adult: Seizure activity associated with pregnancy: 1–4 g IV/IO over 3 minutes; maximum dose of 30–40 g/day. Cardiac arrest due to hypomagnesemia or torsade de pointes: 1–2 g (2–4 mL of a 50% solution) diluted in 10 mL of D_5W IV/IO over 5–20 minutes. Torsade de pointes with a pulse or AMI with hypomagnesemia: Loading dose of 1–2 g mixed in 50–100 mL D_5W over 5–60 minutes IV. Follow with 0.5–1 g/hr IV (titrate to control torsade de pointes). Pediatric: IV/IO infusion: 25–50 mg/kg (maximum dose: 2 g) over 10–20 minutes; faster for torsade de pointes. For asthma: 25–50 mg/kg (maximum dose: 2 g) over 10–20 minutes.

Metoprolol tartrate (Lopressor)

Indications Suspected ACS provided heart rate is > 80 and systolic BP is > 120 mm Hg.

Patients may be taking the tablet form for hypertension or angina. The usual tablet initial dose is 100 mg and effective dose is between 100 and 400 mg daily. Has also been used for ventricular arrhythmias and migraine headaches. Paramedic protocols are usually for the IV dose of the drug.

Contraindications In the context of a suspected MI, the drug is contraindicated in patients with a heart rate < 45 beats/min; second- and third-degree heart block; significant first-degree heart block (P-R interval ≥ 0.24 sec); systolic blood pressure < 100 mm Hg; or moderate-to-severe cardiac failure. Hypersensitivity to the drug, related derivatives, or other beta-blockers (cross sensitivity between beta-blockers can occur).

Dosage and administration Adult: 5 mg slow IV bolus, may be repeated every 2 minutes up to maximum of 15 mg. Pediatric: not recommended.

Midazolam (Versed)

Indications Sedation, anxiolytic prior to endotracheal or nasotracheal intubation; administer for conscious sedation.

Contraindications Glaucoma, shock, coma, alcohol intoxication, overdose, depressed vital signs, concomitant use with other CNS depressants, barbiturates, alcohol, narcotics.

Dosage and administration Adult: 2.0–2.5 mg slow IV over 2–3 minutes; may be repeated to total maximum: 0.1 mg/kg. Pediatric: Not recommended.

Morphine Sulfate (Astramorph/PF and others)

Indications Severe CHF, pulmonary edema, chest pain associated with acute MI, analgesia for moderate to severe acute and chronic pain (use with caution).

Contraindications Head injury, exacerbated COPD, depressed respiratory drive, hypotension, undiagnosed abdominal pain, decreased level of consciousness, suspected hypovolemia, patients who have taken MAOIs within the past 14 days.

Dosage and administration Adult: Initial dose: 2–4 mg IV (over 1–5 minutes) every 5–30 minutes. Repeat dose: 2–8 mg at 5- to 15-minute intervals. Pediatric: 0.1–0.2 mg/kg per dose via IV, IO, IM, or SC; maximum dose of 5 mg.

Nifedipine (Procardia)

Indications Hypertensive crisis, angina pectoris, pulmonary edema (investigational).

Contraindications Compensatory hypertension, hypotension, hypersensitivity.

Dosage and administration Adult: 10 mg SL or buccal (puncture end of capsule with needle and squeeze; may administer SL or buccally or may have patient bite and swallow); may repeat in 30 minutes. Pediatric: Not recommended.

Medication Review

Nitroglycerin (Nitrostat, Tridil, and others)

Indications Acute angina pectoris, ischemic chest pain, hypertension, CHF, pulmonary edema.

Contraindications Hypotension, hypovolemia; intracranial bleeding or head injury; previous administration of Viagra, Revatio, Levitra, Cialis, or similar agents within past 24 hours.

Dosage and administration Adult: Tablets: 0.3–0.4 mg SL; may repeat in 3–5 minutes to maximum of 3 doses. NTG spray: 0.4 mg under the tongue; 1–2 sprays. NTG IV infusion: begin at 10 to 20 µg/min; increase by 5–10 µg/min every 5 minutes until desired effect. Pediatric: Not recommended.

Nitropaste (Nitro-Bid Ointment)

Indications Angina pectoris and chest pain associated with acute MI.

Contraindications Same as NTG.

Dosage and administration Adult: Paste: Apply ½" to ¾" (1–2 cm), 15–30 mg, cover with wrap and secure with tape; maximum, 5" (75 mg) per application. Transdermal: Apply unit to intact skin (usually chest wall) in varying doses. Pediatric: Not recommended.

Norepinephrine Bitartrate (Levophed, Levarterenol)

Indications Cardiogenic shock, significant hypotensive (< 70 mm Hg) states.

Contraindications Hypotensive patients with hypovolemia, pregnancy (relative contraindication).

Dosage and administration Adult: Dilute 8 mg in 500 mL of D_5W or 4 mg in 250 mL of D_5W (16 mg/mL); infuse by IV piggyback at 0.5–1.0 µg/min, titrated to improve blood pressure (up to 30 µg/min). Pediatric: 0.1–1.0 µg/min IV infusion, titrated to patient response.

Ondansetron Hydrochloride (Zofran)

Indications For the prevention or control of nausea or vomiting. Also used in the hospital setting for patients undergoing chemotherapy or surgical procedures.

Contraindications Known allergy to this medicine or other 5-HT3 receptor antagonists.

Dosage and administration Adult: 4 mg IV or IM (may repeat in 10 minutes).

Pediatric: 0.1 mg/kg IV or IM.

Oxygen

Indications Confirmed or expected hypoxemia, ischemic chest pain, respiratory insufficiency, prophylactically during air transport, confirmed or suspected carbon monoxide poisoning, all other causes of decreased tissue oxygenation, decreased level of consciousness.

Contraindications Certain patients with COPD or emphysema who will not tolerate oxygen concentrations over 35%, hyperventilation. Oxygen should never be withheld from a patient who needs it, however. Be prepared to assist with ventilations in a patient with COPD who requires high concentration, as apnea may result.

Dosage and administration Adult: Cardiac arrest and carbon monoxide poisoning: 100%. Hypoxemia: 10–15 L/min via nonrebreathing mask. COPD: 1–6 L/min via nasal cannula or 28%–35% Venturi mask. Be prepared to provide ventilatory support if higher concentrations of oxygen needed. Pediatric: Same as for adult with exception of premature infant.

Medication Review

Procainamide Hydrochloride (Pronestyl, Procanbid)

Indications Stable monomorphic V-tach with normal QT interval, reentry SVT uncontrolled by vagal maneuvers and adenosine, stable wide-complex tachycardia of unknown origin, atrial fibrillation with rapid ventricular rate in patients with Wolff-Parkinson-White syndrome.

Contraindications Torsade de pointes, second- and third-degree AV block (without functional artificial pacemaker), digitalis toxicity, tricyclic antidepressant overdose.

Dosage and administration Adult: Recurrent V-fib/pulseless V-tach: 20 mg/min IV infusion (maximum dose: 17 mg/kg). In urgent situations, up to 50 mg/min may be administered (maximum dose of 17 mg/kg). Other indications: 20 mg/min IV infusion until any one of the following occurs: arrhythmia suppression, hypotension, QRS widens by > 50% of its pretreatment width, or total dose of 17 mg/kg has been given. Maintenance infusion: 1–4 mg/min (dilute in D_5W or normal saline). Pediatric: Loading dose of 15 mg/kg IV/IO over 30–60 minutes.

Promethazine Hydrochloride (Phenergan)

Indications Nausea, vomiting, motion sickness; sedation for patients in labor; potentiation of analgesic effects of narcotics.

Contraindications Hypersensitivity, coma, CNS-depressed patients from alcohol, barbiturates, narcotics, Reye's syndrome.

Dosage and administration Adult: 12.5–25 mg IV, deep IM, PO, rectally. Pediatric: (older than 2 years old) 0.25–0.5 mg/kg dose IM.

Propranolol Hydrochloride (Inderal)

Indications Hypertension, angina pectoris, V-tach and V-fib refractory to lidocaine; selected supraventricular tachycardias.

Contraindications Sinus bradycardia, second- or third-degree AV block, asthma, CHF, COPD.

Dosage and administration Adult: Dilute 1–3 mg in 10–30 mL of D_5W; administer slowly IV at rate of 1 mg/min; maximum, 5 mg. Pediatric: 0.01–0.05 mg/kg/dose slow IV over 10 minutes; maximum, 3 mg.

Sodium Bicarbonate

Indications Mild or moderate metabolic acidosis due to shock, severe dehydration, anoxia, uncontrolled diabetes, renal disease, cardiac arrest, and severe primary lactic acidosis. To treat overdose of aspirin and cyclic-antidepressants.

Contraindications Metabolic and respiratory alkalosis, hypertension, convulsions, CHF, and other situations where sodium can be dangerous.

Dosage and administration 1 mEq per kg IV bolus (may repeat every 10 minutes at ½ initial dose).

Streptokinase (Streptase)

Indications Acute evolving MI, massive pulmonary emboli, arterial thrombosis and embolism, to clear arteriovenous cannulas.

Contraindications Hypersensitivity; active bleeding, recent surgery (within 2–4 weeks), recent CVA; prolonged CPR; intracranial or intraspinal neoplasm, arteriovenous malformation, or surgery; recent significant trauma (particularly head trauma); uncontrolled hypertension.

Dosage and administration Note: Reconstitute by slowly adding 5 mL of sodium chloride or D_5W, directing stream to side of vial instead of into powder. Gently roll and tilt vial for reconstitution; dilute slowly to 45 mL total. Adult: 500,000–1,500,000 IU diluted to 45 mL IV over 1 hour. Pediatric: safety not established.

Medication Review

Succinylcholine (Anectine, Quelicin)

Indications To facilitate intubation, to terminate laryngospasm, to promote muscle relaxation, to facilitate electroconvulsive shock therapy.

Contraindications Acute narrow-angle glaucoma, penetrating eye injuries, inability to control airway or support ventilations with oxygen and positive pressure.

Dosage and administration Adult: 1–2 mg/kg rapid IV; repeat once if needed. Pediatric: 1–1.5 mg/kg dose rapid IV, IO; repeat once if needed.

Tissue Plasminogen Activator (TPA)

Indications Acute evolving myocardial infarction, massive pulmonary emboli, arterial thrombosis and embolism, to clear arteriovenous cannulas.

Contraindications Recent surgery (within 3 weeks), active bleeding, recent CVA, prolonged CPR, intracranial or intraspinal surgery; recent significant trauma, especially head trauma; uncontrolled hypertension (generally BP over 200 mm Hg).

Dosage and administration Adult: 10-mg bolus IV over 2 minutes; then 50 mg over 1 hour, then 20 mg over the second hour and 20 mg over the third hour, for a total dose of 100 mg (other doses may be prescribed through Medical Direction). Pediatric: safety not established.

Vasopressin (Pitressin synthetic)

Indications Alternate vasopressor to the first or second dose of epinephrine in cardiac arrest, may be useful in cases of vasodilatory shock (ie, septic shock).

Contraindications Responsive patients with coronary artery disease.

Dosage and administration Adult: 40-unit one-time dose IV/IO to replace the first or second dose of epinephrine in cardiac arrest. Pediatric: Not recommended.

Verapamil (Calan, Isoptin)

Indications Paroxysmal supra-ventricular tachycardia, paroxysmal atrial tachycardia, atrial fibrillation, and atrial flutter with rapid ventricular response.

Contraindications Wolff-Parkinson-White syndrome, second-degree or third-degree AV block, sick sinus syndrome (unless patient has functioning pacemaker), hypotension, cardiogenic shock, severe CHF, pulmonary edema, patients receiving IV beta-blockers, wide-complex tachycardias, children younger than 12 months of age.

Dosage and administration Adult: 2.5–5.0 mg IV bolus over 2 minutes (over 3 minutes in older patients). Repeat doses of 5–10 mg may be given every 15–30 minutes to a maximum of 20 mg. Pediatric: 0.1–0.2 mg/kg/dose IV, IO push over 2 minutes. Repeat dose in 30 minutes if not effective. (Note: not to be used in children younger than 12 months of age.)

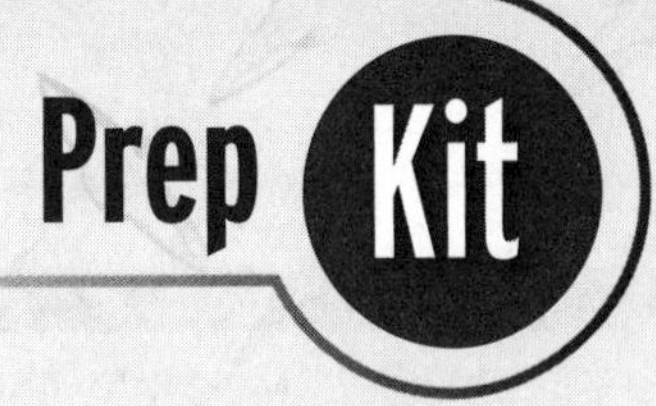

Chapter Summary

- Acute coronary syndromes include conditions such as: unstable angina, non-Q wave MI, Q wave MI, and sudden cardiac death.
- The atypical signs of ACS include: weakness, dyspnea, confusion, syncope, and new-onset congestive heart failure.
- The importance of the window of opportunity for transporting an ACS patient to a facility for reperfusion therapy with clotbusters (fibrinolytics) or coronary catheterization cannot be overstated.
- The precipitating factors to sudden cardiac arrest include: coronary artery disease, valvular disease, congenital heart disease, long Q-T syndrome, Wolff-Parkinson-White syndrome, previous cardiac arrest or heart attack, drug abuse, hyperthyroidism, considerable electrolyte changes, and a low (< 35%) ejection fraction.
- The importance of high-quality CPR and strengthening the links in communities' "chain of survival" cannot be emphasized enough.
- The impedance threshold device is used as an adjunct during CPR to improve perfusion.
- Teamwork divides the task while multiplying the chances of success in the code.
- Since many of the medications used in cardiovascular emergencies are designed to have an effect on the nervous system's adrenergic receptors, the alpha 1, alpha 2, beta 1, and beta 2 receptors are discussed.
- Pacemakers come in three types: external or noninvasive transcutaneous pacer (TCP), transvenous temporary wires, and internal or invasive (surgically implanted).
- The four commonly found tachycardias in the field are sinus tachycardia, atrial flutter, supraventricular tachycardia, and ventricular tachycardia.
- Cardioversion is the use of the defibrillator to terminate arrhythmias other than ventricular fibrillation (V-fib).
- It is helpful to understand the home medications that heart failure patients may be taking (ie, antianginals, beta-blockers, calcium channel blockers, antihypertensives, anticoagulants, ACE inhibitors, and antiarrhythmics).
- Cardiogenic shock is the most serious form of heart failure resulting from insufficient cardiac output due to left ventricular malfunction.
- It is important for the paramedic to recognize the seriousness of patients who present with cardiovascular-related symptoms and hypertension, and who do not have the typical history for you to suspect ACS.
- Patients with elevated blood pressure have an increased risk of aneurysm, TIA, or stroke.
- Hypertensive crisis, which is a significantly elevated blood pressure, should be recognized and managed by the paramedic in consult with medical control.
- Hypertension in the third trimester or postpartum period of pregnancy should indicate to the paramedic that there is a distinct potential for preeclampsia.
- When it comes to medicating hypertensive patients, the adage, "the enemy of good is better" certainly applies.

Vital Vocabulary

Acute myocardial infarction (AMI) A heart attack. A sudden death of heart cells due to the decreased blood supply from a blocked artery. The word "infarction" comes from the Latin "infarcire" meaning "to plug up or cram."

Alpha 1 receptors When stimulated, cause vasoconstriction of the smooth muscle. They also cause vasoconstriction to the blood vessels in the skin, GI system, kidneys, and the brain.

Alpha 2 receptors When stimulated, inhibit the release of insulin by the pancreas, inhibit the release of norepinephrine, contracts sphincters of the GI tract, and induce glucagon release from the pancreas.

Angina pectoris Actually means "pain in the chest." The sudden pain from myocardial ischemia, caused by diminished circulation to the cardiac muscle. The pain is usually substernal and often radiates to the arms, jaw, or abdomen and usually lasts 3 to 5 minutes and disappears with rest.

Atherosclerosis An arteriosclerosis made up of atheromatous deposits in the inner layer of the arteries.

Atrial tachycardia An ECG involving a supraventricular tachycardia (SVT) that does not require the atrioventricular (AV) junction, accessory pathways, or ventricular tissue for initiation and maintenance of the tachycardia.

AV node The primary pacemaker site of the heart.

Beta-adrenergic blocking agent Drugs that block the actions of the beta receptor sites.

Beta 1 receptors When stimulated, are responsible for increasing the cardiac output and increasing the rate and force of myocardial contraction.

Beta 2 receptors When stimulated, relax the smooth muscles (ie, bronchi), dilate the skeletal muscles, relax the urinary sphincter, and contract the sphincters of the GI tract.

Bundle of His Cardiac muscle fibers that pass from the AV node to the ventricles by way of the septum. The bundle is a part of the normal cardiac conduction system.

Cardiac catheterization The insertion of a catheter through the femoral artery in the groin, and carefully moved up and into the heart's coronary arteries. By entering the coronary arteries this allows the physician to inject radiopaque dye so an X-ray can be taken of the heart and its vessels.

Hypertensive crisis A severe increase in blood pressure that can lead to a stroke. Extremely high blood pressure, above 180/110 mm Hg, damages the blood vessels causing them to become inflamed and leak fluid or blood. As a result, the heart may not be able to maintain adequate circulation of blood.

Impedence threshold device (ITD) Used as an adjunct to ventilations during cardiac arrest, the device has been shown to enhance the vacuum in the chest during the recoil phase of the compression. This device helps to create the natural negative pressure in the lungs.

Internodal pathways Lying or extending between the two nodes in the cardiac conduction system.

Junctional tachycardia An ECG which is a tachycardia that is associated with the generation of impulses in a location in the region of the AV node.

P waves The wave on an ECG that precedes the QRS complex and represents the atrial contraction.

P-R interval The duration of time on the ECG between the P wave and the QRS complex. It represents the time it takes for the impulse to make it from the SA node to the ventricle.

Preload The initial stretching of the cardiac muscle cells prior to the contraction.

Prostaglandins Oxygenated, unsaturated cyclic fatty acids that have hormone-like actions such as controlling blood pressure or smooth muscle contraction.

QRS complex/interval On an ECG, the series of three waves, the Q, the R, and the S, which together represent the ventricular contraction of the heart.

Q-T interval The length of time on an ECG that it takes from the beginning of the Q wave, which is the start of ventricular contraction to the T wave, which is the relative refractory period of the cardiac cycle.

R wave In an ECG, the first upright deflection following the P wave.

SA node The sinoatrial node where the heart's normal pacemaker is found.

ST segment On an ECG, the length from the beginning of the S wave to the T wave.

ST segment elevation myocardial infarction (STEMI) A heart attack, or MI, that is caused by a prolonged period of blocked blood supply. It affects a large area of the heart muscle, and thus causes changes on the ECG involving elevation of the ST segments in two or more leads, as well as changes in blood levels of key chemical markers.

Sinus tachycardia A sinus rhythm with a heart rate greater than 100 beats/min.

Sympathomimetics Synthetic analogs of naturally occurring catecholamines that bind to beta or alpha receptors and mimic the actions of the endogenous neurotransmitters. These agents can be divided into direct and indirect acting sympathomimetics. Common examples include amphetamine, ephedrine, and cocaine.

Vasopressor An agent that constricts the blood vessels causing the blood pressure to rise.

Ventricular fibrillation (V-fib) An ECG that is totally erratic and does not produce a heartbeat. V-fib is the most commonly identified arrhythmia in cardiac arrest patients and it usually ends in death within minutes unless corrective measures are promptly taken.

Ventricular tachycardia (V-tach) An ECG rhythm faster than 100 beats/min arising distal from the bundle of His. The patient with V-tach may have a pulse or be pulseless.

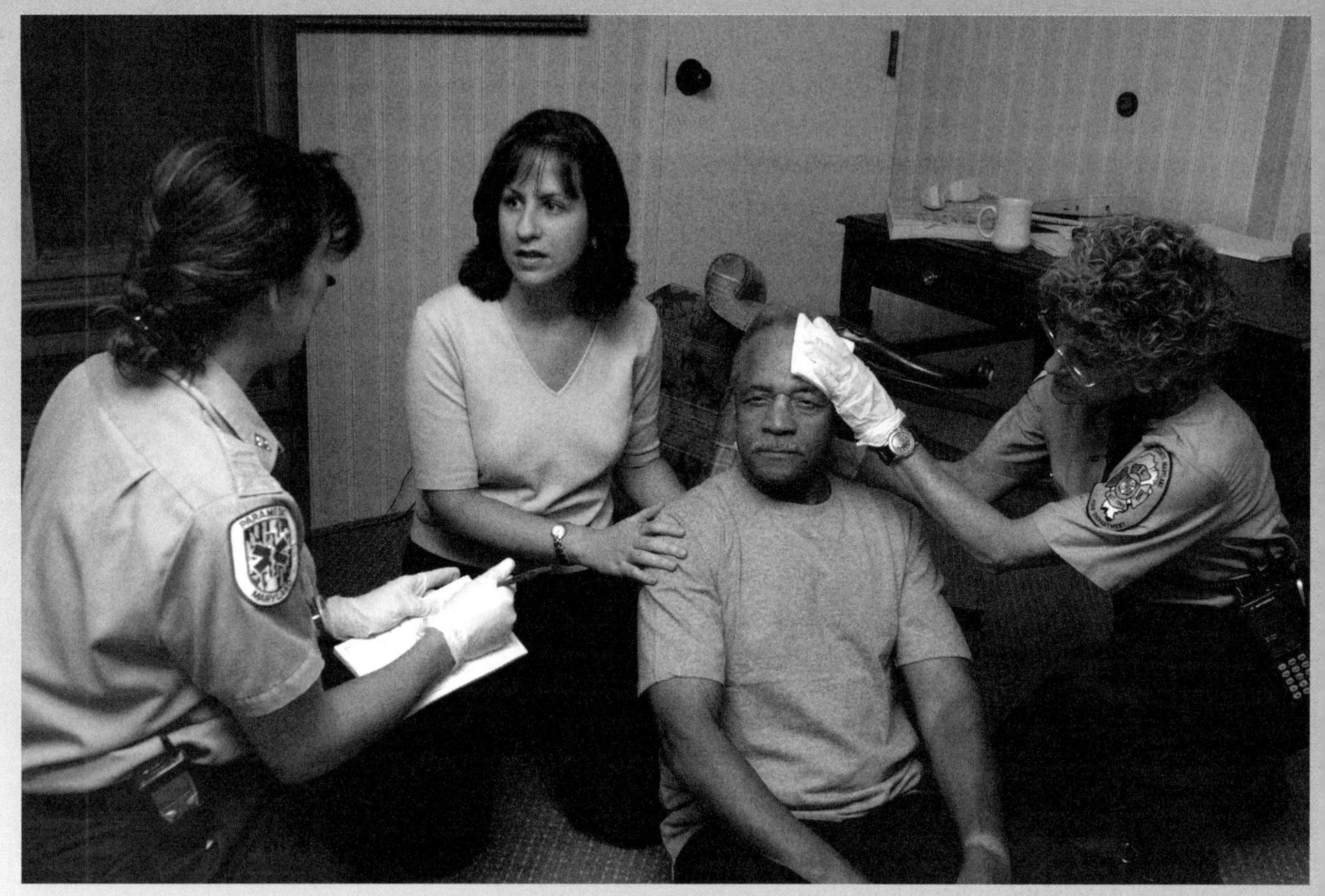

Neurologic Emergencies 5

Objectives

Cognitive

5-3.32 Differentiate among the various treatment and pharmacological interventions used in the management of neoplasms. (page 203)

5-3.41 Differentiate among the various treatment and pharmacological interventions used in the management of abscess. (page 208)

5-3.51 Differentiate among the various treatment and pharmacological interventions used in the management of stroke and intracranial hemorrhage. (pages 190–195)

5-3.60 Differentiate among the various treatment and pharmacological interventions used in the management of transient ischemic attack. (pages 190–197)

5-3.69 Differentiate among the various treatment and pharmacological interventions used in the management of degenerative neurological diseases. (page 208)

Affective

None

Psychomotor

5-3.79 Appropriately manage a patient with coma or altered mental status, including the administration of oxygen, oral glucose, 50% dextrose and narcotic reversal agents. (pages 190–194)

5-3.83 Appropriately manage a patient with seizures, including the administration of diazepam [Valium] or lorazepam [Ativan]. (pages 195–203)

Additional Objectives

5-1 Discuss the acronym FAST and its application to the possible stroke patient. (pages 190–197)

5-2 Discuss the importance of time and bringing the patient to a stroke center if one is designated in your EMS System. (pages 190–195)

5-3 Review the Cincinnati Prehospital Stroke Scale, an assessment tool for possible stroke used by paramedics in the prehospital setting. (page 190)

5-4 Review the fibrinolytic stroke checklist and its usefulness in the field management of the potential stroke patient. (pages 195–197)

5-5 Discuss the following medications used in the prehospital setting for neurologic patients: dextrose 50% ($D_{50}W$), glucagon, diazepam [Valium], lorazepam [Ativan], midazolam [Versed], magnesium sulfate, diazepam gel [Diastat], phenobarbital [Luminal], phenytoin [Dilantin]. (pages 190–208)

5-6 List the medications that a patient with a history of migraines may be taking. (pages 204–207)

Suspected Stroke

A **stroke** is a disruption of blood flow or bleeding into the brain that causes the patient to have potentially permanent brain cell death and long-term physical disabilities (**Figure 5-1**). The "mantra" for stroke is quickly becoming, "FAST." FAST is an acronym used to train the public as well as health care providers:

Face—Be sure to ask the patient to smile. Is there facial droop?

Arms—Be sure to ask the patient to raise both arms. Does one arm drift downward or outward? This is also known as pronator drift.

Speech—Be sure to ask the patient to repeat a simple sentence. Are the words slurred?

Time—If the answer to any of the above questions is yes, time is essential because brain cells may be dying. It is likely the patient may be experiencing a stroke.

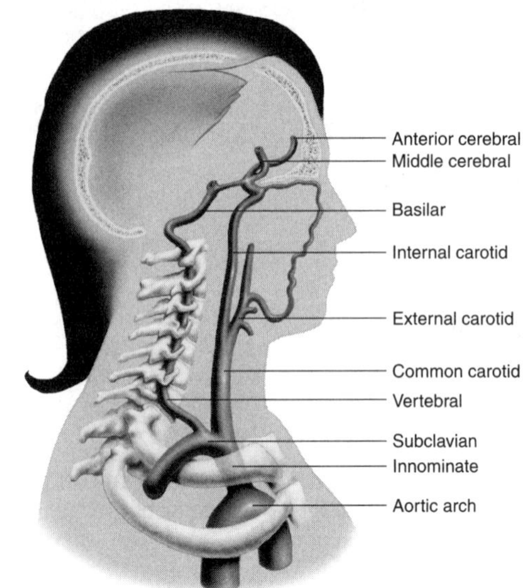

Figure 5-1 Blood supply to the brain.

Health care providers are taught to specifically include the Cincinnati Prehospital Stroke Scale in their assessment of the patient with a neurologic complaint. The research has shown that if a patient has assessment criteria that are abnormal on the Cincinnati Prehospital Stroke Scale, the probability of a stroke is approximately 72% (**Table 5-1**).

The most definitive treatment of a stroke, in its acute phase, involves the use of fibrinolytics which are often only administered in hospitals with stroke programs or a stroke center. Since stroke can involve clots or blockages of the cerebral arteries (ischemic stroke or embolic stroke) as well as intracranial hemorrhage into the brain itself (hemorrhagic stroke), these drugs cannot be administered until a determination has been made as to which type of stroke has occurred. To make the diagnosis, a CT scan or MRI scan is needed. Without first determining the type of stroke before administering clot buster medications, the patient is at risk of having an increased volume of bleeding into the brain if a hemorrhagic stroke has occurred. This accentuates the need for prompt assessment and transport so rapid and accurate diagnosis of the type of stroke can be made prior to initiation of therapy.

The best medicine for a stroke is prevention. The conditions that are treatable risk factors linked to a stroke include: hypertension, cigarette smoking, heart disease, diabetes, and a previous **transient ischemic attack (TIA)**. A TIA usually has all the signs and symptoms of a stroke but they disappear within the first 12 hours or so. It is a warning sign that a major stroke is likely to occur within the next year if the causes leading to the stroke or TIA are not dealt with by the patient and his or her physician. Specific interventions to prevent a stroke include the following:

High blood pressure. *Treat it.* Eat a balanced diet, maintain a healthy weight, and exercise to reduce blood pressure. A wide variety of medicines are available to treat hypertension and should be taken as directed.

Table 5-1 Cincinnati Prehospital Stroke Scale

Assessment	Normal	Abnormal
Facial Droop. Ask the patient to smile and show the teeth.	Both sides of the face move equally well.	One side of the face does not move as well as the other.
Arm Drift. Ask the patient to close the eyes and hold the arms out with palms up for 10 seconds.	Both arms move the same, or both arms do not move.	One arm does not move, or one arm drifts down compared with the other.
Abnormal Speech. Ask the patient to say, "The sky is blue in Cincinnati" or "You can't teach an old dog new tricks."	The patient uses the correct words with no slurring.	The patient slurs words, uses inappropriate words, or is unable to speak.

Interpretation: If any assessment criterion is abnormal, the probability of a stroke is 72%.

Cigarette smoking. *Quit.* Medical help is available to help quit. Some patients may be using a "patch" to help wean them off their nicotine addiction.

Heart disease. *Manage it.* Your doctor can treat your heart disease and may prescribe medication to help prevent the formation of clots or make the red blood cells less "sticky" (ie, aspirin). If you are older than 50 years of age, researchers from the National Institute of Neurological Disorders and Stroke (NINDS) believe you and your doctor should make a decision about aspirin therapy.

Diabetes. *Control it.* Treatment can delay complications that increase the risk of stroke.

Transient ischemic attacks (TIAs). *Seek help.* TIAs are small strokes that last only for a few minutes or hours. They should never be ignored and your physician may choose to treat them with medications, such as antihypertensives, or surgical procedures.

Case Study 1 Possible Stroke

Part 1

Your unit has been dispatched to meet an incoming airplane at the regional airport. The information you have received is a bit vague but an incoming flight has a middle-aged man who has been sick most of the flight. Your ambulance is met at the Crash Fire Rescue building and you and your partner receive an escort onto the landing field where most of the other passengers have already been removed from the plane.

You are met by a flight attendant and she states there is a physician on the flight who is attending to the patient. As you approach the patient, who is seated in the rear of the plane, the physician introduces himself and states emergency medicine is not his specialty. He is a plastic surgeon and states most of his patient care involves reconstructive surgery! He reports that the patient has slurred speech and right-sided weakness that came on suddenly about 30 minutes ago. His pulse was regular and blood pressure was high. Your partner begins a report and conducts an initial assessment of the patient (see **Table 1**).

During the initial assessment the physician reports that the patient's name is Mr. Joe Taylor and he developed slurred speech and right-sided weakness shortly after the onset of nausea and confusion, which occurred at 2:00 p.m. It is now 2:40 p.m. according to your watch so you jot down the time symptoms developed.

Table 1 Initial Assessment

Initial Assessment	Recording Time: 1 Minute
General Impression/ Appearance	Weak and tired looking male in his 50s
Mental Status	"V" verbally responsive (knows his name but confused as to place and day)
Airway	Open but drooling
Breathing	Regular
Circulation	Fast and irregular
Priority/Plan	High due to poor general impression and altered mental status

You question Mr. Taylor's son who is traveling with him. They are returning from a weekend of basketball games.

Question 1: Why is it so important to establish the time when the patient began to experience symptoms?

Question 2: As a part of your assessment of this patient, what physical examination should be conducted?

Case Study 1 Continued

Part 2

Clearly Mr. Taylor is a patient who is a responsive medical patient so you begin your focused history and physical examination (see **Table 2**). To elaborate on the chief complaint of altered mental status and right-sided weakness you use the acronym OPQRST. Many of the questions are quickly answered by the physician who has been attending to the patient. He also states that Mr. Taylor is not a diabetic and has never experienced these symptoms previously. Mr. Taylor does have a history of hypertension and takes medications for it.

Mr. Taylor is able to understand your line of questioning but is slow to respond with answers. You decide in the interest of time to get him packaged and moving.

Table 2 Focused History and Physical Examination

Baseline Vital Signs	Recording Time: 5 Minutes
Skin CTC (color, temperature, condition)	Pale, warm, and clammy
Pulse	Radial pulse of 130 beats/min, strong and irregular
Blood Pressure	168/100 mm Hg
Respirations	24 breaths/min and regular

The son is very helpful and knows all about his dad's medical history. It seems his father had an incident about 3 months ago which the family physician called a transient ischemic attack (TIA).

Question 3: What is the significance of a history of a TIA?

Question 4: What is the significance of asking if the patient has a history of diabetes and should you still check his blood glucose?

Part 3

As you obtain a SAMPLE history your partner obtains a set of baseline vital signs (see **Table 3**). Next you do your physical examination which will consist of a mini-neurologic examination that includes the reassessment of AVPU, the Cincinnati Prehospital Stroke Scale, and determining strength and distal pulses, motor function, and sensory function (PMS) in all four extremities. You recall from your training that the research has shown that if a patient has assessment criteria that are abnormal on the Cincinnati Prehospital Stroke Scale, the probability of a stroke is approximately 72%. It is clear that the patient has slurred speech and an obvious weakness in his right side.

As you transfer him from the stair chair to your stretcher he vomits into a convenience bag. En route to the ED you will provide supplemental oxygen, check his glucose level, get a 12-lead ECG, and start an IV line. At this point medications would generally not be indicated.

Table 3 SAMPLE History

SAMPLE History	Comments
Signs/symptoms	Right-sided weakness, nausea, vomiting, slurred speech
Allergies	Codeine
Medications	Ramipril [Altace] an ACE inhibitor taken for hypertension, verapamil hydrochloride [Calan, Isoptin] a calcium channel blocker that lowers the blood pressure by regulating the heart's strength and rate
Pertinent past medical history	Hypertension, possible TIA, atrial fibrillation
Last oral intake	Orange juice and peanuts an hour ago
Events leading up to the incident	Stress and excitement, was seated on airplane for hours

Case Study I Continued

Treatment Plan

1. Monitor and manage the ABCs.
2. Administer supplemental oxygen therapy.
3. If possible, work to establish the time the patient was last seen normal.
4. Obtain a complete set of baseline vital signs and assess the 12-lead ECG.
5. Start an IV for a keep vein open line of normal saline.
6. The blood glucose should be checked and only treated with $D_{50}W$ if it is below 70 mg/dL.
7. Run through the stroke fibrinolytic checklist to gather information that the ED physician will need before fibrinolytics can be considered (see Table 5-2 on page 197).
8. Transport as soon as possible and give the ED early warning of Mr. Taylor's condition. Preference would be to transfer this patient to a stroke center.
9. Consider treating the nausea and vomiting with promethazine hydrochloride [Phenergan] or ondansetron hydrochloride [Zofran].
10. Medical control may also consider judicious administration of metoprolol tartrate [Lopressor], or nitroglycerin paste.

In this case the medications in the prehospital setting will be: oxygen, promethazine hydrochloride [Phenergan] although some regions may chose to use ondansetron hydrochloride [Zofran], metoprolol tartrate [Lopressor], or nitroglycerin paste, and glucose only if the patient has a documented low blood glucose. Each of these medications has already been discussed in other parts of this book.

You will be running through the fibrinolytic checklist for stroke en route to the ED, and of course you will call in to alert the ED staff of his current condition.

Question 5: What is the significance of the atrial fibrillation?

Question 6: Why is the stroke fibrinolytic checklist needed? Don't all strokes get "clot busters"?

Part 4

The patient's condition remains the same en route to the ED. As you reassess every 5 minutes or so, you do note he is attempting to speak less (see **Table 4**).

You call into the ED with a report of the patient's status and your estimated time of arrival which should be within an hour of the onset of the symptoms. This is important to note as conventional stroke centers have a 3-hour window for the administration of IV fibrinolytics (3-hour window for IV **tissue plasminogen activator (tPA)** (clot buster) in conventional stroke centers; however, the window has been extended to 6 hours in "interventional" centers that use intra-arterial tissue plasminogen activator tPA administration, cerebral angioplasty, or Merci technology). Of course there is still a lot to do in the ED to first determine the type of stroke and if the patient is truly a candidate for thrombolysis.

Question 7: What is an embolic or ischemic stroke?

Question 8: What is the advantage of taking this patient directly to a stroke center?

Table 4 Reassessment and Ongoing Assessment of the Patient

Serial Vital Signs and Relevant Data	Recording Time: 10 Minutes
Skin CTC	Pale, warm, and wet
Pulse	132 beats/min and irregular
Blood Pressure	170/106 mm Hg
Respirations	22 breaths/min and regular
Mental Status	"V" verbal (oriented to name but not to place and day)
ECG	Atrial fibrillation (by definition, AF is all ectopy)
SpO_2	96% on supplemental oxygen by nonrebreathing mask
Lung Sounds	Clear bilaterally
Other (ie, glucose, core body temperature)	Glucose is 100 mg/dL, body temperature is within normal range

Case Study I Continued

Part 5

Experts say that a TIA should not be underplayed and often it is a forerunner of a future stroke. In Mr. Taylor's situation, that is what seems to have occurred and he is experiencing the classic symptoms of a stroke. Fortunately, it was toward the end of his 3-hour flight and his symptoms were recognized right away.

When there is an in-flight medical emergency, the pilot, on advisement of those attending to the patient as well as the medical control, can either 1) return to the originating airport, 2) seek a site for an emergency landing (ie, an unplanned airfield en route), or 3) request air traffic control to clear a path to the final destination airfield. The third choice was the best in this situation and it often can cut 30 minutes of circling in the pattern prior to actually landing the airplane. The time saved helped Mr. Taylor considerably because on arrival at the stroke center he was within the 180-minute window from onset of symptoms to confirmation of ischemic stroke (based on a CT scan). Mr. Taylor was given fibrinolytics and the staff was happy to see the 12-lead ECG, blood glucose, and checklist were completed on arrival at the ED. After a weeklong hospitalization, Mr. Taylor is now in good spirits and receiving outpatient physical therapy and looking forward to a complete recovery.

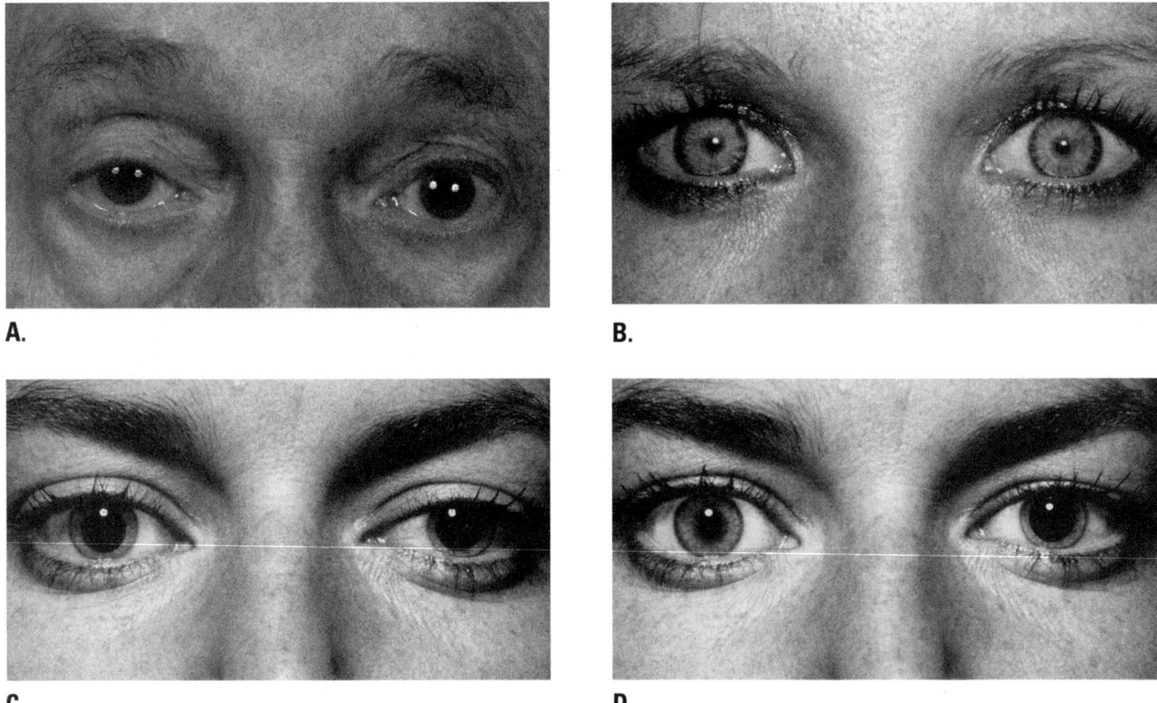

Figure 5-2 Pupil responses. A. Normal. B. Constricted (pinpoint). C. Dilated. D. Unequal.

The symptoms of a stroke include a sudden numbness or weakness of the face, arm, or leg. Usually hemiparesis or hemiplegia (on one side of the body) is present. The patient frequently suffers from confusion, or has trouble speaking. However, it is unusual to see loss of consciousness with acute ischemic stroke. The patient may have difficulty understanding your speech, and may suddenly have difficulty seeing in one or both eyes. It is also important to watch for changes in the pupils (**Figure 5-2**▲). He or she may have trouble walking, experience dizziness, or exhibit loss of balance or coordination. Patients may describe a severe headache with no known cause.

We often think of stroke as a condition that happens to the elderly. The truth is, a stroke can occur at any age. Risk factors for stroke in children include premature birth, trauma during birth, congenital heart disease, sickle cell anemia, coagulation disorders, and arteriovenous disorders. Learn to recognize when a younger person is having signs and symptoms of a stroke.

ACE Inhibitors

Angiotensin converting enzyme (ACE) inhibitors are one of three primary drug classifications used to treat hypertension. Beta-blockers and thiazide diuretics are the other two. ACE inhibitors work by blocking the conversion of angiotensin I to angiotensin II, a potent vasoconstrictor that raises blood pressure. ACE inhibitors work to reduce or control hypertension and may be prescribed with diuretics.

Stroke Management

The two primary causes of stroke are blood clots (approximately 80%) and bleeding in the brain (approximately 20%). The accepted treatments for stroke include medications, surgery, hospital care, and rehabilitation (**Figure 5-3 ▸**). The treatment plan a patient receives will depend on several factors including: the time of onset of symptoms, the type of stroke they are having, age, and health status.

Preventing the stroke, as stated earlier, is the ideal treatment. When one or both carotid arteries in the neck become partially blocked with plaque, this can produce a TIA or mini stroke. TIA is the warning sign of an imminent stroke; however, not every stroke patient has a TIA prodrome. Surgery called endarterectomy might be used to remove the accumulated plaque, helping to reduce the risk of stroke. Cerebral angioplasty is another procedure in which balloons, stents, and coils are used to treat some types of problems with blood vessels in the brain.

When a patient with stroke symptoms is taken to the appropriate facility within the 180 minutes of onset, he or she may be a candidate for reperfusion therapy, also called fibrinolytic therapy or clot buster therapy. The clot-dissolving drug tissue plasminogen activator (tPA) is used to treat thromboembolic stroke. tPA dissolves the clot, restores blood flow to the brain, and has been shown to be effective if given promptly to a select group of patients. tPA carries a risk of fatal bleeding in the brain; therefore, the patient must be screened first using an exclusion criteria checklist that includes noncontrasted CT scanning (**Table 5-2 ▸**).

When a stroke patient is not a candidate for fibrinolytic therapy or surgery, less invasive treatment is the only alternative and includes hospital care followed by rehabilitation. The patient is often left with one or more physical deficits. This is often the case despite the use of IV tPA use as well.

Blood Clots and Travel

People with a history of stroke, TIA, and heart disease are also at risk for developing blood clots in their legs or deep venous thrombosis (DVT). The danger with DVT is that the clot can break away into circulation and become lodged in the lung causing a pulmonary embolism. DVT can also affect healthy people, especially during long periods of sitting associated with travel such as long drives and long flights. This condition has been named "economy class syndrome" or "coach class syndrome" because of the cramped seating and limited leg room for passengers in economy class. This condition can also affect passengers in first or business class because there are other factors in addition to limited mobility in cramped spaces that contribute to developing DVT during long flights. Dehydration, low humidity, and low cabin pressure are constant throughout the plane and appear to be significant contributing factors to the thickening of blood, a condition called "relative polycythemia." The risk for developing DVT during long flights can be reduced by staying well hydrated, standing and moving every hour, and by skipping the drinks that dehydrate (ie, coffee, tea, alcohol) before and during the flight.

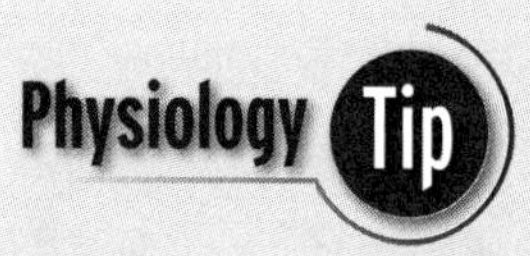

tPA carries a risk of fatal bleeding in the brain; therefore, the patient must be screened first using an exclusion criteria checklist that includes noncontrasted CT scanning.

Seizures

Causes of seizures are numerous and include those such as hypoxia, hypoglycemia, or a rapid change in body temperature. Other causes include structural irregularities or infectious processes within the brain such as: head trauma, tumors, strokes, eclampsia, or brain abscess. The most common cause of seizures is idiopathic epilepsy which is a chronic seizure disorder. The less common or more infrequent causes (ie, tumors or abscess) can signal a potentially fatal disorder that cannot be diagnosed in the prehospital setting. From a management perspective, all seizures are treated in a similar manner (ie, ensuring adequacy of ABCs and protecting the patient from injury). When a patient has **status epilepticus** (two or more back-to-back seizures without the return of consciousness in between episodes or a seizure that lasts for longer than 3 to 5 minutes), pharmacological interventions are appropriate and discussed later in this chapter. Seizure can occur in patients of all ages (**Table 5-3 ▸**).

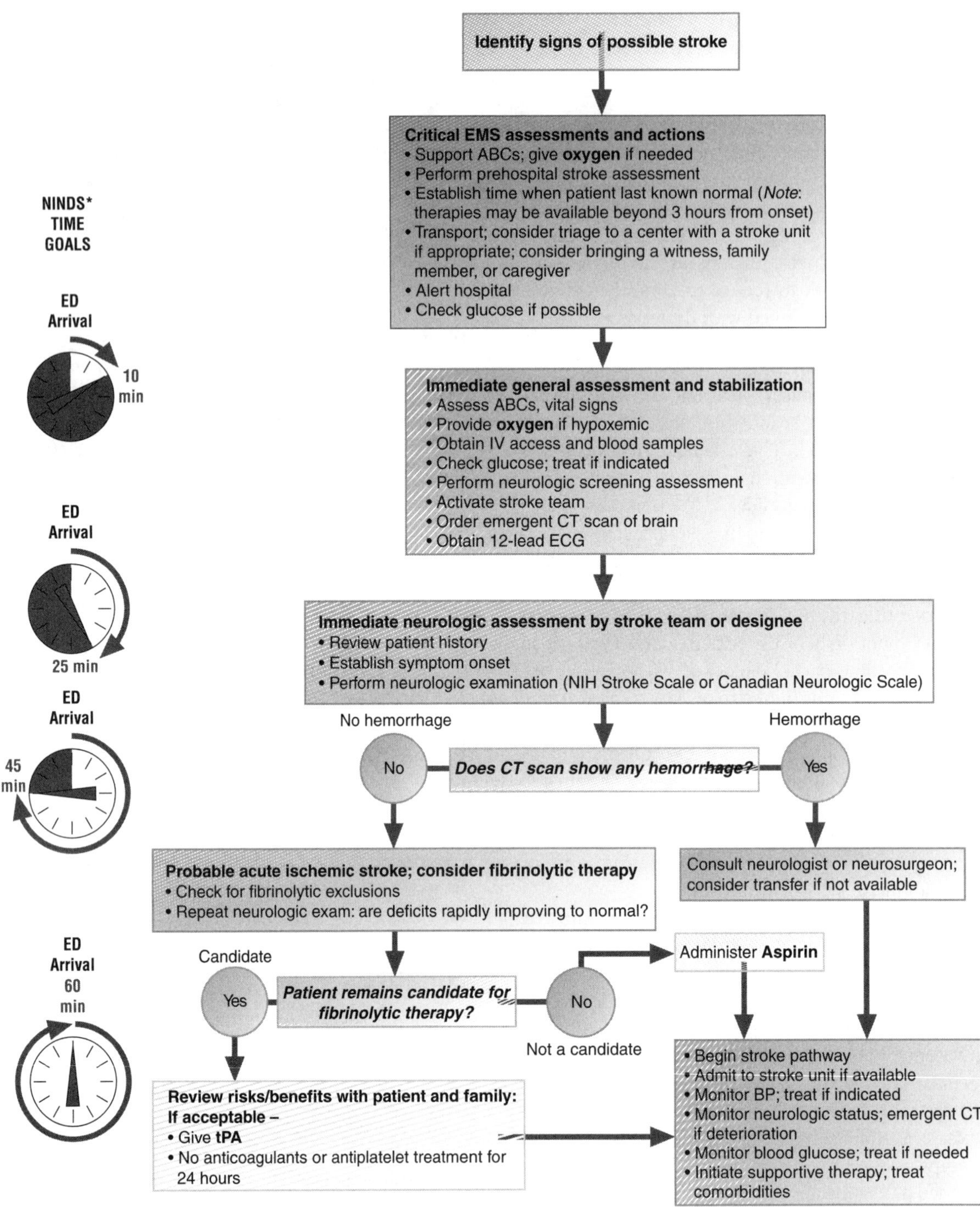

Figure 5-3 Algorithm for management of patients with suspected stroke.

Table 5-2 American Heart Association Fibrinolytic Checklist for Stroke

Use of tissue-type plasminogen activator (tPA) in a patient with acute ischemic stroke. All boxes must be checked before tPA can be given.

Note: The following checklist includes FDA-approved indications and contraindications for tPA administration for acute ischemic stroke. A physician with expertise in acute stroke care may modify this list.

Inclusion Criteria (*all Yes boxes in the section must be checked*)

Yes

- ❑ Age 18 years or older?
- ❑ Clinical diagnosis of ischemic stroke with a measurable neurologic deficit?
- ❑ Time of symptom onset (when patient was last seen normal) well established as < 180 minutes (3 hours) before treatment would begin?

Exclusion Criteria (*all No boxes in "Contraindications" section must be checked*)

Contraindications

No

- ❑ Evidence of intracranial hemorrhage on pretreatment noncontrast head CT?
- ❑ Clinical presentation suggestive of subarachnoid hemorrhage even with normal CT?
- ❑ CT shows multilobar infarction (hypodensity greater than one third cerebral hemisphere)?
- ❑ History of intracranial hemorrhage?
- ❑ Uncontrolled hypertension: At the time treatment should begin, systolic pressure remains > 185 mm Hg or diastolic pressure remains > 110 mm Hg despite repeated measurements?
- ❑ Known arteriovenous malformation, neoplasm, or aneurysm?
- ❑ Witnessed seizure at stroke onset?
- ❑ Active internal bleeding or acute trauma (fracture)?
- ❑ Active bleeding diathesis, including but not limited to
  - Platelet count < 100,000/mm^3
  - Heparin received within 48 hours, resulting in an activated partial thromboplastin time (aPTT) that is greater than upper limit of normal for laboratory?
  - Current use of anticoagulant (eg, warfarin sodium) that has produced an elevated international normalized ratio (INR) > 1.7 or prothrombin time (PT) > 15 seconds.*
- ❑ Within 3 months of intracranial or intraspinal surgery, serious head trauma, or previous stroke?
- ❑ Arterial pressure at a noncompressible site within past 7 days?

Relative Contraindications/Precautions

Recent experience suggests that under some circumstances—with careful consideration and weighing of risk-benefit ratio—patients may receive fibrinolytic therapy despite one or more relative contraindications. Consider the pros and cons of tPA administration carefully if any of these relative contraindications is present.

- *Only minor* or *rapidly* improving stroke symptoms (clearing spontaneously)
- Within 14 days of major surgery or serious trauma
- Recent gastrointestinal or urinary tract hemorrhage (within previous 21 days)
- Recent acute myocardial infarction (within previous 3 months)
- Postmyocardial infarction pericarditis
- Abnormal blood glucose level (< 50 or > 400 mg/dL [< 2.8 or > 22.2 mmol/L])

*In patients without recent use of oral anticoagulants or heparin, treatment with tPA can be initiated before availability of the coagulation study results but should be discontinued if the INR > 1.7 or the partial thromboplastin time is elevated by local laboratory standards.

Source: Reproduced with permission, 2005 *American Heart Association Guidelines for Cardiopulmonary Resuscitation and Emergency Cardiovascular Care.* © 2005, American Heart Association.

Table 5-3 Seizure by Age Group

Age Group	Causes of Seizures
Infant	Childbirth trauma, infection, electrolyte abnormalities, congenital defects, genetic disorders, stroke
Toddler	Trauma, infection, fever, stroke
Preschool/School Age	Trauma, fever, infection, epilepsy, stroke
Adolescent	Trauma, drug or alcohol, epilepsy, hemorrhagic stroke
Young adult	Trauma, acute intoxication or withdrawal, brain tumor, hemorrhagic stroke
Older adult	Stroke, brain tumor, intracerebral hemorrhage, alcoholism, metabolic disorders, embolic stroke

Case Study II Status Epilepticus

Part 1

Your unit has been dispatched to a local motel for a patient who is having a seizure. On arrival, the manager leads you and your partner to a room in the back of the second floor. He states that the woman's boyfriend called the front desk and said his girlfriend, Kim, was watching TV when she suddenly began convulsing. The scene appears safe at this time. You note as you enter that the patient is still seizing and with your response time this would be at least 10 minutes of seizure activity. You perform an initial assessment of Kim (see **Table 1**).

Table 1 Initial Assessment

Initial Assessment	Recording Time: 1 Minute
General Impression/ Appearance	25-year-old female on the couch seizing (general motor type)
Mental Status	"P" posturing with deep pain response
Airway	Open but in need of suctioning due to secretions "foaming" at the mouth
Breathing	Rapid and full
Circulation	The radial pulse feels rapid (tachycardiac)
Priority/Plan	High priority, transport as soon as possible due to potential "status epilepticus"

Kim is not responsive due to active seizing activity. There appears to be no obvious trauma. As your partner gets the baseline vital signs you move from the initial assessment to a focused history and physical examination of an unresponsive medical patient. This will involve a rapid medical assessment and ALS management.

Question 1: What is the significance of the long seizure?

Question 2: What type of seizure is a life-threat and must be taken very seriously?

Part 2

According to the boyfriend, Kim has been feeling ill all day and may have not taken her medications in the past few days since they have been traveling this week. Your focused history and physical examination reveals additional information (see **Table 2**).

Kim's seizure activity is almost over, but she is not waking up. A rapid medical assessment does not produce any significant findings from examining the major body cavities (head, neck, chest, abdomen, pelvis, back, buttocks, and extremities). She does have a minor cut to her tongue which is bleeding.

Table 2 Focused History and Physical Examination

Baseline Vital Signs	Recording Time: 3 Minutes
Skin CTC (color, temperature, condition)	Pale, warm, and clammy
Pulse	110 beats/min and regular
Blood Pressure	140/78 mm Hg
Respirations	24 breaths/min and gurgling (suctioning improves them)

With a chief complaint of a seizure, the OPQRST questions are asked of the boyfriend (see **Table 3**).

Question 3: What are some of the causes of a seizure?

Question 4: Given that this patient has known epilepsy and is prescribed a daily dose of an anticonvulsant, what is the most likely cause of today's seizure activity?

Table 3 OPQRST Questions

Chief Complaint	Lengthy seizure
Onset	Suddenly while watching TV
Provocation	None known aside from medication noncompliance
Quality	Full body movements "generalized"
Region/radiation/ referral	None
Severity	Boyfriend says this is much longer than previous ones
Time	Approximately 15 minutes so far

Case Study II Continued

Part 3

You will need to contact medical control for a drug order so you fill in the SAMPLE history with the aid of Kim's boyfriend (see **Table 4**). Due to her age and sex you inquire if Kim is pregnant and the boyfriend says no. You know it is important to ask if this woman is pregnant. Had she been in her third trimester of pregnancy (> 20 weeks) or up to 2 weeks postpartum and was seizing, you would consult with medical control to consider the administration of magnesium sulfate 4 g IV (mixed in 50 mL of fluid and given over 5 to 10 minutes) [see chapter 11]. Meanwhile, your partner has suctioned the patient, started supplemental oxygen with a nonrebreathing mask at 12–15 L/min, and is now starting an IV.

Table 4 SAMPLE History

SAMPLE History	Comments
Signs/symptoms	Nausea and vomited this afternoon
Allergies	Penicillin and sulfur drugs
Medications	Phenytoin [Dilantin], and divalproex sodium [Depakote] for manic episodes of bipolar disorder
Pertinent past medical history	Epileptic who had last seizure about 2 months ago. History of depression.
Last oral intake	Water and juice 45 minutes ago, tried soup but vomited it up
Events leading up to the incident	Not feeling well all day, very stressful week traveling

Treatment Plan

1. This patient needs a fast track approach involving management of the ABCs including suctioning and possibly insertion of a nasopharyngeal airway and supplemental oxygen therapy. It is important to assess the need for ventilation with a bag-mask device or if a nonrebreathing mask will be adequate at this point.
2. After obtaining a complete set of baseline vital signs, start an IV for a keep vein open line of normal saline.
3. If the patient's blood glucose is less than 80 mg/dL, administer dextrose 50% 25 g (50 mL) slowly into an IV. If no IV site is available, glucagon 1 unit can be administered IM.
4. Next, administer a benzodiazepine, such as diazepam [Valium] 5 mg IV or 5 mg intranasal with a mucosal atomization device as shown in Chapter 1, or 10 mg per rectum (see **Table 5**). Other options include, lorazepam [Ativan] 2 mg IV or 2 mg IM if no IV site is established, or midazolam [Versed] 2 mg IV or 2 mg intranasal with a mucosal atomization device (see **Table 6** and **Table 7**).
5. Monitor the patient closely for respiratory depression.
6. Repeat serial vital signs every 5 minutes on this critical patient.
7. Transport as soon as possible and contact medical control for a single repeat dose of the specific benzodiazepine you selected for this patient.

For your management of the seizing patient you will need to select one of the following three benzodiazepines.

Table 5 Diazepam

Do you know?	Comments
Right drug? Generic name: [**Diazepam**] Trade name: [Valium]	This is a benzodiazepine, antianxiety drug. It is used for relief of anxiety, an adjunct therapy for convulsive disorders, relief of skeletal muscle spasms, and relief of symptomatic acute alcohol withdrawal. It is a controlled substance. In many areas its use requires medical control's authorization.
Right patient?	Yes. The most frequently used drug for status epilepticus in the prehospital setting. It is given in acute anxiety states, acute alcohol withdrawal (delirium tremens), muscle relaxant, and agitation. It can also be given for sedation for medical procedures (ie, fracture reduction or cardioversion).
Right dose?	5–10 mg IV or 5 mg intranasal or 10 mg per rectum (rectal gel)
Right route?	IV is best; IO and rectal are also options
Right time?	As soon as possible after baseline vital signs are taken and if the patient is still seizing
Right documentation?	Clearly document any changes in seizure activity.

continues

Case Study II Continued

Table 5 **Diazepam (*Continued*)**

Do you know?	Comments
Expected action	To stop the seizure activity and sedate the patient. It potentiates effects of inhibitory neurotransmitters. It raises seizure threshold and induces amnesia and sedation.
Side effects	Respiratory depression, hypotension, drowsiness, ataxia, reflex tachycardia, nausea, confusion, thrombosis, and phlebitis.
Contraindications	Hypersensitivity, glaucoma, coma, shock, substance abuse, head injury.
Precautions	Can cause respiratory depression. Watch for it and if needed, be prepared to assist ventilations.
Pharmacokinetics	Onset 5 minutes through IV, more rapid per rectal, 30–60 minutes IM so not a preferred route; peak is 0.5–2 hrs IM, more rapid PR, 15 minutes IV; duration 3 hours; metabolized in the liver and excreted through urine.

Table 6 **Lorazepam**

Do you know?	Comments
Right drug? Generic name: [**Lorazepam**] Trade name: [Ativan]	A benzodiazepine, sedative anticonvulsant. It is used for relief of anxiety and for status epilepticus. Note that it expires in 6 weeks if not refrigerated.
Right patient?	Yes. Used for the initial control of status epilepticus or severe recurrent seizures, severe anxiety, or sedation.
Right dose?	2–4 mg slow IV or IO diluted with equal volume of sterile water or sterile saline. Can give 2 mg/min IM (do not dilute). May repeat in 15–20 minutes to a maximum dose of 8 mg. For sedation 0.05 mg/kg up to 4 mg IM. (Some physicians prefer a lower dose such as 1 to 2 mg IV every 5 minutes until seizure terminates or apnea ensues).
Right route?	IV is best; IM and IO are also options.
Right time?	As soon as possible after baseline vital signs if the patient is still seizing.
Right documentation?	Clearly document any changes in seizure activity on your prehospital care report.
Expected action	To stop the seizure activity and sedate the patient.
Side effects	Respiratory depression, apnea, drowsiness, sedation, ataxia, psychomotor impairment, confusion, restlessness, delirium, hypotension, and bradycardia.
Contraindications	Acute narrow-angle glaucoma, coma, shock, or suspected drug abuse.
Precautions	May precipitate CNS depression if patient is already taking CNS depressant medications.
Pharmacokinetics	Absorbed and eliminated faster than other benzodiazepines. Peak 1–1.5 hrs IM; more rapid IV; metabolized in the liver and excreted through urine.

Table 7 **Midazolam**

Do you know?	Comments
Right drug? Generic name: [**Midazolam**] Trade name: [Versed]	A short-acting benzodiazepine CNS depressant. It is used for relief of anxiety, sedation, and as an adjunct to induction of general anesthesia.
Right patient?	Yes. It has anxiolytic and sedative properties similar to other benzodiazepines, memory impairment.
Right dose?	2.0 to 2.5 mg slow IV over 2–3 minutes or 2.0 to 2.5 mg intranasal (may repeat to a max of 0.1 mg/kg).
Right route?	IV is best; IM and IO are also options.
Right time?	As soon as possible after baseline vital signs if the patient is still seizing.

continues

Case Study II Continued

Table 7 **Midazolam (*Continued*)**

Do you know?	Comments
Right documentation?	Clearly document any changes in seizure activity on your prehospital care report.
Expected action	To stop the seizure activity and sedate the patient. It is an anxiolytic (drug that reduces anxiety) given prior to endotracheal or nasotracheal intubation. It is also administered for conscious sedation.
Side effects	Can cause hiccough, cough, over-sedation, nausea, vomiting, injection site pain, headache, blurred vision, hypotension, respiratory depression, and arrest.
Contraindications	Glaucoma, shock, coma, alcohol intoxication, overdose, depressed vital signs, concomitant use with other CNS depressants, barbiturates, alcohol, narcotics.
Precautions	Can cause respiratory depression so watch for it and if needed be prepared to assist ventilations. Should not be used in patients who have taken a CNS depressant or are hypotensive.
Pharmacokinetics	Onset 1–3 minutes IV and dose dependant, peak effect is variable. Onset 15 minutes IM; peak effect is 45 minutes. Duration 2–6 hours; metabolized in the liver and excreted through urine.

Question 5: Why is oxygen helpful for this patient?

Question 6: Why is a benzodiazepine administered to this patient?

Part 4

After administering oxygen and diazepam [Valium], you reassess the patient (see **Table 8**).

Question 7: Why was it important to check this patient's blood glucose?

Question 8: What other medications might be used to break a seizure in the emergency department?

Table 8 **Reassessment and Ongoing Assessment of the Patient**

Serial Vital Signs and Relevant Data	Recording Time: 10 Minutes
Skin CTC	Pale, warm, and clammy
Pulse	110 beats/min
Blood Pressure	140/70 mm Hg
Respirations	24 breaths/min, regular with no secretions
Mental Status	"P" patient is beginning to withdraw from pain source
ECG	Sinus tachycardia with no ectopy
SpO_2	96% on supplemental oxygen
Lung Sounds	Clear bilaterally
Other (ie, glucose, core temperature)	Glucose is 98 mg/dL and body temperature is normal

Part 5

Due to your rapid assessment and management of this patient's condition as status epilepticus, you have been able to terminate the seizing activity. This was done by quickly managing the life-threats during your initial assessment and quickly moving on the focused history and physical examination of this nonresponsive medical patient. By continuing to manage the ABCs, ruling out hypoglycemia, obtaining IV access, and administering the benzodiazepines selected (diazepam [Valium]), the patient is now resting quietly upon arrival at the ED.

The ED physician states, "Well, it looks like you folks did all of the work and helped this patient save some brain cells. Now it's up to us to figure out exactly why this happened today, although the evidence sure does point to medication noncompliance."

Table 5-4 Field Presentation of Seizure Types

Classification of Partial (Focal) Seizures	Description
Simple Partial Seizure	Tonic/clonic activity localized to one part of the body that may spread and progress to a generalized tonic/clonic seizure. Patients may not lose consciousness nor have an aura. Also called a focal motor or "Jacksonian March" seizure.
Complex Partial Seizure	Often preceded by an aura, manifests as changes in mood and abrupt bouts of rage lasting 1 to 2 minutes. There is no postictal phase. Also called a temporal lobe or psychomotor seizure.
Classification of Generalized Seizures	**Description**
Petit mal (Absence) Seizure	Described as a staring episode during which the patient's activity ceases, there is loss of motor control, and the eyes may blink and lips smack. Most common in children from ages 4 to 12 years old, the spell lasts less than 15 seconds and then there is a return to alert mental status.
Grand mal (Tonic/clonic) Seizure	Generalized full body muscle contraction (tonic phase) alternating with jerking movements (clonic phase). Often preceded by an aura, warning the patient of an impending seizure. Lasts several minutes and is typically followed by a postictal phase involving confusion, agitation, or sleepiness.

Seizures are classified into generalized and partial (focal) seizures (**Table 5-4▲**). The characteristics of a generalized seizure depend on the type of seizure activity the patient exhibits. Typically generalized seizures are further broken down into petit mal (absence) seizure and the grand mal (tonic/clonic) seizure.

Partial or focal seizures are also further broken down into simple partial seizures and complex partial seizures.

Because you are not there when most seizure activity occurs, it is important to question the witnesses about the type of activity they saw and how long it lasted. This will help you to classify the type of seizure. The presence of an aura or warning sensation that a seizure is going to occur is important to question the patient about. Patients who have experienced an aura describe it as a strange taste, smell, visual perception, or abnormal sensation immediately prior to the seizure. The patient may lose control of his or her bladder or bowels during a seizure so do not be surprised if they are very embarrassed when coming to after the seizure. They may also complain of diffuse muscle soreness or fatigue following the seizure, as well as have some degree of trauma to the tongue. Almost all seizures are followed by a postictal phase, the awareness of which is very useful for differentiating seizure from syncope and associated contractions of a muscle or a group of muscles. A very common cause of seizure activity is noncompliance with the prescribed antiseizure medication regimes. Often patients allow their blood level of anticonvulsant medication to drop considerably by missing doses. This is all-important information for you to document on the patient care report for the other members of the health care team.

One type of seizure that has been prioritized as a high priority "true emergency" is the condition called status epilepticus. Status epilepticus is a series of two or more back-to-back seizures without a lucid interval or a prolonged seizure lasting more than 10 minutes. Most EMS agencies define a prolonged seizure as one where a call for a seizing patient is received and the EMS unit arrives on the scene to find that the patient is still actively seizing. Patients who seize for

A patient's baseline level of consciousness (LOC) is not always what you would consider to be normal. Talk to friends and bystanders to determine the baseline LOC of the patient.

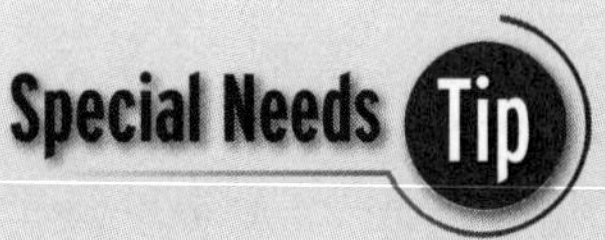

Geriatric patients generally have more than one doctor, medication, and condition.

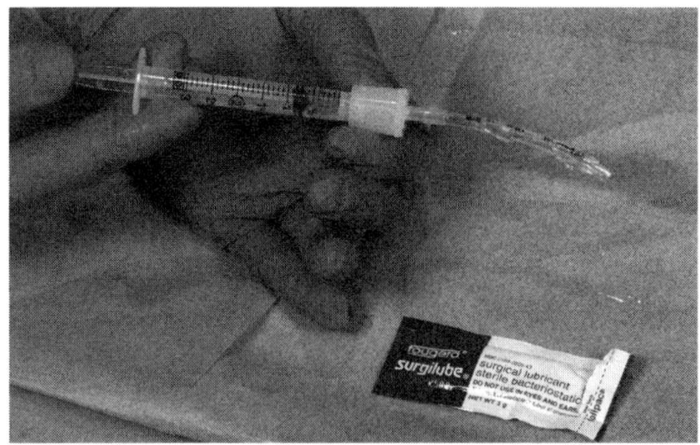

Figure 5-4 Syringe attached to an endotracheal tube.

prolonged periods of time usually do not have a tonic/clonic seizure for that entire time period. Rather, they may experience a period of time with no body movement and have a fixed gaze but not regain consciousness. The potential damage that status epilepticus can cause is damage to the brain cells. This patient needs to be treated right away, ensuring the ABCs are properly managed and that a benzodiazepine is administered to stop the seizure activity.

In pediatric patients who are seizing, diazepam gel [Diastat] can be used for rectal administration (0.5 mg/kg). One way to administer this medication is to use a tiny ET tube attached to the syringe and lubricate with KY jelly (**Figure 5-4▲**). This is also an "option" in the adult patient when an IV or IO site cannot be rapidly obtained. Another option would be to use the syringe without the needle.

Febrile Seizures

Patients who have a fever have been known to seize. This is most common in younger children and infants and can be very scary for the new parent to see. The febrile seizure occurs because of the change in body temperature, and could happen either with rapid elevation or drop in temperature. Aside from managing the patient's ABCs, you should consider the potential source of the fever and always use the appropriate PPE. It is difficult to tell the difference between a sick child with a high body temperature who just had a seizure and a sick child who has a fever as a symptom of a potentially devastating infection such as meningoencephalitis. Also, many patients with prolonged seizures will manifest a degree of hyperthermia from the episode itself and have no underlying infection as a proximate cause of the seizure. Again, that can be a difficult distinction to make in the field. For this reason, most medical treatment protocols require management of the ABCs and transport of the child who has had a seizure with an accompanying fever. As always, keep the child warm during transport even though he or she may feel like they are burning up. In rare instances, the child may have back-to-back or prolonged seizures. If found in the field, this condition is to be treated as status epilepticus and not downplayed as just a febrile seizure!

The combination of medications can result in unexpected neurologic effects.

Neoplasms and Seizure

According to the National Cancer Institute, a **neoplasm** is an abnormal mass of tissue that results when cells divide more than they should or do not die when they should. When a neoplasm develops in the brain tissue, it is called a cerebral neoplasm (brain tumor). Neoplasms may be benign or malignant. The commonly used term for a neoplasm is a tumor. The development of a tumor in the brain usually occurs without symptoms in its earliest stages. As the tumor grows, it is likely to impinge on areas of the brain and may cause seizure activity. If the neoplasm bleeds, it is likely to cause signs and symptoms of a stroke. It is estimated that patients older than the age of 21 who develop a seizure have a one in five likelihood of a cerebral neoplasm.

The treatments of cerebral neoplasms in the prehospital setting are symptomatic when the patient presents with seizure or stroke-like symptoms. Depending on the specific location in the brain and if a tumor is cancerous, the patient usually undergoes radiation therapy or surgery. Without a known history of metastatic cancer or a primary brain mass, it would be difficult to make this diagnosis in the context of seizures without the benefit of neuroimaging, which is why all patients with new onset of seizures or status epilepticus undergo an imaging evaluation.

Other Neurologic Emergencies

There are a number of other neurologic medical emergencies that do not come under the context of "toxicologic" or "infectious." In most cases, presenting problems such as headache, dizziness, vertigo, or nontraumatic problems with the sense organs (ie, eyes, ears, and nose) are symptoms that are not

Table 5-5 Approximated Occurrences of Neurologic Disorders in the United States*

Condition	Estimated Incidence
Abscess	1,500 cases
Acute polio	No new wild poliovirus cases since 1979
Alzheimer's disease	**4,500,000 cases**
Amyotrophic lateral sclerosis	20,000 cases
Bell's palsy	40,000 cases
Cerebral palsy	500,000 cases
Dystonia	300,000 cases
Guillain-Barré syndrome	2,700 cases
Headache	45,000,000 cases with chronic headaches
Multiple sclerosis	300,000 cases
Muscular dystrophy	40,000 cases combining all types
Myasthenia gravis	50,000 cases
Neoplasms	**40,000 cases**
Parkinson's disease	500,000 cases
Peripheral neuropathy	9,000,000 diabetics with neuropathy
Postpolio syndrome	100,000 cases
Seizures	2,500,000 cases
Spina bifida	1,500 new births per year
Stroke	**700,000 cases**
Syncope	3% of emergency department visits nationwide
Trigeminal neuralgia	11,000 cases

*Items in bold type fall into the top 10 causes of death according to the National Center for Health Statistics/National Vital Statistics System. *(Data from 2000–2003)*

generally dealt with in the field. If there are presenting problems that involve threats to the patient's ABCs, the paramedic would be extensively involved. Syncope is an example of a symptom that can be caused by a number of conditions (ie, hypoxia, hypovolemia, and arrhythmias) and should always be taken very seriously in the field. In some cases, patients have been known to have a syncopal episode based solely on the medications they have been prescribed or combinations of multiple medications. Examples of classifications of medications that have been known to cause syncope would include the following: ACE inhibitors, beta-blockers, antihypertensives, antiarrhythmics, digitalis, diuretics, narcotic analgesics, nitrates, and psychiatric medications.

The frequency of occurrences of neurologic disorders in the United States is shown in **Table 5-5▲**.

Table 5-6 Head Pain and Associated Conditions

Location of Pain	Possible Condition
Localized to one side of the head	Cerebral aneurysm
Eye pain	Glaucoma
Back of the head	Meningitis
Bilateral or Unilateral	Migraine
Any area of the head	Stress
Described as worst ever experienced	Subarachnoid bleed
Over temporal artery	Temporal arteritis
Pain with jaw movement	Temporomandibular joint (TMJ) syndrome

Head Pain: Where Does It Hurt?

In patients who have nontraumatic head pain or a headache, the location of the pain does not always give you an indication of the specific cause of the pain. There are some conditions that present with localization of the head pain that you should be aware of in your assessment of the patient (**Table 5-6▲**).

Medications Prescribed for Serious Headaches

Migraine headaches are often debilitating to the patient. Patients may complain of extreme pain, **photophobia**, nausea, vomiting, and other symptoms. Migraines are thought to be caused by dilation and inflammation of the cerebral blood vessels. It is common for patients who experience migraines to be on a medication to prevent the headaches or to take a different medication once the medication has started to treat the pain as well as end the headache (**Table 5-7▶**). Most of these medications do not mix with other medications well so it is always a good idea to refer to a resource if the patient may have taken numerous medications and is experiencing symptoms.

Cluster headaches are different than migraines and are known to occur in rapid succession and then disappear for months at a time. Some of the medications used are very potent anticonvulsants, NSAIDs, or narcotic analgesics.

The nerves that come directly out of the brain and service functions mostly from the shoulders and up are called the cranial nerves. There are twelve cranial nerves (**Table 5-8▶**).

Table 5-7 Medications for Headaches and Migraines

Brand Name	Generic Name	Comments
Topamax	Topiramate	Antiepileptic drug also used for migraine prevention
Zomig	Zolmitriptan	Used to treat migraines by providing vasoconstriction and reducing inflammation
Migranal	Dihydroergotamine mesylate	Nasal spray used to treat an active migraine and not for prevention
Stadol	Butorphanol	Narcotic analog analgesic to treat migraines
Phrenilin, Axocet, Bucet, Bupap	Acetaminophen and butalbital	For tension headaches to relax nervous system and relieve pain
Ergomar	Ergotamine	Causes vasoconstriction of blood vessels and treats vascular headaches
Acular	Ketorolac tromethamine	NSAID that reduces pain and inflammation in the eyes after surgery
Toradol	Ketorolac tromethamine	Anti-inflammatory medication—NSAID
Maxalt	Rizatriptan benzoate	Vasoconstricts the arteries and veins supplying the head. Not for prevention.
Axert	Almotriptan	Selective serotonin receptor agonist for migraines currently in progress
Imitrex	Sumatriptan succinate	Reduces the triggers for the headache (ie, pain, nausea, light sensitivity, and sound). Also used for cluster headaches.
Midrin	Isometheptene mucate, dichloralphenazone, and acetaminophen	Used to treat tension headaches, vascular headaches, and migraines
Fioricet, Esgic, Anolor 300	Butalbital, acetaminophen, caffeine	Strong non-narcotic pain reliever that reduces the muscle contractions that cause tension headaches
Cafergot	Ergotamine tartrate, caffeine	Used for relief or prevention of vascular headaches
Amerge	Naratriptan hydrochloride	Causes vasoconstriction of the arteries and veins in the head during an attack

Table 5-8 Cranial Nerves

Number	Name	Motor vs Sensory	Functions
I	Olfactory	Sensory	Smell
II	Optic	Sensory	Light perception and vision
III	Oculomotor	Motor	Pupil constriction, eye movements
IV	Trochlear	Motor	Eye movements
V	Trigeminal	Motor and sensory	Motor: chewing Sensory: face, sinuses, teeth
VI	Abducens	Motor	Eye movements
VII	Facial	Motor	Facial movements
VIII	Vestibulocochlear	Sensory	Hearing, balance perception
IX	Glossopharyngeal	Motor and sensory	Motor: throat and swallowing, gland secretion Sensory: tongue, throat, ear
X	Vagus	Motor and sensory	Heart, lungs, palate, pharynx, larynx, trachea, bronchi, GI tract, external ear
XI	Spinal accessory	Motor	Shoulder and neck movements
XII	Hypoglossal	Motor	Tongue, throat, and neck movements

Case Study III Head Pain

Part 1

You have been dispatched to a law office building in the late afternoon on a bright sunny summer day. You are met at the elevator of the building where a security officer leads you up to the 6th floor. One of the secretaries of the law firm has been in the break room resting on the couch for the past 2 hours. As you enter the room you notice that the lights are dimmed.

The scene is safe and you and your partner leave the stretcher in the hallway as you enter the room with your first in bag, the ECG monitor, and the drug box. You begin your initial assessment by making a general impression of this woman who is supine on the couch, awake, and probably in her early 40s (see **Table 1**). Next you introduce yourself and find out that the patient's name is Marie.

As you complete your initial assessment you decide that the patient is not a high priority at this point. Additional information may change this early decision. The patient's chief complaint is a severe headache and nausea.

Question 1: When would a headache be a potential life-threat?

Question 2: What is the significance of the dimly lit room?

Table 1 Initial Assessment

Initial Assessment	Recording Time: 2 Minutes
General Impression/ Appearance	Young, female, lying on the couch
Mental Status	Alert (oriented to person, place, and day)
Airway	Open and clear
Breathing	20 breaths/min and normal
Circulation	88 beats/min and regular
Priority/Plan	Low at this point

Part 2

With Marie being a responsive medical patient, you begin the focused history and physical examination (see **Table 2**). Based on the chief complaint of head pain, you proceed with elaboration of the chief complaint by using the OPQRST questions and a focused neurologic examination.

Table 2 Focused History and Physical Examination

Baseline Vital Signs	Recording Time: 5 Minutes
Skin CTC (color, temperature, condition)	Pale, normal temperature, and dry
Pulse	94 beats/min and regular
Blood Pressure	152/84 mm Hg
Respirations	20 breaths/min and regular

The neurologic examination is done as a part of your examination for a medical patient with a complaint of headache. The patient does tell you that this is the worst headache she has had in a long time and she says she gets headaches a couple of times a week.

Question 3: What is the purpose of checking for strength in both arms and legs?

Questions 4: If the patient described the headache as the worst ever, what should you consider?

Part 3

The neurologic examination that you do on Marie is a combination of the mental status examination (AVPU and GCS) and the Cincinnati Prehospital Stroke Score. In addition, it is helpful to check the cranial nerves as well as check for sensation and strength in all four extremities. Be sure to check to see if she has a stiff neck. Yet another cause of the photophobia and headache is meningitis, although she is not complaining of a fever. After your focused history and physical examination, you find no neurologic deficits and Marie has equal strength in all four extremities. All other findings are within normal range. The SAMPLE history reveals additional information (see **Table 3**).

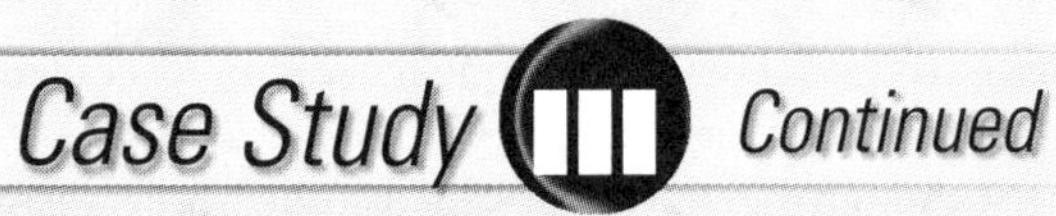

Table 3 SAMPLE History

SAMPLE History	Comments
Signs/symptoms	Nausea
Allergies	Codeine
Medications	Sumatriptan succinate [Imitrex]
Pertinent past medical history	Migraines
Last oral intake	Some water and aspirin 45 minutes ago
Events leading up to the incident	The blinds did not work at her desk so she sat in direct sunlight for 2 hours

Treatment Plan

1. Manage the ABCs and place the patient into the position of comfort. Provide quiet transport with the lights dimmed.
2. Consider supplemental oxygen via a nonrebreathing mask if cluster headaches are a consideration. Offer an ice pack for the forehead or back of the neck.
3. You may want to consider IV fluids and antiemetic medications such as promethazine hydrochloride [Phenergan] or ondansetron hydrochloride [Zofran], as both will help with migraine ablation while en route to the hospital. Some EMS systems have changed their protocols to ondansetron hydrochloride [Zofran] due to the potential for severe tissue damage when promethazine hydrochloride [Phenergan] is inadvertently administered SQ or intraarterial, rather than deep IM or IV routes.
4. Monitor the patient en route and be prepared for a vomiting patient should the ride be a bumpy one.

Question 5: Why would an EMS Medical Director consider using ondansetron hydrochloride [Zofran] over the more traditionally used promethazine hydrochloride [Phenergan]?

Question 6: What is the priority of this patient based on the information you have been given?

Part 4

Your partner provides a quiet ride to the hospital and you have a nice quiet conversation with Marie. It seems that she has been under a lot of stress lately and she is having some marital problems. Since this is not a high priority, you do an ongoing assessment and obtain the serial vital signs every 15 minutes during the ride to the ED (see **Table 4**).

Question 7: Why was the blood glucose checked?

Question 8: Are this patient's vital signs considered "normal"?

Table 4 Reassessment and Ongoing Assessment of the Patient

Serial Vital Signs and Relevant Data	Recording Time: 10 Minutes
Skin CTC	Pale, warm, and dry
Pulse	96 beats/min and regular
Blood Pressure	154/84 mm Hg
Respirations	20 breaths/min and regular
Mental Status	Alert (oriented to person, place, and day)
ECG	Normal sinus rhythm (NSR) with no ectopy
SpO_2	98% on supplemental oxygen
Lung Sounds	Clear bilaterally
Other (ie, glucose, core temperature)	Blood glucose of 126 mg/dL

Part 5

Upon arrival at the ED you provide a verbal report to the nurse who will be taking over the care. Marie's headache is still present but the nausea has subsided. They are likely to give her some medication to curtail the migraine but according to the patient that medication still takes a few hours to work. You wish her well as you complete your paperwork and head out the door on another call.

Nervous System Disorders

There will be times when you are called to care for a patient with a nervous system disorder or degenerative disease (ie, cerebral palsy, multiple sclerosis, Parkinson's disease, spina bifida, or amyotrophic lateral sclerosis (ALS)) that has an acute exacerbation of the disorder, a complication associated with progressive deterioration of the disorder, or when the patient gets injured or sick the same as a healthy individual would. These diseases vary in the severity of debilitation to nerve and muscle tissue. You should keep in mind that many of these conditions cause the patients to have good and bad days. That is to say that the symptoms of the condition can be more or less on any given day and that the baseline for the patient should be obtained in the focused history prior to treating. Problems can occur when the patient neglects or has problems with their scheduled medication, is exposed to extreme temperatures, develops an infection, falls, or aspirates. For example, the patient with spina bifida may have problems with shunts becoming occluded and have latex allergies.

Although the nervous system disorders previously mentioned are not contagious, there are infectious diseases that affect the nervous system (encephalitis, meningitis, brain abscess, poliomyelitis (polio), tetanus, and shingles) that can be contagious. You must take the appropriate precautions. Since you do not routinely administer medications in the prehospital setting to manage many of these neurologic disorders, we have not discussed the specific medications here. For example, in-hospital management of abscess will likely involve antibiotics, seizure precautions, and potentially surgical removal of the abscess. Please see the end of this chapter for specific information regarding the drugs that may be administered to a neurologic patient. It would be helpful to have a resource available in the ambulance to look up prescription medications or OTC medications that the patients may be taking to expand your knowledge base.

Case Study ANSWERS

Case Study 1 Possible Stroke

Question 1: Why is it so important to establish the time when the patient began to experience symptoms?

Answer 1: The timeline for the administration of a fibrinolytic is a 3-hour window and there is a lot to do both prehospital and in-hospital during that time frame.

Question 2: As a part of your assessment of this patient, what physical examination should be conducted?

Answer 2: The mini-neuro examination should be done which includes a reassessment of AVPU, assessment of distal PMS, and the Cincinnati Prehospital Stroke Scale, and begin screening the patient using the exclusion criteria for tPA. Some EMS systems use the Los Angeles Prehospital Stroke Screen.

Question 3: What is the significance of a history of a TIA?

Answer 3: A history of a TIA is a warning of a stroke likely to occur within the next year if the cause of the TIA is not adequately addressed.

Question 4: What is the significance of asking if the patient has a history of diabetes and should you still check his blood glucose?

Answer 4: The signs and symptoms of a stroke may mimic those of a diabetic problem. A blood glucose reading by fingerstick should be obtained on any patient with altered mental status or symptoms of stroke. Ask the SAMPLE questions to determine the patient's medical history. If the patient is a diabetic, the most likely cause of his AMS is hypoglycemia. To determine if in fact he has hypoglycemia, a blood glucose should be done by a fingerstick or using a drop of the blood when the IV is started. Always attempt to minimize punctures in a patient where thrombolysis is anticipated.

Question 5: What is the significance of the atrial fibrillation?

Answer 5: Atrial fibrillation (AF) is a very common arrhythmia in the elderly, and is a well described risk factor for development of stroke. Atrial fibrillation results in incomplete atrial emptying and allows blood to pool in the left atria where it can form clots. These can then be ejected and then embolize via the arterial circulation to either the brain, the gut, or the extremities. This is a principal reason patients with atrial fibrillation are placed on blood thinners. The most worrisome time for atrial thrombi to embolize is when the heart converts from AF to sinus rhythm, which is why patients with relatively new onset of AF are typically anticoagulated from 6 to 8 weeks prior to elective cardioversion. Often the paramedic is the first to diagnose a patient with new-onset atrial fibrillation, and certainly occurs when EMS is called for a patient having a stroke. The atrial fibrillation is discovered during the assessment, yet the patient has no prior history of it.

Question 6: Why is the stroke fibrinolytic checklist needed? Don't all strokes get "clot busters?"

Answer 6: The stroke fibrinolytic checklist will help determine if the patient is a candidate for clot busters. Some patients may not be a good candidate based on recent surgery or bleeding disorders. Not all patients who are having a stroke will get fibrinolytic therapy. They need to meet the physiologic criteria, meet the time constraints, and have a neuroimaging study excluding a hemorrhagic stroke.

Question 7: What is an embolic or ischemic stroke?

Answer 7: There are two types of strokes: thromboembolic or ischemic and hemorrhagic. An ischemic stroke is a narrowing or blockage of a cerebral artery that causes damage to the downstream brain tissue served by the vessel. If the blockage is temporary, it is a TIA. If the blockage is long enough to precipitate cellular necrosis, it is then termed a stroke. This is very similar, from a pathophysiologic standpoint to angina and an acute myocardial infarction. The treatment is to unclog the vessel to reperfuse the downstream brain tissue. A hemorrhagic stroke involves bleeding into the tissue of the brain. In this case, administering a fibrinolytic would simply increase the bleeding into the brain tissue tremendously and lead to death. That is why it is imperative to actually diagnose the type of the stroke prior to making the decision to go ahead with fibrinolytic therapy.

Question 8: What is the advantage of taking this patient directly to a stroke center?

Answer 8: A stroke center has all the right staff and all the right equipment ready to move within the very brief time window so that the patient can be assessed, diagnosed, and managed rapidly. The patient's greatest chance of long-term survival and the best recovery from the stroke is directly tied to the prehospital recognition of stroke symptoms and the care provided in a stroke center or a hospital with a stroke team within the first 3 hours.

Case Study ANSWERS

Case Study II Status Epilepticus

Question 1: What is the significance of the long seizure?

Answer 1: A lengthy seizure (over 3 to 5 minutes long) or two seizures back to back, without a lucid interval, is known as status epilepticus.

Question 2: What type of seizure is a life-threat and must be taken very seriously?

Answer 2: When you suspect a patient is having status epilepticus, you should move quickly to end the seizure activity by medication. The cost of the lengthy seizure activity is dying brain cells. Some EMS systems have standing orders for diazepam [Valium] administration when status epilepticus is suspected.

Question 3: What are some of the causes of a seizure?

Answer 3: A seizure can be caused by many things. Examples would include: tumors, hypoglycemia, fever, sepsis, head trauma, overdose, hypoxemia, alcoholism, withdrawal, electrolyte imbalances, epilepsy, heat stroke, hemorrhagic stroke, and infection.

Question 4: Given that this patient has known epilepsy and is prescribed a daily dose of an anticonvulsant, what is the most likely cause of today's seizure activity?

Answer 4: Anticonvulsants typically work by raising the brain's seizure threshold and preventing breakthrough seizure activity by establishing a specific blood level of the medicine. This often takes a few days to attain and then requires the patient to be compliant in taking his or her daily medicine. When a day or two have been skipped, the blood level of anticonvulsant can significantly drop and seizure activity can occur.

Question 5: Why is oxygen helpful for this patient?

Answer 5: In any situation where there may be a decrease in blood flow to the brain and vital organs, it is helpful to increase the oxygen saturation by providing supplemental oxygen therapy to the patient. In many cases, episodes of seizure are accompanied by periods of apnea and/or hypoventilation, so supplemental oxygenation and/or mechanical ventilations are also useful to consider. Lastly, seizure represents a situation of extreme metabolic work for the brain and body, and additional oxygen is very useful for helping to manage that. Many of the causes of seizure activity are also potential threats to the brain and vital organs so it is appropriate to consider administering oxygen, guided by the improvements in the patient's condition and SpO_2 readings.

Question 6: Why is a benzodiazepine administered to this patient?

Answer 6: The benzodiazepine is administered to the patient because it can rapidly terminate seizure activity. During a lengthy seizure the patient can literally kill brain cells. Thus the seizure should be brought to an end as soon as possible. Select one of the three benzodiazepines listed (your State or Regional treatment protocols may have already narrowed down the choice). If the benzodiazepine administered in the prehospital setting (ie, diazepam [Valium], lorazepam [Ativan], or midazolam [Versed]) does not bring about an end to the seizure activity, medical control may order a second dose. If that does not work, specific IV anticonvulsants will be considered in the in-hospital setting of this patient's care.

Question 7: Why was it important to check this patient's blood glucose?

Answer 7: Hypoglycemia is one of those potential causes of seizure activity that can be treated in the field. Rather than administering the benzodiazepine immediately, if the patient's blood glucose is less than 80 mg/dL it would make more sense to administer 50% dextrose through a large bore IV. With the increase in glucose, it is possible that the seizure activity would cease and there would not be a need for other medications at this point. Glucagon is another option if the patient does not have an IV site and has documented hypoglycemia.

Question 8: What other medications might be used to break a seizure in the emergency department?

Answer 8: If the benzodiazepine you administered does not work, the ED may want to consider other medication choices such as phenobarbital [Luminal], phenytoin [Dilantin], or sodium pentabarbitol.

Case Study ANSWERS

Case Study III Head Pain

Question 1: When would a headache be a potential life-threat?

Answer 1: If the headache is related to a stroke, cerebral hemorrhage, or brain mass, it could be a threat to the patient's life. Always consider a "first-worst" headache to be a "high-risk" headache and react accordingly.

Question 2: What is the significance of the dimly lit room?

Answer 2: Many times a patient who has photophobia, one of the symptoms of meningitis or migraine headache, will ask for the lights to be turned down low.

Question 3: What is the purpose of checking for strength in both arms and legs?

Answer 3: You are checking for equal strength to see if there are any observable neurologic deficits such as a weakness or lack of sensation on one side of the body.

Question 4: If the patient described the headache as the worst ever, what should you consider?

Answer 4: Consider that the patient has a history of headaches. Comparatively speaking, how does this one today rate to the patient's previous experiences? This may be the worst in many months, but not the worst ever. If the headache were to have been described as "the worst ever," you would need to have considered intracerebral hemorrhage or subarachnoid hemorrhage. Both of these conditions can be immediately life-threatening and require prompt diagnosis and management.

Question 5: Why would an EMS Medical Director consider using ondansetron hydrochloride [Zofran] over the more traditionally used promethazine hydrochloride [Phenergan]?

Answer 5: Deep IM injection into a large muscle is the preferred route of administration for promethazine hydrochloride [Phenergan]. It can also be given by the slow IV route and actually, this is very common. Due to the frequency of severe, tragic, local injuries after infiltration or inadvertent intra-arterial injection, the FDA has recently been asked to reexamine the product labeling and consider eliminating the IV route of administration and diluting it when IV administration is used. Some EMS system Medical Directors are currently considering replacing promethazine hydrochloride [Phenergan] with a different antiemetic agent such as ondansetron hydrochloride [Zofran]. Others feel this is merely an education issue about proper administration of the medication. The bottom line is to make sure the IV is in the vein before giving any drug!

Question 6: What is the priority of this patient based on the information you have been given?

Answer 6: Unless you have reason to think the patient could be having a CNS infection, stroke, CNS mass, or cerebral hemorrhage, this is not a high priority patient.

Question 7: Why was the blood glucose checked?

Answer 7: Some of the symptoms could be caused by hypoglycemia so it is helpful to establish the patient's blood glucose level. In this case, her blood glucose is within normal range.

Question 8: Are this patient's vital signs considered "normal"?

Answer 8: The pulse rate and the respirations are normal, but a blood pressure of 154/84 mm Hg is considered hypertensive for a young female such as our patient. Given her degree of discomfort it is not a necessarily unexpected finding.

Medication Review

Aspirin

Indications New onset chest pain suggestive of acute myocardial infarction. Signs and symptoms suggestive of recent cerebrovascular accident.

Contraindications Hypersensitivity. Relatively contraindicated in patients with active ulcer disease or asthma.

Dosage and administration 160 mg to 325 mg PO (chewed if possible).

Dexamethasone Sodium Phosphate (Decadron, Hexadrol)

Indications Anaphylaxis, asthma, croup.

Contraindications Hypersensitivity to product, systemic sepsis, bacterial infection.

Dosage and administration Adult: 10–100 mg IV (1 mg/kg slow IV bolus) (considerable variance through medical control). Pediatric: 0.25–1.0 mg/kg/dose IV, IO, IM.

Dextrose

Indications Hypoglycemia, altered level of consciousness, coma of unknown etiology, seizure of unknown etiology, status epilepticus.

Contraindications Intracranial hemorrhage.

Dosage and administration Adult: 12.5–25 g slow IV; may be repeated as necessary. Pediatric: 0.5–1 g/kg/dose slow IV; may be repeated as necessary.

Diazepam (Valium)

Indications Acute anxiety states, acute alcohol withdrawal (delirium tremens), muscle relaxant, seizure activity, agitation. Analgesia for medical procedures (fracture reduction, cardioversion).

Contraindications Hypersensitivity, glaucoma, coma, shock, substance abuse, head injury.

Dosage and administration Seizure activity: Adult: 5–10 mg IV every 10–15 minutes as needed (5 mg over 5 min) (maximum dose, 30 mg). Seizure activity: Pediatric: 0.2–0.5 mg slowly every 2–5 minutes up to 5 mg (maximum dose, 10 mg/kg). Rectal diazepam: 0.5 mg/kg via rectal catheter and flush with 2–3 mL air after administration. Sedation for cardioversion: 5–15 mg IV over 5–10 minutes prior to cardioversion.

Diltiazem Hydrochloride (Cardizem, Lyo-Ject)

Indications Control of rapid ventricular rates due to atrial flutter, atrial fibrillation, and re-entry SVT; Angina pectoris.

Contraindications Hypotension, sick sinus syndrome, second- or third-degree AV block, cardiogenic shock, wide-complex tachycardias, poison/drug-induced tachycardia.

Dosage and administration Adult: Initial bolus: 0.25 mg/kg (average dose 15–20 mg) IV over 2 minutes. If inadequate response, may re-bolus in 15 minutes: 0.35 mg/kg (average dose 20–25 mg) IV over 2 minutes. Maintenance infusion of 5–15 mg/h. Pediatric: Not recommended.

Diphenhydramine (Benadryl)

Indications Symptomatic relief of allergies, allergic reactions, anaphylaxis, acute dystonic reactions (phenothiazines). Blood administration reactions; used for motion sickness, hay fever.

Contraindications Asthma, glaucoma, pregnancy, hypertension, narrow-angle glaucoma, infants, patients taking monoamine oxidase inhibitors (MAOIs).

Dosage and administration Adult: 25–50 mg IM or IV or PO. Pediatric: 1–2 mg/kg IV, IO slowly or IM. If given PO: 5 mg/kg/24 hours.

Medication Review

Flumazenil (Romazicon)

Indications Reversal of respiratory depression and sedative effects from pure benzodiazepine overdose.

Contraindications Hypersensitivity, tricyclic antidepressant overdose, seizure-prone patients, coma of unknown etiology, benzodiazepine dependence.

Dosage and administration Adult: First dose: 0.2 mg IV/IO over 15 seconds. Second dose: 0.3 mg IV/IO over 30 seconds. If no response, give third dose. Third dose: 0.5 mg IV/IO over 30 seconds. If no response, repeat once every minute until adequate response or a total of 3 mg is given. Pediatric: Not recommended.

Furosemide (Lasix)

Indications CHF, pulmonary edema, hypertensive crisis.

Contraindications Hypovolemia, anuria, hypotension (relative contraindication); hypersensitivity, hepatic coma.

Dosage and administration Adult: 0.5–1.0 mg/kg injected IV over 1 to 2 minutes. If no response, double the dose to 2 mg/kg over 1 to 2 minutes. Pediatric: 1 mg/kg/dose IV, IO.

Glucagon

Indications Altered level of consciousness when hypoglycemia is suspected. May be used as inotropic agent in beta-blocker overdose.

Contraindications Hyperglycemia, hypersensitivity.

Dosage and administration Adult: Hypoglycemia: 0.5–1 mg IM; may repeat in 7–10 minutes. Calcium channel blocker or beta-blocker overdose: 3 mg initially, followed by infusion at 3 mg/hr as necessary. Pediatric: Hypoglycemia: 0.5–1 mg IM (for children < 20 kg). Calcium channel blocker or beta-blocker overdose: Not recommended.

Haloperidol (Haldol)

Indications Acute psychotic episodes.

Contraindications Agitation secondary to shock or hypoxia. Hypersensitivity.

Dosage and administration Adult: 2–5 mg IM every 30–60 minutes until sedation achieved. Pediatric: Not recommended.

Hydroxyzine Hydrochloride (Atarax, Vistaril)

Indications To potentiate the effects of analgesics; to control nausea and vomiting, anxiety reactions, and motion sickness; preoperative and postoperative sedation.

Contraindications Hypersensitivity.

Dosage and administration Adult: 25–100 mg IM. Pediatric: 0.5–1.0 mg/kg/dose IM.

Ketorolac Tromethamine (Toradol IM)

Indications Short-term management of moderate to severe pain.

Contraindications Allergy to salicylates or other NSAIDs; patients with history of asthma; bleeding disorders, especially gastrointestinal (GI) related (peptic ulcer disease); renal failure.

Dosage and administration Adult: 30–60 mg IM. Pediatric: Not recommended.

Labetalol (Normodyne, Trandate)

Indications Moderate to severe hypertension.

Contraindications Bronchial asthma, CHF, cardiogenic shock, second- and third-degree heart block, bradycardia.

Dosage and administration Adult: 5–20 mg slow IV over 2 minutes (additional injections of 10–40 mg can be given at 10-minute intervals). Infusion: 2 mg/min titrated to acceptable supine blood pressure. Pediatric: Safety not established.

Medication Review

Lorazepam (Ativan)

Indications Initial control of status epilepticus or severe recurrent seizures, severe anxiety, sedation.

Contraindications Acute narrow-angle glaucoma. Coma, shock, or suspected drug abuse.

Dosage and administration Note: When given IV or IO, must dilute with equal volume of sterile water or sterile saline; When given IM, lorazepam is not to be diluted. Adult: 2–4 mg slow IV at 2 mg/min or IM; may repeat in 15–20 minutes to maximum dose of 8 mg. For sedation: 0.05 mg/kg up to 4 mg IM. Pediatric: 0.05–0.20 mg/kg slow IV, IO slowly over 2 minutes or IM; may repeat in 15–20 minutes to maximum dose of 0.2 mg/kg.

Magnesium Sulfate

Indications Seizures of eclampsia (toxemia of pregnancy), torsade de pointes, hypomagnesemia, Class IIa agent for V-fib/pulseless V-tach that is refractory to lidocaine.

Contraindications Heart blocks, myocardial damage.

Dosage and administration Adult: Seizure activity associated with pregnancy: 1–4 g IV/IO over 3 minutes; maximum dose of 30–40 g/day. Cardiac arrest due to hypomagnesemia or torsade de pointes: 1–2 g (2–4 mL of a 50% solution) diluted in 10 mL of D_5W IV/IO over 5–20 minutes. Torsade de pointes with a pulse or AMI with hypomagnesemia: Loading dose of 1–2 g mixed in 50–100 mL D_5W over 5–60 minutes IV. Follow with 0.5–1 g/hr IV (titrate to control torsade de pointes). Pediatric: IV/IO infusion: 25–50 mg/kg (maximum dose: 2 g) over 10–20 minutes; faster for torsade de pointes. For asthma: 25–50 mg/kg (maximum dose: 2 g) over 10–20 minutes.

Meperidine Hydrochloride (Demerol)

Indications Analgesia for moderate to severe pain.

Contraindications Hypersensitivity to narcotic agents, diarrhea caused by poisoning, patients taking MAOIs, during labor or delivery of a premature infant, undiagnosed abdominal pain or head injury.

Dosage and administration Adult: 50–100 mg IM, SC or 25–50 mg slowly IV. Pediatric: 1–2 mg/kg/dose IV, IO, IM, SC.

Metoprolol Tartrate (Lopressor)

Indications Suspected ACS provided heart rate is >80 and systolic BP is >120 mm Hg. Patients may be taking the tablet form for hypertension or angina. The usual tablet initial dose is 100 mg and effective dose is between 100 and 400 mg daily. Has also been used for ventricular arrhythmias and migraine headaches. Paramedic protocols are usually for the IV dose of the drug.

Contraindications In the context of a suspected MI, the drug is contraindicated in patients with a heart rate <45 beats/min; second- and third-degree heart block; significant first-degree heart block (P-R interval ≥0.24 sec); systolic blood pressure <100 mm Hg; or moderate-to-severe cardiac failure. Hypersensitivity to the drug, related derivatives, or other beta-blockers (cross sensitivity between beta-blockers can occur).

Dosage and administration Adult: 5 mg slow IV bolus, may be repeated every 2 minutes up to maximum of 15 mg, Pediatric: Not recommended.

Midazolam (Versed)

Indications Sedation, anxiolytic prior to endotracheal or nasotracheal intubation; administer for conscious sedation.

Contraindications Glaucoma, shock, coma, alcohol intoxication, overdose, depressed vital signs, concomitant use with other CNS depressants, barbiturates, alcohol, narcotics.

Dosage and administration Adult: 2.0–2.5 mg slow IV over 2–3 minutes; may be repeated to total maximum: 0.1 mg/kg. Pediatric: Not recommended.

Medication Review

Morphine Sulfate (Astramorph/PF)

Indications Severe CHF, pulmonary edema, chest pain associated with acute MI, analgesia for moderate to severe acute and chronic pain (use with caution).

Contraindications Head injury, exacerbated COPD, depressed respiratory drive, hypotension, undiagnosed abdominal pain, decreased level of consciousness, suspected hypovolemia, patients who have taken MAOIs within the past 14 days.

Dosage and administration Adult: Initial dose: 2–4 mg IV (over 1–5 minutes) every 5–30 minutes. Repeat dose: 2–8 mg at 5- to 15-minute intervals. Pediatric: 0.1–0.2 mg/kg per dose via IV, IO, IM, or SC; maximum dose of 5 mg.

Nalbuphine (Nubain)

Indications Chest pain associated with acute MI; moderate to severe acute pain; pulmonary edema, with or without associated chest pain (morphine remains first line).

Contraindications Head injury or undiagnosed abdominal pain, diarrhea caused by poisoning, hypovolemia, hypotension.

Dosage and administration Adult: 2–5 mg slowly IV; may repeat 2-mg doses as needed to maximum dose of 10 mg. Pediatric: Not recommended.

Naloxone Hydrochloride (Narcan)

Indications Opiate overdose, coma; complete or partial reversal of CNS and respiratory depression induced by opioids; decreased level of consciousness; coma of unknown origin; narcotic agonist for the following: morphine, heroin, hydromorphone (Dilaudid), methadone, meperidine (Demerol), paregoric, fentanyl citrate (Sublimase), oxycodone (Percodan), codeine, propoxyphene (Darvon); narcotic agonist and antagonist for the following: butorphanol (Stadol), pentazocine (Talwin), nalbuphine (Nubain).

Contraindications Use with caution in narcotic-dependent patients; use with caution in neonates of narcotic-addicted mothers.

Dosage and administration Adult: 0.4–2.0 mg IV, IM, SC, or ET (diluted); minimum recommended dose, 0.4 mg; repeat at 5-minute intervals to a maximum dose of 10 mg (medical control may request higher amounts). Infusion: 2 mg in 500 mL of D_5W (4 µg/mL), infuse at 0.4 mg/h (100 mL/h). Pediatric: 0.1 mg/kg/dose IV, IM, SC, ET (diluted); maximum dose of 0.8 mg; if no response in 10 minutes, administer an additional 0.1 mg/kg/dose.

Nifedipine (Procardia)

Indications Hypertensive crisis, angina pectoris, pulmonary edema (investigational).

Contraindications Compensatory hypertension, hypotension, hypersensitivity.

Dosage and administration Adult: 10 mg SL or buccal (puncture end of capsule with needle and squeeze; may administer SL or buccally or may have patient bite and swallow); may repeat in 30 minutes. Pediatric: Not recommended.

Nitroglycerin (Nitrostat, Tridil)

Indications Acute angina pectoris, ischemic chest pain, hypertension, CHF, pulmonary edema.

Contraindications Hypotension, hypovolemia; intracranial bleeding or head injury; previous administration of Viagra, Revatio, Levitra, Cialis, or similar agents within past 24 hours.

Dosage and administration Adult: Tablets: 0.3–0.4 mg SL; may repeat in 3–5 minutes to maximum of 3 doses. NTG spray: 0.4 mg under the tongue; 1–2 sprays. NTG IV infusion: begin at 10 to 20 µg/min; increase by 5–10 µg/min every 5 minutes until desired effect. Pediatric: Not recommended.

Medication Review

Nitropaste (Nitro-Bid Ointment)

Indications Angina pectoris and chest pain associated with acute MI.

Contraindications Same as NTG.

Dosage and administration Adult: Paste: Apply ½" to ¾" (1–2 cm), 15–30 mg, cover with wrap and secure with tape; maximum, 5" (75 mg) per application. Transdermal: Apply unit to intact skin (usually chest wall) in varying doses. Pediatric: Not recommended.

Ondansetron Hydrochloride (Zofran)

Indications For the prevention or control of nausea or vomiting. Also used in the hospital setting for patients undergoing chemotherapy or surgical procedures.

Contraindications Known allergy to this medicine or other 5-HT3 receptor antagonists.

Dosage and administration Adult: 4 mg IV or IM (may repeat in 10 minutes). Pediatric: 0.1 mg/kg IV or IM.

Oxygen

Indications Confirmed or expected hypoxemia, ischemic chest pain, respiratory insufficiency, prophylactically during air transport, confirmed or suspected carbon monoxide poisoning, all other causes of decreased tissue oxygenation, decreased level of consciousness.

Contraindications Certain patients with COPD or emphysema who will not tolerate oxygen concentrations over 35%, hyperventilation. Oxygen should never be withheld from a patient who needs it, however. Be prepared to assist with ventilations in a patient with COPD who requires high concentration, as apnea may result.

Dosage and administration Adult: Cardiac arrest and carbon monoxide poisoning: 100%. Hypoxemia: 10–15 L/min via nonrebreathing mask. COPD: 1–6 L/min via nasal cannula or 28%–35% Venturi mask. Be prepared to provide ventilatory support if higher concentrations of oxygen needed. Pediatric: Same as for adult with exception of premature infant.

Pancuronium Bromide (Pavulon)

Indications Induction or maintenance of paralysis after intubation to assist ventilations.

Contraindications Hypersensitivity, inability to control airway and support ventilations with oxygen and positive pressure, neuromuscular disease (myasthenia gravis), hepatic or renal failure.

Dosage and administration Adult: 0.1 mg/kg slow IV; repeat every 30–60 minutes as needed. Pediatric: 0.1 mg/kg slow IV, IO.

Phenobarbital (Luminal)

Indications Prevention and treatment of seizure activity; prophylaxis for febrile seizures; anxiety, apprehension; status epilepticus.

Contraindications Patients with porphyria, hypersensitivity, severe liver or respiratory diseases.

Dosage and administration Adult: 100–250 mg slow IV, or IM; may repeat as needed in 20–30 minutes. Pediatric: 10–20 mg/kg IV, IO (less than 1 mg/kg/min) or IM; repeat as needed in 20–30 minutes.

Phenytoin (Dilantin)

Indications Prophylaxis and treatment of major motor seizures, digitalis-induced arrhythmias.

Contraindications Hypersensitivity, bradycardia, second- and third-degree heart block.

Dosage and administration Adult: Seizures: 10–20 mg/kg slow IV, not to exceed 1 g or rate of 50 mg/min). Arrhythmias: 50–100 mg (diluted) slow IV every 5–15 min as needed; maximum, 1 g. Pediatric: Seizures: 10–20 mg/kg slow IV (1–3 mg/kg/min). Arrhythmias: 5 mg/kg slow IV; maximum, 1 g.

Medication Review

Promethazine Hydrochloride (Phenergan)

Indications Nausea, vomiting, motion sickness; sedation for patients in labor; potentiation of analgesic effects of narcotics.

Contraindications Hypersensitivity, coma, CNS-depressed patients from alcohol, barbiturates, narcotics, Reye's syndrome.

Dosage and administration Adult: 12.5–25 mg IV, deep IM, PO, rectally. Pediatric: (older than 2 years old) 0.25–0.5 mg/kg dose IM.

Streptokinase (Streptase)

Indications Acute evolving MI, massive pulmonary emboli, arterial thrombosis and embolism, to clear arteriovenous cannulas.

Contraindications Hypersensitivity; active bleeding, recent surgery (within 2–4 weeks), recent CVA; prolonged CPR; intracranial or intraspinal neoplasm, arteriovenous malformation, or surgery; recent significant trauma (particularly head trauma); uncontrolled hypertension.

Dosage and administration Note: Reconstitute by slowly adding 5 mL of sodium chloride or D_5W, directing stream to side of vial instead of into powder. Gently roll and tilt vial for reconstitution; dilute slowly to 45 mL total. Adult: 500,000–1,500,000 IU diluted to 45 mL IV over 1 hour. Pediatric: Safety not established.

Succinylcholine Chloride (Anectine, Quelicin)

Indications To facilitate intubation, to terminate laryngospasm, to promote muscle relaxation, to facilitate electroconvulsive shock therapy.

Contraindications Acute narrow-angle glaucoma, penetrating eye injuries, inability to control airway or support ventilations with oxygen and positive pressure.

Dosage and administration Adult: 1–2 mg/kg rapid IV; repeat once if needed. Pediatric: 1–1.5 mg/kg dose rapid IV, IO; repeat once if needed.

Thiamine Hydrochloride (Vitamin B-1)

Indications Coma of unknown origin, delirium tremens, beriberi, Wernicke's encephalopathy.

Contraindications None.

Dosage and administration Adult: 100 mg slow IV or IM. Pediatric: 10–25 mg slow IV or IM.

Tissue Plasminogen Activator (tPA)

Indications Acute evolving myocardial infarction, massive pulmonary emboli, arterial thrombosis and embolism, to clear arteriovenous cannulas.

Contraindications Recent surgery (within 3 weeks), active bleeding, recent CVA, prolonged CPR, intracranial or intraspinal surgery; recent significant trauma, especially head trauma; uncontrolled hypertension (generally BP over 200 mm Hg).

Dosage and administration Adult: 10-mg bolus IV over 2 minutes; then 50 mg over 1 hour, then 20 mg over the second hour and 20 mg over the third hour, for a total dose of 100 mg (other doses may be prescribed through Medical Direction). Pediatric: Safety not established.

Vecuronium Bromide (Norcuron)

Indications To facilitate intubation, to terminate laryngospasm, to promote muscle relaxation, to facilitate electroconvulsive shock therapy.

Contraindications Acute narrow-angle glaucoma, penetrating eye injuries, inability to control airway or support ventilations with oxygen and positive pressure, newborns, myasthenia gravis, hepatic or renal failure.

Dosage and administration Adult: 0.1 mg/kg IV push; maintenance dose within 25–40 minutes: 0.01–0.05 mg/kg IV push. Pediatric: 0.1 mg/kg IV, IO; maintenance dose within 20–35 minutes: 0.01–0.05 mg/kg IV push.

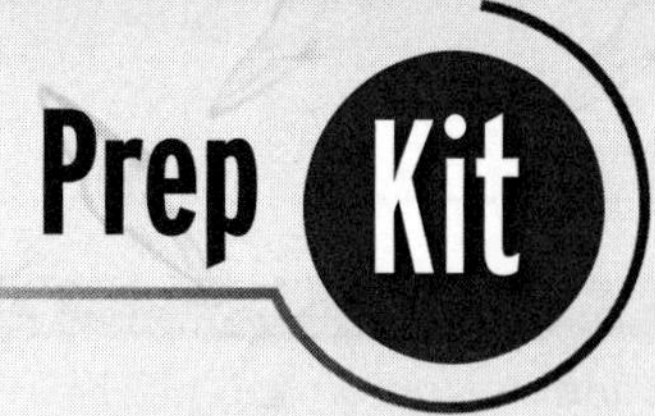

Chapter Summary

- The best medicine for a stroke is prevention.
- The most definitive treatment of a stroke, in its acute phase, involves the use of fibrinolytics and care often only administered in a hospital with a stroke program or a stroke center.
- Angiotensin converting enzyme (ACE) inhibitors are one of three primary drug classifications used to treat hypertension. Beta-blockers and thiazide diuretics are the other two.
- The accepted treatments for stroke include medications, surgery, hospital care, and rehabilitation. The treatment plan a patient receives will depend on several factors including: the time of onset of symptoms, the type of stroke they are having, age, and health status.
- When the patient with stroke symptoms is taken to the appropriate facility within the first 3 hours of onset, he or she may be a candidate for reperfusion therapy, also called fibrinolytic therapy or clot buster therapy.
- All seizures are treated in a similar manner, ensuring adequacy of ABCs and protecting the patient from injury.
- When a patient has status epilepticus (two or more back-to-back seizures), pharmacological interventions are appropriate and a benzodiazepine is administered to stop the seizure activity.
- The treatments of cerebral neoplasms in the prehospital setting are symptomatic when the patient presents with seizure or stroke-like symptoms. Depending on the specific location in the brain and if a tumor is cancerous, the patient usually undergoes radiation therapy or surgery.
- Syncope is a symptom that can be caused by a number of conditions (ie, hypoxia, hypovolemia, and arrhythmias).
- Patients have been known to have a syncopal episode based solely on the medications they have been prescribed or combinations of multiple medications.
- Examples of classifications of medications that have been known to cause syncope include the following: ACE inhibitors, beta-blockers, antihypertensives, antiarrhythmic, digitalis, diuretics, narcotic analgesics, nitrates, and psychiatric medications.
- Patients who experience migraines often take medications to prevent headaches, treat the pain, and end the headache.
- The paramedic does not routinely administer medications to manage many neurologic disorders.

Vital Vocabulary

Angiotensin converting enzyme (ACE) inhibitors One of three primary drug classifications used to treat hypertension. Beta-blockers and thiazide diuretics are the other two.

Neoplasm An abnormal mass of tissue that results when cells divide more than they should or do not die when they should.

Photophobia Unusual sensitivity to light.

Status epilepticus Two or more back-to-back seizures without a lucid interval or a lengthy (3–5 minutes) seizure. This is a very dangerous condition and the seizure needs to be terminated as soon as possible.

Stroke Disruption of blood flow or bleeding into the brain that causes the patient to have potentially permanent brain cell death and long-term physical disabilities.

Tissue plasminogen activator (tPA) Used to treat thromboembolic stroke. tPA dissolves the clot (clot buster) and restores blood flow to the brain and has been shown to be effective if given promptly to a very select group of patients.

Transient ischemic attack (TIA) TIAs are small strokes that last only for a few minutes or hours.

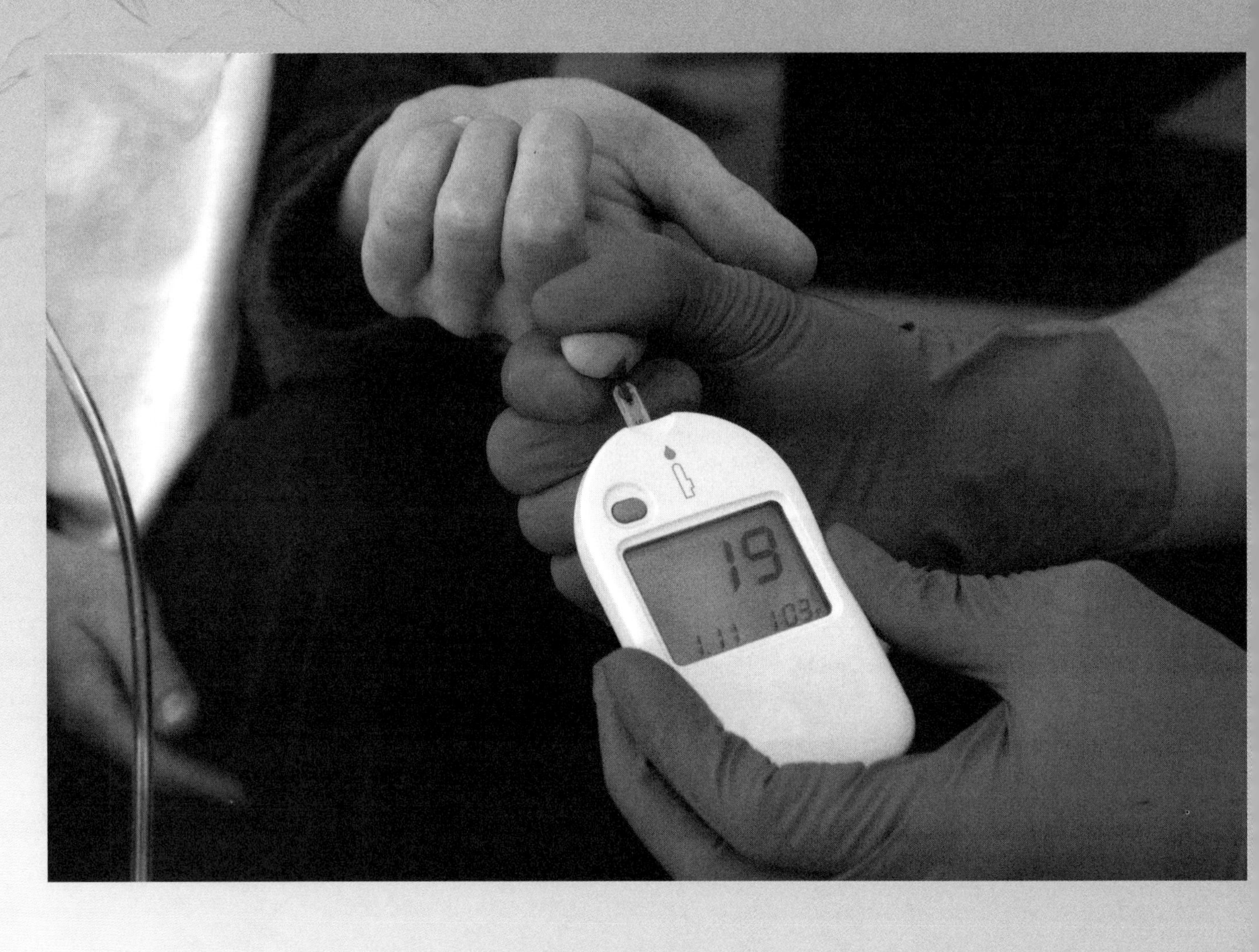
19

Endocrine Emergencies 6

Objectives

Cognitive
None

Affective
None

Psychomotor
None

Additional Objectives

6-1 Describe conditions of the thyroid gland, the pituitary and adrenal gland, and the pancreas. (pages 222–223)

6-2 Discuss the three forms of diabetes mellitus. (pages 223–224)

6-3 Explain the procedure for using a glucometer. (page 230)

6-4 Describe how to administer oral glucose to a patient. (pages 230–231)

6-5 Discuss the physiology of glucagon. (page 232)

6-6 Discuss the physiology and the administration of insulin. (pages 232–233)

6-7 Discuss the following medications used in the prehospital setting for endocrine patients: dextrose 50% ($D_{50}W$), glucagon, insulin. (pages 225–229)

Overview to Endocrine Emergencies

Endocrine diseases can affect hormone production, resulting in levels that are too high or too low, and can interfere with the feedback inhibition systems involving the hypothalamus, pituitary gland, endocrine glands, and the target organs. The most clinically significant endocrine problems result in alterations of the level of consciousness, ABCs, vital signs, glucose level, and fluid balance. The most common emergencies associated with the endocrine system are diabetic problems. Diabetic problems and the complications associated with this disease (ie, blindness, neuropathy, loss of limbs) occur more frequently and account for more health care expenditures than all other endocrine diseases combined. A brief description of diabetes and other endocrine diseases and conditions are listed within this chapter.

Conditions of the Thyroid Gland

Hyperthyroidism is a condition of an overactive thyroid resulting in the release of too many thyroid hormones. Thyrotoxicosis is a toxic condition caused by excessive levels of circulating thyroid hormone. Although hyperthyroidism can cause thyrotoxicosis, the two conditions are not identical. Thyrotoxicosis may also be caused by goiters, autoimmune disease, such as Graves disease which is the most common cause of hyperthyroidism, and thyroid cancer. An exacerbation of this condition can lead to thyroid storm, a rare, life-threatening condition that may occur in patients with thyrotoxicosis. A thyroid storm is often brought on by a stressful event or increased volumes of thyroid hormones in the circulation.

Hypothyroidism is a condition of an underactive thyroid and is far more common. Adult hypothyroidism is sometimes referred to as myxedema. Prolonged states of hypothyroidism lead to myxedema, and if left untreated, it can result in myxedema coma. Neither of these conditions is generally managed in the prehospital setting. Of course, oxygen should be administered if you suspect the patient may be hypoxic. If the patient has diminished respiratory drive or is unable to protect his or her airway, insertion of an advanced airway should be considered. If the patient is hypotensive, consider crystalloid therapy and vasopressive agents such as dopamine [Intropin]. If the patient has a blood glucose level that is less than 60 mg/dL, administer 25 to 50 g of $D_{50}W$ into a large vein. In summary, supportive care and consultation with Medical Direction is usually the most appropriate action.

Conditions of the Pituitary and Adrenal Glands

The secretions of the pituitary gland are responsible for controlling and regulating the secretions of other endocrine glands. The pituitary glands secrete hormones (**Table 6-1▼**). The adrenal glands produce hormones (**Table 6-2▼**). Adrenal insufficiency is defined as the decreased function of the adrenal cortex and the consequent underproduction of the adrenal hormones cortisol and aldosterone. The primary role of cortisol is to assist with the body's response to stress, and aldosterone regulates and maintains the salt and potassium balance in the blood. Adrenal insufficiency is considered either primary or secondary. Primary

Table 6-1 Hormones of the Pituitary Glands

Hormone	Function
Growth hormone (GH)	Regulates metabolic processes related to growth and adaptation to physical and emotional stressors
Thyroid-stimulating hormone (TSH)	Increases production and secretion of thyroid hormone
Adrenocorticotropic hormone (ACTH)	Stimulates the adrenal gland to secrete cortisol and adrenal proteins that contribute to the maintenance of the adrenal gland
Luteinizing hormone (LH)	In women: ovulation, progesterone production In men: regulates spermatogenesis, testosterone production
Follicle-stimulating hormone (FSH)	In women: follicle maturation, estrogen production In men: spermatogenesis
Prolactin	Milk production
Antidiuretic hormone (ADH)	Controls plasma osmolality; increases the permeability of the distal renal tubules and collecting ducts, which leads to an increase in water reabsorption
Oxytocin	Contracts the uterus during childbirth and stimulates milk production

Table 6-2 Hormones of the Adrenal Glands

Hormone	Function
Cortisol	Increases metabolic rate, using fat and protein for energy
Aldosterone	Reabsorbs sodium and water from the urine, and excretes excess potassium
Epinephrine/norepinephrine	Stimulates sympathetic nervous system receptors

adrenalin insufficiency is also referred to as Addison disease. Addison disease is a rare condition in which the adrenal glands produce an inadequate amount of adrenal hormones.

Cushing syndrome is hypersecretion of adrenal hormones and is caused by an excess of cortisol production by the adrenal glands or by excessive use of cortisol or other similar steroid hormones.

Neither of these conditions is managed with medications in the prehospital setting. Supportive care and consultation with Medical Direction are usually the most appropriate actions.

Conditions of the Pancreas

The pancreas is the gland that is responsible for secreting insulin. **Insulin** is the essential chemical that makes it possible for the glucose in the bloodstream to enter the cells of the body. Diabetes mellitus (DM) is a chronic endocrine disease caused by a decreased secretion action of the hormone insulin. **Hyperglycemia** is an elevation of the blood glucose level above normal. **Hyperosmolar hyperglycemia nonketotic coma (HHNC)** is insulin deficiency that leads to hyperglycemia without ketones and acidosis. **Diabetic ketoacidosis (DKA)** is a metabolic condition consisting of hyperglycemia, dehydration, and the accumulation of ketones and ketoacids. **Hypoglycemia** is a decrease in the blood glucose level to the point where it results in symptoms that can quickly become life-threatening. Because diabetic patients are often managed in both the prehospital as well as in the in-hospital setting, the entire next section of this text expands on the emergencies that can occur with a diabetic patient and how you should manage them in the field.

Diabetic Patients

When you encounter a patient with diabetes mellitus, you are expected to integrate the pathophysiological principals of this disease with your patient's assessment findings to help formulate a field impression. Once this is done, you should then proceed to implement a treatment plan for the patient having a diabetic emergency. Therefore, it is essential to understand the pathophysiology of the diabetic emergencies such as hypoglycemia, hyperosmolar hyperglycemia nonketotic coma (HHNC), hyperosmolar nonketotic coma (HONK), hyperglycemia, and diabetic ketoacidosis.

A hypoglycemic patient may experience permanent cell damage from remaining unconscious, with an altered LOC, for an extended period of time. Be ready to act quickly.

Diabetes mellitus is a disease with lifelong implications on the health of the patient. There are three forms of the disease that affect the body's ability to balance the carbohydrate needs of the cells with the endocrine hormone insulin. Insulin is manufactured in the pancreas and is responsible for helping carbohydrates in the form of glucose enter the cells (**Figure 6-1 ▸**). It works like the key to your car. Your car may be sitting in the driveway but without the key you simply cannot go any place with the car. Without a sufficient amount of functional insulin available, the glucose in a patient's bloodstream will not enter the cells. Insulin therefore works to keep blood glucose levels at a relatively stable and low level. By promoting carbohydrate metabolism, insulin also blocks fat metabolism, thereby preventing the breakdown of fat tissue in the body. **Glucagon** and epinephrine, so-called "stress hormones," have the opposite effect, resulting in increased circulating blood glucose. Glucagon, a protein hormone produced in the pancreas, stimulates an increase in glucose in the blood by stimulating the breakdown of glycogen to glucose. During a diabetic emergency, glucagon is often administered by a family member SC or IM prior to the arrival of EMS. It works by stimulating the liver to release glycogen stores which in turn results in increased blood glucose levels.

Types of Diabetes Mellitus

As mentioned above, there are three "types" of diabetes: type 1 (commonly referred to as juvenile-onset diabetes), type 2 (commonly referred to as adult-onset diabetes), and gestational diabetes. The type 1 (insulin-dependent DM) diabetic has a pancreas that cannot produce insulin. These patients have to monitor their blood glucose levels very closely throughout the day and inject themselves with insulin. The type 2 diabetic (non-insulin-dependent DM) has a pancreas that produces insulin but that is relatively nonfunctional, resulting in a state of so-called insulin resistance. Also, cell surface insulin receptors in a type 2 diabetic can, over time, develop resistance to one's own insulin, resulting in the progression of non-insulin-dependence. The net effect is the same as in the case of a type 1 patient. Most of the time a patient with type 2 diabetes can control his or her glucose/insulin balance through a combination of oral anti-diabetic medications and an appropriate diet. Many times insulin resistance is a function of advancing age and/or obesity. The patient with gestational diabetes mellitus (GDM) is a pregnant woman who develops all the symptoms of diabetes during pregnancy. In most

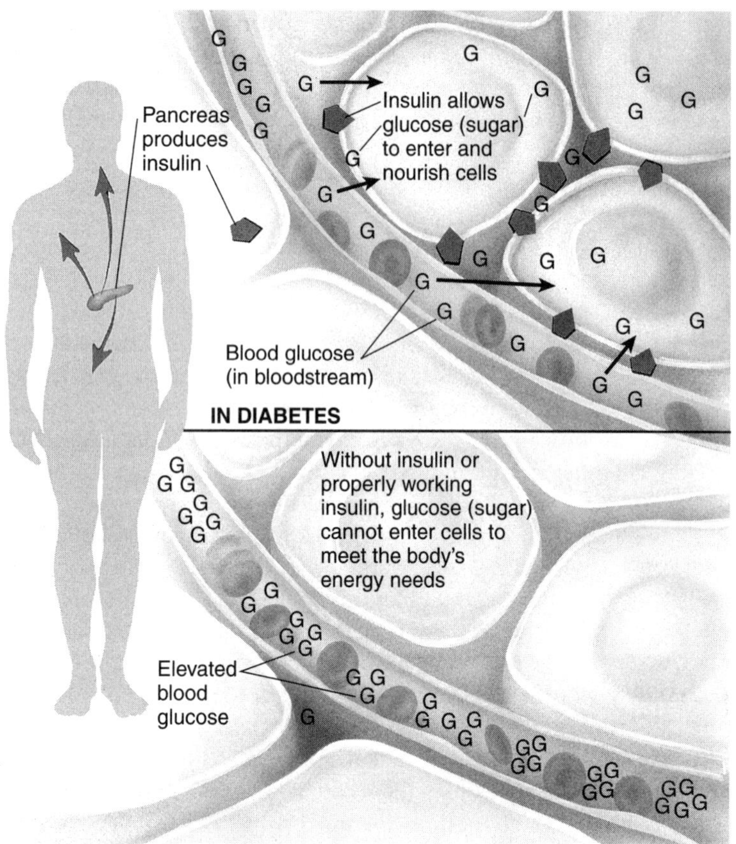

Figure 6-1 Diabetes is defined as a lack of or ineffective action of insulin. Without insulin, cells begin to starve because insulin is needed to allow glucose to enter and nourish the cells.

cases, this resolves itself shortly after the pregnancy. GDM is the inability to process carbohydrates during pregnancy. This produces a high risk pregnancy for both the mother and the fetus, and is also considered a risk factor for the development of type 2 diabetes later in life.

Hyperglycemia and Hypoglycemia

Diabetic emergencies are defined as blood glucose levels that are either too low or too high, and insulin supply is imbalanced relative to carbohydrate demand. A normal blood glucose reading is approximately 70 to 120 mg/dL. The conditions associated with abnormal blood glucose levels include: hypoglycemia, hyperglycemia, diabetic ketoacidosis (DKA), and hyperosmolar hyperglycemic nonketotic coma (HHNC), or hyperosmolar nonketotic coma (HONK). Frequently, mild to moderate hyperglycemia is seen in association with states of physiologic stress such as acute illness or injury.

Hypoglycemia is a state of low blood glucose levels (< 45 mg/dL) with associated clinical symptoms, and is a very common side effect of the treatment for diabetes. It happens when too much insulin is administered, too little food is taken in, or a combination of both occurs. Diabetics can also become hypoglycemic when they do not take in enough carbohydrates for exercise or unplanned activities. The brain's response to hypoperfusion of glucose results in an altered level of consciousness and some patients may also become violent. When hypoglycemia is prolonged, a loss of consciousness results and may lead to permanent brain cell damage or insulin shock.

Hyperglycemia is a state of elevated blood glucose levels (> 120 mg/dL) above the normal range and occurs with or without symptoms. If left untreated, hyperglycemia can progress to diabetic ketoacidosis (DKA). DKA typically involves moderate to severe hyperglycemia, but more specifically is a metabolic condition that also includes fairly profound dehydration and the accumulation of abnormal compounds called ketones and ketoacids. It occurs when a lack of available insulin triggers a change in the body from regular carbohydrate metabolism to fat metabolism, precipitating a dramatic cascade of abnormal physiologic processes. Because glucose must be excreted in the urine in solution, the body loses excess amounts of water and electrolytes (sodium and potassium). When ketoacidosis is not treated adequately, diabetic coma may result. Diabetic coma is a state of unconsciousness, resulting from several problems, including ketoacidosis, dehydration due to excessive urination, and hyperglycemia. Blood glucose levels are often greater than 800 mg/dL when diabetic coma develops.

Hyperosmolar hyperglycemic nonketotic coma (HHNC), or hyperosmolar nonketotic coma (HONK) involves very marked hyperglycemia (often > 1,000 mg/dL), dehydration, and usually coma, and occurs with insulin deficiency but without ketones and acidosis. This occurs principally in patients with type 2 diabetes.

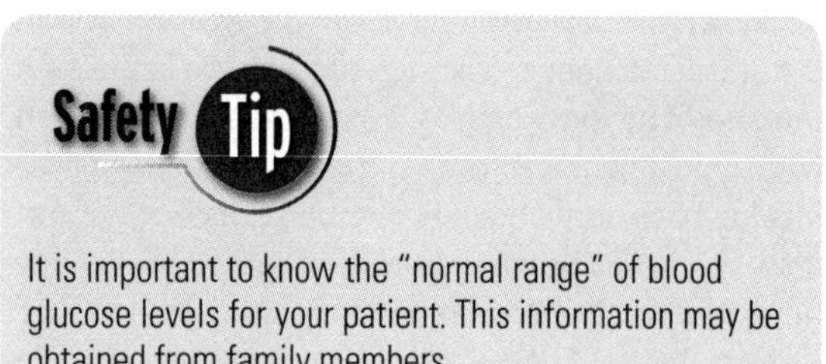

It is important to know the "normal range" of blood glucose levels for your patient. This information may be obtained from family members.

Case Study 1 Hypoglycemia

Part 1

Your unit has been dispatched along with the police to a private residence in the inner city for a combative patient. His wife called 9-1-1 when her 58-year-old husband woke up from a deep sleep and started cursing and flailing his arms. The police arrive moments before you and you find them holding the patient down on the living room floor. The police officers say they have wrestled with this guy before. His wife states that he is an "insulin-dependent" diabetic who skipped his evening snack because he got home late last night from a hockey game. She says that he has gotten this way before and she recognizes the police officers from a previous incident. She says that he is very strong and she cannot control him when he gets this way. Normally she gives him a shot of glucagon [Glucagon] intramuscularly and that works until he eats. Today she has not been able to give him a shot.

You kneel down next to the patient, whose name is Willie McDonald, and quickly begin your initial assessment as your partner pulls out the glucometer and obtains a finger stick blood glucose reading (see **Table 1**).

Table 1 Initial Assessment

Initial Assessment	Recording Time: 2 Minutes
General Impression/ Appearance	Confused, angry, diaphoretic, struggling middle-aged male
Mental Status	"V" verbally responsive with inappropriate statements and slurred speech
Airway	Open and clear
Breathing	Rapid and shallow
Circulation	Rapid and strong radial pulse
Priority/Plan	High priority

Question 1: What did Mr. McDonald's wife mean when she said he was an "insulin-dependent" diabetic?

Question 2: Why is glucagon [Glucagon] administered and how does it work?

Part 2

Based on the information you have about Mr. McDonald at this point, and seeing no apparent trauma, you decide he is a medical patient who will need a rapid medical assessment since he is not responsive enough to answer most of the OPQRST questions. He presents chiefly with an altered mental status. After completing the initial assessment, you decide to wait on providing supplemental oxygen by nonrebreathing mask because he is so combative. Your partner completes the focused history and physical examination and announces that his blood glucose reading is 35 mg/dL (see **Table 2**).

Table 2 Focused History and Physical Examination

Baseline Vital Signs	Recording Time: 5 Minutes
Skin CTC (color, temperature, condition)	Pale, cool, and clammy
Pulse	100 beats/min regular, and strong
Blood Pressure	146/84 mm Hg
Respirations	26 breaths/min and shallow
Blood glucose level	35 mg/dL

The rapid medical assessment does not reveal any relevant findings when the major body regions (head, neck, chest, abdomen, pelvis, back, buttocks, and four extremities) are examined. His lungs are clear bilaterally and he does have some jugular vein distention due to his screaming and struggling. You decide to hold on the OPQRST questions and proceed with inserting an IV because the patient has a great vein that will be easily accessible provided that the police can continue to hold him down.

Your partner is able to get an 18-gauge IV catheter into a good vein; therefore, you opt to give the patient 25 grams of $D_{50}W$. Dextrose in a 50% solution is highly concentrated and very viscous. Smaller diameter IV lines can result in longer times to push the medication in. Accessing smaller veins to give $D_{50}W$ also increases the chance of infiltrating the medicine into the soft tissues surrounding the vessel, greatly increasing the risk of tissue necrosis. Be sure to use the largest bore IV catheter placed into the best available vein prior to pushing $D_{50}W$. It is always a good idea to check line patency by pulling back slightly on your syringe or lowering the IV fluid bag below the venipuncture site to make sure that blood begins to easily back up into the line. Had it been difficult to find a vein you would have given glucagon IM. While starting the IV, a set of blood tubes are taken so you will have some blood for the ED that is taken prior to $D_{50}W$ administration.

Case Study 1 Continued

Mrs. McDonald states that she doesn't think Mr. McDonald took his insulin yet this morning. His only allergy is to sulfate drugs. As soon as the $D_{50}W$ goes in, Mr. McDonald responds.

Question 3: What is a normal blood glucose level and how does Mr McDonald's blood glucose of 35 mg/dL compare?

Question 4: Why is it so important to have a good vein when administering $D_{50}W$ to the patient?

Part 3

As the $D_{50}W$ goes in, Mr. McDonald starts to calm down. When you ask him appropriate questions to determine his mental status he is now able to state his name and where he is, although he is not yet sure what day of the week it is. He is no longer violent and the police are standing by questioning the wife. It is no longer necessary to restrain the patient. He is a little nauseous and states he might vomit so you grab a small garbage can from the bathroom.

While your partner obtains an updated set of vital signs you complete the SAMPLE history (see **Table 3**).

Treatment Plan

1. Ensure an open and clear airway.
2. Assess ventilations and assist as needed, otherwise administer supplemental oxygen via a nonrebreathing mask.
3. Obtain the blood glucose level using a fingerstick.
4. Start an IV and obtain blood for the ED.
5. Administer 25 g of 50% dextrose ($D_{50}W$) if glucose is below the level specified by protocol (see **Table 4**). This number varies widely from region to region, and should always be considered in the context of the patient's clinical picture.
6. Begin transport to the ED.
7. Obtain a 12-lead ECG (remember diabetics have silent MIs), monitor ECG rhythm, obtain serial vital signs, and reassess the blood glucose level en route to the hospital (see **Table 5** and **Table 6**).
8. If mental status decreases en route, reassess the blood glucose level and consider the need for additional $D_{50}W$.

Table 3 SAMPLE History

SAMPLE History	Comments
Signs/symptoms	Aggressive behavior and altered MS
Allergies	Sulfate drugs
Medications	Insulin NPH, hydroclorathiazide, allopurinol
Pertinent past medical history	Type 1 diabetes, hypertension, gout
Last oral intake	Dinner about 12 to 13 hours ago as he skipped his late night snack
Events leading up to the incident	Upset stomach, missed meal, and has not yet eaten in the morning. He got home late and overslept this morning.

One option sometimes suggested by patients but which should be discouraged is to allow the patient to refuse transport. In the specific case of Mr. McDonald, his wife has difficulty controlling him when his blood glucose level is low; therefore, it would not be a good idea to allow him to sign a refusal of medical aid (RMA). If necessary, you will need to use all of your persuasive powers, your partner's, and if necessary your supervisor's, to convince Mr. McDonald he should be checked out in the ED. If that does not work, usually putting the patient on the telephone with the Medical Control physician convinces the patient to allow transport. If in the case of another patient, you are authorized by Medical Control to allow an RMA, you will need to be sure to accurately document everything that was done and all methods you used to persuade the patient to be transported. You will also need to make sure the entire process is witnessed by a credible nonbiased witness (ie, not your partner).

Mr. McDonald responds well to the treatment. He is alert and oriented and no longer violent. He is also able to reliably take medication by mouth (PO), and has done so in your presence. Therefore, your Medical Control agrees that he is theoretically competent to sign off. However, one concern should be that he is at risk for recurrent hypoglycemia despite the initial PO intake. Fortunately, with all the discussion, he decided to go along with his wife's strong recommendation that he needs to go to the hospital to be checked.

Case Study I Continued

Table 4 50% Dextrose

Do you know?	**Comments**
Right drug? Generic name: [**50% Dextrose**] Trade name: [$D_{50}W$]	This is a carbohydrate hypertonic solution. Also called glucose or d-glucose.
Right patient?	Symptomatic hypoglycemia, unable to tolerate oral carbohydrate (ie, insulin shock, alcoholism).
Right dose?	25 grams IV bolus for the adult patient.
Right route?	IV inserted in a good vein with as large a bore IV catheter as can be accommodated.
Right time?	As soon as possible after obtaining baseline vital signs since brain cells may be dying without adequate glucose perfusion.
Right documentation?	The patient care report should state the glucose level, the amount of $D_{50}W$ administered, and the serial vital signs as well as the patient's response to the medication.
Expected action	The patient's mental status should improve within minutes. Each 100 mL of fluid contains 50 g of dextrose which delivers 3.4 kcal/g. Particularly brittle diabetics may take longer to achieve significant clinical improvement after IV dextrose.
Side effects	Virtually none, provided the $D_{50}W$ is administered in a good vein. Redness or pain may occur at the injection site. If the $D_{50}W$ does leak into the surrounding tissue (extravasation), it is so concentrated it can cause tissue necrosis.
Contraindications	Previous hypersensitivity to dextrose solution. Diabetic coma while patient is hyperglycemic. Intracranial or intraspinal hemorrhage.
Precautions	With patients with suspected stroke, check the glucose level prior to administering $D_{50}W$. In an ischemic stroke it has been shown that increased blood glucose concentrations may worsen cerebral ischemic brain damage and impair recovery.
Pharmacokinetics	Onset 1 minute; duration varies with the severity of hypoglycemia.

Table 5 Glucagon

Do you know?	**Comments**
Right drug? Generic name: [**Glucagon**] Trade name: [Glucagon]	This drug is a pancreatic hormone, insulin antagonist. The generic and trade names are the same for this medication. Considered to have a major role in the maintenance of a normal concentration of glucose in the blood. Glucagon is considered to be the opposing factor to insulin in keeping glucose within its normal range.
Right patient?	The diabetic patient with a suspected or confirmed low blood glucose level. It has also been used for esophagitis since it has a theoretical effect of relaxing esophageal smooth muscle.
Right dose?	0.5 to 1 mg that may be repeated in 7 to 10 minutes. The drug comes in a container of liquid and a container of dry powder which needs to be mixed prior to administration.
Right route?	May be administered IV or IM, and it is likely that family members may have administered the medication to the patient prior to calling EMS.
Right time?	As soon as possible after obtaining baseline vital signs since brain cells may be dying without glucose. Family members are usually told to administer the medication while the patient is still conscious.
Right documentation?	The patient care report should state the glucose level, the amount of glucagon administered, the serial vital signs, and the patient's response to the medication. It may not be possible to get a tube of blood prior to administration of the glucagon because the diabetic may have "tough veins," increasing the time it takes to start an IV. In that case, you should obtain a fingerstick glucose reading.

continues

Case Study 1 Continued

Table 5 Glucagon (*Continued*)

Do you know?	Comments
Expected action	Generally effective for up to 17 minutes. A dose of glucagon stimulates an increase in blood concentration of glucose. This should rapidly improve the patient's mental status.
Side effects	Dizziness, lightheadedness, nausea, vomiting (which are also symptoms of hypoglycemia), and sometimes urticaria.
Contraindications	A known hypersensitivity to glucagon or hyperglycemia.
Precautions	There are none in the prehospital setting.
Pharmacokinetics	Onset 1 minute; duration 9–17 minutes. How fast and how effective this drug is will vary on the amount of the patient's glucose reserves.

Table 6 Insulin

Do you know?	Comments
Right drug? Generic name: [**Insulin**] Trade name: [Humulin, NPH, Novolin R, and many more]	This is an insulin product, also called regular, Lente, Ultralente, Semilente, and zinc suspension.
Right patient?	Type 1 (insulin-dependent DM) and type 2 (non-insulin-dependent DM), ketoacidosis.
Right dose?	Individualized.
Right route?	SC, IV, or nasal.
Right time?	Individually structured with meal and exercise regimen.
Right documentation?	Daily glucose readings and all insulin dosages.
Expected action	Decreases blood glucose.
Side effects	Hypoglycemia, blurred vision, urticaria, swelling, redness at injection site.
Contraindications	Hypersensitivity to protamine.
Precautions	Pregnancy.
Pharmacokinetics	Onset 30–60 min SC, 10–30 IV; peak 2–5 hours SC, 15-30 IV, duration 8–12 hours SC, 30–60 minutes IV.

Due to Mr. McDonald's age and history of hypertension, you elect to obtain a 12-lead ECG en route to the hospital. You remember from paramedic school that diabetics can be prone to so-called silent ischemia, meaning they could experience acute coronary syndrome without the associated chest pains. In this case and fortunately for Mr. McDonald, his 12-lead ECG shows no evidence of an infarct and his condition continues to improve during the ride to the ED.

Question 5: In terms of the emergencies that you have learned can occur with the diabetic patient, what do you suspect was Mr. McDonald's problem today?

Question 6: In some cases after administration of $D_{50}W$ the patient becomes alert and refuses transport to the hospital. What would you do if this occurred in Mr. McDonald's situation?

Case Study I Continued

Part 4

As you load Mr. McDonald into the ambulance he seems to be alert and joking about being so strong. Typically he would not go to the hospital after a hypoglycemic event, but this time is different most likely because of the GI upset. He must have apologized to the police officers at least three times and thanked them for their help. His wife will be following along in her car so they will have a way to get home. She has contacted their private physician and told him they will be going to the Eastside ED for treatment. She has taken all of his medications as well as his logbook that shows his daily glucose tests and insulin shots.

En route to the ED you find out that Mr. McDonald has a nasty left hook as he was an amateur boxer when he was a young man. Fortunately no one got to see that punch in action today! You continue to reassess the patient en route (see **Table 7**).

Question 7: Do all patients with hypoglycemia get violent?

Question 8: How can diabetic patients do a better job of managing their disease?

Table 7 Reassessment and Ongoing Assessment of the Patient

Serial Vital Signs and Relevant Data	Recording Time: 15 Minutes
Skin CTC	Pale, warm, and dry
Pulse	88 beats/min and regular
Blood Pressure	140/80 mm Hg
Respirations	20 breaths/min and regular
Mental Status	Alert (oriented to person, place, and day)
ECG	Normal sinus rhythm
SpO_2	98%
Blood glucose level	190 mg/dL
Lung Sounds	Clear bilaterally
Other (ie, core body temperature)	Normal temperature

Part 5

A trip to the McDonald house for a medical call can be a dangerous situation for the emergency services personnel. Fortunately this does not happen too often. The dispatcher has entered a warning notice in the computer to alert the future crews who are not familiar with Mr. McDonald. There are patients like this in most communities and the paramedics have to come to expect this behavior on occasion. With the obesity epidemic contributing to a rise in the number of diabetic patients, these calls are likely to increase. Be careful of the hypoglycemic diabetic patient. Technologies such as insulin pumps and glucometers are accurate and easy to use, improving the life of the diabetic patient.

In this case, the paramedics listened to the information provided by the patient's wife and with assistance by the police officers, they restrained the patient so IV access could be obtained. The $D_{50}W$ quickly turned an angry, violent combative patient to a big thankful Teddy Bear. With a little convincing, they are able to get Mr. McDonald to the ED where a nurse will spend some time reviewing with him the implications of skipping meals and his disease. A little education at the right time will go a long way in helping him to help himself and avoid further complications of his disease.

Using a Glucometer

Diabetic patients use glucometers to measure the level of glucose in the blood (**Figure 6-2**). The reading is in mg/dL (milligrams of glucose per deciliter of blood).

Follow these steps to use a glucometer (**Skill Drill 6-1**):

1. Take BSI precautions.
2. Obtain a focused history and physical examination, and confirm any patient medication allergies.
3. Follow standing orders, or contact medical control for permission.
4. Prepare the blood glucose meter and supplies (ie, lancet, test strip, adhesive bandage, sharps container, alcohol prep).
5. Cleanse the skin with an alcohol prep. Allow the alcohol to dry before performing the finger stick. It is useful to note that many manufacturers and diabetes educators simply state to "wash your hands, dry, and perform the fingerstick."
6. Use the lancet to perform a finger stick. Wipe away the first drop of blood that appears. Squeeze the finger to get a second drop of blood. The newer devices require less blood.
7. Apply the blood to the test strip. This may be done by holding the strip to the finger to draw the blood into the strip.
8. Dispose of the lancet in a sharps container.
9. Read the blood glucose level displayed on the glucose meter. It may take from 15 to 60 seconds for the device to provide a reading. The newer devices take less time.
10. Assess the puncture site and apply direct pressure or an adhesive bandage to control the bleeding.

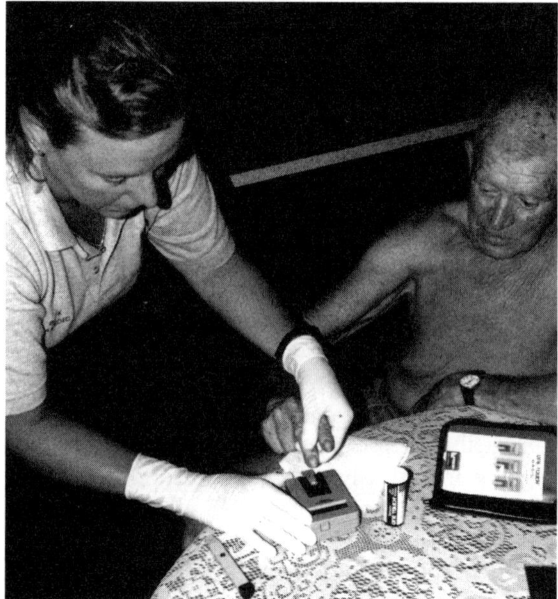

Figure 6-2 A glucometer is a device used by diabetic patients to measure the level of glucose in the blood.

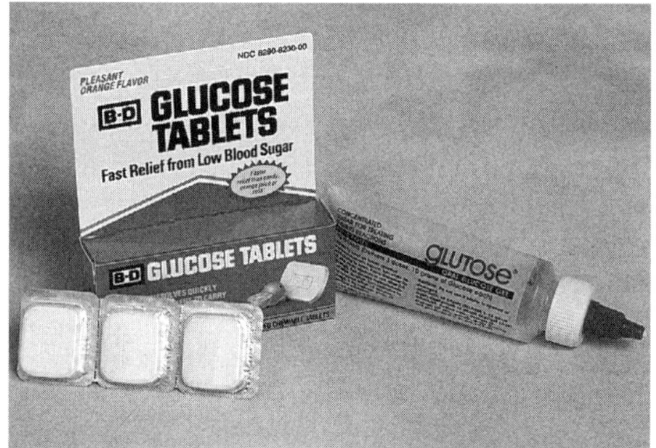

Figure 6-3 Administering glucose is appropriate when the patient is alert enough to eat. Oral glucose gel or glucose tablets may be given to the patient to increase the blood glucose level.

Exercise caution when administering $D_{50}W$ due to its viscosity. The patency of the IV site may be compromised if this drug is given too rapidly.

Oral Glucose Administration

In cases where the patient is alert enough to eat, sweetened drinks, food, oral glucose gel, or glucose tablets may be given to the patient to increase the blood glucose level (**Figure 6-3**).

Increasing the blood glucose level in this way is slower than by the intravenous route, but very effective. Oral glucose gel may be placed under the tongue or in the buccal area of the mouth for the conscious patient. These areas are very vascular and absorb glucose and medications rapidly. Oral medications should never be given to a patient when you are in doubt as to if the patient can protect his or her airway. A good rule of thumb is that if a patient cannot swallow on command, then do not give any substances by mouth until his or her mental status has improved to the point where he/she can follow a simple command. Follow these steps to administer oral glucose

(Skill Drill 6-2 ▼):

1. Take BSI precautions.
2. Obtain a focused history and physical examination, and confirm any patient medication allergies.
3. Follow standing orders, or contact medical control for permission.
4. Examine the tube to ensure that it is not open or broken. Check the expiration date. (**Step 1**)
5. Squeeze a generous amount or the entire tube onto the bottom third of a bite stick or tongue depressor. (**Step 2**)
6. Open the patient's mouth.
7. Place the tongue depressor on the mucous membrane between the cheek and gum, with the gel side next to the cheek. Once the gel is dissolved, or if the patient becomes unresponsive or has a seizure, remove the tongue depressor. (**Step 3**)

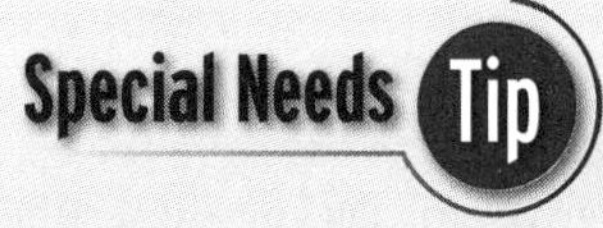

New-onset weakness in a preexisting diabetes patient may be considered an MI until proven otherwise. Remember, due to the incidence of neuropathy in diabetics and elderly patients, "silent" or pain-free MIs often occur.

Skill Drill 6-2 Administering Oral Glucose

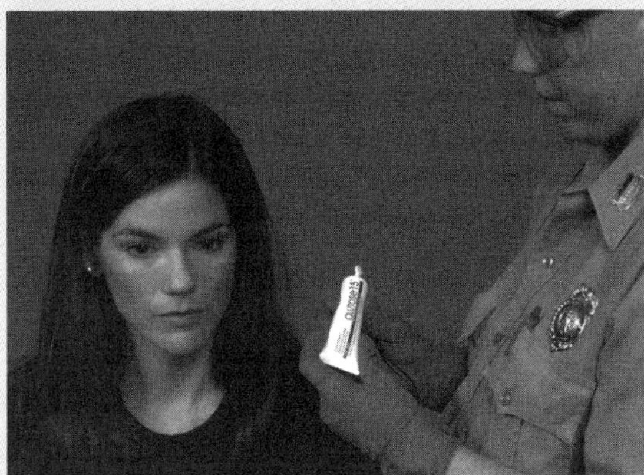

1 Make sure the tube of glucose is intact and has not expired.

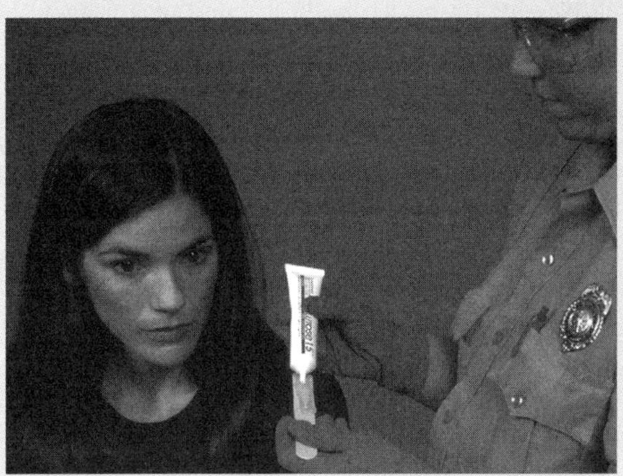

2 Squeeze the entire tube of oral glucose onto the bottom third of a bite stick or tongue depressor.

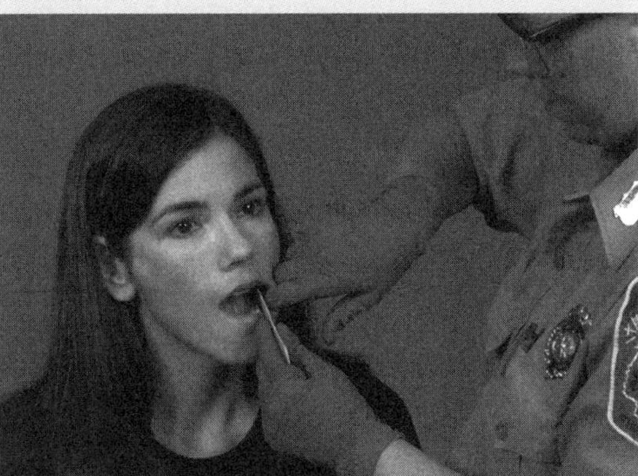

3 Open the patient's mouth. Place the tongue depressor on the mucous membranes between the cheek and the gum with the gel side next to the cheek.

Physiology of Glucagon

Glucagon is a drug that activates two key metabolic processes in the liver: the breakdown of glycogen stored in the liver and **gluconeogenesis**. Gluconeogenesis is the formation of glucose by the liver and kidneys from substances other than carbohydrates (ie, fats or proteins). These two effects stimulate release of glucose to the rest of the body. During periods when blood glucose is high, the liver stores large amounts of sugar. Insulin pressures the liver to store the extra sugar in the form of glycogen. During those times of low blood sugar, glucagon is secreted to act on the hepatocytes. These in turn activate the enzymes designed to depolymerize the stored glycogen and release glucose into the bloodstream. Non-hexose substrates (ie, amino acids) are converted to glucose by a process called gluconeogenesis, thus providing a second source of glucose for the blood.

Release of glucagon can also be triggered by elevated blood levels of amino acids as well as exercise (or possibly the exercise depletion of glucose). Some patients do not typically respond to glucagon (ie, indigent, malnourished, or alcoholic patients and patients that had hypoglycemia reversed by glucagon in the past 2 days).

Insulin

Insulin is required to move glucose from the blood into other body tissues where it is needed. In addition, insulin helps the body to metabolize carbohydrates, fats, and proteins from the diet. Insulin controls, but does not cure DM and must be taken regularly. Over time people with poorly controlled diabetes develop serious nerve, blood vessel, kidney, and vision problems. The amount of insulin needed depends on underlying physiology, as well as diet, exercise, and concurrent diseases, and other medication being taken. The required dose may change with time. Diabetic patients should be instructed to maintain a logbook that contains their daily activities, the food they eat, blood glucose testing results, and insulin taken. When they eat something out of the ordinary that has extra sugar or carbohydrates, they need to accommodate for the food with additional insulin. The same holds true for extraordinary physical activity or sickness. During your assessment, inquire if the patient has a log because it can give you clues as to how closely the patient has been monitoring his or her condition and how much insulin is being taken.

Insulin is classified by its source (which may be one of three): either beef or pork intestines and synthesized (manmade) insulin from human DNA. Insulin preparations are also classified as regular (natural) or modified and differ in their onset of action and the duration they last. Regular insulin is used as insulin would occur naturally. The modified preparations have been developed with additives that produce differing times of absorption and therefore different times of onset, peak activity, and duration of action. These modified preparations are classified as short-acting, intermediate-acting, and long-acting preparations. Rapid onset and short-acting insulin preparations, such as regular insulin and lispro [Humalog], start to work in 15 to 30 minutes, peak within an hour, and are used up within about 4 to 6 hours. There are intermediate preparations like NPH and lente insulins, and slow onset, long-acting insulins, such as Ultralente and glargine [Lantus]; these preparations start to work in 2 to 8 hours and continue working for 24 to 36 hours. All insulin bottles are marked to indicate the type of insulin they contain as well as the strength in units (U). There are two different strengths of insulin: U-100 and U-500. U-100 syringes must be used with U-100 insulin, and different syringes must be used with U-500 insulin.

Insulin cannot be taken orally because stomach enzymes would deactivate it before it could take effect. Regular insulin may be administered IV or SC, while modified insulin is administered SC. Traditionally, the user draws up insulin from a vial into an insulin syringe and self-injects the medication either on a scheduled basis or in response to a fingerstick. Prefilled or refillable insulin-containing pens for personal insulin use now exist and are increasingly popular. An inhaled form of insulin is now available as well. Insulin inhalation is used to treat type 1 and type 2 diabetes. Insulin inhalation is a short-acting, synthesized version of human insulin that starts to work within 10 to 20 minutes after it is inhaled and continues to work for about 6 hours. Insulin inhalation comes as a powder to inhale by mouth using a specially designed inhaler. It is usually taken immediately before meals (within 10 minutes before eating). The primary side effect of any type of insulin is hypoglycemia.

Insulin Pumps

External insulin pumps have made it possible to deliver more precise amounts of insulin than can be injected using a syringe. Tighter control over glucose levels helps to reduce the chance of long-term complications associated with diabetes. This is also referred to as continuous subcutaneous insulin infusion therapy. The use of rapid-acting insulin through the pump offers more freedom from the tightly controlled meal and exercise schedule that patients needed to follow to control blood glucose with the slow-acting form of insulin.

The pump delivers insulin through narrow, flexible plastic tubing that ends with a needle inserted just under the skin near the abdomen. The insulin pump is about the size of a deck of cards, weighs about 3 ounces, and can be worn on a belt or carried in a pocket. Modern technology has advanced the insulin pump by incorporating features such as integration with blood glucose meters, bolus calculators, touch bolus, custom alarms, personal computer interface, remote control, and more. Many users feel the pump is more convenient and discrete compared to injection. However, frequent blood glucose monitoring is necessary to determine insulin dosages and to ensure that insulin is delivered. Diabetics with insulin pumps only use short-acting insulin, so they may be at greater risk of DKA or hyperglycemia quicker than patients without pumps since they have no intermediate or long-acting insulin coverage (on board in their system).

Type 2 Oral Hypoglycemic Agents

A large number of oral hypoglycemic agents currently exist and work in a variety of ways. Some help to lower the blood glucose by helping the pancreas make more insulin, others work by decreasing the amount of glucose the liver produces, and others work by making the cells more sensitive to insulin. Some of the agents work rapidly, while others have a delayed or extended release in which plasma drug concentrations gradually rise reaching maximum concentrations within 6 to 12 hours after administration. Also available are combined medicines such as Glucovance which is glyburide and metformin. These oral agents may also be used in combination with insulin at various times when type 2 diabetics do not respond to diet management and exercise alone. Currently there are five classes of hypoglycemic agents (**Table 6-3**▼).

Examples of Oral Hypoglycemic Agents

Acarbose—class I
Glimepiride—class I
Glipizide—class I
Glyburide—class I
Metformin hydrochloride—class II
Miglitol—class III
Nateglinide—class V
Pioglitazone hydrochloride—class IV
Repaglinide—class V
Rosiglitazone maleate—class IV
Tolazamide—class I
Tolbutamide—class I
Tolbutamide sodium—class I

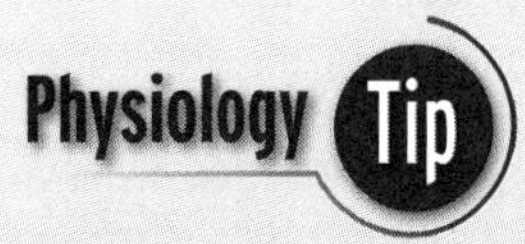

Glucose metabolism may also be affected by illness, alcohol consumption, drug interactions, steroids, and aerobic activity.

Table 6-3 Classes of Hypoglycemic Agents

Class	Medication	Actions
I	**Sulfonylureas**	Help the body increase insulin production.
II	**Biguanides**	Help the body use insulin better by decreasing glucose synthesis and increasing glucose uptake.
III	**Alpha-glucosidase inhibitors**	Slows the intestinal breakdown of carbohydrates which results in lower glucose levels.
IV	**Thiazolinediones**	Help the body use insulin more efficiently which results in more efficient glucose utilization, with less residual glucose available to be converted to fat.
V	**Meglitinides**	Stimulate pancreatic insulin production similar to sulfonylureas but in a short-acting version.

Case Study ANSWERS

Case Study 1 Hypoglycemia

Question 1: What did Mr. McDonald's wife mean when she said he was an "insulin-dependent" diabetic?

Answer 1: Being termed an insulin-dependent diabetic means that Mr. McDonald needs insulin injections to survive. Most likely his pancreas is no longer able to manufacture insulin so the glucose in his bloodstream will not enter the cells of his body without the aid of insulin injections.

Question 2: Why is glucagon [Glucagon] administered and how does it work?

Answer 2: Glucagon is often administered by the family member SC or IM prior to the arrival of EMS. It works by stimulating the liver to release glycogen stores that, in turn, results in increased blood glucose levels.

Question 3: What is a normal blood glucose level and how does Mr. McDonald's glucose of 35 mg/dL compare?

Answer 3: Normal "fasting" blood glucose values (not eating for 8 hours) are less than 100 mg/dL. If the patient has a value of less than 80 mg/dL and is symptomatic, as in Mr. McDonald's case, treatment should be provided following local medical control.

Question 4: Why is it so important to have a good vein when administering $D_{50}W$ to the patient?

Answer 4: Dextrose in a 50% solution is highly concentrated and very viscous. Smaller diameter IV lines can result in longer times to push the medication in. Accessing smaller veins to administer $D_{50}W$ through also increases the chances of infiltrating the medicine into the soft tissues surrounding the vessel, greatly increasing the risk of tissue necrosis. Be sure to use the largest bore IV catheter placed into the best available vein prior to pushing $D_{50}W$. It is always a good idea to check line patency by pulling back slightly on your syringe or lowering the IV fluid bag below the venipuncture site to make sure that blood begins to flow easily back up into the line.

Question 5: In terms of the emergencies that you have learned can occur in the diabetic patient, what do you suspect was Mr. McDonald's problem today?

Answer 5: Mr. McDonald most likely has hypoglycemia. This was confirmed by his blood glucose test that revealed a level of 35 mg/dL.

Question 6: In some cases after administration of $D_{50}W$, the patient becomes alert and refuses transport to the hospital. What would you do if this occurred in Mr. McDonald's situation?

Answer 6: Since Mr. McDonald's wife has trouble controlling him when he gets a low reading, it is not a good idea to let him sign a refusal of medical aid (RMA). You should use all of your persuasive powers, your partner's and, if necessary, your supervisor's to convince Mr. McDonald he should be checked out in the ED. If that does not work, usually putting the patient on the telephone with the Medical Control physician convinces the patient to allow transport. If authorized to allow an RMA, which would not be the case in Mr. McDonald's situation, the paramedic should be sure to accurately document everything that was done and all the methods that were used to persuade the patient to be transported. Also make sure this is witnessed by a credible nonbiased witness (ie, not your partner).

Fortunately, Mr. McDonald is better after your treatment. He is alert and oriented × 3 and no longer violent. He is able to reliably take medication by mouth (PO), and has done so in your presence. However, one concern should be is if he is on oral agents, he is at risk for recurrent hypoglycemia despite the initial PO intake. Mr. McDonald is competent to sign off, with approval from Medical Control. However, in the midst of all the discussion, Mr. McDonald's wife convinced him that it was necessary to go to the hospital to get checked.

Case Study ANSWERS

Question 7: Do all patients with hypoglycemia get violent?

Answer 7: No! It is best to think of it as how your friends react to over-imbibing alcohol. Some get quiet and giddy, some get obnoxious and argumentative, some become the life of the party, and some pass out when they have too much to drink. In the past, diabetics were often confused with intoxicated individuals because of similar behaviors and it was not uncommon for a diabetic found in a public place to be thrown in a jail cell to sleep it off. Of course many of them simply got worse and some actually died. Most communities deal with possibly intoxicated individuals from a medical perspective first and then later on from an enforcement point of view.

Question 8: How can diabetic patients do a better job of managing their disease?

Answer 8: Diabetics should log their daily activities, the foods they eat, and the results of their blood glucose testing. When they eat something out of the ordinary that has extra sugar or carbohydrates, they need to accommodate for the food with additional insulin. The same holds true for extraordinary physical activity or sickness.

Medication Review

Dextrose

Indications Hypoglycemia, altered level of consciousness, coma of unknown etiology, seizure of unknown etiology, status epilepticus.

Contraindications Intracranial hemorrhage.

Dosage and administration Adult: 12.5–25 g slow IV; may be repeated as necessary. Pediatric: 0.5–1 g/kg/dose slow IV; may be repeated as necessary.

Glucagon

Indications Altered level of consciousness when hypoglycemia is suspected. May be used as inotropic agent in beta-blocker overdose.

Contraindications Hyperglycemia, hypersensitivity.

Dosage and administration Adult: Hypoglycemia: 0.5–1 mg IM; may repeat in 7–10 minutes. Calcium channel blocker or beta-blocker overdose: 3 mg initially, followed by infusion at 3 mg/hr as necessary. Pediatric: Hypoglycemia: 0.5–1 mg IM (for children < 20 kg). Calcium channel blocker or beta-blocker overdose: not recommended.

Naloxone Hydrochloride (Narcan)

Indications Opiate overdose, coma; complete or partial reversal of CNS and respiratory depression induced by opioids; decreased level of consciousness; coma of unknown origin; narcotic agonist for the following: morphine, heroin, hydromorphone (Dilaudid), methadone, meperidine (Demerol), paregoric, fentanyl citrate (Sublimase), oxycodone (Percodan), codeine, propoxyphene (Darvon); narcotic agonist and antagonist for the following: Butorphanol (Stadol), pentazocine (Talwin), nalbuphine (Nubain).

Contraindications Use with caution in narcotic-dependent patients; use with caution in neonates of narcotic-addicted mothers.

Dosage and administration Adult: 0.4–2.0 mg IV, IM, SC, or ET (diluted); minimum recommended dose, 0.4 mg; repeat at 5-minute intervals to a maximum dose of 10 mg (medical control may request higher amounts). Infusion: 2 mg in 500 mL of D_5W (4 µg/mL), infuse at 0.4 mg/h (100 mL/h). Pediatric: 0.1 mg/kg/dose IV, IM, SC, ET (diluted); maximum dose of 0.8 mg; if no response in 10 minutes, administer an additional 0.1 mg/kg/dose.

Medication Review

Oral Glucose (Insta-Glucose)

Indications Conscious patients with suspected hypoglycemia.

Contraindications Decreased level of consciousness, nausea, vomiting.

Dosage and administration Adult: Should be sipped slowly by patient until clinical improvement noted. Pediatric: Same as adult.

Oxygen

Indications Confirmed or expected hypoxemia, ischemic chest pain, respiratory insufficiency, prophylactically during air transport, confirmed or suspected carbon monoxide poisoning, all other causes of decreased tissue oxygenation, decreased level of consciousness.

Contraindications Certain patients with COPD or emphysema who will not tolerate oxygen concentrations over 35%, hyperventilation. Oxygen should never be withheld from a patient who needs it, however. Be prepared to assist with ventilations in a patient with COPD who requires high concentration, as apnea may result.

Dosage and administration Adult: Cardiac arrest and carbon monoxide poisoning: 100%. Hypoxemia: 10–15 L/min via nonrebreathing mask. COPD: 1–6 L/min via nasal cannula or 28%–35% Venturi mask. Be prepared to provide ventilatory support if higher concentrations of oxygen needed. Pediatric: Same as for adult with exception of premature infant.

Thiamine Hydrochloride (Vitamin B-1)

Indications Coma of unknown origin, delirium tremens, beriberi, Wernicke's encephalopathy.

Contraindications None.

Dosage and administration Adult: 100 mg slow IV or IM. Pediatric: 10–25 mg slow IV or IM.

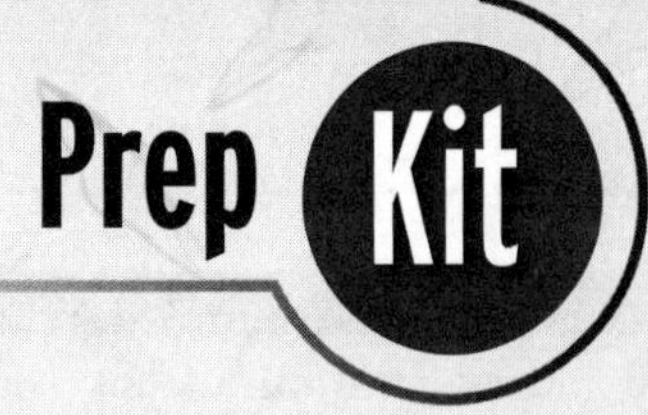

Chapter Summary

- Endocrine diseases can affect hormone production resulting in levels that are too high or too low.
- The most common emergencies associated with the endocrine system are diabetic problems.
- Diabetes mellitus is a chronic endocrine disease caused by a decreased secretion action of the hormone insulin.
- Hyperthyroidism is a condition of an overactive thyroid resulting in the release of too many thyroid hormones.
- Hypothyroidism is a condition of an underactive thyroid and is far more common than hyperthyroidism.
- The pituitary glands secrete hormones. The adrenal glands produce hormones.
- A normal blood glucose reading is approximately 70 to 120 mg/dL.
- Hyperglycemia is an elevation of the blood glucose level above 120 mg/dL.
- Hyperosmolar hyperglycemia nonketotic coma (HHNC) is insulin deficiency that leads to hyperglycemia without ketones and acidosis (often > 1,000 mg/dL).
- If left untreated, hyperglycemia can progress to diabetic ketoacidosis (DKA). Diabetic ketoacidosis (DKA) is a metabolic condition consisting of hyperglycemia, dehydration, and the accumulation of ketones and ketoacids.
- When diabetic ketoacidosis is not treated adequately, diabetic coma may result. Diabetic coma is a state of unconsciousness, resulting from several problems, including ketoacidosis, dehydration due to excessive urination, and hyperglycemia (> 800 mg/dL).
- Hypoglycemia is a decrease in the blood glucose level to the point where it results in symptoms that can quickly become life-threatening (< 45 mg/dL).
- The type 1 (insulin-dependent) diabetic has a pancreas that cannot produce insulin. These patients have to monitor their blood glucose levels very closely throughout the day and inject themselves with insulin.
- The type 2 (non-insulin-dependent) diabetic has a pancreas that produces insulin but that is relatively nonfunctional, resulting in a state of so-called insulin resistance.
- In cases where the patient is alert enough to eat, sweetened drinks, food, oral glucose gel, or glucose tablets may be given to the patient to raise the blood glucose level.
- Glucagon stimulates the breakdown of glycogen to glucose.
- Oral hypoglycemic agents may be used in combination with insulin at various times when type 2 diabetics do not respond to diet management and exercise alone.

Vital Vocabulary

Alpha-glucosidase inhibitors A hypoglycemic agent that slows the intestinal breakdown of carbohyhdrates which results in lower glucose.

Biguanides A hypoglycemic agent that helps the body use insulin better by decreasing glucose synthesis and increasing glucose uptake.

Diabetic ketoacidosis (DKA) A metabolic condition that includes hyperglycemia, dehydration, and the accumulation of abnormal compounds called ketones and ketoacids.

Glucagon A hormone that increases blood glucose levels.

Gluconeogenesis The formation of glucose by the liver and kidneys from substances other than carbohydrates (ie, fats or proteins).

Hyperthyroidism A condition of an overactive thyroid resulting in the release of too many thyroid hormones.

Hypothyroidism A condition of an underactive thyroid. This is far more common than hyperthyroidism.

Hyperglycemia A state of elevated blood glucose levels above the normal range. It occurs with or without symptoms.

Hypoglycemia A state of low blood glucose levels. It is the most common side effect of the treatment for diabetes.

Hyperosmolar hyperglycemia nonketotic coma (HHNC) A condition of hyperglycemia, dehydration, and coma, without ketosis and acidosis.

Insulin A hormone produced in the pancreas required to move glucose from the blood into other body tissues where it is metabolized into energy.

Meglitinides A hypoglycemic agent that stimulates pancreatic insulin production similar to sulfonylureas but in a short-acting version.

Sulfonylureas A hypoglycemic agent that helps the body increase insulin production.

Thiazolinediones A class of oral hypoglycemic agents that enhance insulin sensitivity in the peripheral tissues.

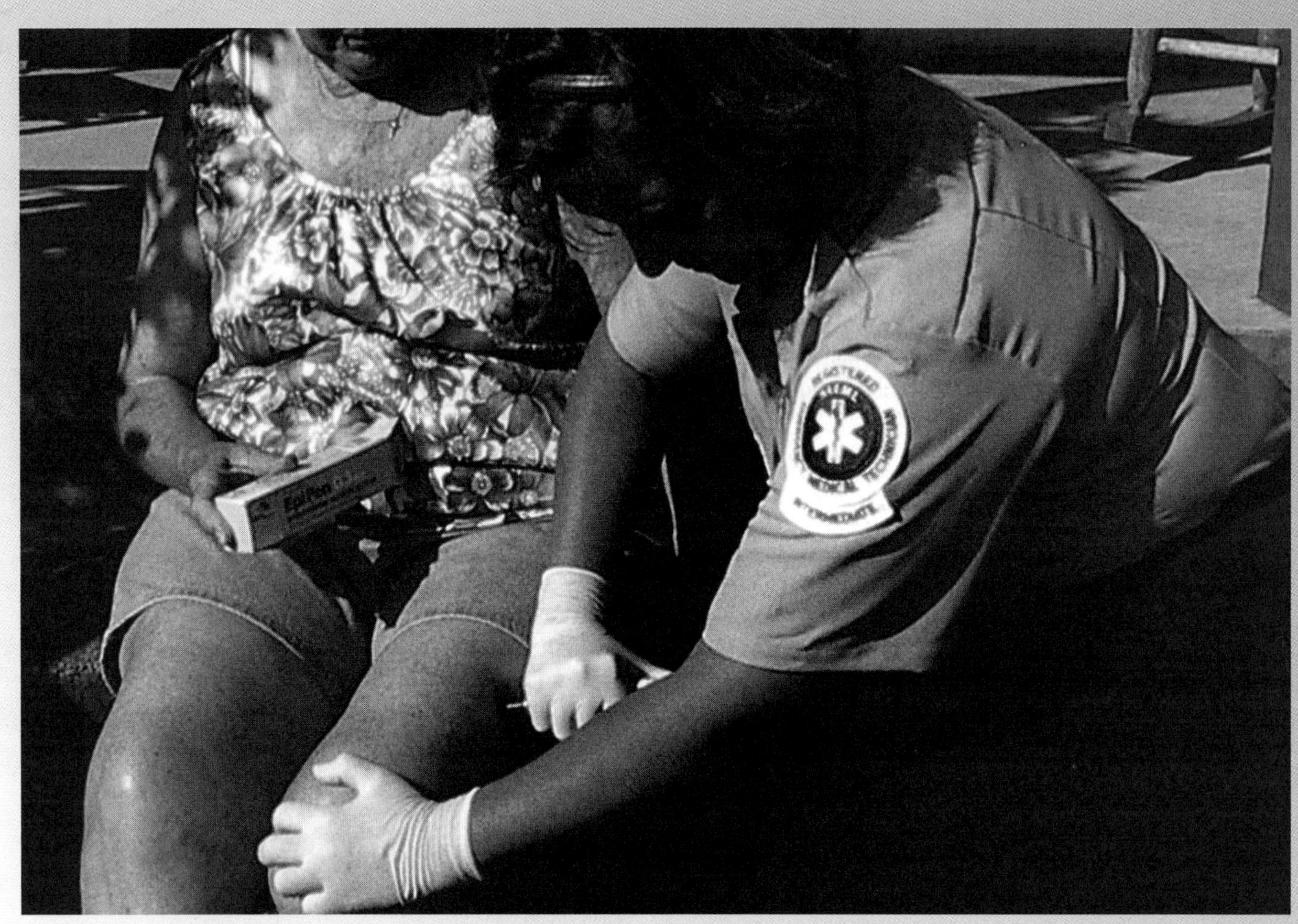
EpiPen
REGISTERED
MEDICAL TECHNICIAN
INTERMEDIATE

Allergic and Anaphylactic Emergencies 7

Objectives

Cognitive

5-5.16 Differentiate among the various treatment and pharmacological interventions used in the management of anaphylaxis. (pages 246–251)

Affective

None

Psychomotor

None

Additional Objectives

7-1 Discuss the following medications used in the prehospital and/or in-hospital setting for the patient experiencing an allergic reaction: epinephrine [Adrenalin], diphenhydramine [Benadryl], albuterol [Proventil], ipratropium bromide [Atrovent], dopamine [Intropin], methylprednisolone sodium succinate [Solu-Medrol], epinephrine infusion. (pages 246–251)

7-2 Discuss the medication Cimetidine [Tagamet] and its extensive drug interaction list. (pages 243–245)

7-3 Discuss and demonstrate the use of the EpiPen. (page 252)

Mild and Severe Reactions

Assessment of the patient having an **allergic reaction** will reveal various signs and symptoms from mild to severe and life-threatening such as bronchospasm, vasoconstriction, decreased cardiac output, decreased coronary flow, vasodilation, leaky blood vessels, pruritis, urticaria, and edema (**Figure 7-1** ▾).

Signs that indicate that a patient may be experiencing a mild allergic reaction include localized itching or swelling, redness, or rash. The key signs that can indicate a patient may be having a severe reaction, or an **anaphylactic reaction**, would be altered mental status, respiratory distress often involving airway swelling, wheezing and chest tightness, and/or hypoperfusion.

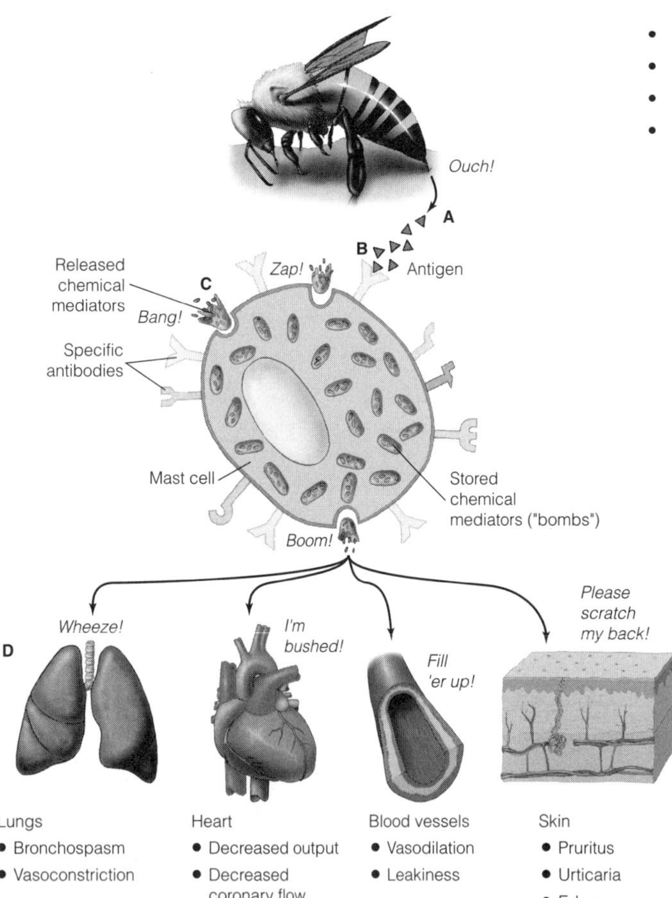

Figure 7-1 The sequence of events in anaphylaxis. A. The antigen is introduced into the body. B. The antigen-antibody reaction at the surface of a mast cell. C. Release of mast cell chemical mediators. D. Chemical mediators exert their effects on end organs.

Mild Reactions

- Local swelling (**angioedema**)
- Local itching (pruritus)
- Local redness or rash

Severe Reactions

- Swelling of lips, tongue, or throat
- Tachypnea
- Difficulty breathing
- Stridor
- Wheezing
- Chest tightness
- Faintness
- Dizziness
- Confusion
- Rapid heartbeat
- Pruritus
- Hives (urticaria)
- Local or systemic angioedema (swelling produced when plasma escapes into the tissues)
- Diaphoresis
- Pallor or cyanosis
- Nausea, cramps, diarrhea, and vomiting
- Hypotension

Pathophysiology of Allergic Reaction

An **antigen** is a substance (including environmental and manufactured substances, pollen, drugs, food, and substances injected during insect stings and insect or other bites) that produces an immune response. **Antibodies** are formed in response to the presence of an antigen to destroy or neutralize the antigen. All antibodies are **immunoglobulins**, a family of proteins with specific functions in the immune system. Approximately 50% of patients with allergies have increased levels of **immunoglobulin E (IgE)**. IgE attaches to **mast cells** in the respiratory and gastrointestinal (GI) tracts and has a significant role in **histamine** release from mast cells. Histamine release by mast cells produces several major effects: (1) severe constriction of the bronchioles (bronchoconstriction), (2) increased tracheobronchial mucus production, (3) widespread dilation of blood vessels in the skin and other tissues, and (4) markedly increased capillary permeability (hypoperfusion and hypotension).

Ensure that the patient has been removed from the suspected source of the antigen.

Each allergic reaction is different and may affect one or more body systems (such as the nervous system, respiratory system, cardiovascular system, skin, and the GI tract), and not every reaction produces all events described or progresses to anaphylaxis, an extreme systemic form of an allergic reaction involving two or more body systems. Subsequent reactions have the potential to be worse than the previous reaction to the particular antigen. Your assessment should always include asking about the severity of the previous reaction. Anaphylactic shock involves any of the signs and symptoms of anaphylaxis and the presence of shock.

When anaphylaxis develops, rapid measures must be taken to reverse the effects or death will occur. The primary treatment in anaphylaxis is the injection of the hormone epinephrine [Adrenalin], which is a potent, rapid-acting bronchodilator and vasoconstrictor. In addition, intravenous (IV) fluids and IV drip medications such as dopamine [Intropin] and epinephrine [Epinephrine] may be helpful for hypotension that does not respond to the initial dose of epinephrine [Epinephrine]. Adjunctive antihistamine medications such as diphenhydramine [Benadryl] are also very useful, as are oxygen supplementation and inhaled bronchodilators. Corticosteroids such as methylprednisolone sodium succinate [Solu-Medrol] are potent anti-inflammatories and ultimately terminate the anaphylactic process. Because corticosteroids require a variable amount of time to begin working and come to full effect, the sooner they are given to a patient with anaphylaxis, the sooner the patient will recover.

Adverse Reactions

Paramedics are often called to the home of a patient who recently started taking a new medication. Not all reactions to medication are full blown anaphylaxis. In some cases the patient may experience an unusual effect or an interaction of the medication with another substance or medication he or she is taking. In this section we will review an example of an adverse reaction to a commonly taken home medication. Since it is not possible to describe all the adverse reactions that may occur, as would be described on the warning labels and in the drug resources, this discussion should serve as an example.

Adverse Reaction to Cimetidine [Tagamet]

One medication you often find patients taking when obtaining the SAMPLE history is cimetidine [Tagamet]. Cimetidine [Tagamet] is a prescribed and an over-the-counter (OTC) medication used by patients for the short-term treatment of active duodenal ulcers and benign gastric ulcers. It also may be prescribed for long-term prophylaxis of GI disorders and their symptoms (such as duodenal ulcer, gastric hypersecretory states, gastroesophageal reflux, and upper GI bleeding in critically ill patients). The OTC preparation of cimetidine [Tagamet] is used for the prevention or relief of heartburn, acid indigestion, and "sour stomach."

This medication works by competitive inhibition of histamine at the H2 receptors of the gastric parietal cells, which results in reduced gastric acid secretion, gastric volume, and hydrogen ion concentration (remember the pH is inversely proportional to the H+ concentration). Adverse reactions occur with cimetidine [Tagamet] in 1% to 10% of patients. Typically, the central nervous system symptoms include dizziness, agitation, headache, and drowsiness. The GI symptoms include diarrhea, nausea, and vomiting. Fewer than 1% of patients experiencing an adverse reaction to cimetidine [Tagamet] have been know to have bradycardia, hypotension, tachycardia, confusion, fever, rash, gynecomastia, edema of the breasts, decreased sexual ability, neutropenia, agranulocytosis, thrombocytopenia, myalgia, or an elevated creatinine level.

Be extra alert when cimetidine [Tagamet] is one of your patient's medications and the patient is exhibiting symptoms. The drug has an extensive drug interaction list, particularly with antiarrhythmics (ie, amiodarone, lidocaine, phenytoin, procainamide hydrochloride, and quinidine) and may also increase the likelihood of toxic effects from theophylline and cyclosporine (**Table 7-1 ▸**). Because of inhibition of warfarin

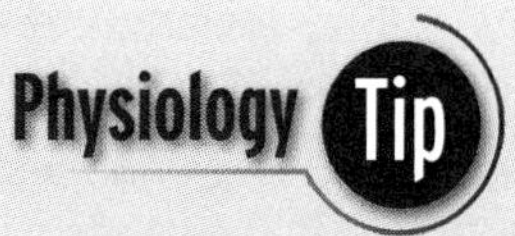

IV fluid therapy can be very helpful in treating hypotension in a patient experiencing an allergic reaction.

Table 7-1 Cimetidine [Tagamet] Drug Interaction Examples

Medication	Interaction with Cimetidine [Tagamet] Examples (The physician should consider an alternative drug or monitor for toxicity!)
Alfentanil	Increased serum concentration
Amiodarone	Increased serum concentration
Benzodiazepines	Increased serum concentration (except with lorazepam, oxazepam, and temazepam)
Beta-blockers	Effects may be increased (except with atenolol, betaxolol, bisoprolol, nadolol, penbutolol)
Calcium channel blockers	Increased serum concentration
Carbamazepine	Possible transient (1 wk) increase in plasma concentration
Carmustine	Increased myelotoxic effects
Cefpodoxime	Oral absorption possibly reduced by increased pH
Cisapride	Increased bioavailability
Citalopram	Increased serum concentration; use of alternative H_2 antagonist or adjustment of citalopram dose recommended
Cyclosporine	Increased serum concentration
CYP1A2* substrates (ie, aminophylline, fluvoxamine, mexiletine, mirtazapine, ropinirole, theophylline, and trifluoperazine)	May increase the levels and effects of CYP1A2 substrates
CYP2C19* substrates (ie, citalopram, diazepam, methsuximide, phenytoin, propranolol, and sertraline)	May increase the levels and effects of CYP2C19 substrates
CYP2D6* substrates (ie, amphetamines, selected beta-blockers, dextromethorphan, fluoxetine, lidocaine, mirtazapine, nefazodone, paroxetine, risperidone, ritonavir, thioridazine, tricyclic antidepressants, and venlafaxine)	May increase the levels and effects of CYP2D6 substrates
CYP2D6* prodrug substrates (ie, codeine, hydrocodone, oxycodone, and tramadol)	May decrease the levels and effects of CYP2D6 prodrug substrates
CYP3A4* substrates (ie, benzodiazepines, calcium channel blockers, cyclosporine, mirtazapine, nateglinide, nefazodone, sildenafil (and other phosphodiesterase inhibitors), tacrolimus, and venlafaxine)	May increase the levels and effects of CYP3A4 substrates; selected benzodiazepines (midazolam and triazolam), cisapride, ergot alkaloids, selected 3-hydroxy-3-methylglutaryl coenzyme A reductase inhibitors (lovastatin and simvastatin), and pimozide are generally contraindicated with strong CYP3A4 inhibitors
Delavirdine	Decreased absorption
Flecainide	Increased serum concentration (especially in patients with renal failure)
Ketoconazole, fluconazole, itraconazole (especially capsule form)	Decreased serum concentration
Lidocaine	Increased serum concentration
Melphalan	Decreased serum concentration
Meperidine	Increased serum concentration
Moricizine	Increased serum concentration
Paroxetine	Increased serum concentration
Phenytoin	Toxic effects; avoid concurrent use
Propafenone	Increased serum concentration
Quinolone	Possible decreased renal elimination of quinolone antibiotics
Tacrine	Increased plasma concentration
Theophylline	Increased serum concentration
Warfarin	Increased international normalized ratio; cimetidine effect is dose-related

*These substances are enzymes in the cytochrome P-450 family that are responsible for catalyzing the chemical reactions of drugs in the body.

metabolism, cimetidine may increase the international normalized ratio (INR) in patients receiving anticoagulation therapy.

Treating Allergies

Patients with known allergies are treated in three ways. First, they are educated about how to avoid exposure. Second, they may be given a variety of medications to use at home, including oral and intranasal antihistamines, inhaled bronchodilators, and inhaled or intranasal steroids. When there is a potential for a severe reaction, an epinephrine self-injection kit [AnaKit] or auto-injector [EpiPen] is prescribed, and the patient is trained in how and when to use it. Even children have been trained and may carry the pediatric dose of epinephrine [Adrenalin] (see Appendix C for more information). Third, immunotherapy via **desensitization** is an excellent treatment option for some patients. In desensitization, patients undergo a series of injections designed to desensitize them to a given set of antigens by gradually increasing the amount of the offending allergen the body receives so that the immune system can learn to defend itself against the specific allergen.

The common causes of anaphylactic reactions include animals (ie, cats and dogs), insect stings (ie, bees, hornets, wasps, and fire ants), foods (ie, peanuts, milk, soy, and shellfish), latex (ie, gloves and other supplies), immunotherapy (such as in skin testing), and drugs. The following illustrates the specific antigens and examples of various drugs that often result in allergies (**Table 7-2**▼).

Consider the allergen that has caused the patient's illness, especially if by contact and *if* you have a similar allergy.

Table 7-2 Drugs that Cause Anaphylaxis in Some Patients

Specific Antigen	Comments or Examples
Beta-lactam antibiotics (cephalosporins)	May be a cross-reaction to penicillin allergy
Biologic extracts and hormones	Insulin and heparin
Colloids	Albumin, Dextran
Enzymes	Chymotrypsin and penicillinase
Iodinated radiocontrast dyes used in medical imaging	Computed tomography scanning
Local anesthetics	Procaine
Mismatched blood transfusions	Type and crossmatch before transfusion
Muscle relaxants, hypnotics, opioids	Acetaminophen with codeine [Tylenol No. 3], morphine, meperidine
Other antibiotics	Ampicillin
Penicillin (antibiotic)	Causes many IgE-mediated drug interactions
Salicylates	Aspirin
Sulfa drugs (antibiotics)	Sulfonamide, sulfisoxazole
Vaccines	Hypersensitivity reactions possible from all vaccines, including polio, measles, diphtheria, pertussis (whooping cough), rubella (German measles), mumps, tetanus, and *Haemophilus influenzae* type b vaccines

Adapted from Dreskin SC, Palmer GW. Anaphylaxis. eMedicine. Available at www.emedicine.com/med/topic128.htm. Accessed 9/15/07.

Case Study I Severe Allergic Reaction

Part 1

Your EMS unit has been dispatched to a call for an allergic reaction with worsening symptoms. The address is a local office building, and the patient is on the third floor. Dispatch advises that the patient has used an EpiPen. With the information provided by dispatch, you anticipate that this call could be a severe allergic reaction or anaphylaxis, so you take all necessary ALS equipment with you on the stretcher. Fortunately, an employee is waiting at the door when you arrive and another is holding the elevator. They tell you that the patient's name is Helen Scampino; she is 32 years old and complaining of difficulty breathing. When you reach the patient, you find a frightened woman sitting upright. She is pale and tells you that "It feels like my throat is swelling closed and I feel dizzy."

You introduce yourself and your partner, and a coworker is quick to tell you that the patient has been receiving a series of allergy shots to determine specific allergies. The patient had received an injection this morning. The patient states that her symptoms began 30 minutes ago and she used her EpiPen for the first time. As part of the initial assessment you listen to her breathing and then examine her face and mouth for swelling (angioedema) (see **Table 1**). You look at her torso and extremities for hives (urticaria) and at the injection site where she administered the EpiPen, while your partner places a nonrebreathing mask on the patient and obtains a set of baseline vital signs.

Question 1: Are the symptoms the patient is having signs of a mild, moderate, or severe allergic reaction?

Question 2: Do all allergic reactions produce respiratory distress?

Table 1 Initial Assessment

Initial Assessment	Recording Time: 2 Minutes
General Impression/ Appearance	Frightened, pale, distressed
Mental Status	Alert
Airway	Open, no swelling
Breathing	Clear lung sounds
Circulation	Strong, regular pulse; tachycardia
Priority/Plan	High priority

Part 2

You look Helen in the eyes to get her attention and then reassure her and ask a few more questions. At the same time, you attach your monitor. She tells you that she also has chest tightness and feels cold. This is the first time she used the auto-injector; she injected it through her pants and held it in place for 10 seconds. Right after using it, she took 50 mg of diphenhydramine [Benadryl] and called her allergist who told her to call 9-1-1.

The focused history and physical examination reveal that there is no visible airway swelling or redness, and Helen's lung sounds are clear in all fields (see **Table 2**). Her distal pulse is strong and regular, the rate is tachycardic, and her hand and wrist are cool. There is no visible urticaria, but there is evidence of an injection from the EpiPen in the upper left thigh. Her SpO_2 reading is 99%, the ECG shows sinus tachycardia at a rate of 118 beats/min, and your partner states that her blood pressure is 134/60 mm Hg, pulse is 120 beats/min, and respirations are 24 breaths/min. Helen has done a good job treating the allergic reaction, and the focused physical assessment is going well. A few more questions reveal that for lunch Helen ate a new product that is part of a new diet plan. She thinks that one of the ingredients, a chemical preservative, may be the culprit in this allergic reaction. She ate the meal 45 minutes ago and saved the package. You ask your partner to look at the package and to keep it away from the patient as to prevent further exposure.

Table 2 Focused History and Physical Examination

Baseline Vital Signs	Recording Time: 4 Minutes
Skin CTC (color, temperature, condition)	Pale, dry, cool extremities
Pulse	Radial pulse of 120 beats/min, regular; tachycardia
Blood Pressure	134/60 mm Hg
Respirations	24 breaths/min and regular

Question 3: Could this allergic reaction be related to the allergy shot that Helen received in the morning?

Question 4: Is it possible to predict the severity of an allergic reaction?

Case Study I Continued

Part 3

Allergic reactions affecting the airway, breathing, and circulation are very serious. The patient must be observed closely because the symptoms can worsen rapidly, and the patient's condition can deteriorate. While you insert an IV line, you ask Helen again how her throat and chest feel and if she is breathing any easier. She tells you that her symptoms feel less intense, but she feels shaky. You explain that epinephrine has side effects [Adrenalin] that can cause her to feel like her heart rate is rapid and to feel shaky. For now you plan to discuss administration of IV methylprednisolone sodium succinate [Solu-Medrol] with medical control, obtain her SAMPLE history, and reassess her airway, breathing, and circulation (see **Table 3**). If bronchospasm develops, you will administer a bronchodilator by nebulizer. Not all EMS Systems use methylprednisolone sodium succinate [Solu-Medrol] in their formulary as this drug can carry with it long-term significant consequences, particularly for a young patient. Always follow your local protocol and consider consulting with medical control first.

Table 3 SAMPLE History

SAMPLE History	Comments
Signs/symptoms	Throat swelling, chest tightness, dizziness, feeling sick and cold
Allergies	Environmental, pollens, mold, and possibly food additives
Medications	Oral birth control pills, Benadryl, EpiPen
Pertinent past medical history	Increased allergy symptoms during the last 18 months
Last oral intake	Processed pasta meal packaged in a microwave dish
Events leading up to the incident	Allergy shot in the morning; ate a new diet product 45 minutes ago

Treatment Plan

1. Ensure an open and clear airway.
2. Assess ventilations and assist as needed, otherwise administer supplemental oxygen via nonrebreathing mask.
3. Determine if the patient has an EpiPen. In this case, Helen does.
4. Implement EMT-B EpiPen protocol.
5. Start an IV, and obtain blood samples for the emergency department (ED).
6. Administer an IV normal saline bolus.
7. Apply the cardiac monitor.
8. Administer the following medications, as needed:
   - Albuterol [Proventil], 2.5 mg in 2 mL of saline, and ipratropium bromide [Atrovent], 0.5 mg in 2.5 mL of saline, mixed together via nebulizer (may repeat up to total of three doses). Make sure the wheezes are from bronchoconstriction and not upper airway swelling.
   - Diphenhydramine [Benadryl], 25 to 50 mg via the IV or intramuscular (IM) route (see **Table 4**)
   - Epinephrine [Adrenalin], 1:1,000, 0.5 mg via the subcutaneous (SC) (considering whether epinephrine [Adrenalin] was already administered in step No. 4) (see **Table 5**)
   - Consider consulting medical control about methylprednisolone sodium succinate, 125 mg IV (see **Table 6**)
   - Epinephrine [Adrenalin], 1:10,000, 0.5 mg via IV, intraosseous (IO), or endotracheal (ET) route if intubated with no vascular access
   - Dopamine infusion, 5 to 20 μg/kg/min (see **Table 7**)
   - Epinephrine infusion (1 mg in 250 mL normal saline) at 5 μg/min (see **Table 8**)

Table 4 Diphenhydramine

Do you know?	Comments
Right drug? Generic name: [**Diphenhydramine**] Trade name: [Benadryl]	Antihistamine with antiemetic, anticholinergic (drying), and sedative effects.
Right patient?	For primary use in patients with mild allergic reactions and secondary use *after epinephrine* in severe allergic reactions or anaphylaxis.

continues

Case Study I Continued

Table 4 Diphenhydramine (*Continued*)

Do you know?	Comments
Right dose?	Adult: 25–50 mg. Pediatric, 6–12 years: 1–2 mg/kg IV or IO slowly or IM. Paramedics do not give the oral (PO) dose, which would be 5 mg/kg/24 h.
Right route?	PO, IM, or IV.
Right time?	In cases of severe allergic reaction, epinephrine is the primary drug of choice. Supplemental diphenhydramine [Benadryl] should to be used as an antihistamine but is not absolutely necessary.
Right documentation?	Always document how and when the drug was administered and the patient's response to the medication on the patient care report.
Expected action	Relief of allergic symptoms, nausea, and dyskinesia symptoms.
Side effects	Drowsiness.
Contraindications	Known sensitivity.
Precautions	Increases effects of metoprolol tartrate [Lopressor].
Pharmacokinetics	Onset, 15–30 minutes; peak, 1 hour; duration, 3–12 hours; metabolized in the liver and excreted in urine.

Table 5 Epinephrine

Do you know?	Comments
Right drug? Generic name: [**Epinephrine**] Trade name: [Adrenalin]	This drug is a sympathomimetic. It has the property (vasopressor) to cause contraction of smooth muscle of arteries and arterioles. Epinephrine is the drug of choice in severe allergic reactions. Epinephrine for self-administration is also known as EpiPen, EpiPen Jr, and AnaKit. Note that if the patient has poor perfusion and the case is severe, the IM, IV, or IO routes may be more effective than SC.
Right patient?	Patients with severe allergic reaction or anaphylaxis.
Right dose?	Adult: Mild allergic reactions and asthma: 0.3–0.5 mg (0.3–0.5 mL of 1:1,000), SC. Anaphylaxis: 0.1 mg (1 mL of 1:10,000) IV/IO over 5 minutes. Pediatric: Mild allergic reactions and asthma: 0.01 mg/kg (0.01 mL/kg) of 1:1,000 solution SC (maximum of 0.3 mL). Note, when administered with a self-injector (EpiPen, EpiPen Jr, or AnaKit), the drug is given IM.
Right route?	SC or IV/IO when peripheral circulation is shut down.
Right time?	As soon as possible after signs and symptoms of severe allergic reaction or anaphylaxis have been recognized.
Right documentation?	Always document how and when the drug was administered and the patient's response to the medication on the patient care report.
Expected action	Relief of bronchoconstriction and improved blood pressure.
Side effects	Tachycardia, anxiety, restlessness, increased myocardial workload, tremors, tachyarrhythmias, loss of consciousness, cerebral or subarachnoid hemorrhage.
Contraindications	None in life-threatening situations.
Precautions	Use with caution in patient older than 50 years and in patients with existing cardiac arrhythmias.
Pharmacokinetics	Onset: immediate by IV, 5–10 minutes by SC and IM; metabolism takes place in the liver and other tissues by monoamine oxidase (MAO) and catechol-*O*-methyl transferase to inactive metabolites.

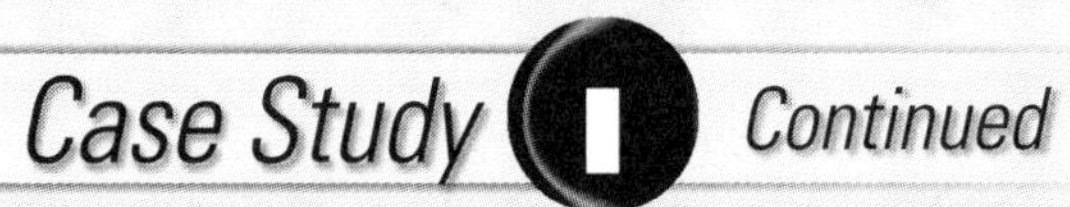

Table 6 Methylprednisolone Sodium Succinate

Do you know?	Comments
Right drug? Generic name: [**Methylprednisolone Sodium Succinate**] Trade name: [Solu-Medrol]	Glucocorticoid used as an acute anti-inflammatory agent.
Right patient?	Respiratory distress due to severe allergic reaction, asthma, and respiratory infection.
Right dose?	Adult: asthma, chronic obstructive pulmonary disease (COPD): 1–2 mg/kg IV. Pediatric: asthma, 1–2 mg/kg per dose IV.
Right route?	Diluted before use and administered IV push.
Right time?	Slow onset with long duration of effects; used after rapid-onset drugs such as albuterol [Ventolin], ipratropium bromide [Atrovent], levalbuterol hydrochloride [Xopenex], and epinephrine [Adrenalin] for patients with acute respiratory distress.
Right documentation?	Always document how and when the drug was administered and the patient's response to the medication on the patient care report.
Expected action	Decreased pain and inflammation; increased smooth muscle relaxation.
Side effects	Hypertension, sodium and water retention, nausea, weakness, substantial immune suppression, decreased bone density, retarded wound healing, hyperglycemia, osteonecrosis of bone (can cause complete collapse of joints in rare circumstances leading to life-long impairment), GI bleeding.
Contraindications	Known sensitivity, suspected bacterial infection with sepsis, gastrointestinal bleeding.
Precautions	Diabetes and GI bleeding.
Pharmacokinetics	Onset, 1–2 hours; peak effects, variable; duration of action: 8–24 hours.

Table 7 Dopamine

Do you know?	Comments
Right drug? Generic name: [**Dopamine**] Trade name: [Intropin]	A sympathomimetic chemically related to epinephrine [Adrenalin] and norepinephrine. Variable doses stimulate alpha-1 and beta-1 receptors. It is used to treat cardiogenic shock due to myocardial infarction, trauma, renal failure, and congestive heart failure.
Right patient?	Hypotension due to cardiac problems.
Right dose?	400 mg diluted in 500 mL of normal saline by continuous IV infusion; Adult: 2–20 μg/kg/min titrated to patient response. Pediatric: 2–20 μg/kg/min titrated to patient response.
Right route?	IV drip.
Right time?	After assessment and recognition of one of the indications for its use.
Right documentation?	Dose, route, time administered, and reassessment should be clearly documented on the patient care report.
Expected action	Improved blood pressure.
Side effects	Tachycardia, bradycardia, ectopy, arrhythmias, hypertension, angina, dyspnea, and headache.
Contraindications	Known sensitivity, uncorrected tachycardia, ventricular fibrillation.
Precautions	Works best when used with volume correction.
Pharmacokinetics	Onset, 5 minutes; metabolized in the liver and excreted in urine.

Case Study I Continued

Table 8 Epinephrine Infusion

Do you know?	Comments
Right drug? Generic name: [**Epinephrine**] Trade name: [Adrenalin]	When used as a drip, stimulates alpha and beta-1 and beta-2 receptors. It is used as a vasopressor in shock.
Right patient?	States of reduced cardiac output.
Right dose?	1 mg diluted in 250 mL of normal saline administered over 15 minutes titrated to effect. Some protocols may also dilute in 500 mL.
Right route?	IV drip.
Right time?	After assessment and recognition of one of the indications for its use.
Right documentation?	Dose, route, time administered, and reassessment should be clearly documented on the patient care report.
Expected action	Improved cardiac output. This drug is a direct-acting alpha and beta agonist. The alpha effect is vasoconstriction, and beta-1 effects are positive inotropic, chronotropic, and dromotropic.
Side effects	Hypertension, tachycardia, arrhythmias, pulmonary edema, anxiety, restlessness, agitation, nausea, headache, angina, ventricular fibrillation, and cerebral or subarachnoid hemorrhage; has many negative interactions with other drugs.
Contraindications	Known sensitivity, narrow-angle glaucoma, hypertension, hypothermia, pulmonary edema, myocardial ischemia, and hypovolemic shock.
Precautions	Use with caution in cases of peripheral vascular disease. EpiPen can potentiate other sympathomimetics. It can be deactivated by alkaline solutions (such as sodium bicarbonate). Use of MAO inhibitors (MAOIs) may potentiate effects, and beta-blockers may blunt its effects.
Pharmacokinetics	Onset, immediate; metabolism takes place in the liver and other tissues by MAO and catechol-*O*-methyl transferase to inactive metabolites.

9. Transport to the ED with notification and serial vital signs.

When the patient is experiencing bronchoconstriction and is wheezing, additional bronchodilators (such as albuterol [Proventil], ipratropium bromide [Atrovent], and levalbuterol hydrochloride [Xopenex]) or additional epinephrine [Adrenalin] may be administered via nebulizer. These medications are discussed further in the respiratory chapter. In the hospital, PO hydroxyzine pamoate [Vistaril] may be used to treat severe itching caused by allergies.

Question 5: How rapidly or slowly can you expect the antihistamine diphenhydramine [Benadryl] to take effect when it is taken orally?

Question 6: Would the use of an antihistamine alone be enough to reverse the effects of a severe allergic reaction?

Part 4

Once the IV line is inserted, you consult with medical control and they agree it would be appropriate to administer methylprednisolone sodium succinate [Solu-Medrol] IV. This drug will take time to become effective but has long-lasting effects that will ultimately end the systemic inflammatory response and get Helen a quicker discharge from the ED if there are no other concerns. You reassess Helen's airway, breathing, and circulation while your partner obtains a second set of vital signs (see **Table 9**). The color in her face is good, the airway is clear of swelling, breath

Case Study I Continued

Table 9 **Reassessment and Ongoing Assessment of the Patient**

Serial Vital Signs and Relevant Data	Recording Time: 10 Minutes
Skin CTC	Good color, dry, cool hands
Pulse	114 beats/min; strong and regular; tachycardia
Blood Pressure	126/68 mm Hg
Respirations	22 breaths/min and not labored
Mental Status	Alert but anxious
ECG	Sinus tachycardia
SpO_2	100%
Lung Sounds	Clear
Other (ie, glucose, core temperature)	Normal body temperature

sounds are clear and her breathing effort is good, and the vital signs are recorded. It is time to move Helen to the stretcher and out to the ambulance. Coworkers are concerned and helpful. They have written down Helen's demographic information and notified her husband. Your partner has placed the food container in a plastic bag, which will be taken to the hospital. En route, you contact medical control to advise about the patient and discuss any additional orders.

Question 7: What is an EpiPen, and how does it work?

Question 8: When would an SC injection of epinephrine [Adrenalin] be ineffective in reversing the effects of an allergic reaction?

Part 5

En route to the hospital, Helen is feeling better. She asks you if you think she administered the EpiPen correctly, and you tell her she did well in administering the epinephrine [Adrenalin], taking the diphenhydramine [Benadryl], and calling 9-1-1. You also reinforce how important it is to call EMS when signs and symptoms of an allergic reaction develop, even when she takes the emergency medications. The transport time is less than 15 minutes, and when you arrive, Helen's heart rate is less than 100 beats/min and the shaky feeling is gone.

Allergic reactions can quickly become life-threatening events. The most serious reactions occur when the antigen reacts with the IgE antibody, which can then produce bronchoconstriction and vascular dilation. You must be able to rapidly recognize when signs and symptoms are progressing from mild to severe and to take necessary actions to reverse the potentially fatal effects. Epinephrine [Adrenalin] is the first drug of choice because it has alpha and beta effects, which will relax smooth muscle (lungs), increase the heart rate, and cause vascular constriction, thus increasing the blood pressure. Signs and symptoms will vary with each patient and each episode, so the patient may also require the use of IV fluids and additional medications such as antihistamines, bronchodilators, vasopressors, and occasionally steroids. Whenever possible, attempt to determine the offending antigen and keep the patient from repeated exposure during care and transport. Consider contacting medical control early before the patient's condition becomes critical to discuss possible treatment options beyond your standing orders and to give ED personnel sufficient time to prepare for the patient.

The EpiPen

An EpiPen is often prescribed to patients who have known serious allergic reactions. Patients are advised to carry these "pens" in purses or backpacks when they might be in situations with a high risk of exposure to the offending allergen, such as gardening, camping, or hiking. Once activated, the EpiPen delivers a dose of epinephrine [Adrenalin] within 10 seconds and works rapidly to reverse the effects of a hypersensitivity reaction that could be fatal. The pens come in two standard doses: the adult auto-injector, which contains 0.3 mg of medicine, and the pediatric auto-injector, which contains 0.15 mg (**Figure 7-2 ▸**).

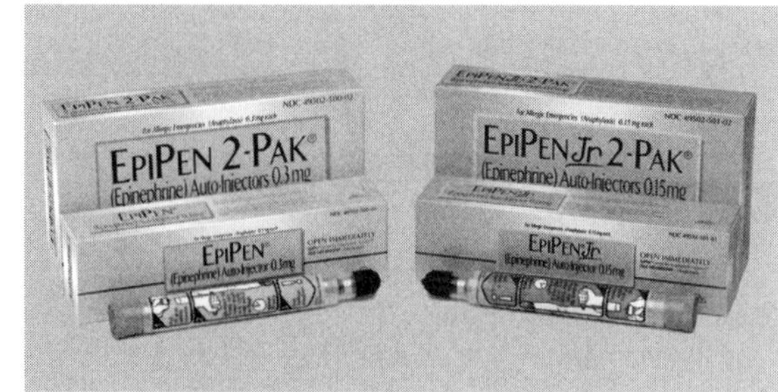

Figure 7-2 EpiPen auto-injectors (adult and pediatric sizes).

Steps for Using an EpiPen and a Typical Regional Protocol

Most states have treatment protocols that describe how medical direction will authorize the use of an EpiPen by trained EMS providers. Follow the steps in **Skill Drill 7-1 ▾** to use an auto-injector.

1. Prepare the injection site with an alcohol wipe or other antiseptic, if there is time. (**Step 1**)
2. Remove the cap from the auto-injector.
3. Place the tip against the patient's thigh. (**Step 2**)
4. Push the auto-injector firmly against the thigh until it activates (needle stick). (**Step 3**)
5. Hold the auto-injector in place for 10 seconds.
6. Dispose of the pen in a sharps container.

Skill Drill 7-1 Using an Auto-injector

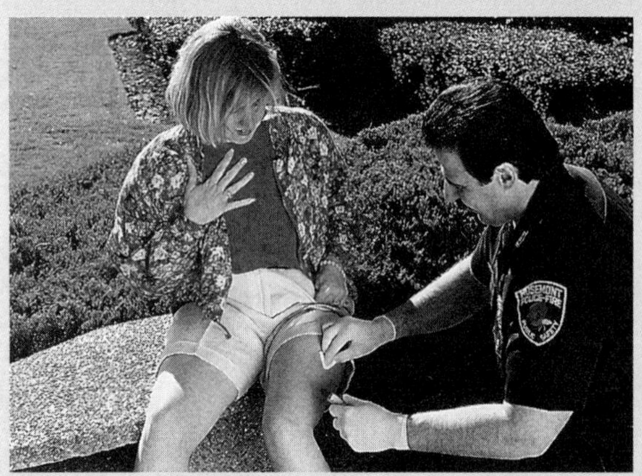

1 Wipe the thigh with antiseptic if time allows.

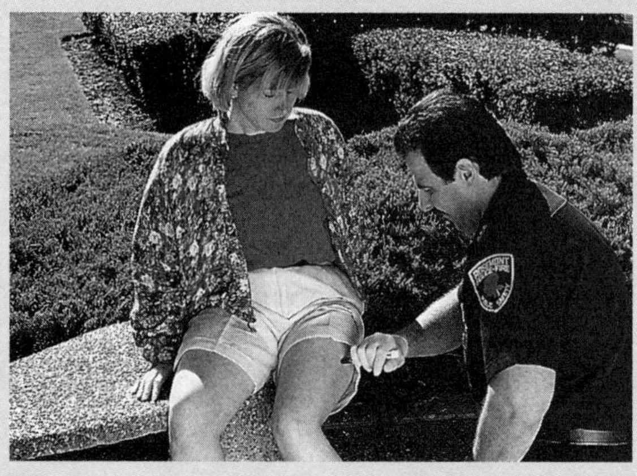

2 Place the tip of the auto-injector against the lateral part of the thigh.

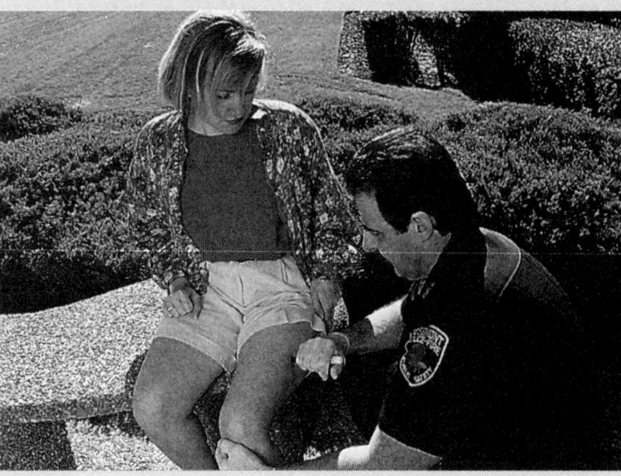

3 Push the auto-injector firmly against the thigh and hold in place until all of the medication has been injected.

Peanut Allergies

According to the Mayo Clinic Web site, peanut allergies are the most common cause of anaphylaxis and account for 80% of fatal or near-fatal reactions each year. It is the binding of the protein to IgE that can trigger severe reactions in sensitized people. Exposure can occur in three ways: direct contact, cross contact, and inhalation. Peanuts may be present in many not-so-obvious foods, such as oils, salad dressings, and candies. The Food Allergy Labeling Consumer Protection Act, passed in 2004, requires labels to be marked such that a 7-year-old child could read and understand the ingredients and that all allergens are declared even if they are in the spices or flavorings. This act went into effect January 1, 2006.

Latex Allergies in Health Care Providers

Health care providers have a higher risk of developing latex allergies than the general public because of the repeated use of gloves and other medical equipment containing latex. Latex is the milky fluid derived from the lactiferous cells of the rubber tree. The reaction is mediated by an IgE response specific for latex proteins. The people who are allergic to latex may also react to various foods because the plants contain proteins that are similar enough to latex proteins to react with the allergy-producing antibodies to latex. Some of these foods include banana, avocado, kiwi fruit, chestnut, plum, peach, cherry, apricot, fig, papaya, tomato, potato, and some other plant foods. Life-threatening anaphylactic latex reactions seem to be rare compared with peanut and other food allergies.

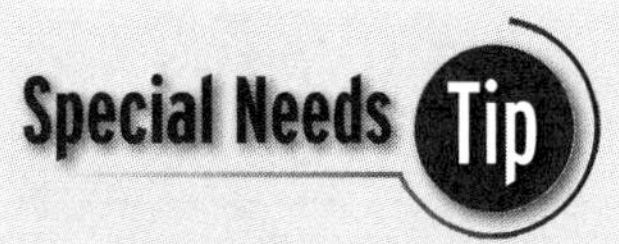

Patients with special health care needs also have a high incidence of latex allergies.

Case Study ANSWERS

Case Study I Severe Allergic Reaction

Question 1: Are the symptoms the patient is having signs of a mild, moderate, or severe allergic reaction?

Answer 1: Helen is complaining of difficulty breathing, throat swelling, and dizziness. Allergic reactions affecting the airway, breathing, and circulation are the most serious and may quickly become life threatening. Be careful to assess wheezing because it can be upper airway swelling or lower airway bronchoconstriction.

Question 2: Do all allergic reactions produce respiratory distress?

Answer 2: No, mild reactions may include only local redness, rash, hives, or angioedema, and severe reactions may occur without respiratory distress.

Question 3: Could this allergic reaction be related to the allergy shot that Helen received in the morning?

Answer 3: Yes, the signs and symptoms Helen is experiencing may be caused by the allergy shot she received earlier. Despite the precautions used in the desensitizing process, reactions occasionally occur. The reaction may have also been caused by the new food product she ate 45 minutes earlier or another unknown substance. Severe reactions typically occur shortly after an exposure (within 30 minutes); however, this is not always the case, so the patient must be observed and any information related to possible antigens should be communicated to ED personnel.

Question 4: Is it possible to predict the severity of an allergic reaction?

Answer 4: Generally, it is impossible to predict how severe any given reaction will be. This is why it is necessary to treat and transport the patient for continued observation. In general, a patient who has had a severe reaction in the past is at an increased risk for other increasingly severe reactions with subsequent antigen exposures. Always ask about previous reactions to similar antigens.

Question 5: How rapidly or slowly can you expect the antihistamine diphenhydramine [Benadryl] to take effect when it is taken orally?

Answer 5: Medications taken orally have the slowest onset, taking an average of 20 to 40 minutes. Mild or severe allergic reactions can produce symptoms of GI upset, which can further delay the onset of effects from medications taken orally. For this reason, paramedics rarely administer diphenhydramine hydrochloride [Benadryl] by the PO route.

Question 6: Would the use of an antihistamine alone be enough to reverse the effects of a severe allergic reaction?

Answer 6: In severe allergic reactions, histamine and other mediators are involved and must be blocked. Once the cascade of events in anaphylaxis has begun, all of the reactions produced by these mediators have the potential to proceed to cardiovascular collapse. Epinephrine [Adrenalin] is the drug of choice. The use of an antihistamine alone is insufficient and may be dangerous and potentially fatal.

Question 7: What is an EpiPen, and how does it work?

Answer 7: An EpiPen is a medication-filled autoinjector prescribed to patients with known severe allergic reactions. These injectors allow patients to rapidly self-administer epinephrine [Adrenalin] when severe allergic reactions are present.

Question 8: When would an SC injection of epinephrine [Adrenalin] be ineffective in reversing the effects of an allergic reaction?

Answer 8: There are two occasions when SC epinephrine [Adrenalin] may not be effective: (1) when the EpiPen is used incorrectly so that the medication is not administered properly and (2) when peripheral perfusion is so severely compromised that the medication is not circulated adequately to reach the target organs and organ systems.

Medication Review

Albuterol (Proventil, Ventolin)

Indications Treatment of bronchospasm in patients with reversible obstructive airway disease (COPD/asthma). Prevention of exercise-induced bronchospasm.

Contraindications Known prior hypersensitivity reactions to albuterol. Tachycardia arrhythmias, especially those caused by digitalis. Synergistic with other sympathomimetics.

Dosage and administration Adult: Administer 2.5 mg (0.5 mL of the 0.5% solution) added to 2 mL of normal saline for inhalation by nebulizer treatment and administer over 10–15 minutes. May repeat every 20 minutes up to three times. MDI: 1–2 inhalations (90–180 µg). Five minutes between inhalations. Pediatric: (between the ages of 2 and 12) administer 2.5 mg (0.5 mL of the 0.083% solution) added to 2 mL of normal saline for inhalation by nebulizer treatment and administer over 10–15 minutes. May repeat every 20 minutes up to three times.

Dexamethasone Sodium Phosphate (Decadron, Hexadrol)

Indications Anaphylaxis, asthma, croup.

Contraindications Hypersensitivity to product, systemic sepsis, bacterial infection.

Dosage and administration Adult: 10–100 mg IV (1 mg/kg slow IV bolus) (considerable variance through medical control). Pediatric: 0.25–1.0 mg/kg/dose IV, IO, IM.

Diphenhydramine (Benadryl)

Indications Symptomatic relief of allergies, allergic reactions, anaphylaxis, acute dystonic reactions (phenothiazines). Blood administration reactions; used for motion sickness, hay fever.

Contraindications Asthma, glaucoma, pregnancy, hypertension, narrow-angle glaucoma, infants, patients taking monoamine oxidase inhibitors (MAOIs).

Dosage and administration Adult: 25–50 mg IM or IV or PO. Pediatric: 1–2 mg/kg IV, IO slowly or IM. If given PO, 5 mg/kg/24 hours.

Dopamine (Intropin)

Indications Cardiogenic, septic, or spinal shock, hypotension with low cardiac output states, distributive shock.

Contraindications Hypovolemic shock, pheochromocytoma, tachyarrhythmias, V-fib.

Dosage and administration Adult: 2–20 µg/kg/min titrated to patient response. Pediatric: 2–20 µg/kg/min titrated to patient response.

Epinephrine (Adrenalin)

Indications Cardiac arrest (V-fib/pulseless V-tach, asystole, PEA), symptomatic bradycardia as an alternative infusion to dopamine, severe hypotension secondary to bradycardia when atropine and transcutaneous pacing are unsuccessful, allergic reactions, anaphylaxis, asthma.

Contraindications Hypertension, hypothermia, pulmonary edema, myocardial ischemia, hypovolemic shock.

Dosage and administration Adult: Mild allergic reactions and asthma: 0.3–0.5 mg (0.3–0.5 mL of 1:1,000) SC. Anaphylaxis: 0.1 mg (1 mL of 1:10,000) IV/IO over 5 minutes. Cardiac arrest: IV/IO dose: 1 mg (10 mL of 1:10,000 solution) every 3–5 minutes during resuscitation. Follow each dose with 20 mL flush and elevate arm for 10 to 20 seconds after dose. Higher dose: Higher doses (up to 0.2 mg/kg) may be used for specific indications (beta-blocker or calcium channel blocker overdose). Continuous infusion: Add 1 mg (1 mL of 1:1,000 solution) to 500 mL normal saline or D_5W. Initial infusion rate of 1 µg/min titrated to effect (typical dose: 2–10 µg/min). Endotracheal (ET) dose: 2–2.5 mg diluted in 10 mL normal saline. Profound bradycardia or hypotension: 2–10 µg/min; titrate to patient response. Pediatric: Mild allergic reactions and asthma: 0.01 mg/kg (0.01 mL/kg) of 1:1,000 solution SC (maximum of 0.3 mL). Cardiac arrest: IV/IO dose: 0.01 mg/kg (0.1 mL/kg) of 1:10,000 solution every 3–5 minutes during arrest. All endotracheal (ET) doses: 0.1 mg/kg (0.1 mL/kg) of 1:1,000 solution. Symptomatic bradycardia: IV/IO dose: 0.01 mg/kg (0.1 mL/kg) of 1:10,000 solution. Continuous IV/IO infusion: Begin with rapid infusion, then titrate to response. Typical initial infusion: 0.1–1 µg/min. Higher doses may be effective.

Medication Review

Hydrocortisone Sodium Succinate (Solu-Cortef)

Indications Shock due to acute adrenocortical insufficiency.

Contraindications None if given as single dose.

Dosage and administration Adult: 4 mg/kg slow IV bolus. Pediatric: 0.16–1.0 mg/kg slow IV bolus.

Ipratropium Bromide (Atrovent)

Indications Maintenance treatment of bronchospasm in patients with reversible obstructive airway disease (COPD/asthma). Can be used alone or in combination with other bronchodilators (especially beta-adrenergics).

Contraindications Known prior hypersensitivity reactions to ipratropium bromide. Hypersensitivity to atropine or any anticholinergic derivatives or to soya lecithin or related food products.

Dosage and administration Adult: Administer 500 µg (1 Unit-Dose vial) administered three to four times a day by oral nebulization, with doses 6 to 8 hours apart. Ipratropium Bromide Inhalation Solution Unit-Dose vials contain 500 µg ipratropium bromide anhydrous in 2.5 mL of normal saline. Ipratropium Bromide Inhalation Solution can be mixed in the nebulizer with albuterol or metaproterenol if used within 1 hour. Pediatric: Safety and effectiveness in the pediatric population younger than the age of 12 have not been established.

Methylprednisolone Sodium Succinate (Solu-Medrol)

Indications Acute spinal cord trauma, anaphylaxis, bronchodilator for unresponsive asthma.

Contraindications Premature infants, systemic fungal infections; use with caution in patients with gastrointestinal bleeding, sepsis, local infection.

Dosage and administration Adult: Acute spinal cord injury: 30 mg/kg IV over 30 minutes followed by infusion: 5.4 mg/kg/h. Asthma, COPD: 1–2 mg/kg IV. Pediatric: Acute spinal cord trauma: 30 mg/kg IV over 30 minutes; infusion: 5.4 mg/kg/h. Asthma: 1–2 mg/kg/dose IV.

Ondansetron Hydrochloride (Zofran)

Indications For the prevention or control of nausea or vomiting. Also used in the hospital setting for patients undergoing chemotherapy or surgical procedures.

Contraindications Known allergy to this medicine or other 5-HT3 receptor antagonists.

Dosage and administration Adult: 4 mg IV or IM (may repeat in 10 minutes). Pediatric: 0.1 mg/kg IV or IM.

Oxygen

Indications Confirmed or expected hypoxemia, ischemic chest pain, respiratory insufficiency, prophylactically during air transport, confirmed or suspected carbon monoxide poisoning, all other causes of decreased tissue oxygenation, decreased level of consciousness.

Contraindications Certain patients with COPD or emphysema who will not tolerate oxygen concentrations over 35%, hyperventilation. Oxygen should never be withheld from a patient who needs it, however. Be prepared to assist with ventilations in a patient with COPD who requires high concentration, as apnea may result.

Dosage and administration Adult: Cardiac arrest and carbon monoxide poisoning: 100%. Hypoxemia: 10–15 L/min via nonrebreathing mask. COPD: 1–6 L/min via nasal cannula or 28%–35% Venturi mask. Be prepared to provide ventilatory support if higher concentrations of oxygen needed. Pediatric: Same as for adult with exception of premature infant.

Promethazine Hydrochloride (Phenergan)

Indications Nausea, vomiting, motion sickness; sedation for patients in labor; potentiation of analgesic effects of narcotics.

Contraindications Hypersensitivity, coma, CNS-depressed patients from alcohol, barbiturates, narcotics, Reye's syndrome.

Dosage and administration Adult: 12.5–25 mg IV, deep IM, PO, rectally. Pediatric: (older than 2 years old) 0.25–0.5 mg/kg dose IM.

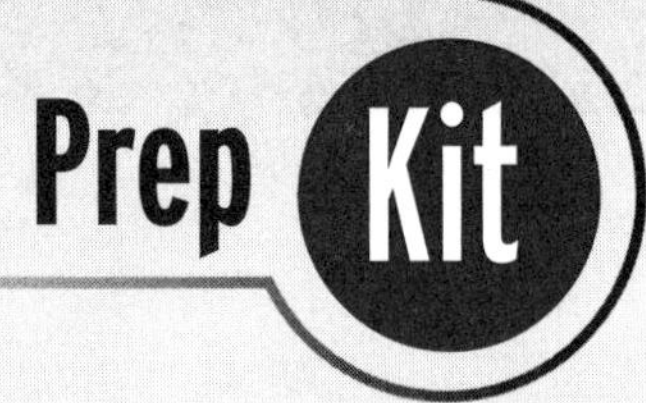

Chapter Summary

- Assessment of the patient having an allergic reaction will reveal various signs and symptoms from mild to severe.
- Signs that indicate that a patient may be experiencing a mild allergic reaction include localized itching or swelling, redness, or rash.
- The key signs that can indicate a patient may be having a severe, or anaphylactic, reaction are altered mental status; respiratory distress often involving airway swelling, wheezing, and chest tightness; and/or hypoperfusion.
- The primary treatment in anaphylaxis is the injection of the hormone epinephrine [Adrenalin].
- The SAMPLE history includes "allergies" and "medications." An example of a home medication many patients take that may precipitate an adverse reaction is cimetidine [Tagamet], commonly taken for GI disorders.
- Cimetidine [Tagamet] has an extensive drug interaction list, particularly with antiarrhythmics (ie, amiodarone, lidocaine, phenytoin, procainamide hydrochloride, and quinidine) and may also increase the likelihood of toxic effects of theophylline and cyclosporine.
- Patients with known allergies are treated in three ways. First, they are educated about how to avoid exposure; second, they may be given a variety of medications to use at home, including oral and intranasal antihistamines, inhaled bronchodilators, and inhaled or intranasal steroids; and third, immunotherapy via desensitization is performed by gradually increasing the amount of offending allergen the body receives so that the immune system can learn to defend itself against that specific allergen.
- The common causes of anaphylactic reactions include animals, insect stings, foods, latex, immunotherapy (such as in skin testing), and drugs.

Vital Vocabulary

Allergic reaction A hypersensitivity reaction to an antigen.

Anaphylactic reaction Also called anaphylaxis; an IgE-medicated hypersensitivity reaction involving bronchoconstriction and cardiovascular collapse in the case of anaphylactic shock.

Angioedema Localized tissue edema caused by an allergic-like process.

Antibodies Substances that destroy or neutralize antigens.

Antigen A substance that produces an immune response.

Desensitization Also called hyposensitization; a process of exposing a patient to the offending antigen in small increments in an effort to minimize systemic immune response to the antigen.

Histamine A chemical substance that causes blood vessels to dilate and become leaky and promotes increased production of mucus in the respiratory tract.

Immunoglobulins A family of proteins with specific functions in the immune system.

Immunoglobulin E (IgE) One of the five major classes of immunoglobulins that is present primarily in the skin and mucous membranes.

Mast cells Basophils that are located in the tissues.

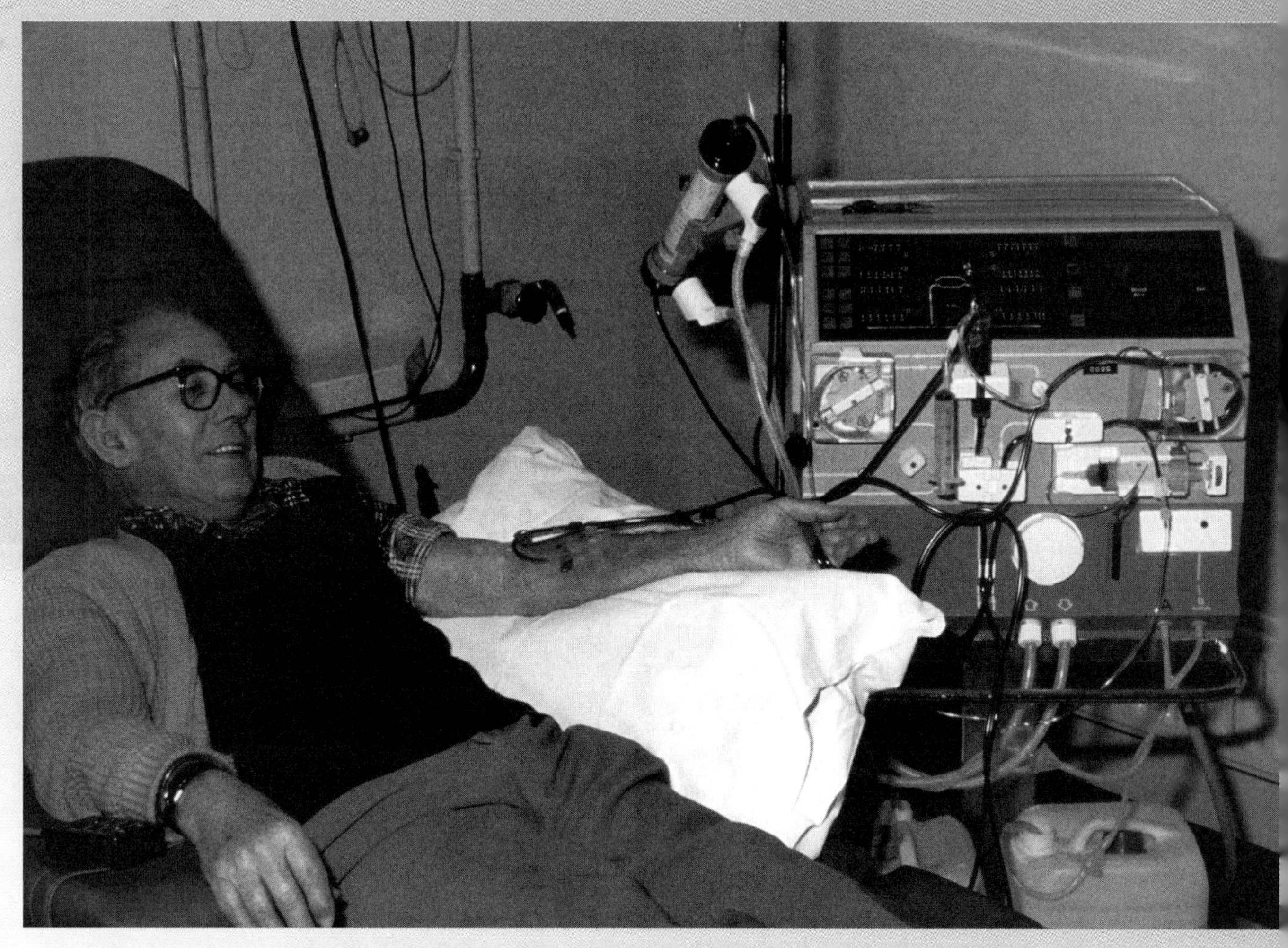

Renal and Urologic Emergencies

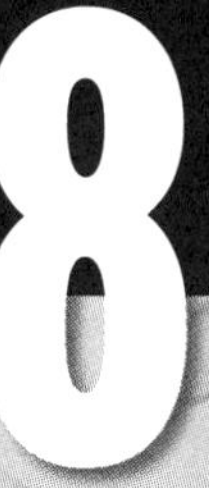

Objectives

Cognitive

None

Affective

None

Psychomotor

None

Additional Objectives

8-1 Discuss the following medications used in the prehospital setting for the patient with severe pain: morphine sulfate [Astramorph PF] and fentanyl citrate [Sublimase]. (pages 261–266)

8-2 Describe the pathophysiology of the following renal conditions: kidney stones, acute renal failure and chronic renal failure. (pages 260–267)

8-3 Describe the prehospital and in-hospital management of the patient with kidney stones. (pages 261–266)

Pathophysiology of Renal and Urologic Conditions

The most common causes of renal and urologic-related calls in the prehospital setting include **kidney stones**, **urinary tract infection (UTI)**, **pyelonephritis**, acute urinary retention, **epididymitis**, **prostatitis**, **torsion of the testicle**, and complications of renal failure. The primary focus of paramedics involves supportive care with assessment and management of the symptoms of these conditions. The majority of the management is performed in the hospital.

Be cautious with undiagnosed abdominal pain. A wise paramedic performs a complete and thorough patient assessment before medicating any patient in pain, especially a patient with abdominal pain.

Kidney Stones

Kidney stones, or **renal calculi**, result when an excess of insoluble salts and uric acid crystallizes in the urine. These small, rocklike concretions are generally 1 to 5 mm in diameter (**Figure 8-1**▼). Kidney stones are typically due to water intake that is insufficient to dissolve the salts. The stones originate in the renal pelvis and are excreted with urine. Most of the stones can travel down the ureter to the bladder and eventually exit via the urethra. This is a shorter journey in women than in men (**Figure 8-2**▼). In some cases, a limited number of the stones become impacted and will require surgical removal. The passage of the stone is very painful. Patients with kidney stones often have associated ureteral colic and cannot find a comfortable position because of the severe pain. Patients often are pacing or squirming, which is often referred to as "the dance."

Other causes of abdominal pain can result in severe pain requiring medication. These causes include abdominal ascites, peritonitis, ruptured ulcer, appendicitis, urinary retention, kidney infection, urinary tract infection, ruptured ovarian cyst, ruptured ectopic pregnancy, and abdominal cramping associated with menstruation. You should perform a proper assessment and inquire about the patient's history.

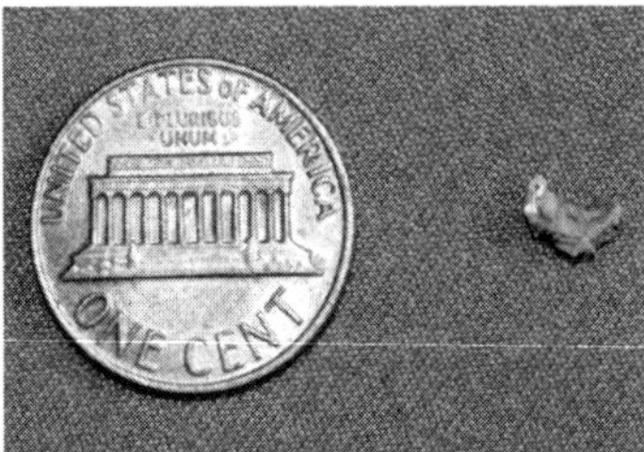

Figure 8-1 A kidney stone.

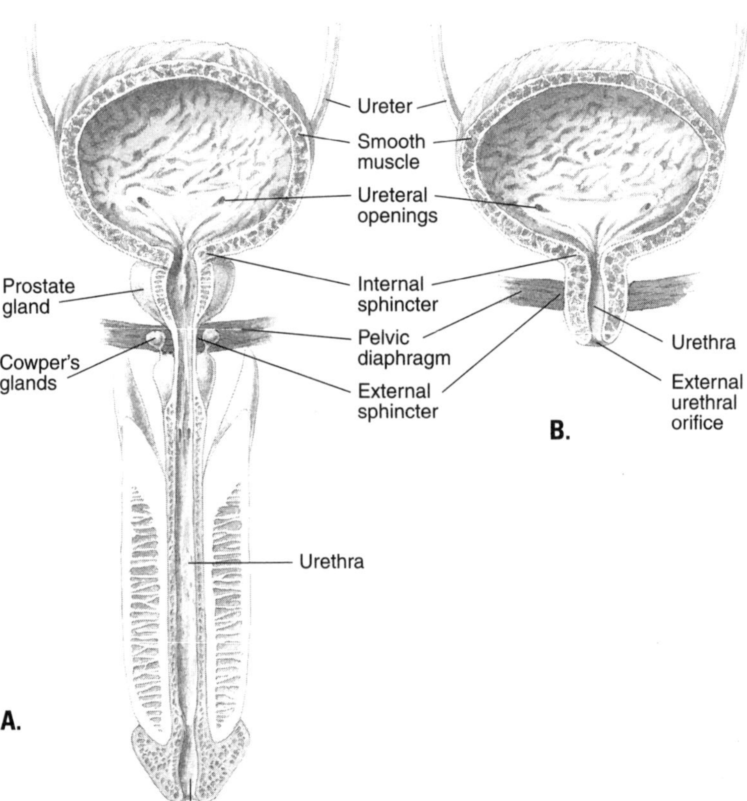

Figure 8-2 The differences in the urethras of (A) men and (B) women.

Case Study 1 Possible Kidney Stones

Part 1

Your unit has been dispatched to a private residence for a man in his 40s who is having severe pain. It is early evening, and his wife called 9-1-1 because she said he "simply could not stand the pain anymore." On arrival at a private home in a residential area, you are met by his wife at the door. The scene appears safe, and you don your body substance isolation apparel as you approach the patient. He is pacing the room. His wife says he cannot find a comfortable position and he has vomited twice in the last few hours. She introduces you to Bill, who begins to tell you that he has been sick for the last day or so. Bill states he thinks he might have another kidney stone and that it was not this painful the last time.

You perform a quick initial assessment to make sure you do not miss any priorities (see **Table 1**).

Table 1 Initial Assessment

Initial Assessment	Recording Time: 2 Minutes
General Impression/ Appearance	Pacing, very fidgety, in obvious pain
Mental Status	"A" alert (oriented to person, place, and day)
Airway	Open and clear
Breathing	Rapid breaths, normal depth
Circulation	Tachycardia; pale, clammy, normal-temperature skin
Priority/Plan	High priority owing to severe pain

The patient is a responsive medical patient. After completing the initial assessment, you plan to proceed with the focused history and physical examination, elaborating on the chief complaint by using the OPQRST acronym. Your partner is obtaining vital signs and mentions under his breath that the patient is "doing the dance."

Question 1: What does your partner mean by "doing the dance?"

Question 2: With no other life threats at this point, why is the patient a high priority?

Part 2

As your partner completes the vital signs, you ask the patient a few questions about his pain (see **Table 2**). It is helpful that he seems to know the cause; however, you want to be careful not to take a myopic view of the situation by immediately focusing on one specific working diagnosis. Be careful to rule out other more serious causes (ie, acute myocardial infarction [AMI] or shock). The patient states the pain has come on during the last few hours, although he has not felt well all day. He says he usually carries a water bottle and drinks plenty of fluids but has been so busy traveling the last week that he seems to have stopped. He describes the pain as flank pain on the right and says it radiates to the abdomen and groin. It is intermittent, crampy, and often intense. On a scale of 1 to 10 he gives it a 7 and states that it is worse than the last stone 3 years ago.

Table 2 Focused History and Physical Examination

Baseline Vital Signs	Recording Time: 8 Minutes
Skin CTC (color, temperature, condition)	Pale, warm, and clammy
Pulse	110 beats/min and regular
Blood Pressure	138/82 mm Hg
Respirations	24 breaths/min and regular

Question 3: Comparing the present situation with a prior incident is helpful. What question should you follow up with?

Question 4: If you asked this patient if any position made the pain feel better, what would you suspect he might say?

Case Study I Continued

Part 3

You will check to make sure that his blood pressure is stable before administering morphine sulfate [Astramorph/PF] titrated to achieve pain control. This may require contact with medical control in some regions. In the meantime, you insert an IV line for fluid administration and begin the SAMPLE history (see **Table 3**). Fluids are helpful in promoting movement of the stone through the system. The patient recalls that he had vomited earlier in the day, but denies nausea at the moment. He is fidgety and not thrilled about sitting on the stretcher for the examination or transport. His lung sounds are clear, and his SpO_2 is 98%. He states he is healthy aside from the fact that he had his gallbladder removed 4 years ago.

Table 3 SAMPLE History

SAMPLE History	Comments
Signs/symptoms	Intermittent, crampy pain in right flank radiating to the groin
Allergies	Penicillin
Medications	Cimetidine [Tagamet], aspirin
Pertinent past medical history	Gallbladder removed; previous kidney stones
Last oral intake	A can of soda about 2 hours ago
Events leading up to the incident	Uncomfortable most of the day

Treatment Plan

1. Ensure an open and a clear airway.
2. Assess ventilations, and assist as needed; otherwise administer supplemental oxygen via nonrebreathing mask.
3. Monitor the electrocardiogram (ECG), consider a 12-lead ECG and vital signs.
4. Rule out life-threatening causes of the pain.
5. Insert an IV line, and obtain blood samples for the emergency department (ED).
6. Administer an IV bolus of normal saline to help flush the stone through the system.
7. Administer one of the following medications, as needed, and authorized by medical control:
   a. Morphine sulfate [Astramorph/PF], 0.05 mg/kg, by the IV, intramuscular (IM), or subcutaneous (SC) route or according to your local protocol (ie, 2–4 mg IV over 1–5 minutes every 5–30 minutes); second dose of 2–8 mg at 5- to 15-minute intervals; have naloxone hydrochloride [Narcan] on standby (see **Table 4** and **Table 5**)
   b. Fentanyl citrate [Sublimase], 0.5-1.0 µg/kg by IM or slow IV route (see **Table 6**)
   c. Ondansetron hydrochloride [Zofran], 4–8 mg, by IV or IM route (see **Table 7**)
8. Transport the patient in a position of comfort to the ED with notification of ED staff of the patient's condition and serial vital signs.

Many medications for pain management can cause respiratory depression, so you should consider the end tidal carbon dioxide ($EtCO_2$) value. Knowing the patient's $EtCO_2$ value will provide better assessment information than a pulse oximetry reading. The pulse oximetry reading will drop 2 to 5 minutes after the patient is already hypoxic, but the $EtCO_2$ value is sensitive on a second-to-second basis. By using $EtCO_2$ results, you can tell the patient to take a deep breath rather than having to assist ventilations with a bag-mask device when the patient has respiratory compromise.

Table 4 Morphine Sulfate

Do you know?	Comments
Right drug? Generic name: [**Morphine Sulfate**] Trade name: [Astramorph PF]	This drug is an opioid analgesic (schedule II narcotic) used for relief of severe pain, anxiety, sedation, to reduce left ventricular work, and for treating dyspnea caused by left ventricular failure and pulmonary edema.
Right patient?	For severe congestive heart failure (CHF), pulmonary edema, chest pain associated with AMI, analgesia for moderate to severe acute and chronic pain (as in this case).
Right dose?	Initial dose of 0.05 mg/kg IV (usually 2–4 mg) over 1–5 minutes every 5–30 minutes; second dose can be 2–8 mg at 5- to 15-minute intervals.
Right route?	Slow IV, IM, SC.
Right time?	When the patient has severe pain as long as the patient is in hemodynamically stable condition.

continues

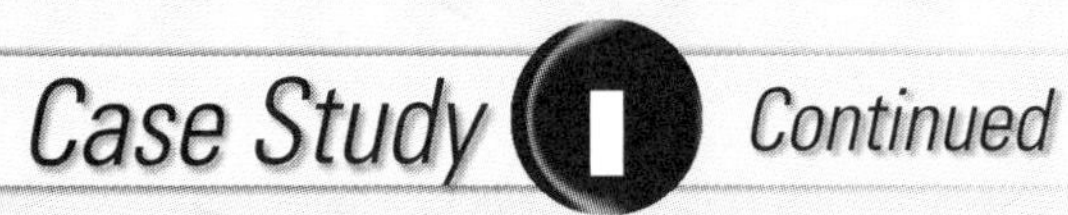

Table 4 Morphine Sulfate (*Continued*)

Do you know?	Comments
Right documentation?	Always document how and when the drug was administered and the patient's response to the medication on your patient care report.
Expected action	Alleviate pain through central nervous system (CNS) receptors, suppress fear and anxiety centers in the brain, depress brain stem respiratory centers, increase peripheral venous capacitance and decrease venous return, and decrease preload and afterload, which decreases myocardial oxygen demand.
Side effects	Respiratory depression, hypotension, decreased level of consciousness, nausea, vomiting, bradycardia, tachycardia, syncope, facial flushing, euphoria, bronchospasm, and dry mouth.
Contraindications	Head injury, exacerbated chronic obstructive pulmonary disease (COPD), depressed respiratory drive, hypotension, decreased level of consciousness, suspected hypovolemia, use of monoamine oxidase inhibitors (MAOIs) within the past 14 days.
Precautions	Potentiates sedative effects of phenothiazines. CNS depressants may potentiate effects of morphine sulfate. MAOIs may cause paradoxical excitation.
Pharmacokinetics	Onset: immediate by IV, 15–30 minutes by IM/SC; peak, 20 minutes by IV, 60 minutes by IM/SC; duration 2–7 hours; metabolized in the liver by glucuronidation and excreted in urine.

Table 5 Naloxone Hydrochloride

Do you know?	Comments
Right drug? Generic name: [**Naloxone Hydrochloride**] Trade name: [Narcan]	This drug is a narcotic antagonist and will precipitate immediate opiate withdrawal. When you suspect that the patient's respiratory depression is due to an overdose of a narcotic or opiate, such as morphine, heroin, or methadone, the drug of choice to reverse the effects of the narcotic or opiate is naloxone hydrochloride [Narcan].
Right patient?	Patients who have depressed respirations or altered mental status from too high a dose of a narcotic or opiate.
Right dose?	The dose is 0.4 to 2 mg; it is best to titrate (increments of 0.4 mg) to desirable effect of improved respirations.
Right route?	Can be given by IV, IO, IM, intranasal, or endotracheal (ET) routes, although the ET route is the least effective and not generally recommended if other routes are available.
Right time?	If the patient has respiratory depression, assist the ventilations with the bag-mask device. Before administering the naloxone hydrochloride [Narcan], properly position and restrain the patient on the stretcher, in case the patient wakes up in an argumentative or violent mood.
Right documentation?	Always document how and when the drug was administered, the patient's response to the medication on your patient care report, and if humane restraint was applied before administration of the drug.
Expected action	Antagonistic to narcotic or opiate medications. Expect it to reverse the effect of the overdose. Small doses should improve the patient's ventilations. Larger doses may cause the patient to wake up, which is generally not necessary; the patient may wake up in an argumentative or violent mood.
Side effects	Nausea, upset stomach, or drowsiness. More serious side effects include withdrawal symptoms: vomiting, sweating, tremors, seizures, and rapid and pounding irregular pulse.
Contraindications	None, aside from the precautions.
Precautions	Administer drug slowly and give only enough to improve respirations. Rapid administration of the entire dose is likely to awaken the patient, who will have withdrawal symptoms and be aggressive.
Pharmacokinetics	Onset: < 2 minutes by IV, < 5 minutes by IM and SC; peak, 5–15 minutes; duration depends on dose and route; metabolized in the liver and excreted in urine.

Case Study I Continued

Table 6 Fentanyl Citrate

Do you know?	Comments
Right drug? Generic name: [**Fentanyl Citrate**] Trade name: [Sublimase]	This is drug is a narcotic analgesic (schedule II narcotic) used to treat severe pain and is used with anesthesia. It has actions similar to morphine sulfate [Astramorph/PF] and meperidine hydrochloride [Demerol].
Right patient?	Relief of severe pain; adjunct to sedation.
Right dose?	0.5–1 μg/kg IM or IV.
Right route?	IV or IM.
Right time?	After assessment and contraindications have been considered.
Right documentation?	Always document how and when the drug was administered and the patient's response to the medication on your patient care report.
Expected action	Pain relief.
Side effects	Skeletal and thoracic muscle rigidity reported in cases of large doses administered via rapid IV push, bradycardia, seizures, and diaphoresis.
Contraindications	Myasthenia gravis.
Precautions	Hypoventilation when given via rapid IV push.
Pharmacokinetics	Onset: immediate by IV, 5–15 minutes by IM; peak, 30 minutes by IM; duration, 20–40 minutes by IV, 1–2 hours by IM; metabolized in the liver and excreted in urine.

Table 7 Ondansetron Hydrochloride

Do you know?	Comments
Right drug? Generic name: [**Ondansetron Hydrochloride**] Trade name: [Zofran]	This drug is an antiemetic used to relieve or prevent nausea and vomiting in a variety of situations.
Right patient?	Nausea in suspected cases of acute coronary syndrome (ACS) and ST-segment elevation MI.
Right dose?	4-mg initial dose; may be repeated in 10 minutes. Follow local protocol.
Right route?	IV or IM.
Right time?	Adjunct treatment in suspected ACS after treating with acetylsalicylic acid [Aspirin], nitrates, and/or morphine sulfate.
Right documentation?	Document the administration of the medication and ongoing assessment findings, including lung sounds on the patient care report.
Expected action	Relief of nausea.
Side effects	Typically, chest pain, wheezing, or hives or skin rash; other side effects include seizures, tachycardia, bradycardia, MI, sedation, blurred vision, hypokalemia, and fever. Acute dystonic reactions, involving painful muscular twisting and twitching, may occur.
Contraindications	Known sensitivity.
Precautions	May worsen preexisting symptoms.
Pharmacokinetics	Onset: 30 minutes; peak effect, 2 hours; duration, 3–6 hours; metabolized in the liver and excreted in urine.

Question 5: Why is it helpful to have naloxone hydrochloride [Narcan] and $EtCO_2$ monitoring handy for this patient?

Question 6: Will this patient remain a high priority for a lights-and-siren ride to the hospital?

Case Study 1 Continued

Part 4

Bill is loaded into the ambulance. He has calmed down, and you are having a conversation about the neighborhood and his line of work. It is clear that although he has not forgotten the pain, it is relieved at this moment. However, you know that pain requiring prehospital narcotic administration demands in-hospital evaluation. As you prepare to do a radio report for the ED, you review your assessment findings and obtain another set of vital signs (see **Table 8**). Because Bill is alert, you know it is not essential that you take his temperature again, but you do anyway.

Questions 7: This patient was originally warm. Is it essential to take his temperature in the field?

Question 8: Because this patient's pain is basically gone at this point, would it be reasonable to allow him to "sign off" and stay at home?

Table 8 Reassessment and Ongoing Assessment of the Patient

Serial Vital Signs and Relevant Data	Recording Time: 10 Minutes
Skin CTC	Pale, warm, and dry
Pulse	106 beats/min and regular
Blood Pressure	134/80 mm Hg
Respirations	22 breaths/min and regular
Mental Status	Alert (oriented to person, place, and day)
ECG	Sinus tachycardia
SpO_2	97%
Lung Sounds	Clear bilaterally
Other (ie, glucose, core body temperature (CBT)	CBT is unchanged

Part 5

Bill was having a bad day, and, despite his pain and insistence on not calling the paramedics, his wife was smart enough to call. The possible kidney stone was very painful, and Bill seemed to have renal colic, he was unable to find a comfortable position and was "doing the kidney stone dance." After the assessment you decided that the most appropriate course of action was to administer analgesics (morphine sulfate [Astramorp/PF] and fentanyl citrate [Sublimase]), an antiemetic (ondansetron hydrochloride [Zofran]), and IV fluids. Bill will continue to be assessed and treated until his condition is appropriate for discharge and likely will have urologic follow-up.

Consider psychological techniques for reducing pain. These techniques include distracting patients by keeping them talking; providing music (of the patient's choice) in the back of the unit; positioning patients on their side or another comfortable position for transport; and providing warmth to the area. These measures should help patients to relax and facilitate safe and successful transport.

Management of Kidney Stones

The prehospital treatment plan for a patient you suspect has kidney stones involves the ABCs, monitoring serial vital signs, inserting an intravenous (IV) line for fluid infusion and administration of pain medications (ie, morphine sulfate [Astramorph/PF] or fentanyl citrate [Sublimase]. Allow the patient to assume a position of comfort. If your region is one of the few that has access to a facility with a lithotripsy unit, medical control may consider a secondary transport after the patient's condition is stabilized. **Lithotripsy** is an in-hospital method of breaking up, or disintegrating, kidney stones (**Figure 8-3**▼).

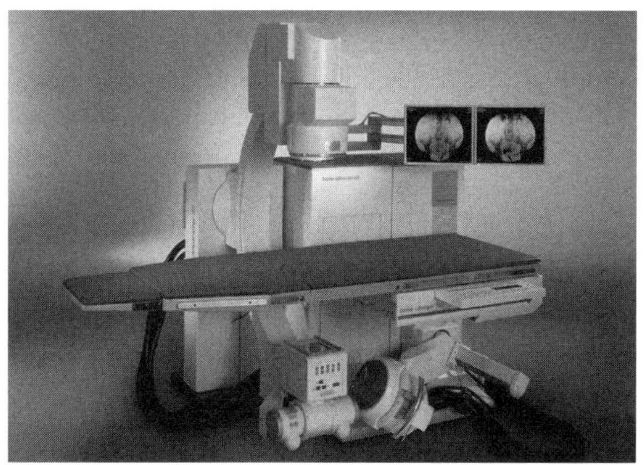

Figure 8-3 Kidney stones are disintegrated using a lithotripsy unit.

For many years, analgesics or painkillers were underused in the prehospital setting because of a number of situations, such as the complications involved in having narcotics available, attitudes about the "need" for pain medication, and the perception that patients could wait until arrival at the ED. Most EMS systems have refined their view of prehospital analgesia. Because in most situations (as long as the patient's vital signs are stable) it is best to alleviate severe pain, many regional ALS protocols now authorize the use of medication for pain, particularly for extremity fractures and severe burns. The medication of choice in most EMS systems is morphine sulfate [Astramorph/PF]. There is still an attitudinal component about the need for pain medication that must be addressed when paramedics are trained in the use of analgesia. Some EMS providers have not experienced severe pain and, so, have little experience to help them understand the patient's pain. In addition, the pain from the abdomen is vague, crampy, and visceral. Once you have lived through the pain of a kidney stone, appendicitis, or an ovarian cyst, the paramedic may have a better understanding for the need of pain medication. Therefore, it is best to believe when the pain is significant as described by the patient. In some EMS systems this may be a standing order and in another system it may involve early contact with medical control for permission to administer a pain reliever.

It is important to consider alternative or additional diagnoses of medication when managing a patient with suspected **renal colic**. In the case of an older patient, a patient with underlying cardiovascular risk factors, or a patient who appears to be in unstable condition, the possibility of serious vascular disease must be addressed, specifically myocardial, aortic, or aortoiliac catastrophe (narrowing or blockage of the main arteries in the pelvis, which supply blood to the legs). Also, hepatobiliary disease (having to do with the liver, the gallbladder, bile ducts, or bile) is sometimes difficult to differentiate from renal colic. Occasionally, a patient with renal colic actually has an upper UTI. Pyelonephritis is inflammation of the kidney lining, often caused by a UTI in the upper urinary tract. Evidence of pyelonephritis in conjunction with a kidney stone is a serious medical problem, one that is treated most often by hospitalization, IV antibiotics, and prompt urologic intervention to remove the obstruction.

Acute Renal Failure

Acute renal failure (ARF) is a sudden decrease in filtration through the glomeruli, the capillaries in the kidneys that serve as the main filter for the blood in the kidneys. ARF may result from many causes including inadequate perfusion, trauma, a surgical or medical procedure, malignant hypertension, bacterial infection, drug reaction, metabolic disorder, and obstruction. ARF is classified into three types, based on the area where the failure occurs: prerenal, intrarenal, and postrenal. Signs and symptoms are related to the severity of renal dysfunction, the loss of excretory function, the rate of renal failure, and the cause (**Table 8-1** ▲). Findings may be as subtle as dark urine followed by diminished urination (oliguria) or absence of urination (anuria). The immediate complications associated with acute renal failure are fluid retention, hyperkalemia, metabolic acidosis, uremia, and bleeding.

Table 8-1 Signs and Symptoms of Acute Renal Failure

Prerenal acute renal failure	Hypotension Tachycardia Dizziness Thirst
Intrarenal acute renal failure	Flank pain Joint pain Oliguria Hypertension Headache Confusion Seizure
Postrenal acute renal failure	Pain in lower flank, abdomen, groin, and genitalia Oliguria Distended bladder Hematuria Peripheral edema

Management of Acute Renal Failure

Treatment is to manage the ABCs, administer high-flow oxygen, provide ventilatory support with a bag-mask device as needed, and consider administration of an IV bolus of normal saline if there are signs of shock. A priority is to establish normal urine flow and correct the cause of ARF, but this is likely to be dealt with in the hospital setting. Treatment may include the use of vasopressors, diuretics, sodium bicarbonate, and dialysis. Always consult medical control because some of the treatments often given by paramedics, such as analgesics and antibiotics, may cause nephrotoxic effects in a patient with ARF.

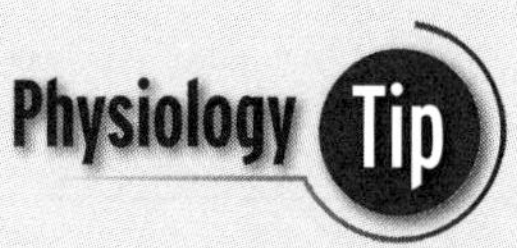

Because patients in chronic renal failure already have serum electrolyte imbalances, be conservative with the treatment plan.

Chronic Renal Failure

Chronic renal failure is progressive and irreversible inadequate kidney function due to permanent loss of nephrons, the structural and functional units of the kidneys that form urine. Chronic renal failure can occur from any renal dysfunction, most commonly diabetic neuropathy. Uremia, severe hyperkalemia, and CHF are life-threatening conditions associated with chronic renal failure. Uremia is a toxic condition that occurs when nitrogenous substances that are normally excreted in the urine are retained owing to renal insufficiency. Hyperkalemia is caused by the failure of the kidneys to excrete potassium adequately. This condition can develop in end-stage renal failure when a scheduled dialysis is delayed. When severe hyperkalemia develops, ECG findings include peaked T waves, prolonged P-R interval, QRS widening, and, eventually, ventricular fibrillation. CHF is most commonly a result of sodium and fluid retention.

Management of Chronic Renal Failure

Uremia requires **renal dialysis** or kidney transplantation. Calcium chloride or calcium gluconate may be helpful to treat severe hyperkalemia before dialysis to counteract toxic effects of the excessive potassium to the cardiac membrane. Diuretics are usually effective, and angiotensin-converting enzyme (ACE) inhibitors can be used if left ventricular function is depressed. The treatment of chronic renal failure is similar to that for ARF in that it includes management of the ABCs, administration of high-flow oxygen, and provision of ventilatory support with a bag-mask device as needed. Consider administration of an IV bolus of normal saline if there are signs of shock but no signs of pulmonary edema. Treatment should focus on the regulation of fluid imbalances and cardiovascular function. If hypotension occurs, a vasopressor may be administered or medical control may order the administration of sodium bicarbonate. Patients with chronic renal failure will ultimately require dialysis (**Table 8-2**▼).

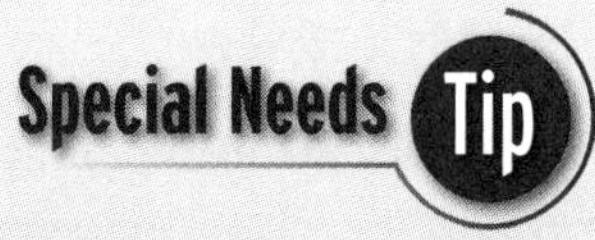

Be prepared to adjust the dose and frequency of medication administration for elderly people. Because the kidneys and the liver are the primary routes of drug elimination, age-related changes in the functions of these organs can have a major impact on the effects of the drugs.

Table 8-2 Medical Emergencies in Dialysis Patients

Problem	Prehospital Management
Problems related to dialysis itself:	
Hypotension	Give 50 mL of normal saline IV
Hemorrhage from the shunt	If the shunt cannot be reconnected, clamp it off; check for signs of shock
Potassium imbalance	For hypokalemia: treat bradycardia with atropine
	For hyperkalemia: calcium and bicarbonate may be considered
Disequilibrium syndrome	Supportive treatment only
Air embolism	Left lateral recumbent position in about 10° of head-down tilt
Machine dysfunction	Turn off machine; clamp ends of shunt; disconnect patient from machine; transport
Problems to which dialysis patients are more vulnerable:	
Congestive heart failure	Oxygen; sitting position; rapid transport to dialysis facility
Myocardial infarction and cardiac dysrhythmias	Treat as any other patient, but use caution in administering any medications
Hypertension	Transport only; the treatment is dialysis
Pericardial tamponade	Emergency transport as soon as detected
Uremic pericarditis	Oxygen; position of comfort; transport
Subdural hematoma	Oxygen; urgent transport

Case Study ANSWERS

Case Study 1 Possible Kidney Stones

Question 1: What does your partner mean by "doing the dance"?

Answer 1: Patients with kidney stones often have associated ureteral colic and cannot find a comfortable position. The patients often are pacing or squirming around (ie, the dance). This case is a classic, straightforward presentation of renal calculi. Keep in mind that many times the patients have an incredible amount of pain and are sweating like they are having an AMI, making the two conditions difficult to differentiate.

Question 2: With no other life threats at this point, why is the patient a high priority?

Answer 2: The high priority is because of the severity of the patient's pain. The pain severity may change after an assessment and administration of the appropriate medication, but, initially, he is a high priority.

Question 3: Comparing the present situation with a prior incident is helpful. What question should you follow up with?

Answer 3: Ask him what treatment he received the last time.

Question 4: If you asked this patient if any position made the pain feel better, what would you suspect he might say?

Answer 4: He would probably say there was no comfortable position and would ask to go to the hospital and have medication for the pain.

Question 5: Why is it helpful to have naloxone hydrochloride [Narcan] and $EtCO_2$ monitoring handy for this patient?

Answer 5: In some patients, respiratory depression may result after administration of narcotics. It generally does not occur at low doses, but naloxone hydrochloride [Narcan] is antagonistic to the narcotic. If respiratory depression occurs, it can be reversed by the administration of naloxone hydrochloride [Narcan]. $EtCO_2$ monitoring is helpful because many medications used for pain management can cause respiratory depression. Knowing the patient's $EtCO_2$ will provide better assessment information than a pulse oximetry reading. The pulse oximetry reading will drop 2 to 5 minutes after the patient is already hypoxic. The $EtCO_2$ reading is sensitive on a second-to-second basis. By using $EtCO_2$ readings, you can simply tell the patient to take a deep breath rather than having to assist ventilations with a bag-mask device because hypoxia is already present.

Question 6: Will this patient remain a high priority for a lights-and-siren ride to the hospital?

Answer 6: Few patients require a lights-and-siren ride to the hospital, which increases the likelihood of a serious collision and injury to the rescuers. In this case, once the patient's pain is reduced or resolved, he should rest comfortably for the quiet ride to the hospital, and his priority changes to low. Regardless of whether the pain is alleviated, a case of renal colic does not justify lights-and-siren transport to the hospital.

Questions 7: This patient was originally warm. Is it essential to take his temperature in the field?

Answer 7: It would be helpful to take his temperature since his skin is warm. He may have a fever which could indicate he is fighting an infection. It would not be considered "essential" since the patient's mental status is still alert.

Question 8: Because this patient's pain is basically gone at this point, would it be reasonable to allow him to "sign off" and stay at home?

Answer 8: Absolutely not. Pain requiring prehospital narcotic administration demands in-hospital evaluation. After a narcotic has been administered to relieve a patient's pain, it would not be appropriate to allow the patient to sign a refusal of medical assistance. The narcotic will ultimately wear off, the patient's pain will recur, and the underlying process will have gone unaddressed. If the patient wants to sign-off, most EMS systems would involve consultation with medical control.

Medication Review

Diazepam (Valium)

Indications Acute anxiety states, acute alcohol withdrawal (delirium tremens), muscle relaxant, seizure activity, agitation. Analgesia for medical procedures (fracture reduction, cardioversion).

Contraindications Hypersensitivity, glaucoma, coma, shock, substance abuse, head injury.

Dosage and administration Seizure activity: Adult: 5–10 mg IV every 10–15 minutes as needed (5 mg over 5 min) (maximum dose, 30 mg). Seizure activity: Pediatric: 0.2–0.5 mg slowly every 2–5 minutes up to 5 mg (maximum dose, 10 mg/kg). Rectal diazepam: 0.5 mg/kg via rectal catheter and flush with 2–3 mL air after administration. Sedation for cardioversion: 5–15 mg IV over 5–10 minutes prior to cardioversion.

Meperidine Hydrochloride (Demerol)

Indications Analgesia for moderate to severe pain.

Contraindications Hypersensitivity to narcotic agents, diarrhea caused by poisoning, patients taking MAOIs, during labor or delivery of a premature infant, undiagnosed abdominal pain or head injury.

Dosage and administration Adult: 50–100 mg IM, SC or 25–50 mg slowly IV. Pediatric: 1–2 mg/kg/dose IV, IO, IM, SC.

Morphine Sulfate (Astramorph/PF and others)

Indications Severe CHF, pulmonary edema, chest pain associated with acute myocardial infarction, analgesia for moderate to severe acute and chronic pain (use with caution).

Contraindications Head injury, exacerbated COPD, depressed respiratory drive, hypotension, undiagnosed abdominal pain, decreased level of consciousness, suspected hypovolemia, patients who have taken MAOIs within the past 14 days.

Dosage and administration Adult: Initial dose: 2–4 mg IV (over 1–5 minutes) every 5–30 minutes. Repeat dose: 2–8 mg at 5- to 15-minute intervals. Pediatric: 0.1–0.2 mg/kg per dose via IV, IO, IM, or SC; maximum dose of 5 mg.

Naloxone Hydrochloride (Narcan)

Indications Opiate overdose, coma; complete or partial reversal of CNS and respiratory depression induced by opioids; decreased level of consciousness; coma of unknown origin; narcotic agonist for the following: morphine, heroin, hydromorphone (Dilaudid), methadone, meperidine (Demerol), paregoric, fentanyl citrate (Sublimase), oxycodone (Percodan), codeine, propoxyphene (Darvon); narcotic agonist and antagonist for the following: butorphanol tartrate (Stadol), pentazocine (Talwin), nalbuphine (Nubain).

Contraindications Use with caution in narcotic-dependent patients; use with caution in neonates of narcotic-addicted mothers.

Dosage and administration Adult: 0.4–2.0 mg IV, IM, SC, or ET (diluted); minimum recommended dose, 0.4 mg; repeat at 5-minute intervals to a maximum dose of 10 mg (medical control may request higher amounts). Infusion: 2 mg in 500 mL of D_5W (4 µg/mL), infuse at 0.4 mg/h (100 mL/h). Pediatric: 0.1 mg/kg/dose IV, IM, SC, ET (diluted); maximum dose of 0.8 mg; if no response in 10 minutes, administer an additional 0.1 mg/kg/dose.

Medication Review

Nitroglycerin (Nitrostat, Tridil, and others)

Indications Acute angina pectoris, ischemic chest pain, hypertension, CHF, pulmonary edema.

Contraindications Hypotension, hypovolemia; intracranial bleeding or head injury; previous administration of Viagra, Revatio, Levitra, Cialis, or similar agents within past 24 hours.

Dosage and administration Adult: Tablets: 0.3–0.4 mg SL; may repeat in 3–5 minutes to maximum of 3 doses. NTG spray: 0.4 mg under the tongue; 1–2 sprays. NTG IV infusion: begin at 10 to 20 µg/min; increase by 5–10 µg/min every 5 minutes until desired effect. Pediatric: Not recommended.

Ondansetron Hydrochloride (Zofran)

Indications For the prevention or control of nausea or vomiting. Also used in the hospital setting for patients undergoing chemotherapy or surgical procedures.

Contraindications Known allergy to this medicine or other 5-HT3 receptor antagonists.

Dosage and administration Adult: 4 mg IV or IM (may repeat in 10 minutes). Pediatric: 0.1 mg/kg IV or IM.

Oxygen

Indications Confirmed or expected hypoxemia, ischemic chest pain, respiratory insufficiency, prophylactically during air transport, confirmed or suspected carbon monoxide poisoning, all other causes of decreased tissue oxygenation, decreased level of consciousness.

Contraindications Certain patients with COPD or emphysema who will not tolerate oxygen concentrations over 35%, hyperventilation. Oxygen should never be withheld from a patient who needs it, however. Be prepared to assist with ventilations in a patient with COPD who requires high concentration, as apnea may result.

Dosage and administration Adult: Cardiac arrest and carbon monoxide poisoning: 100%. Hypoxemia: 10–15 L/min via nonrebreathing mask. COPD: 1–6 L/min via nasal cannula or 28%–35% Venturi mask. Be prepared to provide ventilatory support if higher concentrations of oxygen needed. Pediatric: Same as for adult with exception of premature infant.

Promethazine Hydrochloride (Phenergan)

Indications Nausea, vomiting, motion sickness; sedation for patients in labor; potentiation of analgesic effects of narcotics.

Contraindications Hypersensitivity, coma, CNS-depressed patients from alcohol, barbiturates, narcotics, Reye's syndrome.

Dosage and administration Adult: 12.5–25 mg IV, deep IM, PO, rectally. Pediatric: (older than 2 years old) 0.25–0.5 mg/kg dose IM.

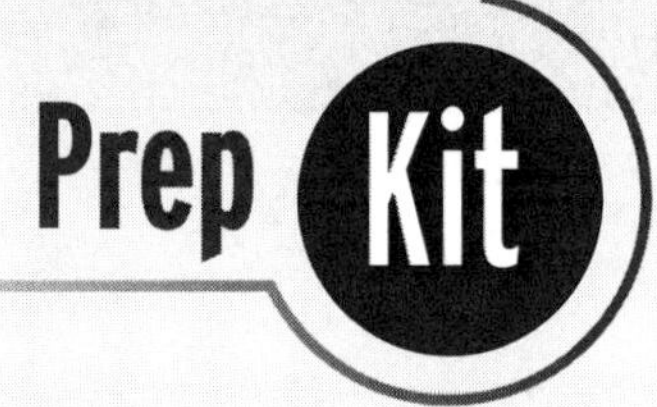

Chapter Summary

- Your primary focus for urologic diseases involves supportive care with assessment and management of the symptoms of these conditions.
- Kidney stones originate in the renal pelvis and are excreted with urine. The passage of the stone is very painful.
- Kidney stones are typically due to water intake that is insufficient to dissolve the salts.
- The prehospital treatment plan for a patient you suspect has kidney stones involves the ABCs, monitoring serial vital signs, and inserting an IV line for fluid infusion and administration of pain medications (analgesics).
- Most EMS systems have refined their view of prehospital analgesia because in most situations, as long as the patient's vital signs are stable, it is best to alleviate severe pain.
- Acute renal failure (ARF) may result from many causes including inadequate perfusion, trauma, a surgical or medical procedure, malignant hypertension, bacterial infection, drug reaction, metabolic disorder, and obstruction.
- Chronic renal failure can occur from any renal dysfunction, most commonly diabetic neuropathy.
- The primary treatments for acute and chronic renal failure are to manage the ABCs, administer high-flow oxygen, provide ventilatory support with a bag-mask device as needed, and consider administering an IV bolus of normal saline if there are signs of shock.

Vital Vocabulary

Acute renal failure (ARF) A sudden decrease in filtration through the glomeruli; acute urinary retention.

Chronic renal failure Progressive and irreversible inadequate kidney function due to permanent loss of nephrons.

Epididymitis An inflammation of the epididymis, which is the system of ductules that emerge from the testicles.

Kidney stones Solid crystalline masses formed in the kidneys, resulting from an excess of insoluble salts or uric acid crystallizing in the urine; may become trapped anywhere along the urinary tract. Also see *renal calculi*.

Lithotripsy An in-hospital method of breaking up kidney stones.

Prostatitis An inflammation of the prostate gland.

Pyelonephritis An inflammation of the kidney lining often caused by a urinary tract infection in the upper urinary tract.

Renal calculi Kidney stones that involve the formation of small rocklike concretions, generally 1 to 5 mm in diameter. Also see *kidney stones*.

Renal colic A type of pain caused by kidney stones and other disorders affecting the kidney, such as thrombosis of the renal artery or renal vein.

Renal dialysis A technique for "filtering" the blood of toxic wastes, removing excess fluids, and restoring the normal balance of electrolytes.

Torsion of the testicle The most common pediatric urologic emergency. Torsion means that the testicle (testis) itself has been twisted.

Urinary tract infection (UTI) Infection, usually of the lower urinary tract (urethra and bladder), which occurs when normal flora bacteria enter the urethra and grow.

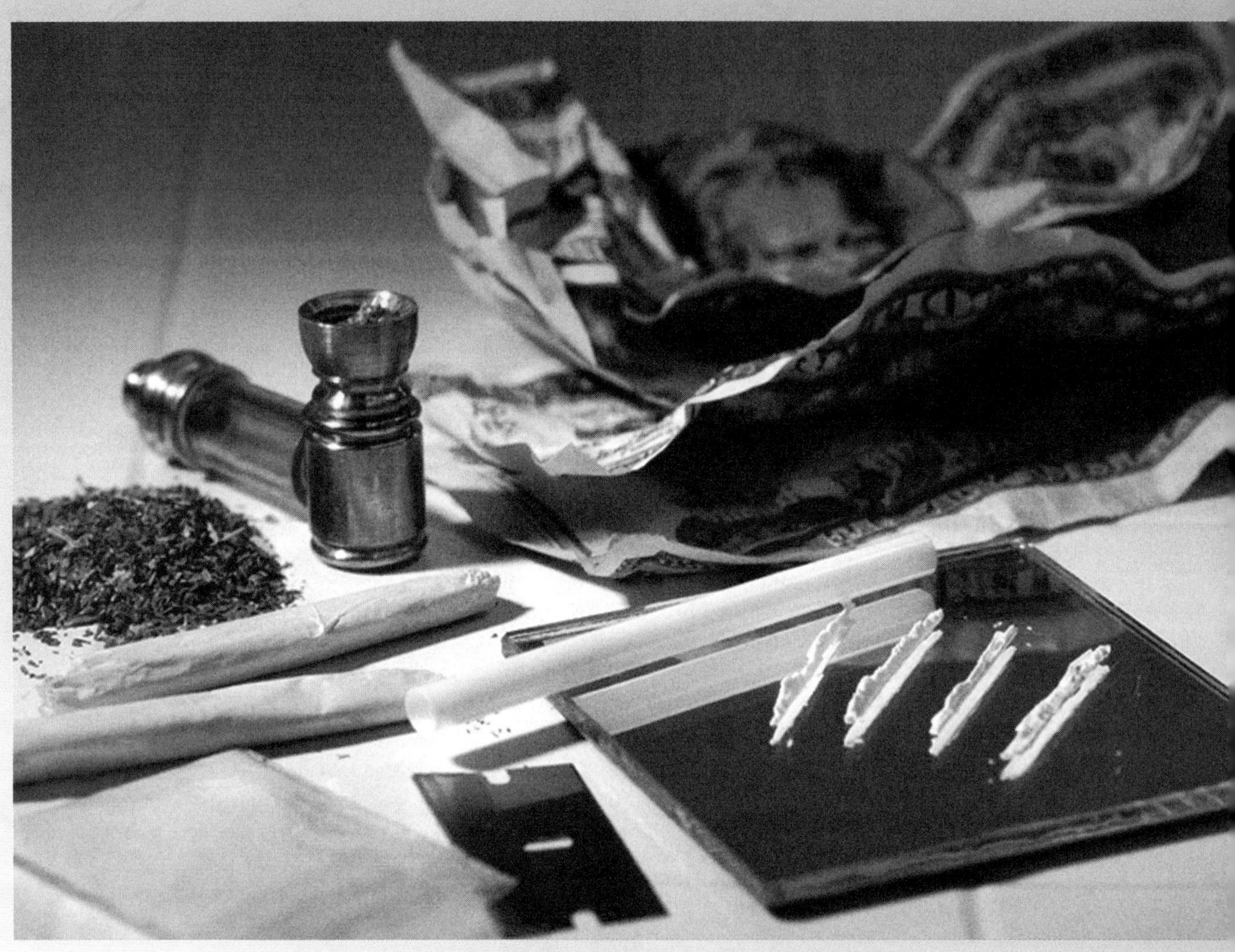

Toxicology and Behavioral Emergencies

9

Objectives

Cognitive

5-8.16 Differentiate among the various treatments and pharmacological interventions in the management of the most common poisonings by ingestion. (pages 274, 278)

5-8.24 Differentiate among the various treatments and pharmacological interventions in the management of the most common poisonings by inhalation. (pages 274, 283)

5-8.31 Differentiate among the various treatments and pharmacological interventions in the management of the most common poisonings by injection. (pages 274, 278–282)

5-8.38 Differentiate among the various treatments and pharmacological interventions in the management of the most common poisonings by surface absorption. (pages 274, 283)

5-8.45 Differentiate among the various treatments and pharmacological interventions in the management of the most common poisonings by overdose. (pages 274–284)

5-8.54 Differentiate among the various treatments and pharmacological interventions in the management of the most commonly abused drugs. (pages 274–284)

5-8.57 Discuss common causative agents, pharmacology, assessment findings, and management for a patient with food poisoning. (page 278)

5-8.58 Discuss common offending organisms, pharmacology, assessment findings, and management for a patient with a bite or sting. (page 278)

Affective

None

Psychomotor

None

Additional Objectives

9-1 Discuss the following medications used in the prehospital setting: activated charcoal [Liqui-Char], naloxone hydrochloride [Narcan], Mark 1 kits (atropine and 2-PAM), haloperidol [Haldol], Midazolam [Versed]—for chemical restraint. (pages 281, 284, 289)

9-2 Discuss patient restraint. (pages 287–291)

9-3 Discuss the SICRAS scale and its use. (pages 285–286)

9-4 Discuss the medications that a patient with a behavioral condition may be taking. (page 286)

Toxicology

The four routes of poisoning are: ingestion, inhalation, injection, and absorption (**Table 9-1**). In this chapter we often use the terminology poisoning and overdose interchangeably. To be accurate, with the exception of food poisoning, poisonings usually involve substances that are not typically intended for human consumption and overdoses usually involve substances (most frequently medicines) that are designed for human consumption but have been taken, either accidentally or purposefully, in excess.

The syndrome-like symptoms of a poisonous agent exposure/ingestion are termed a **toxidrome**. Toxidromes assist us in remembering the assessment and management of different substances that fall under the same clinical umbrella. The major toxidromes are produced by narcotics, cholinergics, anticholinergics, sympathomimetics, stimulants, and sedatives and hypnotics (**Table 9-2**). Some of the common signs and symptoms of poisoning may include peculiar odors, and changes in the pupils, mouth, or skin (**Table 9-3**).

The facts on poison exposures, as collected by the American Association of Poison Control Centers, reveal interesting data on the problem in the U.S. On average, poison centers handle one poison exposure

Table 9-1 Common Poison/Overdose Management and Their Most Common Routes of Exposure

Poison/OD	Common Route	Treatment
Alcohol	Ingestion	Maintain ABCs and be prepared for a vomiting patient. Always assess for the combination of alcohol and other substances that may have a synergistic effect leading to respiratory depression.
Cleaning agents	Inhalation	The scene usually contains clues to help identify the toxin. Assistance from the poison control center and medical control is a must. Administer high-concentration oxygen to correct hypoxia, establish vascular access, apply an ECG monitor, and perform pulse oximetry and capnography.
Heroin	Injection	Maintain ABCs and administer naloxone hydrochloride [Narcan] if necessary to reverse respiratory depression.
Pesticides/organophosphates	Absorption	Do not get the substance on you! Maintain ABCs, administer oxygen, monitor for arrhythmia, and consult with medical control.

Table 9-2 Major Toxidromes

Toxidrome	Drug Examples	Signs and Symptoms
Stimulant	Amphetamine, methamphetamine, cocaine, diet aids, nasal decongestants	Restlessness, agitation, incessant talking, insomnia, anorexia, dilated pupils, tachycardia, tachypnea, hypertension or hypotension, paranoia, seizures, cardiac arrest
Narcotic (opiate and opioid)	Heroin, opium, morphine, hydromorphone (Dilaudid), fentanyl, oxycodone-aspirin combination (Percodan), zolpidem tartrate (Ambien), secobarbital	Constricted (pin-point) pupils, marked respiratory depression, needle tracks (IV abusers), drowsiness, stupor, coma
Sympathomimetic	Pseudoephedrine, phenylephrine, phenylpropanolamine, amphetamine, methamphetamine	Hypertension, tachycardia, dilated pupils (mydriasis), agitation and seizures, hyperthermia
Sedative and hypnotic	Phenobarbital, diazepam (Valium), thiopental	Drowsiness, disinhibition, ataxia, slurred speech, mental confusion, respiratory depression, progressive central nervous system depression, hypotension
Cholinergic	Diazinon, orthene, parathion, sarin, tabun, VX	Increased salivation, lacrimation, gastrointestinal distress, diarrhea, respiratory depression, apnea, seizures, coma
Anticholinergic	Atropine, scopolamine, antihistamines, antipsychotics	Dry, flushed skin, hyperthermia, dilated pupils, blurred vision, tachycardia, mild hallucinations, dramatic delirium

Table 9-3 Common Signs and Symptoms of Poisoning

Sign or Symptom	Type	Possible Causative Agents
Odor	Bitter almonds	Cyanide
	Garlic	Arsenic, organophosphates, phosphorus
	Acetone	Methyl alcohol, isopropyl alcohol, aspirin, acetone
	Wintergreen	Methyl salicylate
	Pears	Chloral hydrate
	Violets	Turpentine
	Camphor	Camphor
	Alcohol	Alcohol
Pupils	Constricted	Narcotics, organophosphates, Jimson weed, nutmeg, propoxyphene (Darvon)
	Dilated	Barbiturates, atropine, amphetamine, glutethimide (Doriden), lysergic acid diethylamide (LSD), cyanide, carbon monoxide (CO)
Mouth	Salivation	Organophosphates, arsenic, strychnine, mercury, salicylates
	Dry mouth	Atropine (belladonna), amphetamines, diphenhydramine (Benadryl), narcotics
	Burns in mouth	Formaldehyde, iodine, lye, toxic plants, phenols, phosphorous, pine oil, silver nitrate, acids
Skin	Pruritis	Jimson weed, belladonna, boric acid
	Dry, hot skin	Atropine (in belladonna), botulism, nutmeg
	Sweating	Organophosphates, arsenic, aspirin, amphetamines, barbiturates, mushrooms, naphthalene
Respiratory	Depressed respirations	Narcotics, alcohol, propoxyphene, CO, barbiturates
	Increased respirations	Aspirin, amphetamines, boric acid, cyanide, kerosene, methyl alcohol, nicotine
	Pulmonary edema	Organophosphates, petroleum products, narcotics, CO
Cardiovascular	Tachycardia	Alcohol, amphetamines, arsenic, atropine, aspirin, cocaine, some anti-asthma drugs
	Bradycardia	Digitalis, gasoline, nicotine, mushrooms, narcotics, cyanide, mistletoe, rhododendron
	Hypertension	Amphetamines, lead, nicotine, antiasthma drugs
	Hypotension	Barbiturates, narcotics, tranquilizers, house plants, mistletoe, nitroglycerin, antifreeze
Central nervous system	Seizures	Amphetamines, camphor, cocaine, strychnine, arsenic, CO, petroleum products, scorpion sting
	Coma	All depressant drugs (such as narcotics, barbiturates, tranquilizers, alcohol), CO, cyanide
	Hallucinations	Atropine, LSD, mushrooms, organic solvents, phencyclidine (PCP), nutmeg
	Headache	CO, alcohol, disulfiram (Antabuse)
	Tremors	Organophosphates, CO, amphetamine, tranquilizers, poisonous marine animals
	Weakness or paralysis	Organophosphates, botulism, eel, hemlock, puffer fish, pine oil, rhododendron
Gastrointestinal	Cramps, nausea, vomiting, and/or diarrhea	Many, if not most, ingested poisons

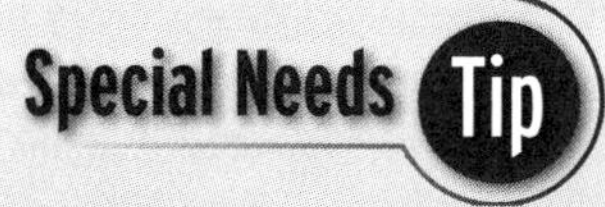

It is becoming more common for people to overdose on multiple medications. Whether it is accidental (combining the wrong medications) or intentional is of no consequence. Multi-pharmacopeia overdose commonly consists of pain medications, anti-anxiety medications, and/or one of the following: alcohol, muscle relaxants, illicit drugs, or over-the-counter preparations. Care should be taken to prevent severe withdrawal effects such as seizures when narcotic or benzodiazepine reversal agents (naloxone hydrochloride [Narcan] and flumazenil [Romazicon]) are administered. The first priority in any patient is to ensure patency of the airway. If you feel that the patient is unable to protect their airway and is at high risk for aspiration, then secure the airway using either nasal intubation or pharmacologic-assisted intubation.

every 13 seconds. In 2005 alone, there were over two million poison exposures reported to local poison centers. Most poisonings involve everyday household items (ie, medicines, cleaning supplies, cosmetics, personal care items). Here are some interesting general facts on poisoning exposures:

- 92.7% of all poison exposures occur in the home.
- 91.3% of exposures involve only one poisonous substance.
- 83.8% of poison exposures are unintentional.
- 76.7% of poison exposures involve ingestion of a poisonous substance. Other causes include breathing in poison gas, getting foreign substances in the eyes or on the skin, and bites and stings.
- 73.5% of all exposures are treated on the site where they occurred, generally the patient's home with phone advice and assistance from local poison control experts.

Specific to children, 50.7% of poison exposures occur in children younger than age 6 years with the most common forms of poison exposure for this age group being cosmetics and personal care products (13.4%), cleaning substances (9.8%), analgesics (8.2%), and foreign bodies (7.4%). The data also show that although children younger than 6 years were involved in more than 50% of poisoning reports, they account for just 1.9% of the fatalities. In the teenage (adolescent) years, there were more than 171,000 cases of poison exposure reported in 2005. The data also reveal that in children between ages 13 and 19, the majority of poison exposures (54.5%) involve girls. In children younger than age 13, the reverse is true, with the majority of these exposures involving boys. Of the reported adolescent deaths from poison exposure, 89.6% were due to intentional poison exposure such as suicide or drug abuse.

As far as the most severe of the poisoning exposures, more than 70% of all poison fatalities occur in adults ages 20 to 59. In the elderly population (age 60 and over), this group accounts for just over 5% of poison exposures; however, they account for 16.3% of the fatalities.

[Data from the 2005 Annual Report of the American Association of Poison Control Centers National Poisoning and Exposure Database, which is compiled by the American Association of Poison Control Centers in cooperation with the majority of U.S. poison centers.]

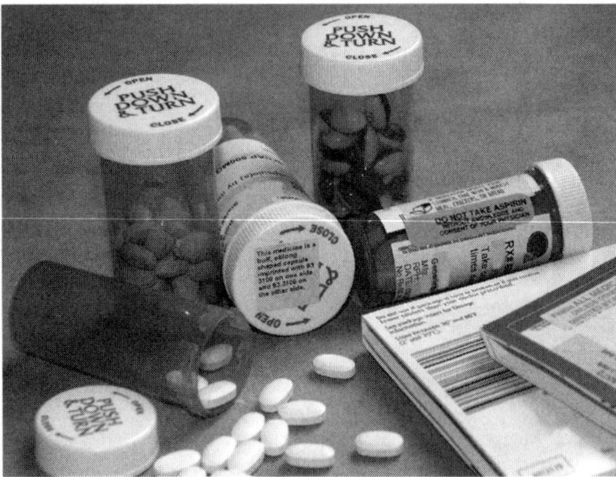

Figure 9-1 Medications are legal substances that can be abused.

Accidental or Purposeful Poisoning by Overdose

The inappropriate use of prescription medications has been the leading cause of drug-related ED visits over the past few years (**Figure 9-1** ◀).

According to figures collected by the Substance and Mental Health Services Administration (SAMHSA), from data collected by the Drug Abuse Warning Network, the number of overdoses from prescription medications is very close to the number of overdoses from cocaine and heroin. It was found that the ED visits for abuse or misuse of prescription drugs such as narcotics (ie, oxycodone hydrochloride [Roxicodone], hydrocodone [Vicodin], methylphenidate hydrochloride [Ritalin], and methadone hydrochloride [Dolophine]) increased 21% from 2004 to 2005. ED visits from abuse or misuse of anti-anxiety drugs (ie, alprazolam [Xanax] and diazepam [Valium]) increased 19%. The greatest increase was from overdoses of methylphenidate (a stimulant and the primary ingredient in the drug **Ritalin** [methylphenidate hydrochloride]), which doubled from 2004 to 2005. Of the illicit drugs, the rate of abuse remained basically stable from 2004 to 2005, cocaine abuse accounted for 448,481 ED visits, followed by marijuana with 242,200 visits, and heroin at 164,572 visits.

Table 9-4 Signs and Symptoms of Polysubstance Abuse

Central Nervous System	Respiratory	Cardiovascular	GI
AMS	Tachypnea	Tachycardia	Nausea
Anxiety	Noncardiogenic pulmonary edema	Palpitations	Vomiting
Restlessness		Chest pain	Abdominal pain or cramping
Headache		Arrhythmias	Dry mouth
Vision disturbances			Anorexia
Ataxia			
Seizure			
Hyperthermia			
Hypertensive crisis			

Table 9-5 CNS Stimulants and Depressants

Stimulants	Depressants
Cocaine	Alcohol
Methamphetamines	Benzodiazepines: (ie, alprazolam [Xanax], chlordiazepoxide [Librium], clorazepate [Tranxene], diazepam [Valium], halazepam [Paxipam], lorazepam [Ativan], oxazepam [Serax], and prazepam [Centrax])
3,4-methylenedioxymethamphetamine (MDMA), also known as Ecstasy	gamma-hydroxybutyrate (GHB)*
Khat	flunitrazepam (Rohypnol)*
ketamine (Ketalar)	Narcotics: (ie, heroin, codeine, darvon, methadone)

*GHB and Rohypnol are also known as the "date rape" drugs.

Recreational and Club Drugs

The recreational use of **CNS stimulants** and depressants continues to result in increasing numbers of overdose cases. The rave or club drugs 3,4-methylenedioxymethamphetamine (MDMA), otherwise known as **Ecstasy**, **gamma-hydroxybutyric acid (GHB)**, flunitrazepam (**Rohypnol**), and **ketamine** (Ketalar) are typically combined with alcohol, marijuana, cocaine, **methamphetamines**, and **Khat**.

Polysubstance abuse tends to be the rule rather than the exception with these drugs (**Table 9-4**▲). Patients often have mixed toxidromic presentations. This is due to the coingestion of CNS stimulants with depressants (**Table 9-5**▲). The primary concern when treating a patient who has used club drugs is supporting the cardiovascular systems. There is no standard treatment regimen for club drug polysubstance overdose; rather management should consist of support of the ABCs, oxygenation, monitoring for arrhythmia, and consultation with medical control as needed.

Treatment of Overdose

Close observation with supportive care is the approach in treating overdose. When the predominant symptoms are controlled, the symptoms of a second underlying drug may surface. Most hallucinogens are CNS stimulants. In overdose, patients may present with tachycardia, anxiety, agitation, hypertension, and hyperthermia. The focused examination should concentrate on the neurologic status and vital signs. Observe for hypertension, hyperthermia, and seizures which must be treated. If pharmacologic treatment is needed, IV barbiturates or diazepam [Valium] may be useful in the patient experiencing seizures.

Patients who are unconscious or otherwise disoriented for an uncertain reason should be treated as if they have a spinal injury until such injury can otherwise be ruled out. To be prudent, you should assess mechanism of injury (MOI), look for distracting injuries, and assess the potential for intoxication with alcohol, controlled substances, or over-the-counter medications.

Standard practice for clearing cervical spine injuries in the field consists of the following components:

1. Patient older than 6 years of age.
2. NO altered mental status or decreased level of consciousness.
3. NO suspected alcohol intoxication or other physically or mentally impairing substance used by the patient recently.
4. NO presence of neurologic deficit or complaint.
5. NO presence of C-spine pain or point tenderness.
6. NO distracting injuries of any kind. Examples of this include long bone deformity, abdominal or chest injury, crushing injuries, or extensive body surface area burns.
7. NO language barrier between the paramedic and the patient.
8. NO significant mechanism of injury creating a high index of suspicion of spinal injury. This may include high-speed motor vehicle collision, vehicle ejection, vehicle rollover, or falls from a height of greater than 20 feet.

Vital signs should no longer just consist of pulse rate, blood pressure, and respiratory rate. Consider with every patient obtaining a blood glucose level, temperature, and cardiac assessment early in your patient assessment algorithm. Additionally end-tidal carbon dioxide ($EtCO_2$) is an excellent tool to use when evaluating the respiratory status of patients with COPD and CHF, as well as a "Gold Standard" for continual evaluation of endotracheal tube placement.

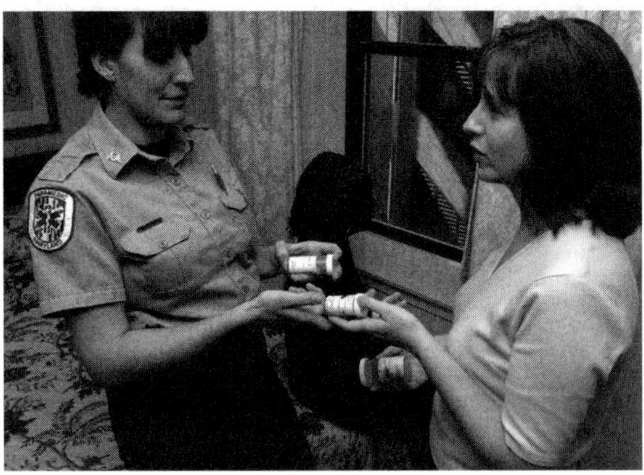

Figure 9-2 Take any bottles, containers, and their remaining contents found at the scene with you to the ED.

Poison by Ingestion and Injection

In terms of assessment and management, injection and ingestion poisonings are often dealt with in a similar manner. That is to say, you will attempt to determine what the patient may have ingested or injected, whether it was drugs, food or plants eaten, or a bite or sting injection, as well as how much of the substance was ingested or injected (**Table 9-6**▼).

Management of Poison by Ingestion and Injection

The management of ingestion or injection is generally supportive and always revolves around the safety of the crew, management of the ABCs, and considering the need for a specific antidote if one is available (ie, naloxone hydrochloride [Narcan] for the narcotic overdose). Pain management can be administered in the prehospital setting for a bite or a sting, per local protocol. If the patient has food poisoning, consider the administration of antiemetics per local protocol. The definitive care of the poisoned or overdosed patient occurs in the ED setting and often involves evacuation of the stomach. If found at the scene, be sure to take bottles, containers, and their remaining contents with you to the ED (**Figure 9-2**▲).

Table 9-6 Common Offenders of Ingestion and Injection Poisoning

Source of Poison	Typical Route	Examples
Plants	Ingestion	Dieffenbachia, Caladium, Lantana, Castor beans, and Foxglove
Food Toxin	Ingestion	*Salmonella, Listeria,* and *Toxoplasma*
Creatures	Injection (caused by a bite or sting)	Snakes, spiders, and scorpions
Drugs	Ingestion and Injection	Mushrooms, heroin

Case Study 1 Poison by Injection

Part 1

Your unit has been dispatched to the schoolyard playground in an inner city district. Apparently a teacher called 9-1-1 when her students began peering out the window at a man in his 20s sleeping in the schoolyard. No one knows the man so the police have also been dispatched.

As you arrive you and your partner are met by the school's custodian, a police officer, and hundreds of pairs of children's eyes peering out the windows. The scene is safe and there does not appear to be any trauma. You decide it would be prudent to manually stabilize the patient's head and neck in a neutral position while beginning your initial assessment (IA) (see **Table 1**). You ask your partner to do so.

According to the custodian he has chased this "drug addict" off the school grounds before. You kneel next to the patient and try to determine if he responds to verbal stimuli, which he does not, so you try a sternal rub. You quickly pull out an oropharyngeal airway and the bag-mask device to hook it up to supplemental oxygen.

After completing the IA and deciding that there does not seem to be any cause for trauma, your partner releases the head and neck and begins to assist the patient's ventilations with the bag-mask device. This will help increase both his tidal volume and the rate, and increase the oxygen concentration in the blood.

Table 1 **Initial Assessment**

Initial Assessment	Recording Time: 1 Minute
General Impression/ Appearance	Unconscious, sloppy, and dirty clothing
Mental Status	"P" responds to painful stimuli by withdrawal
Airway	Open but snoring
Breathing	Very slow and shallow with some breaths being difficult to see
Circulation	Radial pulse is weak and fast
Priority/Plan	High due to the respiratory depression

You begin your focused history and physical examination with a rapid medical examination since the patient is not responsive. Just as you begin your examination, a first responder arrives to assist you.

Question 1: What are some of the causes of shallow respirations in a medical patient?

Question 2: Should the custodian's comment that the patient is a "drug addict" be taken into account in your assessment?

Part 2

Since the patient is not responsive, you begin the rapid medical examination (RME) with a hands-on assessment of the major body regions (ie, head, neck, chest, abdomen, pelvis, back, buttocks, and the four extremities). This examination reveals track marks on both arms as well as a number of bumps and bruises and old scars on his legs. His lungs are clear and his abdomen is soft. You continue with a focused history and physical examination (see **Table 2**).

Table 2 **Focused History and Physical Examination**

Baseline Vital Signs	Recording Time: 5 Minutes
Skin CTC (color, temperature, condition)	Pale, cool, clammy
Pulse	Rapid and thready
Blood pressure	108/72 mm Hg
Respirations	28 breaths/min and very shallow

At this point you are working with a chief complaint of altered mental status although you do suspect that drugs may be a contributing factor. His pupils are pinpoint. You do note that he does not have a Medic Alert bracelet and the police are looking through his wallet for additional information.

You remember from paramedic school that is it not a good idea to search through a patient's pockets, especially if they may have drug paraphernalia such as sharps in their pockets, so you refrain from doing so.

Question 3: What is the significance of the pinpoint pupils?

Question 4: What is the significance of the track marks and bruising on both arms on this patient?

Case Study I Continued

Part 3

The custodian locates a dirty needle, spoon, and rubber tourniquet on the ground about 20 feet from where the patient is located. This adds more evidence to the story that this patient has injected himself with a drug. The pinpoint pupils peak your interest since they are often evidence of a narcotic or opiate overdose. The OPQRST questions and SAMPLE history questions are difficult to obtain since he is in no condition to speak for himself (see **Table 3**). Your partner manages to start an IV, and tests some of the patient's blood revealing a glucose level of 108 mg/dL. You both agree that a dose of naloxone hydrochloride [Narcan] would be appropriate in this situation.

Table 3 SAMPLE History

SAMPLE History	Comments
Signs/symptoms	Altered mental status, pale, clammy, depressed respirations, occasional raspy cough (may have aspirated prior to your arrival), and constricted pupils
Allergies	Unknown at this time
Medications	Unknown at this time
Pertinent past medical history	Unknown except possible IV drug abuser
Last oral intake	Unknown
Events leading up to the incident	You suspect a drug injection

Your protocols require you to restrain the patient in a semi-Fowler's position before the administration of this drug because it could cause the patient to become violent. You move the patient to the stretcher. You quickly apply tape and roller gauze restraints to his extremities as well as place a sheet across his chest, while your partner draws up the naloxone hydrochloride [Narcan]. After you have administered the naloxone hydrochloride [Narcan], you will consider the need for an advanced airway. You know it is important to administer the naloxone hydrochloride first in order to avoid an angry patient waking up with a tube down his throat!

All the while the first responder has been assisting with the ventilations to ensure that each breath he takes is a full one.

Treatment Plan

1. Assist ventilations.
2. Restrain the patient.
3. Administer 0.4 to 2.0 mg of naloxone hydrochloride [Narcan] titrated to effect (see **Table 4**).
4. Continue to assist ventilations and evaluate the need for an advanced airway.
5. Monitor serial vital signs and ECG en route to the ED.
6. Consider the need for more naloxone hydrochloride [Narcan] in consult with medical control while en route to the ED.

Case Study I Continued

Table 4 Naloxone Hydrochloride

Do you know?	Comments
Right drug? Generic name: [**Naloxone Hydrochloride**] Trade name: [Narcan]	This drug is a narcotic antagonist and will precipitate immediate opiate withdrawal. When the paramedic suspects that the patient's respiratory depression is due to an overdose of a narcotic or opiate, such as morphine, heroin, or methadone, the drug of choice to reverse the effects of the narcotic or opiate is naloxone hydrochloride [Narcan].
Right patient?	Patients who have depressed respirations or an altered mental status from too high a dose of a narcotic or opiate.
Right dose?	The dose is 0.4 mg to 2.0 mg and it is best to titrate (increments of 0.4 mg) to desirable effect of improved respirations.
Right route?	Can be given by IV, IO, IM, intranasal, SC, or ET routes, although the ET route is the least effective and not generally recommended if other routes are available.
Right time?	If the patient has respiratory depression, assist the ventilations with your bag-mask device while properly positioning and restraining the patient on your stretcher in the event the patient wakes up in an argumentative or violent mood. Then it is time to administer the naloxone hydrochloride [Narcan].
Right documentation?	Always document how and when the drug was administered as well as the patient's response to the medication on your patient care report.
Expected action	Antagonistic to narcotic or opiate medications. Expect it to reverse the effect of the overdose. Small doses should improve the patient's ventilations. Larger doses may cause the patient to actually wake up, which is generally not necessary since they wake up in an argumentative or violent mood.
Side effects	Nausea, upset stomach, or drowsiness can occur. More serious side effects from naloxone hydrochloride [Narcan] include withdrawal symptoms including: vomiting, diaphoresis, tremors, seizures, and a rapid and pounding irregular pulse.
Contraindications	Use with caution in narcotic-dependent patients; use with caution in neonates of narcotic-addicted mothers.
Precautions	Administer this drug slowly and only administer enough to improve his respirations. If you administer the entire dose the patient is likely to awaken with withdrawal symptoms and be very aggressive. You will have just spoiled his high!
Pharmacokinetics	Onset: within 2 minutes; peak effect: variable; duration: 30–60 minutes; metabolized in the liver and excreted in urine.

Question 5: Why is it a policy in some regions to restrain a patient before administering naloxone hydrochloride [Narcan]?

Question 6: Why is it important to wait on the insertion of an advanced airway until after the first dose of naloxone hydrochloride [Narcan]?

Case Study I Continued

Part 4

After administering the naloxone hydrochloride [Narcan] to the patient, his respirations have improved to the point where you are comfortable switching from the bag-mask to a nonrebreathing mask at 12 L/min of supplemental oxygen. The patient is arousable with a strong sternal rub, but he does push your hand away when painful stimuli are applied. His pupils have changed to PEARRL (Pupils Equal and Round, Regular in Size, React to Light) and are no longer pinpoint. You and your partner discuss the need for more naloxone hydrochloride [Narcan] and you both decide to monitor the patient closely but feel he is very manageable at this point (see **Table 5**). Just to be on the safe side, one of the first responders agrees to ride in the back of the ambulance with you in case anything changes. However, at this point, things are looking good. Of course you are keeping the naloxone hydrochloride [Narcan] nearby because you remember from your training that often the naloxone hydrochloride [Narcan] can wear off before the narcotic wears off and the patient can slip back into his prior respiratory depression.

Question 7: The patient's lung sounds are like a bad "smoker's cough." What is this most likely the result of?

Table 5 Reassessment and Ongoing Assessment of the Patient

Serial Vital Signs and Relevant Data	Recording Time: 6 Minutes
Skin CTC	Pale, warm, and dry
Pulse	100 beats/min and regular
Blood Pressure	116/78 mm Hg
Respirations	24 breaths/min and normal depth
Mental Status	Responds to painful stimuli by withdrawal
ECG	Normal sinus rhythm
SpO_2	96% on supplemental oxygen
Lung Sounds	Some rhonchi, like a bad smoker's cough (the rhonchi may be due to the patient having aspirated prior to your arrival on the scene)
Other (ie, glucose, core body temperature)	Glucose is within normal range

Question 8: Some patients with a narcotic overdose have been known to have acute pulmonary edema. If that were the case with this patient, from your knowledge of acute pulmonary edema patients, what other signs would you expect to see?

Part 5

This case is one example of a patient overdose on opioids. It easily could have been further complicated by numerous substances, including alcohol, but the scenario was kept simple to illustrate the important teaching points. You need to be diligent about airway management and ventilation, and rule out other causes of the altered mental status such as head injury, hypoxia, or hypoglycemia. In this case, realize that it is helpful to use medication to lighten the patient's mental status to the point where an adequate respiratory effort is restored rather than rapidly giving excessive amounts of naloxone hydrochloride [Narcan], thus causing the patient to experience an instantaneous total withdrawal. After all, it is easier to manage the patient when he is sleepy with adequate ventilations compared to a patient who is awake, spitting, argumentative, or potentially violent. In addition, overdosed patients put into withdrawal are at risk of fleeing the scene. As the half-life of a single dose of naloxone hydrochloride [Narcan] is typically less than the agent being reversed, these patients are inadvertently placing themselves at risk of relapsing in an unmonitored environment. This in turn may place the provider in some degree of medico-legal jeopardy.

Although this is a typical case, it is important to note that there are atypical patients who overdose on narcotics in all communities. Addiction does not limit itself to any specific race, social class, or economic standing. Chronic care patients who are being managed for chronic pain in skilled nursing facilities have also been known to overdose and can present with similar symptoms to those discussed in this case.

One final important point about the use of naloxone hydrochloride [Narcan] is that you will often need to administer additional doses since the half-life of the medication is shorter than the narcotic that is causing the respiratory depression. Most EMS systems that encounter narcotic or opiate overdoses frequently have a policy that states that the patient should be restrained and must be transported to the ED. Allowing the patient to "sign off" once he awakens in an angry condition is not appropriate and may mean another call at a later time to care for the patient who has again become unconscious and possibly aspirated. As with any medication you administer, an ongoing assessment is essential since the patient's condition is dynamic and ever changing.

Poison by Surface Absorption and Inhalation

Many drugs are designed to be absorbed slowly through the surface of the skin such as nitroglycerin paste and the numerous transdermal patches (ie, nicotine cessation, birth control, estrogen, and pain relievers). Many chemicals that are not designed to be used in this method (ie, pesticides, plant oils) also dissolve easily in the fat of the skin. In the latter case, the patient may not realize that a poison has been absorbed through the skin.

The easiest way to be poisoned is to simply breathe in, or inhale, the toxic substance in the form of a gas. The most common inhalation poisoning is carbon monoxide (CO) poisoning because it displaces the oxygen on the red blood cell's hemoglobin receptor sites. Since this gas is highly toxic, colorless, and odorless, it accounts for a significant number of inhalation poisonings and may present as a danger to the rescuers.

Management of Poison by Surface Absorption and Inhalation

Treatment of surface absorption or inhalation poisoning must always first include ensuring that the scene is safe for the rescuer and limiting the potential for exposure to the substance. For situations that involve possible inhalation of poisonous substances, this may involve the use of self-contained breathing apparatus by appropriately trained personnel. Identification of the substance and its dangers is paramount to rescuer safety, and if there is a need to call for local expertise before proceeding, that would be a smart approach.

Once the substance that was inhaled or absorbed is identified, your field management should focus on supporting the ABCs. For incidents involving absorption, and without exposing yourself to the agent, remove any remaining paste, patches, powder, spray, oils, etc. Wash the affected area with soap and water. Aside from oxygen, most paramedic services do not carry antidotes for poisoning by inhalation or absorption in their typical formulary. This may not be the case in areas where it has been determined that there is an increased exposure to specific chemicals due to local industry. The use of any pharmacological intervention will depend on the agent involved (ie, fentanyl patch on a child, nitroglycerine powder absorbed thru the skin, or carbon monoxide inhaled). Additional information on the specific management required can be obtained by consulting with the poison center and medical control.

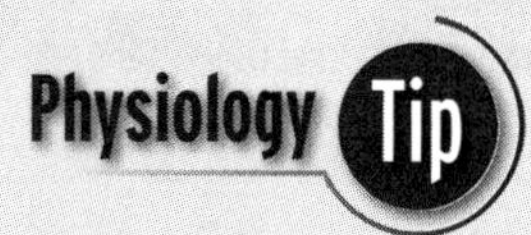

Is there a difference between venous versus capillary draw for obtaining a blood sample to test for a blood glucose level? Yes, there is a difference between the samples! There is also a huge exposure risk from either the needle (no EMS personnel would ever touch a test strip to the tip of the needle) or from excessive blood leaking from the IV site. According to one manufacturer (Bayer), there can be an average +/– 10 mg/dL variance in the blood glucose level between the two types of samples. Most glucometers are calibrated for capillary samples only. Some of the newer devices can be calibrated for either type of sample, dependent on the type of test strip used.

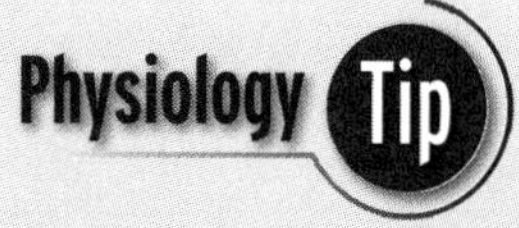

Alcohol can dilute the blood sample that is used in the glucometer. When preparing the skin prior to the use of a lancet, make sure the alcohol dries before piercing the skin. Alcohol mixed with the blood can actually cause a falsely low blood glucose reading. Make sure that you are using the appropriate type of sample for the glucometer being used. And when in doubt, repeat the test. It only takes 60 to 90 seconds!

Other Medications Used in Poisoning Cases

The following are additional medications carried in some EMS systems for use in the prehospital care of the poisoned patient (**Table 9-7 ▸** and **Table 9-8 ▸**). The medication haloperidol [Haldol] is discussed later in this chapter in the behavioral section.

Table 9-7 Activated Charcoal

Do you know?	Comments
Right drug? Generic name: [**Activated Charcoal**]	This is an adsorbent. When a patient has ingested an excessive dose of one or more drugs or poison, activated charcoal can be used to adsorb the agent.
Right patient?	The patient must be alert enough to drink the dose and protect his or her own airway if vomiting should occur or be intubated prior to administration.
Right dose?	If not in a premixed slurry, dilute with 1 part charcoal to 4 parts water. Adult: 1–2 g/kg by mouth (PO) or via NGT.
Right route?	By mouth (PO) in the alert patient and by orogastric or nasogastric tube in the intubated patient.
Right time?	After the patient has been assessed and precautions taken to prevent accidental aspiration (ie, positioning, maintaining the airway, and consideration for intubation).
Right documentation?	Always document how and when the drug was administered and the patient's response to the medication on your patient care report.
Expected action	Activated charcoal adsorbs certain poisons which can keep them from being absorbed through the GI tract (gastric dialysis). Gastric dialysis is considered to be more effective than inducing vomiting in the overdose patient.
Side effects	May induce nausea and vomiting; possible constipation; may cause black stools.
Contraindications	It does not absorb ethyl alcohol (ETOH), lithium, iron, or lead.
Precautions	Activated charcoal can deactivate the effects of ipecac (a medicinal preparation made from the dried roots and rhizomes of a shrub that is used to induce vomiting). Activated charcoal should be administered first if they are used together.
Pharmacokinetics	Depends on gastrointestinal function; duration is continuous while in the GI tract.

Table 9-8 Atropine-Pralidoxime

Do you know?	Comments
Right drug? Generic name: [**Atropine—Pralidoxime (2-PAM Chloride)**] Trade name: [Mark I Kit]	This kit contains two drugs, atropine sulfate and pralidoxime chloride (2-PAM Chloride). When a patient has been exposed to an organophosphate pesticide or nerve agent, the chemical causes overstimulation and excessive release of chemical neurotransmitters, causing the signs and symptoms of cholinergic poisoning.
Right patient?	Patient exposed to organophosphate pesticide or nerve agent with signs and symptoms of cholinergic poisoning.
Right dose?	2 mg atropine, 600 mg pralidoxime chloride. Repeat dosing will vary depending on the severity of symptoms.
Right route?	Auto-injectors, IV
Right time?	As soon as possible after assessment and recognition of exposure to organophosphate nerve agent.
Right documentation?	Always document how and when the drug was administered and the patient's response to the medication on your patient care report.
Expected action	Atropine blocks the overstimulation and subsequent release of neurotransmitters, relaxes smooth muscle in the lungs and GI tract, and dries respiratory secretions. 2-PAM-Chloride enhances the action of atropine.
Side effects	Atropine—tachycardia, dizziness, dilated pupils, blurred vision; Pralidoxime chloride—tachycardia, dizziness, blurred vision, speech problems, muscle weakness or stiffness.
Contraindications	No contraindications when exposure produces moderate to severe symptoms.
Precautions	Do not use prophylactically.
Pharmacokinetics	Onset rapid; metabolism rapid; potentiates the effects of atropine.

The Subject In-Custody Risk Assessment Scale (SICRAS)

The following information is well known in law enforcement and in the corrections community and is used to determine the risk for subjects in custody with a potential for cardiac arrest (**Table 9-9▼**). EMS providers are beginning to also use the SICRAS, which provides a means to rapidly assess an in-custody subject's risk of sudden death based on known symptoms and risk factors.

Table 9-9 The SICRAS

Directions:
Begin at the first observed sign or symptom. Add the numbers for each sign or symptom that applies. A score of 16 or above indicates the subject is at extreme risk for Sudden In-Custody Death Syndrome (SICDS). Immediate medical attention is necessary.

Alcohol Intoxication	1
Acute Alcohol Intoxication (BAC 0.25 or above)	3
History of Alcoholism	2
Cocaine Intoxication	4
Methamphetamine Intoxication	3
Drug Intoxication (other)	2
Bizarre Behavior	2
Aggressive Behavior	2
Shouting	2
Paranoia	3
Violence Against Others	2
Above Normal Physical Strength	3
Sudden Tranquility/Lethargy	2
Moderate Physical Activity	3
Intense Physical Activity	3
Obesity	1
"Big Bellies"	2
Hyperthermia	4
Hypotonicity of Skeletal Muscles	4
Antipsychotic Drug Use	2
History of Schizophrenia	2
Male	1
Ineffectiveness of OC Spray (pepper spray)	2
Cyanosis of Lips/Nail Beds	5
Confusion—Disorientation	3

Score 10–16
Subject is at HIGH risk for Sudden In-Custody Death Syndrome (SICDS). Immediate evaluation by EMS personnel is necessary. Medical treatment may be warranted. Subject should be closely monitored.

Score 5–10
Subject is at MODERATE risk for SICDS. Subject should be reevaluated by another officer/provider familiar with the SICRAS system and SICDS. Subject should be monitored by police, corrections, and/or EMS personnel.

Score 0–5
Subject is at LOW risk for SICDS based on known risk factors. Personnel should be watchful for any signs of distress that would preclude the SICRAS score.

continues

Table 9-9 The SICRAS (*Continued*)

The following conditions or circumstances represent serious, or immediate, threats to safety that necessitate immediate medical treatment or evaluation and supersede the Subject In-Custody Risk Assessment Scale.

Loss of consciousness	Severe headache
Seizure	Medical shock (any cause)
Anaphylactic shock	Chest pain
Respiratory rate < 6 breaths/min	Gagging, gasping, or choking > 4 minutes after OC ingestion
Resting heart rate < 40 or > 140 beats/min	Obvious respiratory distress

The SICRAS and other guidelines presented here cover only conditions and circumstances known to date. It is impossible for us to cover all circumstances that personnel may face. All public safety and health care professionals should rely on his or her common sense, experience, and training. A good rule of thumb is that when conducting an ABCs survey of a subject, any obvious impairment of the airway, breathing, or circulation requires immediate evaluation by medical personnel. When in doubt, have it checked out.

* NOTE: The information regarding the SICRAS scale is taken directly from the Montgomery, New York, County Hospital district EMS protocols.

Behavioral Emergencies

Patients who suffer from psychiatric illness may have conditions such as bipolar disorder, schizophrenia, paranoia, and psychosis. They are often on medications intended to heighten the "lows" (depression) and lower the "highs" (mania). Many of the medications that these patients may be taking are listed in **Table 9-10▼**. An overdose of these medications can produce a multitude of effects, including lethal arrhythmias. Always be sure to carefully assess and monitor the potentially psychiatrically ill patient with an altered mental status or abnormalities in the vital signs.

Table 9-10 Medications Behavioral Patients May Be Taking

Class	Name
Antidepressants	Citalopram [Celexa]
	Escitalopram [Lexapro]
	Fluoxatine [Prozac]
	Fluvoxamine [Luvox]
	Paroxetine [Paxil]
	Sertraline [Zoloft]
	Phenelzine [Nardil]
	Venlafaxine [Effexor]
Atypical antipsychotic agents	Clozapine [Clozaril]
	Olanzapine [Zyprexa]
	Quetiapine [Seroquel]
	Risperidone [Risperidal]
	Ziprasidone [Geodon]
	Aripiprazole [Abilify]
Traditional antipsychotics	Chlorpromazine [Thorazine]
	Chlorprothixene [Taractan]
	Fluphenazine [Prolixin, Permitil]
	Haloperidol [Haldol]
	Loxapine [Loxitane, Daxolin]
	Mesoridazine [Serentil]
	Molindone [Moban]
	Perphenazine [Trilanfon]
	Thioridazine [Mellaril]
	Thiothixene [Navane]
	Trifluoperazine [Stelazine]
Anxiolytics	Alprazolam [Xanax]
	Chlordiazepoxide [Librium]
Anxiolytics	Clonazepam [Klonopin]
	Clorazepate [Tranxene]
	Diazepam [Valium]
	Lorazepam [Ativan]
	Buspirone [BuSpar]
Antihistamines	Hydroxyzine [Atarax, Vistaril]
Beta-blockers	Propanolol [Inderol]
Anticonvulsants	Carbamazepine [Tegretol]
	Gabapentin [Neurontin]
	Valproic acid [Depakote]
Cyclic antidepressants	Amitriptyline [Amitril, Endep, Elavil]
	Amoxapine [Asendin]
	Desipramine [Norpramin, Pertofrane]
	Doxepin [Adapin, Sinequan]
	Imipramine [Imavate, Janimine, Pramine, Presamine, Tofranil]
	Maprotiline [Ludiomil]
	Nortriptyline [Aventyl, Pamelor]
	Protriptyline [Vivacil]
	Trimipramine [Surmontil]
MAO inhibitors	Isocarboxazid [Marplan]
	Phenelzine [Nardil]
	Tranylcypromine [Parnate]
Serotonin reuptake inhibitors	Bupropion [Wellbutrin]
	Fluoxetine [Prozac]
Antimanic agents	Lithium carbonate [Eskalith, Lithane, Lithobid, Lithonate, Lithotabs]

Case Study II Patient Restraint

Part 1

Your unit has been dispatched to an office in the city for a call involving a patient who has been acting very aggressive toward his co-workers. Apparently he came to work today and has been arguing since he arrived. Hearing that there was screaming in the background when taking the call information, the dispatcher has alerted the two nearest police officers and told you to stage the ambulance until the scene is secure.

After a few minutes the police advise that you should respond into the scene without lights and siren. They said you should bring in your stretcher and some form of restraints. You consider your options and know that having the ability to chemically restrain a patient helps decrease the risk of rescuer and patient injury. It also helps to calm the patient and prevents the patient from worsening an already potentially serious associated medical problem. As an alternative, you hope that you are able to use gauze and bandages to restrain the patient.

As you arrive on the scene, a number of the office workers are standing outside the building. It is obvious that there are more than two police officers at the scene. You can see through the windows where a couple of officers are talking with the patient. Although it seems to be calm at this moment, you know from prior experience that there was a reason you were told to park the vehicle at a safe distance and location from the patient and wait for further instructions, otherwise known as stage. It is likely to not remain safe. You do not drop your guard.

After being oriented to the situation by an officer, you slowly approach the patient to begin your initial assessment (see **Table 1**).

Table 1 **Initial Assessment**

Initial Assessment	Recording Time: 2 Minutes
General Impression/ Appearance	Angry expression on face
Mental Status	Alert (oriented to person, place, and time) but not thrilled about even talking to you
Airway	Open and clear
Breathing	Rapid and shallow
Circulation	Has a radial pulse that is rapid and bounding
Priority/Plan	Low at this point because there is no obvious life-threat to the patient

Since there is no obvious trauma you decide the patient will need a focused history and physical examination for a responsive medical patient. However, it is clear that he is very angry and is not going to be very cooperative in answering your questions. The police advise that his wife was sent for and should be arriving on the scene in a few minutes. She may have more information about his history and the medications he is taking. A co-worker states that he has been having a lot of emotional problems for the past year since his father died suddenly.

Question 1: Is the scene ever really safe or secure?

Question 2: What does it mean when your unit is advised to stage?

Part 2

The chief complaint in this situation is aggressive behavior and it is clear that the patient is very upset and in need of evaluation in an ED with mental health facilities. The police have agreed to ride along and follow in their patrol car and the wife agrees that this is the best course of action at this time. It seems the patient, whose name is Joey, and his wife have gone this route before, and he ended up staying in the hospital mental health unit for about 2 weeks. According to his wife, when Joey is noncompliant with his medications, his "bipolar disorder" causes him to go through periods of depression and then manic periods where he is sometimes aggressive.

Since the field diagnosis of a behavioral disorder is a "diagnosis of exclusion," it is your responsibility to try to determine if there is an injury or other medical problem that could be causing his current condition. You have seen diabetics who were hypoglycemic become very combative, as well as head-injured patients, and drug overdose patients. Of course the hypoxic patient can act in an agitated manner as well.

After asking a series of questions to elaborate on the chief complaint and performing a focused history and physical examination, it is clear to you and your partner that Joey has no apparent trauma and most likely does not have a medical problem causing his anger and agitation (see **Table 2**). He has not been very

Case Study II Continued

helpful in answering your questions and you sense he is suffering from building agitation that is soon going to boil over. You predict he will need transport to the ED with the use of humane restraint and the help of law enforcement.

Question 3: What should be your next plan of action with Joey?

Question 4: What types of restraint are used in the field?

Table 2 Focused History and Physical Examination

Baseline Vital Signs	Recording Time: 5 Minutes
Skin CTC (color, temperature, condition)	Red skin, normal temp, slightly sweaty
Pulse	96 beats/min and regular
Blood Pressure	148/82 mm Hg
Respirations	22 breaths/min and regular

Part 3

Next you obtain the patient's SAMPLE medical history from his wife (see **Table 3**). Joey hears her description of what has been going on in his life since his dad died and all the doctors he has been seeing. He blurts out, "that's not true, she's lying again!" It is obvious that the discussion about his history upsets Joey. His wife says he has been on a couple of forms of lithium carbonate [Eskalith] and a few other medications such as valproic acid [Depakote]. She adds that he does not always take his medications. Medication noncompliance is almost always a key component to these kinds of presentations.

Table 3 SAMPLE History

SAMPLE History	Comments
Signs/symptoms	Argumentative and aggressive behavior, swearing, and loud voice
Allergies	No known allergies
Medications	Noncompliant with lithium carbonate [Eskalith] and valproic acid [Depakote]
Pertinent past medical history	Diagnosed manic and bipolar disorder
Last oral intake	A glass of milk 20 minutes ago
Events leading up to the incident	Very agitated all day

Your partner and a police officer bring the stretcher into the office. Joey senses that he is going to have to go to the hospital and states, "I am NOT going anywhere . . . you all should just leave me alone and let me get back to my work. Tell my wife to go back home . . . leave me alone!" At this point it is obvious that this will not be easy and you confer with the police on the best approach to restrain Joey on the stretcher if that becomes necessary.

Treatment Plan

1. Assess and manage the ABCs.
2. Obtain baseline vital signs.
3. Airway management with supplemental oxygen (if tolerated).
4. Check blood glucose level (if abnormal, treat as hypoglycemia).
5. Start an IV and draw blood if safe for you to do so.
6. Contact medical control to consider the following medications:
   a. If patient is younger than 70 years old—haloperidol [Haldol] 5 mg mixed with midazolam [Versed] 2 mg IM (see **Table 4** and **Table 5**).
   b. If patient is older than 70 years old—haloperidol [Haldol] 5 mg IM.
   c. Consult with Medical Control for additional doses of either medication.
7. Transport the patient (restrained in a semi-Fowler's position on the stretcher).

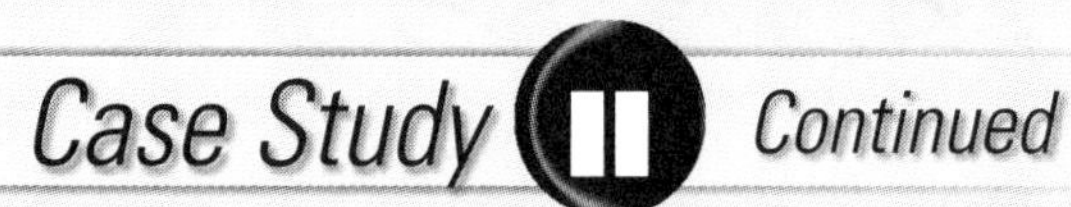

Table 4 Haloperidol

Do you know?	Comments
Right drug? Generic name: [**Haloperidol**] Trade name: [Haldol]	A tranquilizer and antipsychotic drug. Used for managing patients with excited or agitated delirium and who are extremely aggressive. It inhibits central nervous system (CNS) catecholamine receptors; it is strongly antidopaminergic and weak anticholinergic. Acts on CNS to depress subcortical areas, mid-brain, and ascending reticular activating systems in the brain.
Right patient?	Used for managing patients with excited or agitated delirium and who are extremely aggressive.
Right dose?	Adults are typically given 2 to 5 mg IM every 30 to 60 minutes until sedation is achieved.
Right route?	IM.
Right time?	As soon as possible provided you have ruled out the contraindications for the medication.
Right documentation?	Always document how and when the drug was administered as well as the patient's response to the medication on your patient care report.
Expected action	Calming the patient experiencing an acute psychotic episode.
Side effects	Extrapyramidal signs and symptoms, restlessness, spasms. Parkinson-like symptoms, drooling, dystonia, hypotension, orthostatic, hypotension, nausea, vomiting, blurred vision.
Contraindications	Agitation secondary to shock or hypoxia. Hypersensitivity.
Precautions	Enhanced CNS depression and hypotension in combination with alcohol. Antagonized amphetamines and epinephrine. Other CNS depressants may potentiate effects.
Pharmacokinetics	Onset: 10 minutes; peak effect: 30–45 minutes; duration: variable; metabolized in the liver and excreted in urine and feces.

Table 5 Midazolam

Do you know?	Comments
Right drug? Generic name: [**Midazolam**] Trade name: [Versed]	This drug is a short-acting benzodiazepine CNS depressant. Anxiolytic and sedative properties similar to other benzodiazepines, memory impairment.
Right patient?	Indicated in a patient in need of sedation, anxiolytic prior to endotracheal or nasotracheal intubation; administer for conscious sedation.
Right dose?	Adult dose is 2.0 to 2.5 mg slow IV over 2–3 minutes. May be repeated to a total maximum of 0.1 mg/kg.
Right route?	IV slow over 2–3 minutes; IM.
Right time?	Can be given to restrain the patient in concert with haloperidol [Haldol].
Right documentation?	Always document how and when the drug was administered as well as the patient's response to the medication on your patient care report.
Expected action	Sedation and anxiolytic reaction similar to other benzodiazepines.
Side effects	Memory impairment.
Contraindications	Glaucoma, shock, coma, alcohol intoxication, overdose, depressed vital signs, concomitant use with other CNS depressants, barbiturates, alcohol, narcotics.
Precautions	Should not be used in patients who have taken a CNS depressant as it may have a synergistic effect and make the respiratory depression significantly worse.
Pharmacokinetics	Onset: 1–3 minutes IV and dose dependent. Peak effect: variable. Duration: 2–6 hours, dose dependent; metabolized in the liver and excreted in urine.

Question 5: If the patient was on a CNS depressant, how would that affect your chemical restraint?

Question 6: Is it true that the patient might not remember the fight to be restrained?

Case Study II Continued

Part 4

Just as you suspected, as soon as it becomes clear to Joey that he is going to go to the ED, he explodes! Fortunately, the police were prepared and you are able to wheel the stretcher into the office with the least amount of damage to the patient, the officers, and the office. He is placed on the stretcher while being held in place. Gauze and the straps on the stretcher are used to secure his extremities and his chest, and a blanket is tightly wrapped around the patient. Of course you attached pulse oximetry and are careful to not make the chest strap too tight so as to not impede his ability to breathe.

Remember what your paramedic instructor taught you in class. Although a patient has a medical history of behavioral problems, he is having a medical problem and needs to be evaluated by medical and mental health professionals in the most appropriate ED setting. It has been shown repeatedly that handcuffing an agitated and delirious patient and leaving him or her in the back of a squad car puts the patient at great risk medically and exposes all other persons interacting with that patient to potential legal peril.

There was a lot of screaming and commotion and the other office workers are very concerned. Your partner has contacted medical control and received an order to administer haloperidol [Haldol] 5 mg mixed with midazolam [Versed] 2 mg IM to sedate the patient. By the time you are rolling the stretcher out of the office he is calming down and much more quiet. This allows you to do a reassessment and an ongoing assessment of the patient (see **Table 6**).

Question 7: Why not just let the police handcuff the patient and put him in the squad car?

Question 8: What is the value of chemical restraint in the field?

Table 6 **Reassessment and Ongoing Assessment of the Patient**

Serial Vital Signs and Relevant Data	Recording Time: 15 Minutes
Skin CTC	Red, warm, and dry
Pulse	108 beats/min and regular
Blood Pressure	140/80 mm Hg
Respirations	24 breaths/min and shallow
Mental Status	Alert
ECG	Sinus tachycardia with no ectopy
SpO_2	98%
Lung Sounds	Clear bilaterally
Other (ie, glucose, core body temperature)	Glucose is 120 mg/dL

Part 5

The patient calmed down en route to the hospital and started to talk to you about why he has been so upset. This time he was talking and not just screaming. His wife followed you to the hospital in her own car and did not ride in the ambulance so as to not further aggravate the situation. Upon arrival the ED triage nurse motions to room 7, where a few security guards are available to assist the ED staff in helping transfer the patient to their stretcher. One nurse comments that "Is all this restraint necessary?" and you pull her aside and explain what was going on a half hour earlier!

While cleaning up the back of the ambulance one of the officers stops by to say thank you and notes that it was a lot smoother this time since they started practicing these "take-downs" and "drugs are available to calm these guys down" methods.

Restraints should be treated with respect! The purpose of naloxone hydrochloride [Narcan] is to improve ventilation status and tidal volume, not to completely arouse the patient. Additionally, naloxone hydrochloride [Narcan] can cause severe withdrawal effects that may result in agitation and emesis, increasing the risk for aspiration.

Restraints should be used only when personnel have been thoroughly trained on their use and application. Restraints should allow for rapid release if necessary for emergency patient care but should afford protection to health care providers. Even restraining a patient with gauze requires proper training of personnel. A certain amount of cautious respect should be used when considering restraints. Patients in restraints have a higher incidence of dying in custody or when restrained. (See the discussion on SICRAS in this chapter). Documentation regarding the use of restraints should consist of, at a minimum: location of restraints, valid reason for restraint use, time and duration the patient was restrained, and the patient's mental status while restrained.

Obtaining a history from the patient with a psychiatric problem can be challenging but is not impossible. The following are some general principles that can be helpful in your approach to the interview:

- Be calm and direct with the patient.
- Exclude disruptive people from the interview.
- Sit down to interview the patient, giving the patient plenty of personal space.
- Always maintain a nonjudgmental attitude.
- Provide honest reassurance.
- After listening to the patient, develop a plan of action.
- Stay with the patient at all times.
- Bring all of the patient's medications to the ED.
- Never assume that it is impossible to talk to a patient until you have tried!

It is imperative that before you restrain any patient, regardless of how violent, noncompliant, or cooperative he or she may be, you have a plan to restrain. In the worst case scenario, a patient experiencing a psychotic break may be rapid cycling between mania and depression. The patient may have "super-human" strength and pose a threat to themselves and others. They may also require conscious sedation to prevent them from harming themselves or others. Oftentimes appropriate verbal interventions on the part of EMS or police personnel will be adequate to redirect and calm an agitated patient. That strategy should always be initially employed. When a caregiver resorts to chemical restraint, it is with two goals in mind: protecting the patient as well as protecting the caregivers. Chemical restraint mandates a very aggressive approach to caring for the patient once an adequate level of cooperation or sedation is achieved. You must then initiate a comprehensive advanced life support work-up as soon as it is safe to do so. Simply injecting and then neglecting a patient suffering from any form of agitated delirium constitutes a serious breach of the patient-provider relationship.

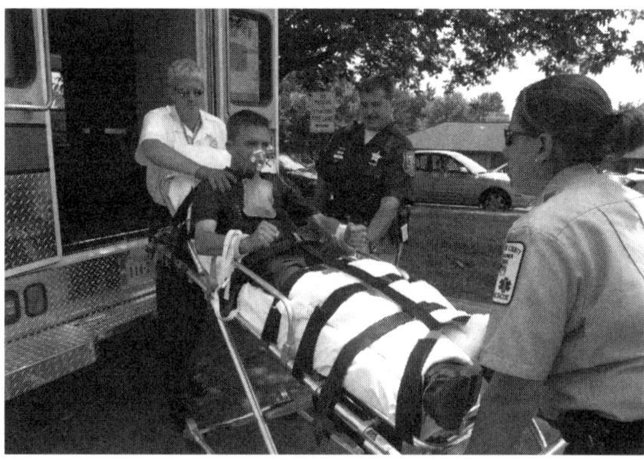

Figure 9-3 Physical restraints are used to prevent harm to personnel and the patient.

Patient physical restraint can be very dangerous to the patient as well as the rescuers. The ability to chemically sedate or restrain a patient is helpful but as with all medications being administered, these actions need to be carefully applied and monitored. Early EMS horror stories of hog-tying and facedown restraint in Reeves stretchers have caused various EMS leadership organizations to develop policies opposing these dangerous techniques due to the potential for positional asphyxia. EMS textbooks no longer show potentially dangerous techniques and strongly recommend safe and humane interventions and restraint (**Figure 9-3▲**).

If a patient is handcuffed and needs to be transported, the cuffs should be switched to the front of the patient and restraint should be accomplished with the use of sheets, tape, towels, and roller gauze. If the patient has ankle shackles because he or she is being transported from a correctional facility, insist that an officer (with the key) travels along with the ambulance. Discuss the procedure for humane restraint with the Service Medical Director and practice the technique with the police so that the next time you need to restrain a patient you will have experience working together as a team. Proper planning, personnel, and process will allow for a positive outcome, with the patient being restrained, and proper medical care obtained for the patient with no harm to emergency personnel.

Case Study ANSWERS

Case Study I Poison by Injection

Question 1: What are some of the causes of shallow respirations in a medical patient?

Answer 1: There are many causes of shallow or depressed respirations in the medical patient ranging from upper or lower airway obstructions to neurologic emergencies, endocrine emergencies, or drug intoxication.

Question 2: Should the custodian's comment that the patient is a "drug addict" be taken into account in your assessment?

Answer 2: You should absolutely take it into account but be careful not to take a myopic approach to your patient assessment by tunneling in on only drugs! Other very serious conditions can cause respiratory depression or altered mental status and you do not want to miss those potential presumptive diagnoses because you focused only on one single condition. Then of course, even drug addicts do get sick and have strokes, heart attacks, diabetic emergencies, and are commonly subject to various kinds of traumatic injury.

Question 3: What is the significance of the pinpoint pupils?

Answer 3: Pinpoint pupils are almost always characteristic (pathognomonic) of the signs of an opiate intoxication. Be sure to always look in the eyes of patients with altered mental status.

Question 4: What is the significance of the track marks and bruises on both arms on this patient?

Answer 4: Track marks are bruising and scars formed by repeated intravenous injections and should always point in the direction of potential IV drug abuse. They also indicate that it could be difficult to find a good peripheral IV site (drug abusers do not generally use up their IO sites). Also, remember that although BSI precautions are taken with all patients, in particular, the behaviors of IV drug abusers make them a substantially higher risk than the general population to carry various bloodborne diseases (eg, hepatitis B, HIV).

Question 5: Why is it a policy in some regions to restrain a patient before administering naloxone hydrochloride [Narcan]?

Answer 5: Many EMS systems have learned that if too much naloxone hydrochloride [Narcan] is administered to a patient they may not only wake up but wake up in a very aggressive mood. This increases the likelihood that the paramedics or other EMS providers can be injured by the patient as well as providing the opportunity for the patient to attempt to "escape." Medical sign-offs for a refusal of medical transport are not appropriate in this particular situation!

Question 6: Why is it important to wait on the insertion of an advanced airway until after the first dose of naloxone hydrochloride [Narcan]?

Answer 6: If the respiratory depression can be managed by assisting with an OPA/NPA, bag-mask ventilation, and supplemental oxygen, this is the best approach. Inserting an advanced airway (ie, ET tube, LMA, or Combitube) prior to the administration of naloxone hydrochloride [Narcan] can produce an angry or potentially vomiting patient with an ET tube in his or her mouth!

Question 7: The patient's lung sounds are like a bad "smoker's cough." What is this most likely the result of?

Answer 7: Although the patient may very well be a smoker or have a history of inhalational drug use, the rhonchi may be due to the patient having aspirated prior to your arrival on the scene. Proper airway management should prevent the possibility of the patient aspirating once you are on the scene.

Question 8: Some patients with a narcotic overdose have been known to have acute pulmonary edema. If that were the case with this patient, from your knowledge of acute pulmonary edema patients, what other signs would you expect to see?

Answer 8: Patients in acute pulmonary edema present with wet lung sounds, hypoxia, and may have pink frothy sputum.

Case Study ANSWERS

Case Study II Patient Restraint

Question 1: Is the scene ever really safe or secure?

Answer 1: No scene is ever truly secure and safety is something that needs to be considered throughout each and every call.

Question 2: What does it mean when your unit is advised to stage?

Answer 2: In most EMS systems when a paramedic unit is advised to stage, that usually means the unit should be parked at a safe distance and location from the patient and the EMS providers should wait until the police advise that it is appropriate to proceed into the scene.

Question 3: What should be your next plan of action with Joey?

Answer 3: Joey will need to be transported to the ED and he is not likely to go willingly. Discuss the approach to restraint with the police first, devise your plan, and then make sure you have enough help so no one gets hurt.

Question 4: What types of restraint are used in the field?

Answer 4: Fortunately it is not often that you need to restrain patients in the field. When restraints are needed, you must first comply with the local and state laws regarding this procedure, and then make sure you have plenty of help (including and especially involving law enforcement). The restraint used by paramedics is referred to as humane restraint and is generally done with sheets, tape, towels, and roller gauze on the stretcher with the patient in the semi-Fowler's position. Isolation precautions should be taken for patients who are spitting or when there is other potential body fluid exposure. Some EMS systems have adopted a chemical restraint protocol that involves medication administration to more safely help manage the patient.

Question 5: If the patient was on a CNS depressant, how would that affect your chemical restraint?

Answer 5: If the patient has taken a CNS depressant, using a chemical restraint could be dangerous as you could very easily overdose the patient by adding additional CNS depressant.

Question 6: Is it true that the patient might not remember the fight to be restrained?

Answer 6: Due to the memory impairment qualities of the medications, a patient may not remember the fight to be restrained.

Question 7: Why not just let the police handcuff the patient and put him in the squad car?

Answer 7: This patient has a medical history of behavioral problems. He is having a medical problem and needs to be evaluated by medical and mental health professionals in the most appropriate ED setting. It has been shown repeatedly that handcuffing an agitated and delirious patient and leaving him or her in the back of a squad car puts the patient at great risk medically and exposes all other persons interacting with that patient to significant legal risk.

Question 8: What is the value of chemical restraint in the field?

Answer 8: Having the ability to chemically restrain a patient helps decrease the risk of injury to the rescuer and the patient. It also helps to calm the patient and prevents the patient from worsening an already potentially serious associated medical problem.

Medication Review

Activated Charcoal

Indications Most oral poisonings and medication overdoses; can be used after evacuation of poisons.

Contraindications Oral administration to comatose patient; after ingestion of corrosives, caustics, or petroleum distillates (ineffective and may induce vomiting); simultaneous administration with other oral drugs.

Dosage and administration Note: if not in premixed slurry, dilute with 1 part charcoal/4 parts water. Adult: 1–2 g/kg PO or via NGT. Pediatric: 1–2 g/kg PO or via NGT.

Amyl Nitrite, Sodium Nitrite, Sodium Thiosulfate (Cyanide Antidote Kit)

Indications Cyanide or hydrocyanic acid poisoning.

Contraindications Not applicable.

Dosage and administration Adult: Amyl nitrite: breathe 30 seconds out of every minute. Sodium thiosulfate and sodium nitrite: IV per antidote kit directions. Pediatric: Same as adult.

Atropine Sulfate

Indications Hemodynamically unstable bradycardia, asystole, bradycardic (< 60 beats/min) pulseless electrical activity (PEA), organophosphate poisoning, bronchospastic pulmonary disorders.

Contraindications Tachycardia, hypersensitivity, unstable cardiovascular status in acute hemorrhage and myocardial ischemia, narrow-angle glaucoma.

Dosage and administration Adult: Asystole or bradycardic PEA: 1 mg IV/IO push. May repeat every 3–5 minutes (if asystole or PEA persists) to a maximum of 0.04 mg/kg. Endotracheal administration: 2–3 mg diluted in 10 mL of water or normal saline. Unstable bradycardia: 0.5 mg IV/IO every 3–5 minutes as needed, not to exceed total dose of 0.04 mg/kg. Use shorter dosing interval (3 minutes) and higher doses in severe clinical conditions. Organophosphate poisoning: Extremely large doses (2–4 mg or higher) may be needed. Pediatric: 0.02 mg/kg via IV/IO push; may double this dose for second IV/IO dose. Minimum single dose: 0.1 mg. Maximum doses: child single dose: 0.5 mg, child total dose: 1 mg, adolescent single dose: 1 mg, adolescent total dose: 2 mg. Endotracheal administration: 0.03 mg/kg (absorption may be unreliable).

Calcium Chloride

Indications Hypocalcemia, hyperkalemia, magnesium sulfate overdose, calcium channel blocker overdose, adjunctive therapy in treatment of insect bites and stings.

Contraindications Hypercalcemia, V-fib, digitalis toxicity.

Dosage and administration Adult: 500 mg to 1,000 mg (5–10 mL of a 10% solution) IV/IO push for hyperkalemia and calcium channel blocker overdose. May be repeated as needed. Pediatric: 20 mg/kg (0.2 mL/kg) slow IV/IO push. Maximum 1 g dose; may repeat in 10 minutes.

Diazepam (Valium)

Indications Acute anxiety states, acute alcohol withdrawal (delirium tremens), muscle relaxant, seizure activity, agitation. Analgesia for medical procedures (fracture reduction, cardioversion).

Contraindications Hypersensitivity, glaucoma, coma, shock, substance abuse, head injury.

Dosage and administration Seizure activity: Adult: 5–10 mg IV every 10–15 minutes as needed (5 mg over 5 min) (maximum dose, 30 mg). Seizure activity: Pediatric: 0.2–0.5 mg slowly every 2–5 minutes up to 5 mg (maximum dose, 10 mg/kg). Rectal diazepam: 0.5 mg/kg via rectal catheter and flush with 2–3 mL air after administration. Sedation for cardioversion: 5–15 mg IV over 5–10 minutes prior to cardioversion.

Medication Review

Diphenhydramine (Benadryl)

Indications Symptomatic relief of allergies, allergic reactions, anaphylaxis, acute dystonic reactions (phenothiazines). Blood administration reactions; used for motion sickness, hay fever.

Contraindications Asthma, glaucoma, pregnancy, hypertension, narrow-angle glaucoma, infants, patients taking monoamine oxidase inhibitors (MAOIs).

Dosage and administration Adult: 25–50 mg IM or IV or PO. Pediatric: 1–2 mg/kg IV, IO slowly or IM. If given PO: 5 mg/kg/24 hours.

Flumazenil (Romazicon)

Indications Reversal of respiratory depression and sedative effects from pure benzodiazepine overdose.

Contraindications Hypersensitivity, tricyclic antidepressant overdose, seizure-prone patients, coma of unknown etiology.

Dosage and administration Adult: First dose: 0.2 mg IV/IO over 15 seconds. Second dose: 0.3 mg IV/IO over 30 seconds. If no response, give third dose. Third dose: 0.5 mg IV/IO over 30 seconds. If no response, repeat once every minute until adequate response or a total of 3 mg is given. Pediatric: Not recommended.

Glucagon

Indications Altered level of consciousness when hypoglycemia is suspected. May be used as inotropic agent in beta-blocker overdose.

Contraindications Hyperglycemia, hypersensitivity.

Dosage and administration Adult: Hypoglycemia: 0.5–1 mg IM; may repeat in 7–10 minutes. Calcium channel blocker or beta-blocker overdose: 3 mg initially, followed by infusion at 3 mg/hr as necessary. Pediatric: Hypoglycemia: 0.5–1 mg IM (for children < 20 kg). Calcium channel blocker or beta-blocker overdose: not recommended.

Haloperidol (Haldol)

Indications Acute psychotic episodes.

Contraindications Agitation secondary to shock or hypoxia. Hypersensitivity.

Dosage and administration Adult: 2–5 mg IM every 30–60 minutes until sedation achieved. Pediatric: Not recommended.

Lorazepam (Ativan)

Indications Initial control of status epilepticus or severe recurrent seizures, severe anxiety, sedation.

Contraindications Acute narrow-angle glaucoma. Coma, shock, or suspected drug abuse.

Dosage and administration Note: When given IV or IO, must dilute with equal volume of sterile water or sterile saline; when given IM, lorazepam is not to be diluted. Adult: 2–4 mg slow IV at 2 mg/min or IM; may repeat in 15–20 minutes to maximum dose of 8 mg. For sedation: 0.05 mg/kg up to 4 mg IM. Pediatric: 0.05–0.20 mg/kg slow IV, IO slowly over 2 minutes or IM; may repeat in 15–20 minutes to maximum dose of 0.2 mg/kg.

Midazolam (Versed)

Indications Sedation, anxiolytic prior to endotracheal or nasotracheal intubation; administer for conscious sedation.

Contraindications Glaucoma, shock, coma, alcohol intoxication, overdose, depressed vital signs, concomitant use with other CNS depressants, barbiturates, alcohol, narcotics.

Dosage and administration Adult: 2.0–2.5 mg slow IV over 2–3 minutes; may be repeated to total maximum: 0.1 mg/kg. Pediatric: Not recommended.

Medication Review

Naloxone Hydrochloride (Narcan)

Indications Opiate overdose, coma; complete or partial reversal of CNS and respiratory depression induced by opioids; decreased level of consciousness; coma of unknown origin; narcotic agonist for the following: morphine sulfate, heroin, hydromorphone (Dilaudid), methadone, meperidine (Demerol), paregoric, fentanyl citrate (Sublimase), oxycodone (Percodan), codeine, propoxyphene (Darvon); narcotic agonist and antagonist for the following: Butorphanol (Stadol), pentazocine (Talwin), nalbuphine (Nubain).

Contraindications Use with caution in narcotic-dependent patients; use with caution in neonates of narcotic-addicted mothers.

Dosage and administration Adult: 0.4–2.0 mg IV, IM, SC, or ET (diluted); minimum recommended dose, 0.4 mg; repeat at 5-minute intervals to a maximum dose of 10 mg (medical control may request higher amounts). Infusion: 2 mg in 500 mL of D_5W (4 µg/mL), infuse at 0.4 mg/h (100 mL/h). Pediatric: 0.1 mg/kg/dose IV, IM, SC, ET (diluted); maximum dose of 0.8 mg; if no response in 10 minutes, administer an additional 0.1 mg/kg/dose.

Ondansetron Hydrochloride (Zofran)

Indications For the prevention or control of nausea or vomiting. Also used in the hospital setting for patients undergoing chemotherapy or surgical procedures.

Contraindications Known allergy to this medicine or other 5-HT3 receptor antagonists.

Dosage and administration Adult: 4 mg IV or IM (may repeat in 10 minutes). Pediatric: 0.1 mg/kg IV or IM.

Oxygen

Indications Confirmed or expected hypoxemia, ischemic chest pain, respiratory insufficiency, prophylactically during air transport, confirmed or suspected carbon monoxide poisoning, all other causes of decreased tissue oxygenation, decreased level of consciousness.

Contraindications Certain patients with COPD or emphysema who will not tolerate oxygen concentrations over 35%, hyperventilation. Oxygen should never be withheld from a patient who needs it, however. Be prepared to assist with ventilations in a patient with COPD who requires high oxygen concentrations as apnea may result.

Dosage and administration Adult: Cardiac arrest and carbon monoxide poisoning: 100%. Hypoxemia: 10–15 L/min via nonrebreathing mask. COPD: 1–6 L/min via nasal cannula or 28%–35% Venturi mask. Be prepared to provide ventilatory support if higher concentrations of oxygen needed. Pediatric: Same as for adult with exception of premature infant.

Phenobarbital (Luminal)

Indications Prevention and treatment of seizure activity; prophylaxis for febrile seizures; anxiety, apprehension; status epilepticus.

Contraindications Patients with porphyria, hypersensitivity, severe liver or respiratory diseases.

Dosage and administration Adult: 100–250 mg slow IV, or IM; may repeat as needed in 20–30 minutes. Pediatric: 10–20 mg/kg IV, IO (less than 1 mg/kg/min) or IM; repeat as needed in 20–30 minutes.

Medication Review

Pralidoxime Chloride (2-PAM Chloride, Protopam)

Indications As an antidote in the treatment of poisoning by organophosphate pesticides and chemicals. In the prehospital arena, is used when atropine is or has become ineffective in management of organophosphate poisoning.

Contraindications Use with caution in patients with reduced renal function; patients with myasthenia gravis and organophosphate poisoning.

Dosage and administration Note: If Protopam is to be used, it should be administered almost simultaneously with atropine. Adult: Initial dose of 1–2 g as an IV infusion with 100 mL saline over 15–30 minutes. Pediatric: 20–40 mg/kg as IV infusion over 15–30 minutes. Doses may be repeated every 1 hour if muscle weakness persists. If IV administration is not feasible, IM or SC injection may be utilized.

Promethazine Hydrochloride (Phenergan)

Indications Nausea, vomiting, motion sickness; sedation for patients in labor; potentiation of analgesic effects of narcotics.

Contraindications Hypersensitivity, coma, CNS-depressed patients from alcohol, barbiturates, narcotics, Reye's syndrome.

Dosage and administration Adult: 12.5–25 mg IV, deep IM, PO, rectally. Pediatric: (older than 2 years old) 0.25–0.5 mg/kg dose IM.

Thiamine Hydrochloride (Vitamin B-1)

Indications Coma of unknown origin, delirium tremens, beriberi, Wernicke's encephalopathy.

Contraindications None.

Dosage and administration Adult: 100 mg slow IV or IM. Pediatric: 10–25 mg slow IV or IM.

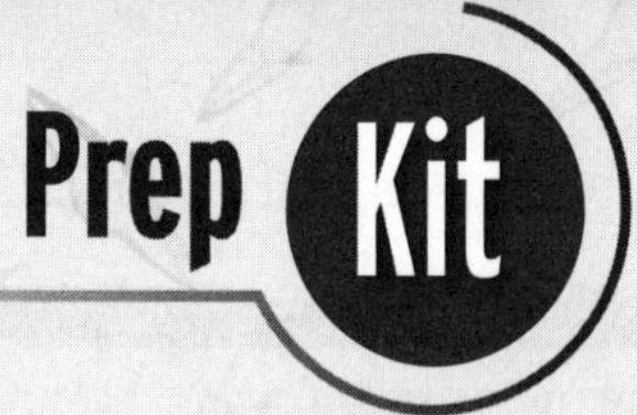

Chapter Summary

- The four routes of poisoning are: ingestion, inhalation, injection, and absorption.
- Some of the common signs and symptoms of poisoning may include peculiar odors, and changes in the pupils, mouth, or skin.
- Although treated in the same manner, it is important to identify what the patient may have ingestion or injected as well as how much of the substance was ingested or injected.
- Management of ingestion or injection poisoning is generally supportive.
- The most common inhalation poisoning is carbon monoxide poisoning.
- There are many chemicals, not intended to be absorbed through the skin, that dissolve easily in the fat of the skin.
- Treatment of surface absorption or inhalation poisoning must always first include ensuring that the scene is safe for the rescuer and limiting the potential for exposure to the substance.
- Once a substance that was inhaled or absorbed is identified, the paramedic field management focuses on supporting the ABCs and contacting medical control and the poison center.
- The SICRAS provides a means to rapidly assess an in-custody subject's risk of sudden death based on known symptoms and risk factors.
- Patients who suffer from behavioral conditions often take many medications intended to heighten the "lows" (depression) and lower the "highs" (mania).
- EMS personnel must always have a plan in place to restrain the patient.

Vital Vocabulary

CNS stimulants Drugs that stimulate the central nervous system.

Ecstasy A synthetic amphetamine used illicitly for its mood-enhancing and hallucinogenic properties (ie, *MDMA, methylenedioxymethamphetamine, XTC*).

Gamma-hydroxybutyric acid (GHB) A depressant of the central nervous system; is used illicitly to produce sedative and euphoric effects or to stimulate release of growth hormone to increase muscle mass (ie, *gamma hydroxybutyrate*).

Ketamine A widely used animal tranquilizer which when taken inappropriately by humans can be a powerful hallucinogen. (Also called "Special K.")

Khat Contains the alkaloid cathinone, an amphetamine-like stimulant that causes excitement and euphoria.

Methamphetamines A drug used medically in the form of its crystalline hydrochloride to treat attention deficit disorder and obesity and that is often abused illicitly as a stimulant (ie, *meth, methedrine, methylamphetamine, speed*).

Polysubstance abuse Mixing multiple medications either purposely or accidentally to achieve greater effects.

Ritalin A medication, chemically related to amphetamine, which acts as a mild CNS stimulant. It is used to treat narcolepsy in adults and hyperkinetic disorders in children.

Rohypnol A preparation of flunitrazepam, formerly a US registered trademark. Has been abused and referred to as a "date rape" drug.

Toxidrome The syndrome-like symptoms of a poisonous agent exposure/ingestion.

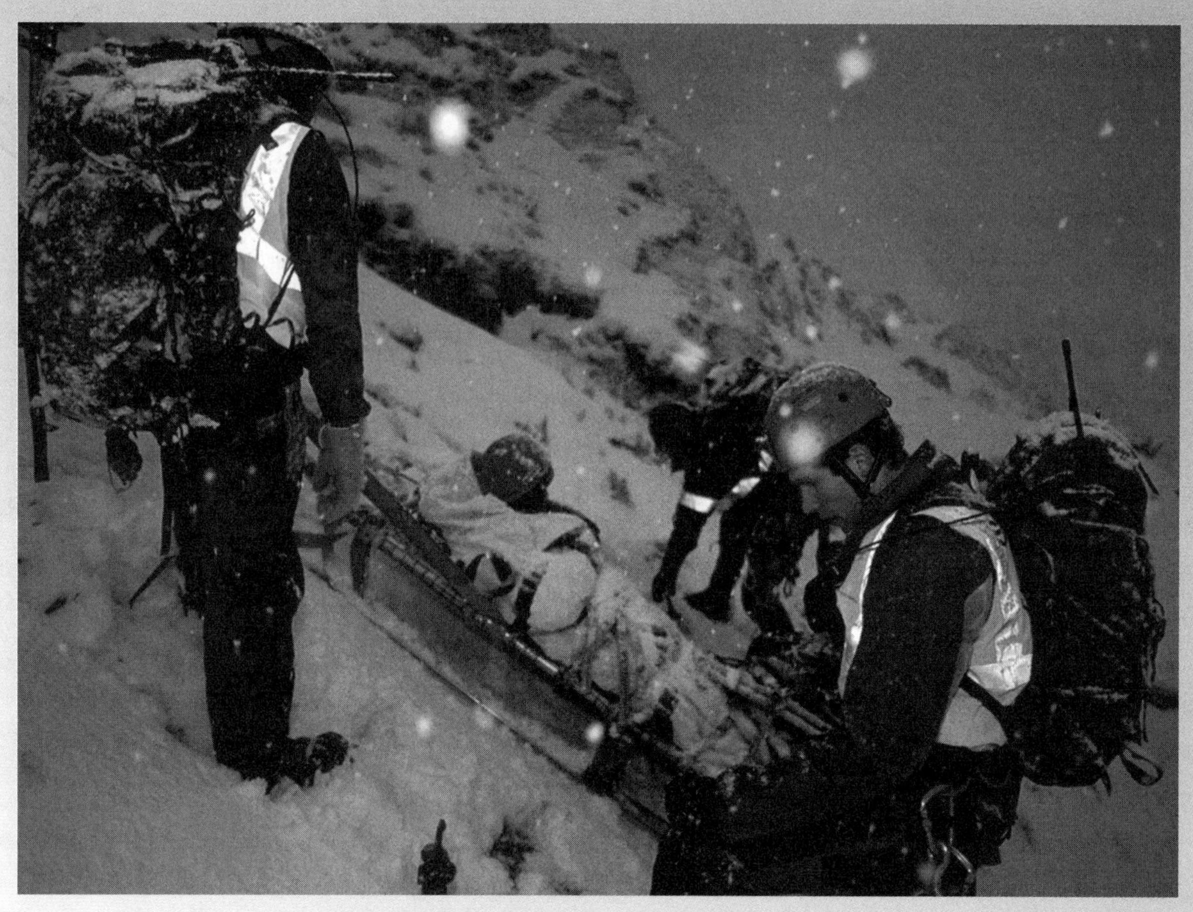

10 Environmental Emergencies

Objectives

Cognitive

5-10.85 Discuss the pharmacology appropriate for the treatment of altitude illnesses. (page 310)

Affective

None

Psychomotor

None

Additional Objectives

10-1 Discuss the signs and symptoms of heat illnesses such as heat cramps, heat exhaustion, and heat stroke. (page 302)

10-2 List 10 medications that may contribute to a patient's reaction to a heat illness. (page 303)

10-3 Discuss the treatment of heat stroke. (pages 303–307)

10-4 Discuss the signs and symptoms of mild and severe hypothermia. (page 308)

10-5 List the types of medications that can predispose a person to a cold illness. (page 308)

10-6 Discuss the treatment of hypothermia. (page 309)

10-7 Discuss the three types of altitude sickness (ie, AMS, HAPE, HACE) and their treatments. (pages 308, 310).

10-8 Discuss conditions that may develop from diving with compressed gas that the paramedic may begin management of while in the field (ie, barotrauma, decompression sickness (the bends), nitrogen narcosis, and arterial gas embolism [AGE]) and their treatment. (page 311–312)

Environmental Conditions

Medical conditions can be caused by extremes in weather, terrain, atmospheric pressure, and other local factors. These conditions are usually referred to as environmental emergencies or conditions. The most common causes of environmental conditions are extremes in temperature as illustrated in **Figure 10-1 ▸**.

Less common causes of environmental emergencies are associated with altitude, submersion or drowning, and diving with compressed air. Age, general health, obesity, alcoholism, debility, and many drugs increase a person's susceptibility to cold and heat disorders (ie, hypothermia, frostbite, heat cramps, heat exhaustion, and heat stroke). An indication of the severity of the environmental emergency can be gained by assessing the patient's mental status. The more altered the mental status, the more severe the condition is likely to be. Care for patients who have become ill due to an environmental cause almost always includes safely removing them from the extreme environment (**Figure 10-2 ▸**).

You will need to recognize the need for prompt evaluation and treatment while constantly focusing on the mental status, airway, breathing, and circulation.

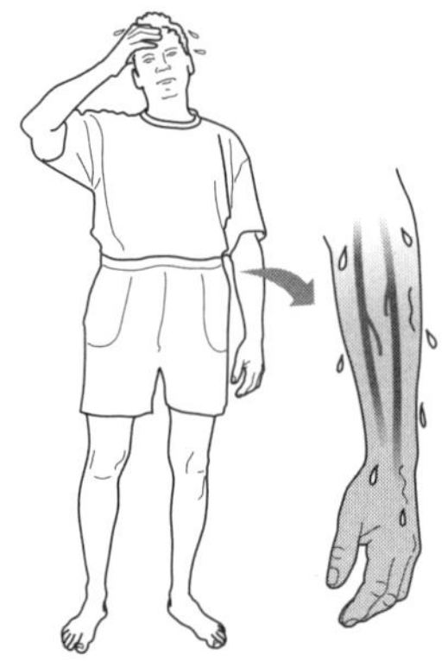

Hot Environment

- Hypothalamus stimulated
- Blood vessels dilate, maximizing heat loss from skin
- Body sweats, causing evaporation and cooling

Body temperature *decreases*

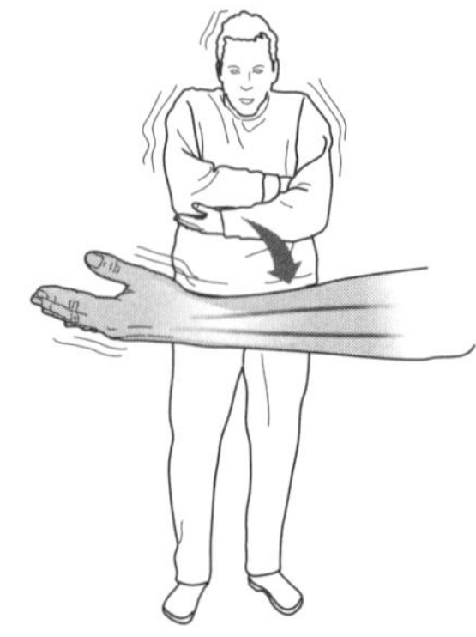

Cold Environment

- Hypothalamus stimulated
- Blood vessels constrict, minimizing heat loss from skin
- Muscles shiver, generating heat

Body temperature *increases*

Figure 10-1 Like a car thermostat, the hypothalamus notes a rise or fall in core body temperature and elicits responses to regulate it.

Heat Illnesses

Heat illness, or heat stress, occurs when the body cannot disperse heat sufficiently and develops an increased **core body temperature (CBT)**. The three major types of emergencies associated with heat illness are **heat cramps**, **heat exhaustion**, and **heat stroke**. Of these three conditions, heat stroke is the most severe.

Increased CBT produces signs and symptoms ranging from mild to severe (**Table 10-1 ▾**).

There are many factors that can contribute to a patient's heat illness (**Table 10-2 ▸**).

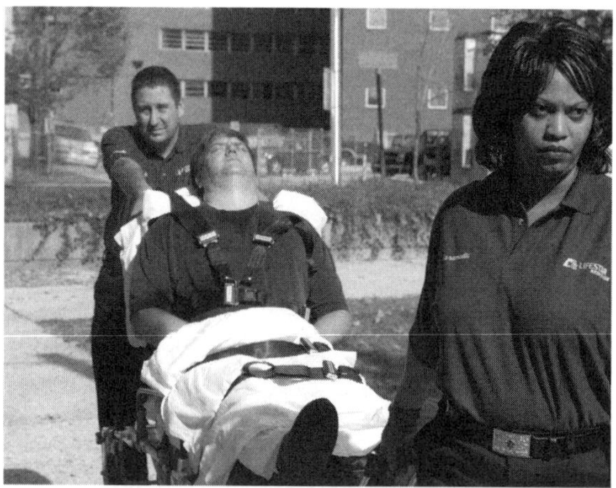

Figure 10-2 Remove the patient from the extreme environment.

Table 10-1 Comparing Conditions Resulting From Heat Illness

Variable	Heat Cramps	Heat Exhaustion	Heat Stroke
Pathophysiology	Sodium and water loss	Sodium and water loss, hypovolemia	Failure of heat-regulating mechanisms
Mental status	Normal	Normal or mild confusion	Altered, delirium, seizures
Temperature	May be mildly elevated	Usually mildly elevated	> 104°F (40°C)
Skin	Cool, moist	Pale, cool, moist	Dry, hot, but sweating may persist, especially with exertional heat stroke
Muscle cramping	Severe	May or may not be present	Absent

Table 10-2 Factors Contributing to Heat Illness

- Alcohol
- Alpha agonists
- Amphetamines
- Anticholinergic medications (atropine sulfate, scopolamine, benztropine mesylate, belladonna, and synthetic alkaloids)
- Antihistamines
- Antiparkinsonian agents
- Antipsychotics (such as haloperidol)
- Beta-blockers
- Calcium channel blockers
- Cocaine
- Diuretics (furosemide, hydrochlorothiazide, bumetanide)
- Heroin
- Laxatives
- Lithium
- Lysergic acid diethylamide (LSD)
- Monoamine oxidase inhibitors
- Phencyclidine hydrochloride
- Phenothiazines (prochlorperazine, chlorpromazine, promethazine)
- Sympathomimetic medicines (amphetamines, epinephrine, ephedrine, cocaine, norepinephrine)
- Thyroid agonists (levothyroxine)
- Tricyclic antidepressants (amitriptyline, imipramine, nortriptyline, protriptyline)

Case Study 1 Heat Stroke

Dispatch has sent you to a residence for an elderly patient who is unresponsive. The police are already on the scene. Upon arriving at the address, you see a small bungalow-style home with an overgrown yard. A policeman is talking to a letter carrier outside of the residence. The letter carrier noticed that Mrs. Whitting has not taken in her mail for 3 days and he found this unusual. He rang the doorbell and, when he did not get a response, looked in the window and saw Mrs. Whitting lying on the floor. That is when he called 9-1-1. Another policeman is inside with Mrs. Whitting, who is sitting on the floor propped up with pillows. The officer says that she is confused, and her answers to his questions do not make sense. The room is extremely warm and smells of urine. Mrs. Whitting is flushed, and hot to the touch. Her respirations are rapid and shallow, and her distal pulses are rapid and weak. Her right leg is shortened and rotated inward. When you palpate her hip, she moans. The priority is to get her out of the hot house as soon as possible. Your partner goes back to the ambulance for the backboard.

During the initial assessment, you confirm that this call is both medical and trauma-related (see **Table 1**). Mrs. Whitting has an altered mental status, a possible hip injury, and may have been in a hot environment for up to 3 days with no food or water. She is a high priority due to these findings. A focused history and physical examination will be completed after removing her from the hot environment.

Table 1 Initial Assessment

Initial Assessment	Recording Time: 2 Minutes
General Impression/ Appearance	Elderly woman who is sick and debilitated in a hot environment
Mental Status	Verbally responsive but confused
Airway	Open
Breathing	Rapid and shallow
Circulation	Flushed, hot skin; rapid, weak distal pulse
Priority/Plan	High priority due to altered mental status in an extreme environment

Question 1: What is the first priority in caring for Mrs. Whitting?

Question 2: What are the three major types of emergencies associated with heat illness?

Case Study 1 Continued

Part 2

First responders have arrived to assist, and just in time too. Mrs. Whitting has started to seize just as you were carefully moving her to a long back board. You will use the backboard as a splint for her hip. Her jaw is clenched and her eyes have rolled up and back; she is now not breathing. Your partner tosses you a bag-mask device and you begin ventilations as the first responders lift the backboard outside to the stretcher. You ask one of the responders to go back inside to get the patient's name from the officer and to find out if any medication bottles were found. Once in the ambulance, the air conditioning is turned up high. The seizure is continuing and the jaw remains clenched. You insert a nasal airway and continue ventilations. You consider the possible reasons why Mrs. Whitting is seizing as you perform the focused history and physical examination (see **Table 2**). You know **hypoxia** and **hypoglycemia** must be ruled out first in any patient with an altered mental status. This is due to the severity of the two conditions and because both can be identified and corrected quickly. Another reason for her seizing could be medications, as well as the most obvious reason in this case—her high CBT. Your partner performs a fingerstick to get a glucose reading and to rule out hypoglycemia. Another responder helps to get vital signs and attaches the monitor to the patient. The pulse is 140 beats/min and regular, and blood pressure is 90/50 mm Hg. Respirations are being assisted because she became apneic with the seizure.

Table 2 Focused History and Physical Examination

Baseline Vital Signs	Recording Time: 3 Minutes
Skin CTC (color, temperature, condition)	Dry, hot, flushed
Pulse	140 beats/min and regular
Blood Pressure	90/50 mm Hg
Respirations	Assisted with bag-mask device

Question 3: Which heat emergency is Mrs. Whitting most likely experiencing?

Question 4: What are the two causes of altered mental status that should be ruled out first?

Part 3

The blood glucose is 385 mg/dL, the ECG is sinus tachycardia, and the SpO_2 is 94%. The seizure is still continuing, but with less physical movement. Airway maintenance and ventilation remain the high priority, and the patient needs to be cooled quickly, rehydration needs to be instituted, and the seizure needs to be stopped. The air conditioning is blowing on high and next the clothing will be removed. The responder is back with information for you to complete the SAMPLE history (see **Table 3**). The patient is 85 years old and has three pill bottles: donepezil hydrochloride [Aricept], tolterodine tartrate [Detrol], and docusate sodium [Colace].

Table 3 SAMPLE History

SAMPLE History	Comments
Signs/symptoms	Confusion; incontinence to urine; skin that is hot, moist, and flushed; and seizure activity
Allergies	Unknown
Medications	Donepezil hydrochloride [Aricept], tolterodine tartrate [Detrol], and docusate sodium [Colace]
Pertinent past medical history	Medications indicate possible dementia, bladder control problem, and constipation. There is no one else to provide information, and the patient is unable to.
Last oral intake	Unknown, possibly 3 days since oral intake
Events leading up to the incident	May have been on the floor for up to 3 days with no food or water and may have a hip injury

Treatment Plan

She has limited IV access on first assessment, and because of the prolonged seizure, the treatment plan is to administer diazepam gel [Diastat] PR (see **Table 4**). But watch that injured hip when positioning the patient to place the gel! This can be done quickly and the rectal route is highly vascular, so medication is absorbed rapidly.

1. Administer diazepam gel [Diastat] PR to the patient.*
2. Consider inserting an advanced airway if the patient does not regain consciousness.
3. Evaluate ventilations and oxygenate the patient.
4. Continue cooling the patient.
5. Begin transport.

*You should note that there is another choice of medication that could be administered in this situation, such as a benzodiazepine IM (ie, midazolam [Versed]), but in this scenario it is not immediately available in your EMS system as yet (see **Table 5**).

Table 4 Diazepam

Do you know?	Comments
Right drug? Generic name: [**Diazepam**] Trade name: [Diastat, Valium]	This drug is a benzodiazepine. It is used to treat anxiety and convulsive disorders (seizure in this specific case).
Right patient?	Status epilepticus.
Right dose?	5–10 mg IV; PR dose is 0.5 mg/kg via rectal catheter.
Right route?	IV, PR.
Right time?	Seizing patient after airway and ventilation are managed and contraindications have been considered.
Right documentation?	Always document how and when the drug was administered as well as the patient's response to the medication on your patient care report.
Expected action	Relief of seizure activity.
Side effects	Potentiates antihypertensive effects of thiazides and other diuretics.
Contraindications	Known sensitivity, narrow-angle glaucoma.
Precautions	May worsen seizure activity.
Pharmacokinetics	Onset: 1–5 minutes: peak effect: within minutes; duration: 20–50 minutes; metabolized in the liver and excreted in urine.

Table 5 Midazolam

Do you know?	Comments
Right drug? Generic name: [**Midazolam**] Trade name: [Versed]	A short-acting benzodiazepine CNS depressant. It is used for relief of anxiety, sedation, and as an adjunct to induction of general anesthesia.
Right patient?	It has anxiolytic and sedative properties similar to other benzodiazepines, memory impairment.
Right dose?	2.0–2.5 mg slow IV over 2–3 minutes or 2.0–2.5 mg intranasal (may repeat to a max of 0.1 mg/kg).
Right route?	IV is best; IM and IO are also options.
Right time?	As soon as possible after baseline vital signs if the patient is still seizing.
Right documentation?	Clearly document any changes in seizure activity on your patient care report.
Expected action	To stop the seizure activity and sedate the patient. It is an anxiolytic (drug that reduces anxiety) given prior to endotracheal or nasotracheal intubation. It is also administered for conscious sedation.
Side effects	Can cause hiccough, cough, oversedation, nausea, vomiting, injection site pain, headache, blurred vision, hypotension, respiratory depression, and arrest.
Contraindications	Glaucoma, shock, coma, alcohol intoxication, overdose, depressed vital signs, concomitant use with other CNS depressants, barbiturates, alcohol, narcotics.
Precautions	Can cause respiratory depression, so watch for it and if needed be prepared to assist ventilations. Should not be used in patients who have taken a CNS depressant or are hypotensive.
Pharmacokinetics	Onset: 1–3 minutes IV and dose-dependent; peak effect: variable. Onset: 15 minutes IM; peak effect: 45 minutes. Duration: 2–6 hours; metabolized in the liver and excreted in urine.

Case Study 1 Continued

The diazepam worked and the seizure has stopped. The patient is not awake, but now the airway can be opened and suctioned. She is breathing adequately, so a nonrebreathing mask is put on her. The physical examination reveals numerous abrasions on the face, elbows, hands, knees, and feet, as if she tried to crawl and/or get up to call for help but could not. Her skin is still flushed, dry, very warm, and tents easily, and there is no jugular vein distension, all of which indicate profound dehydration. The lung sounds are clear, the abdomen is soft without masses, her back has abrasions, her right leg remains shortened and rotated inward, and there is no peripheral edema. She smells of urine and there is no fecal matter on her body. It is unclear how long she has been on the floor.

Question 5: Why was the diazepam given PR rather than IV or IM?

Question 6: Based on your understanding of the effects of heat on the CBT, how high would you estimate the patient's CBT to be?

Part 4

En route, Mrs. Whitting has had no further seizure activity. She is very groggy and maintaining a good respiratory effort with the nasal airway and nonrebreathing mask. It will be interesting to see what the ED gets for a CBT. On the third attempt, an IV is placed and rehydration is started with a bolus of normal saline solution. Vital signs are reassessed, and you look her over from head to toe again to be sure you did not miss anything the first time (see **Table 6**). With your attention on the airway during the seizure activity, it is possible that you missed something on the physical examination. Her skin is still flushed and warm, lung sounds remain clear with a good effort and a rate of 22 breaths/min, distal pulse is weak and tachycardic at 136 beats/min, blood pressure is 106/54 mm Hg, and SpO_2 is 100%. The rotation of the right leg may be a new injury or a preexisting condition. Until she is awake or a radiograph is taken, there is no way to know if she also sustained a hip fracture, so it was good you had her on the long backboard.

You contact the ED and let them know about Mrs. Whitting so they can be prepared for your arrival.

Table 6 Reassessment and Ongoing Assessment of the Patient

Serial Vital Signs and Relevant Data	Recording Time: 15 Minutes
Skin CTC	Dry, flushed, and warm
Pulse	Tachycardic, weak 136 beats/min
Blood Pressure	106/54 mm Hg
Respirations	Good effort with a rate of 22 breaths/min
Mental Status	Groggy/responds to pain stimuli
ECG	Sinus tachycardia
SpO_2	100% on high flow oxygen
Lung Sounds	Clear
Other (ie, blood glucose, CBT)	385 mg/dL, the patient's body temperature is definitely elevated by comparison to your own

Question 7: Are the prescription medications found in Mrs. Whitting's home a possible cause of a heat illness?

Question 8: What is the most likely cause of the heat-related emergency for Mrs. Whitting?

Part 5

One of the most common causes of environmental emergencies is heat. The very young, elderly, and debilitated are at high risk for developing illness related to heat and cold. In the initial assessment (IA) of Mrs. Whitting, there appears to be both a medical and trauma aspect to this call. Mrs. Whitting has an altered mental status, a possible hip injury, and may have been in a hot environment for up to 3 days with no access to food or water. She is a high priority due to these findings. One of the first priorities in an environmental emergency is to safely remove the patient from the source of the illness. As this was being accomplished, she experienced a seizure. Completing a rapid trauma and medical examination was delayed briefly as the focus of care changed to reestablishing an adequate airway and ventilations, and stopping the seizure activity.

Case Study 1 Continued

The causes of both altered mental status and seizure were considered; the two most important possibilities, hypoxia and hypoglycemia, were quickly assessed and ruled out. That left the most obvious factor, the extreme heat, as the most likely cause. Diazepam [Valium] was administered PR. This is the drug of choice to correct ongoing seizure activity or status epilepticus. The seizure activity stopped and Mrs. Whitting's airway and breathing become less of a problem, allowing for completion of the assessment. Her mental status remained altered, but stable for the duration of the transport. Thank goodness for the observant letter carrier noticing the uncollected mail at Mrs. Whitting's home, leading to the 9-1-1 call.

Special Needs Tip

Elderly patients are more prone to heat-related disorders. This is due to medications that the patients may be taking and slower central nervous system processing. As we age, we tend to lose body mass. This contributes to a slower systemic response to environmental changes, speech, and cognition. Since the elderly patient's brain may process sensory information slower, the brain may not be able to detect subtle and slow ambient temperature changes. Oftentimes the elderly will feel cold, even when the ambient temperature is above 80°F.

After ensuring the scene is safe and completing your initial assessment, a key concept when confronted with a patient with an altered mental status is to perform an appropriate focused assessment, obtain a SAMPLE history (including medication history) and baseline vital signs as well as blood glucose evaluation, obtain an ECG, and ask about the patient's usual and customary mental status. It is a BEST PRACTICE to strive to have obtained all of this information within your first 5 minutes of patient contact. Remember that the causes of altered mental status are recalled using the pneumonic AEIOU-TIPS.

A = Alcohol/Acidosis
E = Epilepsy
I = Insulin (Hypo or Hyperglycemia)
O = Overdose
U = Uremia (Sepsis)
T = Trauma
I = Infection
P = Psychosis
S = Stroke/Seizure

Heat Stroke

Heat stroke is a life-threatening heat emergency that must be recognized and corrected quickly. When the body can no longer adequately rid itself of heat, causing the CBT to rise over 104°F (40°C), the patient may develop confusion or lose consciousness. If the cooling measures are not promptly initiated, seizures, brain damage, and death may follow. Some patients develop heat stroke over several days with vague symptoms (ie, fatigue, weakness, nausea, vomiting), while others develop heat stroke rapidly. Those who develop heat stroke rapidly become confused, and then experience a loss of consciousness following long periods of exertion in warm or hot temperatures.

Cold Illness

There are many factors that predispose a patient to cold illness (**Table 10-3 ▸**).

Hypothermia

When the body experiences heat loss in which the CBT drops to less than 95°F (35°C), signs and symptoms will develop ranging from mild to severe. In **hypothermia**, there is no direct or reliable correlation between the CBT and the signs and symptoms. There are, however, common progressive findings that can be observed as hypothermia becomes more severe (**Table 10-4 ▸**). It is the change in mental status that indicates the severity of hypothermia.

Table 10-3 Factors That Predispose to Cold Illness

Factors That Increase Heat Loss	Factors That Impair Thermoregulatory Mechanisms	Factors That Decrease Heat Production	Miscellaneous Causes
• Cold water drowning • Wet clothes • Windchill • Impaired judgment from drugs or alcohol • Vasodilatation from: –Alcohol –Acute spinal cord injury • Diabetic peripheral neuropathies	• Dehydration • Parkinson's disease or dementias • Multiple sclerosis • Anorexia nervosa • Central nervous system bleeding or ischemic cerebrovascular accident • Multisystem trauma • Drugs interfering with vasoconstriction: –Alcohol –Benzodiazepines –Phenothiazines –Tricyclic antidepressants	• Hypothyroidism • Age extremes • Hypoglycemia • Malnutrition • Inability to shiver and immobility	• Sepsis • Meningitis • Overzealous heat stroke treatment

Table 10-4 Signs and Symptoms of Hypothermia

Loss of Coordination	Loss of fine motor control Increased loss of movement
Altered Mental Status	Confusion Loss of consciousness
Cardiac Arrhythmias	Atrial fibrillation Bradycardia Ventricular fibrillation Asystole

The 2005 Advanced Cardiac Life Support (ACLS) Guidelines divided hypothermia into the three classes most paramedic protocols focus on (ie, mild, moderate, and severe). The course of treatment based on these classes, the CBT, and the presence or absence of a perfusing rhythm are shown in (**Figure 10-3** ▸) on the next page.

Altitude Sickness

The pressure in the atmosphere and the amount of oxygen in the atmosphere decreases as the altitude increases. There are many activities that place people in high altitudes. Physical exertion is one risk factor for altitude illness (**Figure 10-4** ▸).

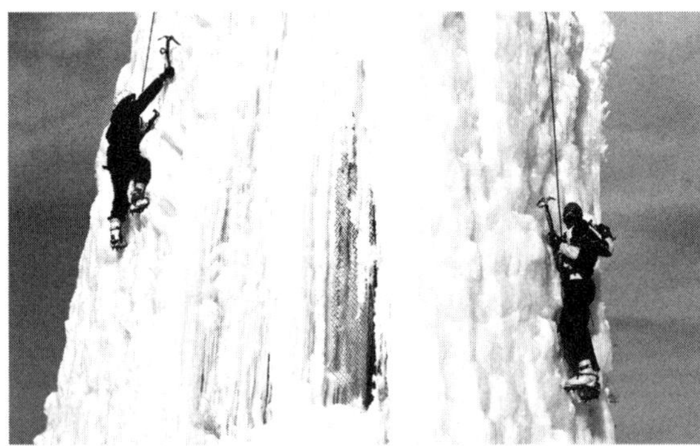

Figure 10-4
Physical exertion is a risk factor for altitude illness.

At altitudes of greater than 8,000 feet above sea level, the body may manifest signs or symptoms of decreased atmospheric oxygen, which can increase the chance of developing **altitude sickness**. The most common disorders are **acute mountain sickness (AMS)**, **high-altitude pulmonary edema (HAPE)**, and **high-altitude cerebral edema (HACE)**. The signs and symptoms range from mild to severe, and the treatment of each varies (**Table 10-5** ▸).

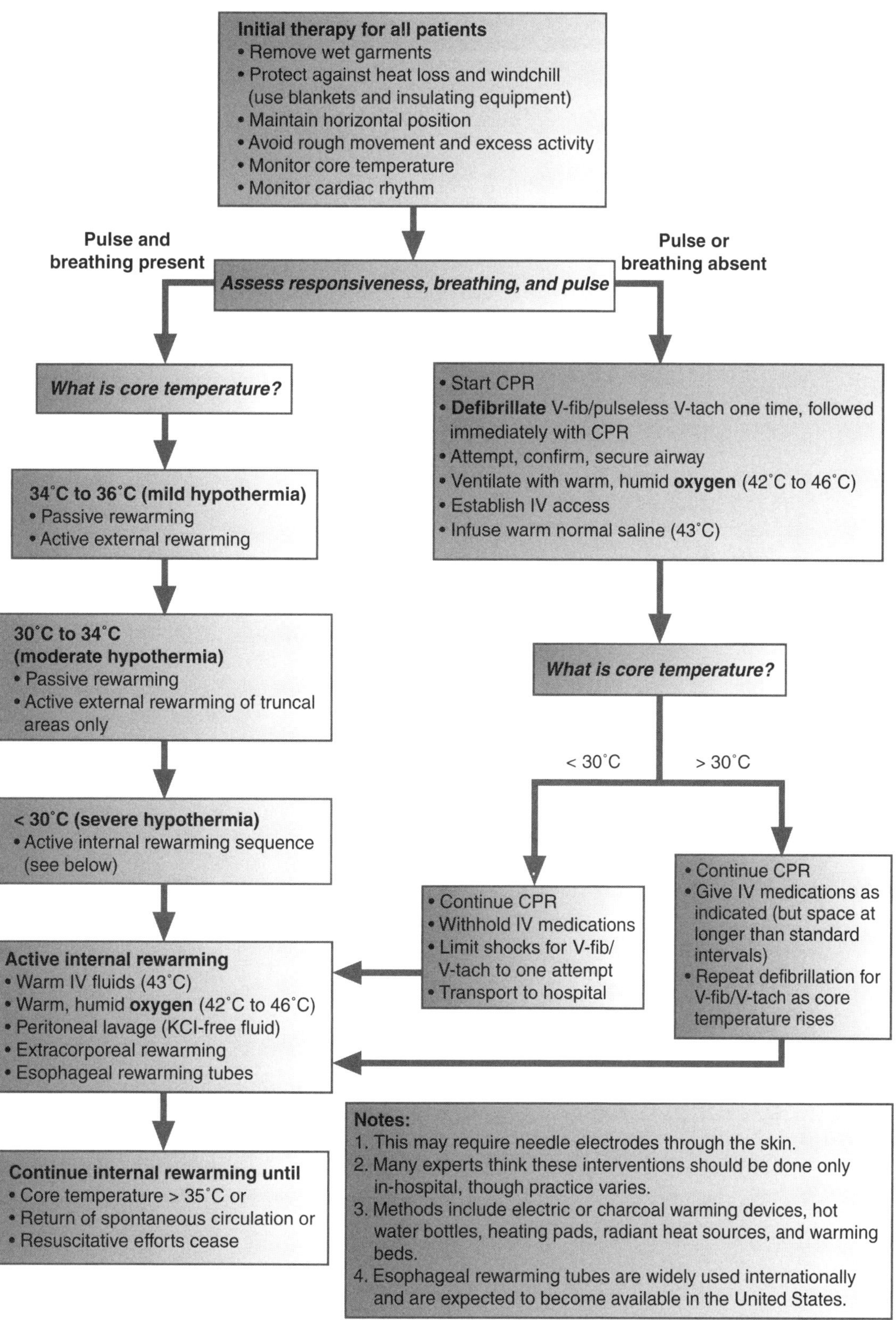

Reproduced with permission, *Handbook of Emergency Cardiovascular Care for Healthcare Providers.* © 2005, American Heart Association.

Figure 10-3 Prehospital hypothermia treatment algorithm.

Table 10-5 Management and Prevention of Altitude Illnesses

Clinical Condition	Signs and Symptoms	Management	Prevention
Mild AMS	Headache with nausea, dizziness, and fatigue during first 12 h after rapid ascent to high altitude (> 8,000′); "hung over"	Descend ≥ 1,600′; or rest, and acclimatize; or speed acclimatization with acetazolamide (125–250 mg twice daily); or treat symptoms with analgesics and antiemetics; or use a combination of above.	Slower ascents; spend a night at an intermediate altitude; avoid overexertion; avoid direct transport to ≥ 9,000′; consider taking acetazolamide (125–250 mg twice daily) beginning 1 day before ascent and continuing for 2 days at high altitude.
Moderate AMS	Worsening headache with marked nausea, dizziness, poor sleep, fluid retention at high altitude > 12 h	Descend ≥ 1,600′; if unable, use a portable hyperbaric chamber or low-flow supplemental oxygen (1–2 L/min);if descent is not possible and oxygen is not available, give acetazolamide (250 mg twice daily), dexamethasone (4 mg orally or intramuscularly every 6 h), or both until symptoms resolve; treat symptoms; or use a combination of above.	Same as above but treat and monitor AMS early.
High-altitude cerebral edema	AMS for ≥ 24 h, ataxia, severe **lassitude**, mental confusion	Initiate immediate descent or evacuation; if not possible, use a portable hyperbaric chamber; give supplemental oxygen (2–4 L/min); give dexamethasone (8 mg orally, intramuscularly, or intravenously initially, and then 4 mg every 6 h); administer acetazolamide if descent is delayed.	Avoid direct transport ≥ 9,000′; slower ascents; avoid overexertion; consider taking acetazolamide (125–250 mg twice daily) beginning 1 day before ascent and continuing for 2 days at high altitude; treat and monitor AMS early.
High-altitude pulmonary edema	Dyspnea at rest and cough, severe weakness, drowsiness; later may see cyanosis, tachycardia, tachypnea, rales	Give supplemental oxygen (4–6 L/min until condition improves, and then reduce to conserve supplies); descend as soon as possible, with minimal exertion, or use a portable hyperbaric chamber; if descent is not possible or no oxygen, give nifedipine (10 mg orally then 30 mg of extended release orally every 2–24 h); add dexamethasone if neurologic deterioration occurs. No evidence for furosemide or morphine.	Slower ascents; avoid overexertion; consider using nifedipine (20–30 mg of extended release every 12 h) in persons with repeated episodes; long-acting beta-2 agonists.

Source: Adapted from Hackett PH, Roach RC. High-altitude illness. *N Engl J Med* 2001; 345:107–114.

Anytime a patient is given a benzodiazepine, be alert for deterioration in ventilatory status. Any patient receiving a benzodiazepine in a prehospital environment should be on a cardiac monitor. Furthermore, pulse oximetry status and heart rate should be closely watched for possible oxygen desaturation. An increase or decrease of pulse rate of 10 from baseline and a reduction on pulse oximetry levels to less than 92% indicate a hypoxic state, requiring immediate and prompt intervention by EMS personnel. This may include supplemental oxygen by nonrebreathing mask, assisting ventilations with a bag-mask device, or intubation as a last resort.

Table 10-6 Management of Drowning or Submersion

- Rescuers trained and practiced in doing so should perform the water rescue.
- Ensure basic life support measures are being carried out with an emphasis on airway and oxygenation.
- Anticipate vomiting.
- Administer supplemental oxygen and intubate if needed.
- Establish IV access.
- Measure core temperature, and prevent or treat hypothermia.
- Give a beta-2 adrenergic by metered-dose inhaler or nebulizer for wheezing.
- Monitor end-tidal carbon dioxide and pulse oximetry.
- Insert a nasogastric tube in intubated patients.
- Transport every submersion patient to the hospital, including patients who seem to recover at the scene.

Drowning or Submersion

Drowning is the process of experiencing respiratory impairment from submersion/immersion in liquid. The management of drowning or submersion involves emphasis on airway management and oxygenation (**Table 10-6** ▸).

Diving Injuries

The lower one descends underwater, the greater the atmospheric pressure becomes. The pressure from descending underwater increases much more rapidly than the inverse pressure, which decreases with altitudes above sea level. To compensate for this significant change in pressure when ascending or descending underwater, pressurized (compressed) air is used. Divers learn to breathe slowly and constantly so that they are always equalizing the pressure within their lungs. If a diver were to hold his or her breath and rapidly ascend, the volume of air within the lungs would quickly expand in volume and cause **barotraumas (pressure injury)** to the lungs themselves. Typically, sports divers are taught to dive to less than 100 feet of depth. Diving conditions get significantly more complicated at depths below 100 feet and require specialized training and equipment. When a sports diver is diving in an area with great depth and there is a problem with disorientation or the depth gauge computer, it is possible that the diver may continue to dive deeper rather than ascend. This can be disastrous, and it is one reason why it is always essential that divers, like firefighters entering a burning building, stay in pairs. Many problems can occur when using compressed air, such as barotrauma, **decompression sickness** (the bends), **nitrogen narcosis**, and **arterial gas embolism (AGE)** (**Table 10-7** ▸).

Table 10-7 Diving Injuries

Mechanisms and Pathophysiology	Body Region	Condition	Clinical Features	Treatment
Barotrauma				
During *descent:* compression of gas in closed spaces	Ear	External ear squeeze (*barotitis externa*)	Otalgia, bloody otorrhea	Keep ear canal dry; no swimming or diving until healed
		Middle ear squeeze (*barotitis media*)	Severe ear pain, tympanic membrane can rupture; emesis, vertigo, nystagmus	Decongestants; no diving until healed, may need IV antinausea medications
		Inner ear squeeze	Tinnitus, vertigo, hearing loss; emesis, pallor, diaphoresis	May need IV antinausea medications, surgical repair
	Paranasal sinuses	Sinus squeeze	Severe pain over affected sinuses and upper teeth, epistaxis	Topical and oral decongestants; antibiotics
	Face	Face mask squeeze	Ecchymoses and petechiae of skin beneath face mask; scleral/conjunctival hemorrhage	Cold compresses, prevent by forced exhalation through nose
During *ascent:* expansion of gas in closed spaces	Gastrointestinal tract	"Gas in gut" (*aerogastralgia*)	Colicky belly pain, belching, flatulence	Rare reports of rupture; usually, no care needed
	Lungs	Pulmonary barotrauma "burst lung," pulmonary overpressurization syndrome (POPS)	Dyspnea, dysphagia, hoarseness, substernal pain; subcutaneous emphysema around neck; pneumothorax, syncope	100% oxygen; decompress pneumothorax
		Arterial gas embolism (AGE)—complication of POPS	Altered mental status, vertigo, dizziness, seizures, dyspnea, pleuritic chest pain, sudden loss of consciousness on surfacing; sudden death	100% oxygen; transport supine; hyperbaric therapy; steroids
Decompression sickness	Skin		Pruritus, subcutaneous emphysema, swelling, rashes	Symptomatic; observe for complications
	Joints and muscles	Bends ("pain-only bends")	Arthralgias, especially in elbows and shoulders, relieved by pressure	Analgesia; observe
	Cerebrum		Multiple sensory and motor disturbances	Hyperbaric therapy; IV fluids
	Cerebellum	The "staggers"	Unsteadiness, incoordination, vertigo	Corticosteroids for all patients with anything more than skin and musculoskeletal involvement
	Spinal cord		Paraplegia, paraparesis, bladder dysfunction (inability to void), back pain	See above
	Lungs	Venous air embolism (the "chokes")	Chest pain, cough, dyspnea, signs of pulmonary embolism	See above
Dissolved nitrogen	Central nervous system	Nitrogen narcosis ("rapture of the deep")	Symptoms like those of alcohol intoxication	Ascent to shallower water

Case Study ANSWERS

Case Study 1 Heat Stroke

Question 1: What is the first priority in caring for Mrs. Whitting?

Answer 1: Mrs. Whitting needs to be rapidly but safely removed from the hot environment. If there will be a delay in extricating the patient, then take the time to open windows and doors, turn on any available air conditioning or fans, bring fans to the patient, and expose/cool the patient using any available means.

Question 2: What are the three major types of emergencies associated with heat illness?

Answer 2: Heat cramps, heat exhaustion, and heat stroke.

Question 3: Which heat emergency is Mrs. Whitting most likely experiencing?

Answer 3: Mrs. Whitting is most likely experiencing heat stroke. She was found debilitated in a hot environment with an altered mental status followed by seizure activity.

Question 4: What are the two causes of altered mental status that should be ruled out first?

Answer 4: Hypoxia and hypoglycemia must be ruled out first in any patient with altered mental status. These two conditions are the most severe and in most cases can be identified and corrected quickly.

Question 5: Why was the diazepam given PR rather than IV or IM?

Answer 5: In addition to an elevated CBT, prolonged seizure activity can cause brain damage and must be stopped as soon as possible. There was difficulty rapidly establishing IV access, so the PR route was chosen as a fast, safe alternative to get needed medication into the patient. The rectum is very vascular, so medications tend to be absorbed rapidly.

Question 6: Based on your understanding of the effects of heat on the CBT, how high would you estimate the patient's CBT to be?

Answer 6: Based on the patient's mental status in this case and feeling that the patient is hot compared to your own body temperature, you know that the CBT is elevated. There may certainly be other contributing factors, some of which you will attempt to rule out (eg, blood glucose level). However, the CBT alone may be a cause of the altered mental status. That being said, this mental status could indicate that the CBT has risen to over 104°F or 40°C. Therefore, treatment is urgent because if the body is not cooled rapidly, seizures, brain damage, and death can follow.

Question 7: Are the prescription medications found in Mrs. Whitting's home a possible cause of a heat illness?

Answer 7: Most likely not; drugs that predispose a person to hyperthermia or heat illness include drugs such as antihistamines, antipsychotics, and phenothiazines. She is on three drugs and if you are not familiar with these medications, as most providers may well not be, it is important to take the time to look them up in your pocket reference or the drug book in the ambulance en route to the hospital as time permits. She is taking donepezil hydrochloride [Aricept], tolterodine tartrate [Detrol], and docusate sodium [Colace].

Question 8: What is the most likely cause of the heat-related emergency for Mrs. Whitting?

Answer 8: For any number of reasons (eg, loss of balance, dizziness, chest pain) she could have fallen and not been able to get up or get to a phone. She appears to have sustained an injury in the course of the fall, and as a result she was not able to remove herself from the heat, or to drink, eat, get her medications, or summon help.

Medication Review

Dexamethasone Sodium Phosphate (Decadron, Hexadrol)

Indications Anaphylaxis, asthma, croup.

Contraindications Hypersensitivity to product, systemic sepsis, bacterial infection.

Dosage and administration Adult: 10–100 mg IV (1 mg/kg slow IV bolus) (considerable variance through medical control). Pediatric: 0.25–1.0 mg/kg/dose IV, IO, IM.

Diazepam (Valium)

Indications Acute anxiety states, acute alcohol withdrawal (delirium tremens), muscle relaxant, seizure activity, agitation. Analgesia for medical procedures (fracture reduction, cardioversion).

Contraindications Hypersensitivity, glaucoma, coma, shock, substance abuse, head injury.

Dosage and administration Seizure activity: Adult: 5–10 mg IV every 10–15 minutes as necessary (5 mg over 5 min) (maximum dose, 30 mg). Seizure activity: Pediatric: 0.2–0.5 mg slowly every 2–5 minutes up to 5 mg (maximum dose, 10 mg/kg). Rectal diazepam: 0.5 mg/kg via rectal catheter and flush with 2–3 mL air after administration. Sedation for cardioversion: 5–15 mg IV over 5–10 minutes prior to cardioversion.

Diphenhydramine (Benadryl)

Indications Symptomatic relief of allergies, allergic reactions, anaphylaxis, acute dystonic reactions (phenothiazines). Blood administration reactions; used for motion sickness, hay fever.

Contraindications Asthma, glaucoma, pregnancy, hypertension, narrow-angle glaucoma, infants, patients taking monoamine oxidase inhibitors (MAOIs).

Dosage and administration Adult: 25–50 mg IM or IV or PO. Pediatric: 1–2 mg/kg IV, IO slowly or IM. If given PO: 5 mg/kg/24 hours.

Dopamine (Intropin)

Indications Cardiogenic, septic or spinal shock, hypotension with low cardiac output states, distributive shock.

Contraindications Hypovolemic shock, pheochromocytoma, tachyarrhythmias, V-fib.

Dosage and administration Adult: 2–20 µg/kg/min titrated to patient response; Pediatric: 2–20 µg/kg/min titrated to patient response.

Medication Review

Epinephrine (Adrenalin)

Indications Cardiac arrest (V-fib/pulseless V-tach, asystole, PEA), symptomatic bradycardia as an alternative infusion to dopamine, severe hypotension secondary to bradycardia when atropine and transcutaneous pacing are unsuccessful, allergic reactions, anaphylaxis, asthma.

Contraindications Hypertension, hypothermia, pulmonary edema, myocardial ischemia, hypovolemic shock.

Dosage and administration Adult: Mild allergic reactions and asthma: 0.3–0.5 mg (0.3–0.5 mL of 1:1,000) SC. Anaphylaxis: 0.1 mg (1 mL of 1:10,000) IV/IO over 5 minutes. Cardiac arrest: IV/IO dose: 1 mg (10 mL of 1:10,000 solution) every 3–5 minutes during resuscitation. Follow each dose with 20 mL flush and elevate arm for 10 to 20 seconds after dose. Higher dose: Higher doses (up to 0.2 mg/kg) may be used for specific indications (beta-blocker or calcium channel blocker overdose). Continuous infusion: Add 1 mg (1 mL of 1:1,000 solution) to 500 mL normal saline or D_5W. Initial infusion rate of 1 µg/min titrated to effect (typical dose: 2–10 µg/min). Endotracheal (ET) dose: 2–2.5 mg diluted in 10 mL normal saline. Profound bradycardia or hypotension: 2–10 µg/min; titrate to patient response. Pediatric: Mild allergic reactions and asthma: 0.01 mg/kg (0.01 mL/kg) of 1:1,000 solution SC (maximum of 0.3 mL). Cardiac arrest: IV/IO dose: 0.01 mg/kg (0.1 mL/kg) of 1:10,000 solution every 3–5 minutes during arrest. All endotracheal (ET) doses: 0.1 mg/kg (0.1 mL/kg) of 1:1,000 solution. Symptomatic bradycardia: IV/IO dose: 0.01 mg/kg (0.1 mL/kg) of 1:10,000 solution. Continuous IV/IO infusion: Begin with rapid infusion, then titrate to response. Typical initial infusion: 0.1–1 µg/min. Higher doses may be effective.

Midazolam (Versed)

Indications Sedation, anxiolytic prior to endotracheal or nasotracheal intubation; administer for conscious sedation.

Contraindications Glaucoma, shock, coma, alcohol intoxication, overdose, depressed vital signs, concomitant use with other CNS depressants, barbiturates, alcohol, narcotics.

Dosage and administration Adult: 2.0–2.5 mg slow IV over 2–3 minutes; may be repeated to total maximum: 0.1 mg/kg. Pediatric: Not recommended.

Morphine Sulfate (Astramorph/PF and Others)

Indications Severe CHF, pulmonary edema, chest pain associated with acute MI, analgesia for moderate to severe acute and chronic pain (use with caution).

Contraindications Head injury, exacerbated COPD, depressed respiratory drive, hypotension, undiagnosed abdominal pain, decreased level of consciousness, suspected hypovolemia, patients who have taken MAOIs within the past 14 days.

Dosage and administration Adult: Initial dose: 2–4 mg IV (over 1–5 minutes) every 5–30 minutes. Repeat dose: 2–8 mg at 5- to 15-minute intervals. Pediatric: 0.1–0.2 mg/kg per dose via IV, IO, IM, or SC; maximum dose of 5 mg.

Naloxone Hydrochloride (Narcan)

Indications Opiate overdose, coma; complete or partial reversal of CNS and respiratory depression induced by opioids; decreased level of consciousness; coma of unknown origin; narcotic agonist for the following: morphine sulfate, heroin, hydromorphone (Dilaudid), methadone, meperidine (Demerol), paregoric, fentanyl citrate (Sublimase), oxycodone (Percodan), codeine, propoxyphene (Darvon); narcotic agonist and antagonist for the following: butorphanol (Stadol), pentazocine (Talwin), nalbuphine hydrochloride (Nubain).

Contraindications Use with caution in narcotic-dependent patients; use with caution in neonates of narcotic-addicted mothers.

Dosage and administration Adult: 0.4–2.0 mg IV, IM, SC, or ET (diluted); minimum recommended dose, 0.4 mg; repeat at 5-minute intervals to a maximum dose of 10 mg (medical control may request higher amounts). Infusion: 2 mg in 500 mL of D_5W (4 µg/mL), infuse at 0.4 mg/h (100 mL/h). Pediatric: 0.1 mg/kg/dose IV, IM, SC, ET (diluted); maximum dose of 0.8 mg; if no response in 10 minutes, administer an additional 0.1 mg/kg/dose.

Medication Review

Ondansetron Hydrochloride (Zofran)

Indications For the prevention or control of nausea or vomiting. Also used in the hospital setting for patients undergoing chemotherapy or surgical procedures.

Contraindications Known allergy to this medicine or other 5-HT3 receptor antagonists.

Dosage and administration Adult: 4 mg IV or IM (may repeat in 10 minutes). Pediatric: 0.1 mg/kg IV or IM.

Oral Glucose (Insta-Glucose)

Indications Conscious patients with suspected hypoglycemia.

Contraindications Decreased level of consciousness, nausea, vomiting.

Dosage and administration Adult: Should be sipped slowly by patient until clinical improvement noted. Pediatric: Same as adult.

Oxygen

Indications Confirmed or expected hypoxemia, ischemic chest pain, respiratory insufficiency, prophylactically during air transport, confirmed or suspected carbon monoxide poisoning, all other causes of decreased tissue oxygenation, decreased level of consciousness.

Contraindications Certain patients with COPD or emphysema who will not tolerate oxygen concentrations over 35%, hyperventilation. Oxygen should never be withheld from a patient who needs it, however. Be prepared to assist with ventilations in a patient with COPD who requires high oxygen concentrations as apnea may result.

Dosage and administration Adult: Cardiac arrest and carbon monoxide poisoning: 100%. Hypoxemia: 10–15 L/min via nonrebreathing mask. COPD: 1–6 L/min via nasal cannula or 28%–35% Venturi mask. Be prepared to provide ventilatory support if higher concentrations of oxygen needed. Pediatric: Same as for adult with exception of premature infant.

Phenytoin (Dilantin)

Indications Prophylaxis and treatment of major motor seizures, digitalis-induced arrhythmias.

Contraindications Hypersensitivity, bradycardia, second- and third-degree heart block.

Dosage and administration Adult: Seizures: 10–20 mg/kg slow IV, not to exceed 1 g or rate of 50 mg/min. Arrhythmias: 50–100 mg (diluted) slow IV every 5–15 min as needed; maximum, 1 g. Pediatric: Seizures: 10–20 mg/kg slow IV (1–3 mg/kg/min). Arrhythmias: 5 mg/kg slow IV; maximum, 1 g.

Promethazine Hydrochloride (Phenergan)

Indications Nausea, vomiting, motion sickness; sedation for patients in labor; potentiation of analgesic effects of narcotics.

Contraindications Hypersensitivity, coma, CNS-depressed patients from alcohol, barbiturates, narcotics, Reye's syndrome.

Dosage and administration Adult: 12.5–25 mg IV, deep IM, PO, rectally. Pediatric: (older than 2 years old) 0.25–0.5 mg/kg dose IM.

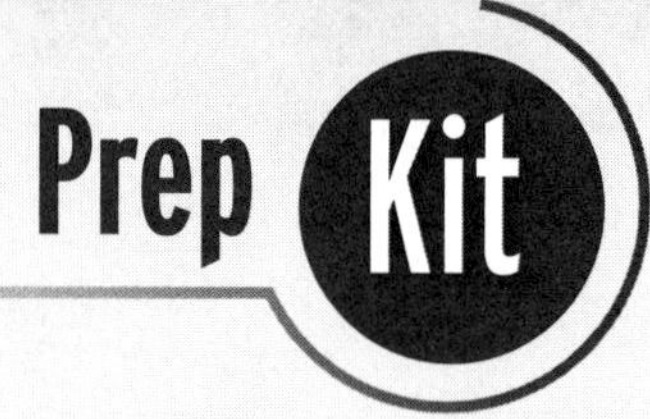

Chapter Summary

- The most common causes of environmental conditions involve cold and heat.
- The severity of the environmental emergency can be assessed by the patient's mental status. The more altered the patient, the more severe the condition is likely to be.
- The three major types of emergencies associated with heat illness are heat cramps, heat exhaustion, and heat stroke. Of the three illnesses, heat stroke is the most severe.
- Heat stroke occurs when the body can no longer adequately rid itself of heat, causing the CBT to rise over 104°F (40°C).
- Hypothermia is a cold illness that occurs when the body experiences heat loss in which the CBT drops to less then 95°F (35°C).
- Altitude sickness becomes a risk at altitudes of greater than 8,000 feet above sea level.
- The most common altitude sickness disorders are acute mountain sickness (AMS), high-altitude pulmonary edema (HAPE), and high-altitude cerebral edema (HACE).
- The lower one descends underwater, the greater the atmospheric pressure becomes. To compensate for this significant change in pressure when ascending or descending underwater, pressurized (compressed) air is used.
- Many problems can occur when using compressed air, such as barotrauma, decompression sickness (the bends), nitrogen narcosis, and arterial gas embolism (AGE).

Vital Vocabulary

Acute mountain sickness (AMS) An altitude illness characterized by headache plus at least one of the following: fatigue or weakness, gastrointestinal symptoms (nausea, vomiting, or anorexia), dizziness or lightheadedness, or difficulty sleeping.

Altitude sickness Conditions caused by the effects of hypobaric (low atmospheric pressure) hypoxia on the CNS and pulmonary systems as a result of nonacclimatized people ascending to altitude; range from acute mountain sickness to high-altitude cerebral edema (HACE) and high-altitude pulmonary edema (HAPE).

Arterial gas embolism (AGE) The resultant gaseous emboli from the forcing of gas into the pulmonary vasculature from barotrauma.

Barotrauma (pressure injury) Injury resulting from pressure disequilibrium across body surfaces.

Core body temperature (CBT) The temperature in the part of the body comprising the heart, lungs, brain, and abdominal viscera.

Decompression sickness A broad range of signs and symptoms caused by nitrogen bubbles in blood and tissues during a rapid ascent.

Drowning The process of experiencing respiratory impairment from submersion or immersion in liquid.

Heat cramps Acute and involuntary muscle pains, usually in the lower extremities, the abdomen, or both, that occur because of profuse sweating and subsequent sodium losses in sweat.

Heat exhaustion A clinical syndrome characterized by volume depletion and heat stress that is thought to be a milder form of heat illness and on a continuum leading to heat stroke.

Heat illness The increase in core body temperature due to inadequate thermolysis.

Heat stroke The least common and most deadly heat illness, caused by a severe disturbance in thermoregulation, usually characterized by a core temperature of more than 104°F (40°C) and altered mental status.

High-altitude cerebral edema (HACE) An altitude illness in which there is a change in mental status and/or ataxia in a person with acute mountain sickness (AMS) or the presence of mental status changes and ataxia in a person without AMS.

High-altitude pulmonary edema (HAPE) An altitude illness characterized by dyspnea at rest, cough, severe weakness, and drowsiness that may eventually lead to central cyanosis, audible rales or wheezing, tachypnea, and tachycardia.

Hypoglycemia A deficiency of glucose in the blood caused by too much insulin or too little glucose.

Hypothermia Condition in which the core body temperature is significantly below normal.

Hypoxia A lack of oxygen to the body's cells and tissues.

Lassitude Condition of listlessness and fatigue.

Nitrogen narcosis A state resembling alcohol intoxication produced by nitrogen gas dissolved in the blood at high ambient pressure; also called rapture of the deep.

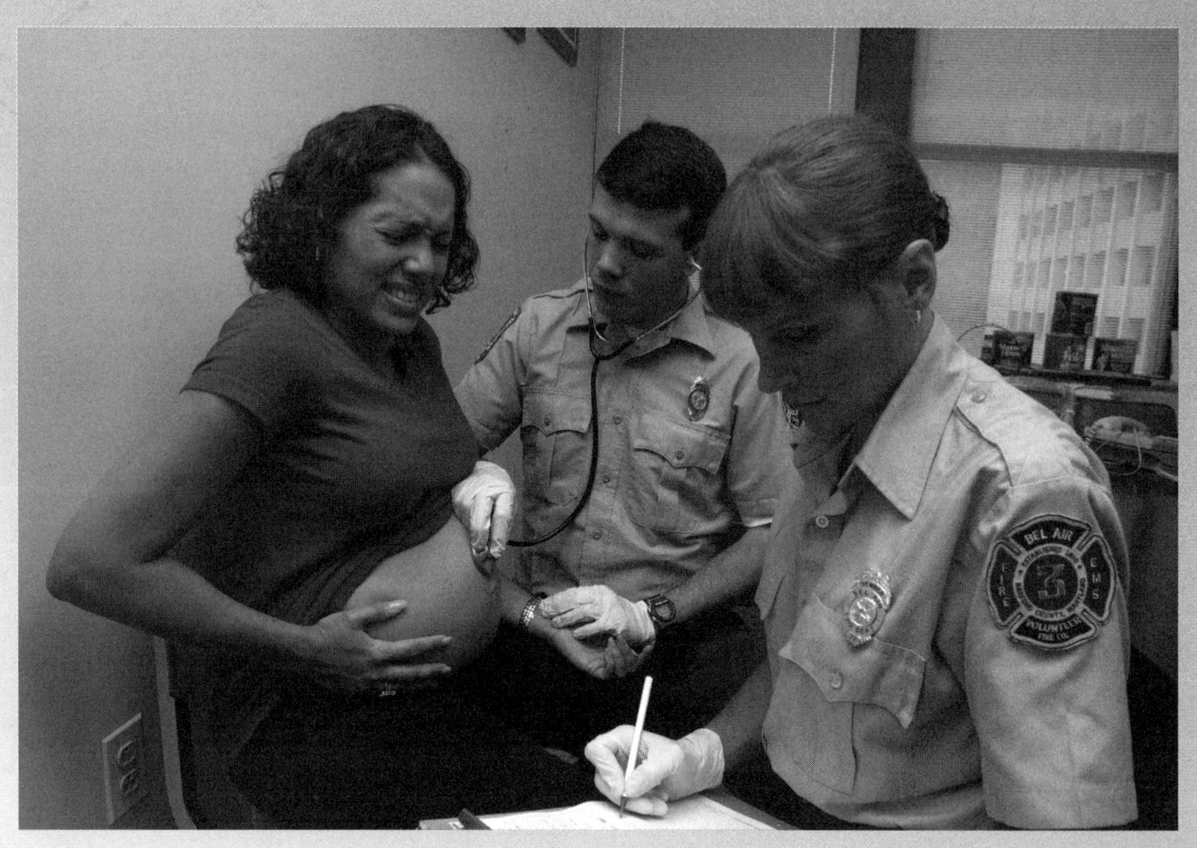
BEL AIR

11 Obstetric Emergencies

Objectives

Cognitive
None

Affective
None

Psychomotor
None

Additional Objectives

11-1 Discuss the following medications used in the prehospital setting for the pregnant patient during labor or its complications: oxytocin [Pitocin, Syntocinon], magnesium sulfate, diazepam [Valium], midazolam [Versed], metoprolol tartrate [Lopressor]. (pages 323, 332–333)

11-2 Discuss assessment of an obstetrical patient and identify the stages of labor. (pages 320–325)

11-3 Identify and describe complications associated with pregnancy and delivery and how they might be managed with a medication. (pages 328–329)

11-4 Identify predelivery emergencies. (pages 329–335)

11-5 Describe the management of the mother post-delivery. (pages 321–324)

11-6 Describe the procedures for handling abnormal deliveries. (pages 327–328)

11-7 Describe the procedure for handling maternal complications of labor involving a medication. (pages 325–326)

Delivery in the Field

There are three stages of labor. The **first stage of labor** begins with contractions and ends with the crowning of the infant and full dilation and effacement of the uterine cervix. Birth is considered imminent when the contractions are strong and very close in time, the baby's head is crowning, and the mother feels the urge to move her bowels. This means that the fetus has moved down into the birth canal, with the head pushing back on the rectum, and is therefore likely to be delivered very soon. The **second stage of labor** starts with full dilation of the cervix (10 cm) and ends with the delivery of the infant. The **third stage of labor** begins after the birth of the child when contractions resume and the placenta is delivered. The *average* amount of time for each of these stages is as follows:

- First stage of labor: from 8 to 12 hours (as long as 12–24 hours for the first pregnancy)
- Second stage of labor: from minutes to an hour
- Third stage of labor: about 5 to 60 minutes.

With each subsequent birth, the duration of the first and second stage of labor become shorter.

PREPARE:

Stretcher: Blankets work best to absorb blood and fluids, not sheets. Additionally, placing several blankets under the mother's buttocks will provide some elevation and cushion for her hips. Placing blankets under the mother will also allow for an easier transfer of the mother from the EMS stretcher to the labor and delivery bed.

Patient: If delivery is imminent, perform the delivery either in the residence or other appropriate area. The back of an ambulance is small and can be confining when several personnel are there providing care for the patient. Place the mother supine, with knees flexed and hips elevated. You can consider draping the legs with the sterile drapes from the obstetric (OB) kit; however, delivering a child is NOT a sterile procedure. You do want to limit the infant's exposure to general pathogens as much as possible.

Equipment:

a. Oxygen for the mother. A nonrebreathing mask is fine; however, a nasal cannula at 4–6 L/min is appropriate unless you suspect severe fetal distress.
b. Oxygen for the infant. Prepare an infant bag-mask device but also have a simple face mask ready.
c. Bulb syringe. Wrap the bulb syringe, from the OB kit, several times with roller gauze. Since you will have gloves on when delivering the infant, and they may be wet or have fluids from delivery on them, the bulb syringe will literally "squirt" from your hands when squeezed. The roller gauze on the bulb syringe will reduce the likelihood of it slipping out of your hand when squeezed. As soon as the head has been delivered, wipe the face and nose, being observant for meconium, and suction the mouth and then the nose. Newborns are obligatory nose breathers.
d. Meconium aspirator. Have a meconium aspirator connected to a 2.0 or 2.5 ET tube and a laryngoscope.
e. Sterile blankets and other drying and warming products to dry and wrap the baby in. Infants are especially prone to loss of heat and you must keep them warm. By drying them, you are stimulating them, warming them, and removing excessive moisture from their skin. This procedure will help the infant achieve a good 1-minute APGAR.

ASSESS:

1. Inspect the perineum visually for bulging or crowning.
   a. DO NOT check for CERVICAL DILATION.
   b. The only times you should place your hand into the vaginal canal is for a breech birth to create an air passage for the child to breathe after the torso has delivered, and for a prolapsed cord to lift the baby off the cord during delivery.
2. Evaluate frequency, duration, and the feel of the contractions.
   a. Distinguish between false labor and true labor.
   b. Contractions that are less than 2 minutes apart are indicative of impeding delivery.

Case Study 1 Normal Childbirth

Part 1

It is 5:00 am and you are watching the morning news when a call comes in for a woman in labor on the interstate. As you and your partner get into the ambulance, you continue to receive additional information. There is a state trooper on the scene and the car is on the side of the road just before the exit 4 southbound ramp. According to the state trooper, birth is imminent.

As you pull past the two vehicles and carefully park on the side of the road, you are waved over to a small sedan. Aside from the occasional car driving by, it looks like the scene is safe. You pull out the stretcher, the first-in kit, and the OB kit and quickly proceed to the vehicle.

As you approach the car you can hear the woman moaning in pain. The trooper is clearly thrilled you have arrived, and says the couple was on their way to the medical center. This is her third pregnancy and second child. Her first pregnancy ended in a miscarriage but the last pregnancy was smooth.

You introduce yourself and your partner to the woman. She tells you to call her Betsy. Betsy tells you that her water broke 20 minutes ago and she had hoped they could make it to the hospital. Unfortunately, things were happening just too fast, compared to the last time. It is obvious that her airway is open and clear and her breathing is just fine. You reach down to check her radial pulse as part of the initial assessment, and just then she begins to have another contraction (see **Table 1**).

Table 1 **Initial Assessment**

Initial Assessment	Recording Time: 2 Minutes
General Impression/ Appearance	Woman in her 30s who is conscious, excited, anxious, and in pain
Mental Status	Alert (oriented to person, place, and day)
Airway	Open and clear
Breathing	Rapid, shallow, and interrupted by contractions
Circulation	Strong radial pulse, no external bleeding (yet)
Priority/Plan	Guarded at the moment

The chief complaint is labor pains, and you use the OPQRST questions to elaborate and determine if the delivery will happen in the car, on your stretcher en route, or at the hospital. It is important to assess if there are any potential complications you should be aware of. From talking to the patient, it is clear that she has had good prenatal care. Betsy tells you she was at the doctor's office late yesterday afternoon and yesterday was her due date. Knowing the patient has been going to her doctor is always a relief, as you know from previous training that women who lack prenatal care are likely to have a substantially increased risk of pregnancy or delivery-related complications.

Question 1: What is the significance of learning that Betsy has been going for prenatal care?

Question 2: If this was Betsy's first pregnancy, how long would labor be expected to take?

Part 2

The patient's initial assessment is unremarkable, so you proceed to the focused history and physical examination of a responsive medical patient (see **Table 2**). You will need to continue with your line of questioning as you try to help Betsy into a comfortable position on your stretcher. She has the urge to move her bowels and when the contractions are timed, they are strong and very close in time (1- to 2-minute intervals lasting 45 to 60 seconds). To determine this, you count the time from the start of the strong contraction to the end of the contractions or cramps. Then count the interval length between the end of one labor pain and the start of the next.

Table 2 **Focused History and Physical Examination**

Baseline Vital Signs	Recording Time: 5 Minutes
Skin CTC (color, temperature, condition)	Pale, warm, clammy
Pulse	100 beats/min and regular
Blood Pressure	120/80 mm Hg
Respirations	24 breaths/min and shallow

Betsy tells you that she is carrying one baby, a boy, and he is in the right position. She states that her pregnancy has been normal with the exception of a lot of morning sickness in the first trimester. Actually this is one of the days she does not feel nauseous!

Case Study I Continued

You drape her appropriately with a sheet, discreetly help her remove her underwear, then assess for crowning as your partner gets a full set of vital signs. The trooper has pulled the husband aside and is advising him of where to park his vehicle while he rides in the ambulance to the hospital with his wife.

Question 3: What is the significance of the urge to move her bowels?

Question 4: How do you count the labor pains?

Part 3

Based on the SAMPLE history taken so far and the fact that Betsy is definitely crowning, birth is imminent (see **Table 3**). You barely have enough time to assist her onto the stretcher when she starts to push the baby out. Quickly your partner opens up the OB kit since you will need the umbilical clamps, the bulb syringe, the scalpel, and the plastic bag for the afterbirth. The rest of the contents of the kit (ie, drapes, napkins, and the wipes) will probably not be needed due to the rush. The delivery may involve bleeding and certainly plenty of amniotic fluid and secretions. You will prepare to suction the infant right away and resuction at a later point to avoid aspiration of the secretions as the baby takes his first breaths. You and your partner quickly move the stretcher behind a tree in order to block the view of onlookers.

Table 3 SAMPLE History

SAMPLE History	Comments
Signs/symptoms	Active labor, pale and clammy, denies any nausea
Allergies	None
Medications	Vitamins
Pertinent past medical history	Second pregnancy, good prenatal care, no expected complications
Last oral intake	Glass of juice about 30 minutes ago
Events leading up to the incident	Has had labor pains for the past few hours but had expected to make it until the morning and then drive to the hospital

Treatment Plan

1. Don the appropriate PPE for BSI precautions.
2. Assess and manage the ABCs and provide supplemental oxygen as needed.
3. Obtain a set of baseline vital signs.
4. Determine by history and examination if birth is imminent.
5. Place the mother in the preferred delivery position (supine) and drape if birth is imminent.
6. When crowning occurs, place gentle pressure on the baby's head with the palm of your gloved hand to prevent an explosive delivery.
7. If the membranes cover the head after it emerges, tear the sac with your gloved fingers or forceps. Suction the oropharynx and then the nostrils with the bulb syringe **(Figure 11-1)**.
8. Gently guide the head downward to allow delivery of the shoulder under the pubic bone, then guide the head upward to allow the other shoulder to deliver **(Figure 11-2)**.
9. If the cord is around the neck, unwrap or clamp twice and then carefully cut between the clamps.

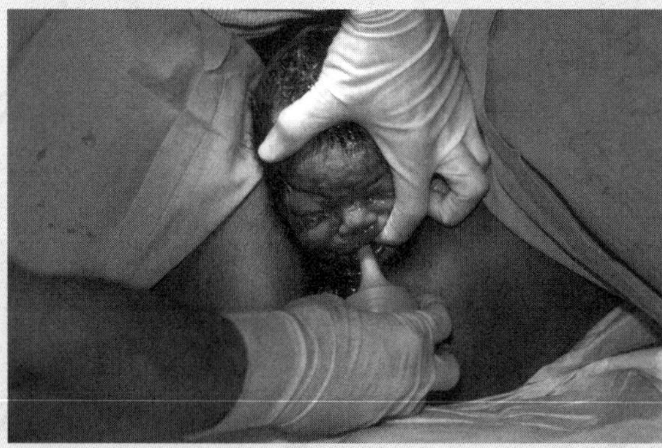

Figure 11-1 Suction the infant's airway.

10. Once the infant is delivered, clamp the cord twice (around 9" and 7" from the baby) and then cut between the clamps.
11. Warm, position, and dry the baby; resuction and assess the APGAR score at 1 and 5 minutes.
12. Reassess the mother and take serial vital signs.

Medications for Consideration:

Based on the normal delivery, Betsy does not need any medications aside from possibly some supplemental oxygen and an IV of normal saline, which should be run during and following her labor. Some EMS systems

Case Study I Continued

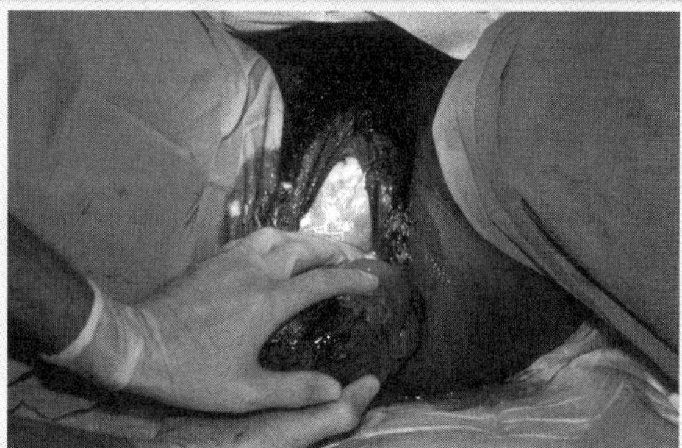

Figure 11-2 Gently guide the infant's head to allow shoulder delivery.

carry oxytocin [Pitocin], which is a potent, smooth-muscle stimulant and is used to strengthen contractions and induce or enhance labor in the in-hospital setting (see **Table 4**). It is also used following delivery to stimulate the uterus to contract and slow down any postpartum hemorrhage. It is similarly indicated for this problem in the prehospital setting as well.

The husband realizes that the time has actually come and he stands by his wife's head in order to be supportive. You note that the bulb syringe is placed nearby where you left it and then begin to provide gentle counterpressure on the infant so Betsy does not have an explosive delivery. It takes two or three good pushes and the infant's head is out. The cord is wrapped around the head but it is easily flipped over the head. You begin to suction the mouth and then the nose. The infant is now out, lying on the stretcher. You quickly dry, warm, position, and suction once more. You think to yourself, "that was easy!" You were taught to place the first clamp about 8″ to 9″ from the infant and 6″ to 7″ away from the mother in order to allow plenty of room to place a third clamp in the event that after the cord is clamped, the cord continues to bleed. You clamp the cord between the two clamps, away from the infant.

Question 5: Why is it so important to suction the infant, even before delivery is complete?

Question 6: Why are the umbilical cord clamps placed so far from the infant?

Table 4 Oxytocin

Do you know?	Comments
Right drug? Generic name: [**Oxytocin**] Trade name: [Pitocin]	This is an oxytocic drug, a naturally occurring hormone that is produced by the hypothalamus and stored in the pituitary. It stimulates contraction of the uterus and smooth muscle.
Right patient?	In-hospital to get the labor moving and strengthen the contractions. Prehospital to improve the contractions of the uterus during and after the third stage of labor as an effort to stop excessive bleeding.
Right dose?	3 to 10 units IM (after delivery of placenta) or IV by mixing 10 to 40 units in 1,000 mL of normal saline. Then infuse at 20–40 milliunits/min titrated to severity of bleeding and uterine response.
Right route?	IM or IV drip.
Right time?	Antepartum use is indicated in certain conditions. Postpartum use to improve the contractions of the uterus during and after the third stage of labor to help stop excessive bleeding.
Right documentation?	Always document how and when the drug was administered and the patient's response to the medication on your patient care report.
Expected action	Stimulates rhythmic contractions of the uterus, increases frequency of existing contractions, and increases the tone of uterine musculature.
Side effects	Nausea and vomiting, tachycardia, seizures, and cardiac arrhythmias.
Contraindications	Known sensitivity, fetal distress where delivery is prolonged or not imminent, history of previous traumatic deliveries.
Precautions	Can induce coma or result in uterine rupture and hypertension if administered in excess.
Pharmacokinetics	Onset IM: 3–5 minutes; IV: immediate. Peak effect: variable. Duration IM: 30–60 minutes; IV: 20 minutes after infusion discontinued; metabolized in the kidney and liver, small amounts excreted unchanged in urine.

Case Study I Continued

Part 4

As you tell Betsy her baby boy is looking good, she asks to hold him. This is a good time to quickly move everyone into the ambulance. Next up will be a quick APGAR score and a set of vitals as part of the reassessment and ongoing assessment (see **Table 5**). Once in the back of the ambulance you are able to get both mother and baby settled and obtain a full set of vital signs.

The decision is made to get rolling toward the hospital as you can always pull over if necessary to assist in the delivery of the placenta. In about 15 minutes after the delivery, Betsy has a couple of strong contractions and out comes the placenta—just as you expected, when you expected. You are able to place it in a plastic bag so it can be examined by the physician.

Although bleeding is not excessive, you place Betsy on a nasal cannula. She did not want a nonrebreathing mask as she really wanted to call her mother on her cell phone. Seeing that her vitals are all normal and her color is improving, you agree that would be a great idea so you go with the cannula. You are thankful, because the outcome could have been a lot different.

Table 5 Reassessment and Ongoing Assessment of the Patient

Serial Vital Signs and Relevant Data	Recording Time: 15 Minutes
Skin CTC	Normal color, warm, dry
Pulse	100 beats/min and regular
Blood Pressure	110/70 mm Hg
Respirations	22 breaths/min and regular
Mental Status	Alert (oriented to person, place, and day)
ECG	Borderline normal sinus rhythm to sinus tachycardia with no ectopy. (It would be acceptable to skip this step on this patient unless you have reason to believe it is a problem.)
SpO_2	98%
Lung Sounds	Clear bilaterally
Other (ie: glucose, core body temperature)	n/a

If Betsy had excessive postpartum bleeding, there are not a lot of treatment options. You would have first treated her for shock by raising her legs, keeping her warm, and administering supplemental oxygen by nonrebreathing mask; you would have then run the IV wide open and checked serial vital signs. You would have quickly notified the ED and asked Betsy to attempt to nurse her child. This would help stimulate release of the body's own oxytocin. An external uterine massage and the administration of IV oxytocin [Pitocin] would increase the strength of the uterine contractions that could help control excessive bleeding.

Question 7: If Betsy's placenta was not delivered within a few minutes, is that a problem?

Question 8: If there is excessive bleeding as Betsy's placenta is being delivered, what treatment strategies are available to you in the field?

Part 5

The happy family is delivered to the ED. Upon arrival, you are told to bring them right up to the obstetrics unit. Having one child already, this is not new territory to Betsy. Of course, the excitement of delivering her baby boy—who they have decided to name after the paramedic who assisted—on the side of a major highway shortly before the start of rush hour traffic does not compare to their first experience. Fortunately, everything went well, everyone is happy and healthy, and after the paperwork and a quick final visit, you are off to the station for change of shift and a shower. Today was a great day and you were graced to be in the right place at the right time to help make it that way!

Table 11-1 Questions to Ask the Pregnant Patient

Information	Question	Ask
Current pregnancy	1	What week are you in? (gestation is 38–42 weeks for "full term")
	2	What is your estimated due date?
	3	Have you been going to prenatal care?
	4	Do you have multiple fetuses?
	5	Did you use fertility drugs?
	6	Is the fetus in the normal position?
	7	Have you had preterm labor, either "real" or "false" (eg, Braxton Hicks contractions)?
Prior pregnancies	1	How many pregnancies have you had? (**gravida**)
	2	How many previous births? (**parity**)
	3	Number of preterm pregnancies?
	4	Any previous abortions or miscarriages?
	5	Types of previous deliveries (ie, vaginal, spontaneous, induced, or cesarean section)?
	6	Any complications during your pregnancy?
	7	Length of the labor(s)?
	8	Any postpartum complications?
Specific past medical history	1	Do you have hypertension (preexisting or pregnancy-induced)?
	2	Diabetes (preexisting or gestational)?
	3	Are you taking any medications (prenatal vitamins, OTC or prescribed medications, herbals or recreational drugs)?
	4	Do you have any allergies?
	5	Any alcohol or drug use during your pregnancy?

Assessment of the Patient

Assessment of the obstetrical patient focuses around obtaining the patient's significant history, determining if birth is imminent, and examining for crowning when necessary. This will reduce the chances of an abnormal delivery and its potential complications. In addition to the OPQRST questions, be sure to ask the laboring patient about discharge (ie, presence, amount, and appearance), cramping and pain, syncope (ie, lightheadedness or dizziness), and the urge to move the bowels. The line of questioning should also include determining the status of the current pregnancy including prenatal care and any concerning issues surrounding it, the number of total pregnancies including this one, total live births, and specific past medical history (**Table 11-1** ▲). It is also important to ask the patient how frequent and intense the contractions are because you will need to distinguish between false labor and real labor (**Table 11-2** ▶).

Table 11-2 False Labor Versus True Labor

Parameter	True Labor	False Labor
Contractions	Regularly spaced	Irregularly spaced
Interval between contractions	Gradually shortens	Remains long
Intensity of contractions	Gradually increases	Stays the same
Effects of analgesics	Do not abolish the pain	Often abolish the pain
Cervical changes	Progressive effacement and dilation	No changes

The FDA Pregnancy Labeling System

Since 1975, the Food and Drug Administration (FDA) has required drug labeling to include a subsection on a drug's ability to cause birth defects and other effects on reproduction and pregnancy. Products also must be classified under one of five letter categories—A, B, C, D, and X (**Table 11-3** ▶). Since 1997, the FDA has been developing a new regulation that will revamp the pregnancy labeling system. The proposed regulation would replace the letter categories with more detailed, narrative descriptions. Information on fertility, pregnancy, and breast feeding would be included.

Table 11-3 The FDA's Current Categories for Drug Use During Pregnancy

Category	Description
A	Adequate, well-controlled studies in pregnant women have not shown an increased risk of fetal abnormalities.
B	Animal studies have revealed no evidence of harm to the fetus; however, there are no adequate and well-controlled studies in pregnant women. **or** Animal studies have shown an adverse effect, but adequate and well-controlled studies in pregnant women have failed to demonstrate a risk to the fetus.
C	Animal studies have shown an adverse effect and there are no adequate and well-controlled studies in pregnant women. **or** No animal studies have been conducted and there are no adequate and well-controlled studies in pregnant women.
D	Studies, adequate well-controlled or observational, in pregnant women have demonstrated a risk to the fetus; however, the benefits of therapy may outweigh the potential risk.
X	Studies, adequate well-controlled or observational, in animals or pregnant women have demonstrated positive evidence of fetal abnormalities. The use of the product is contraindicated in women who are or may become pregnant.

Medications to Treat Nausea and Vomiting

During pregnancy, nausea and vomiting is common for many women. For some it may become very severe, requiring treatment with medication, IV fluids, and hospitalization. **Hyperemesis gravidarum** is a severe form of pregnancy-induced nausea characterized by persistent vomiting, **ketonuria**, and severe weight loss and dehydration. In-hospital medications used to treat nausea and vomiting in the pregnant patient can be given rectally, orally, or through an IV line. These drugs include promethazine [Phenergan], prochlorperazine [Compazine], and chlorpromazine [Thorazine]. Antiemetics such as ondansetron hydrochloride [Zofran] were designed for cancer patients, but also work for pregnant women.

Prochlorperazine [Compazine] is currently the most commonly prescribed medication in the United States for the treatment of nausea and vomiting in pregnancy.

Drugs Used During Labor and Delivery

Drugs used during labor and delivery can cause fetal CNS depression and bradycardia and must be given carefully to avoid toxicity in the fetus. That is why paramedics do not give medications to the patient during transport, with the exception of oxygen. After the cord is cut, the newborn metabolizes any medications transferred from the mother more slowly, due to its immature metabolic and excretory processes.

Teratogens

Drugs taken by the mother during pregnancy can cross the placental barrier and adversely affect the development of the fetus by producing developmental deformities, physical dependency, and/or toxic or lethal effects. Anything that harms normal cellular development in the embryo or fetus is called a **teratogen**. Examples of known teratogens include drugs, chemicals, radiation, and intrauterine viral infections.

Common teratogenic drugs:

- Analgesics and antipyretics (ie, aspirin, salicylates, and narcotics)
- Antibiotics (powerful medicines used to fight bacterial infections [ie, tetracycline])
- Antifungals (medications used to kill fungus)
- Antiparasitics (medications used to kill parasites)
- Antiviral (medications used to eradicate a virus)
- Anticoagulants (warfarin [Coumadin] and its derivatives)
- Anticonvulsants (medications used in seizure disorders)
- Antidiabetics (oral hypoglycemics)
- Antihypertensives (ie, ACE inhibitors, diazoxide, thiazide diuretics, and reserpine)
- Antineoplastics (used in the treatment of tumors, lymphoma, and leukemia)
- Antithyroids (medications used for treatment of thyroid diseases)
- Disulfiram [Antabuse] (used in alcoholism)
- Folic acid antagonists (ie, methotrexate and aminopterin)
- Ergot alkaloids (ie, ergotamine, which works together with caffeine to prevent blood vessels in the head from expanding and causing headaches)
- Hormones (ie, androgens, testosterone derivatives, estrogens, progestins, diethylstilbestrol [DES])

- Isotretinoin [Accutane]
- NSAIDs (nonsteroidal anti-inflammatory drugs)
- Psychoactives (ie, benzodiazepines, lithium, and amitriptyline)
- Valproic acid [Depakene] (used for migraine headaches or convulsions)

Other teratogens:
- Alcohol (probably the most commonly abused substance during pregnancy)
- Aspertame (a noncaloric artificial sweetener used in diet soda)
- Caffeine (from coffee, tea, soda, etc)
- Crack cocaine (an illegal drug of abuse)
- Infections (ie, hepatitis, mumps, rubella, varicella, toxoplasmosis, coxsackievirus, cytomegalovirus)
- Intrauterine viral infections (such as STDs)
- Lead (from paint or old water pipes)
- Organic mercury (from a large quantity of fish and possible industrial exposure)
- Radiation (x-rays, industrial accidents)
- Tobacco (smoking or chewing)
- Trimethadione (used for the control of petit mal seizures) and paramethadione (an anticonvulsant)

Fetal Alcohol Syndrome (FAS)

The consumption of alcohol (a known teratogen) in any amount during pregnancy has the potential to cause serious effects on the developing fetus. It is the most common cause of drug-induced teratogenesis. Fetal alcohol syndrome can be recognized by certain congenital abnormalities. The diagnosis is usually made after birth. The birth weight is low, and shortly after birth the baby may exhibit signs of withdrawal with respiratory depression requiring immediate resuscitation. Physical characteristics include a small head, small eye openings, receded upper jaw, and a wide, flat nose bridge. The most serious consequences of maternal alcohol use are mental retardation, cardiovascular defects, and death.

Drug-Induced Teratogenesis

Crack cocaine is a stimulant that has potent vasoconstrictive effects on the placenta, profoundly limiting circulation to the fetus and resulting in periods of **hypoxia** during development. It also causes acute hypertension, a red flag in your assessment of the pregnant patient. Preterm delivery is the highest complication associated with crack cocaine use. Other complications include slowed fetal growth, **abruptio placenta**, stillbirth, CNS deformities, genitourinary deformities, skeletal defects, behavioral disturbances, and learning defects.

Smoking During Pregnancy

Carbon monoxide causes hypoxia, and nicotine causes **uteroplacental vasoconstriction**. This produces problems in bringing the pregnancy to term. In other words, smoking reduces the supply of oxygenated blood to the developing fetus. Smokers have a higher incidence of spontaneous abortions, stillbirths, abruptio placenta, **placenta previa**, premature births, and premature rupture of membranes. Babies of smoking mothers have a higher incidence of lower birth weights, congenital heart defects, and orofacial clefts. Maternal smoking is also associated with sudden infant death syndrome (SIDS), deficits in physical growth, and abnormal intellectual development and behavior. Studies have shown a 25% to 50% higher rate of fetal and infant deaths among women who smoke during pregnancy compared with those who do not.

[U.S. Food and Drug Administration, FDA Consumer Magazine, May–June 2001]

Abnormal Deliveries

During childbirth, the fetus or umbilical cord can exhibit abnormal presentation (**Table 11-4**▾). There are no pharmacologic remedies for these abnormalities that are carried in the paramedic's drug box.

Table 11-4 Abnormal Presentations

Abnormality	Description
Breech presentation	Anything other than a cephalic presentation. Most often buttocks or lower extremities.
Limb	Single arm or foot presentation
Nuchal cord	Umbilical cord wrapped around the infant's neck
Prolapsed cord	Umbilical cord presents before the baby
Multiple births	Two or more babies, often premature
Premature	Childbirth before 37 weeks of gestation (increased risk for complications in delivery and in infancy)
Shoulder dystocia	Condition during delivery in which the baby's head is out but the shoulder gets stuck against the mother's symphysis pubis. Often results in a fractured collar bone.
Face presentation (sunny side up)	Typically the baby's head is delivered with the face down toward the mother's perineum, but may present face up or "sunny side up."

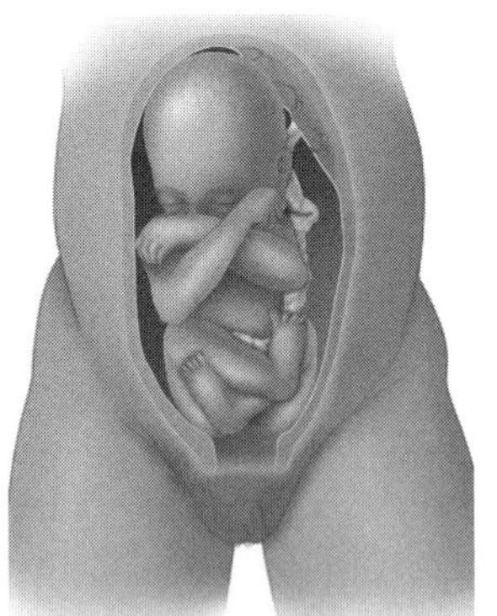

Figure 11-3 In a breech presentation, the buttocks are usually delivered first.

Breech Presentation

In a breech presentation, the presenting part of the infant is anything other than the head, most commonly the legs or the buttocks (**Figure 11-3**).

A patient with a breech presentation cannot deliver in the field. All efforts to slow the labor process should be employed, such as raising the mother's hips and having her pant during a contraction to diminish the strength of the contraction. In this case, put her on your stretcher and head for the ED, making sure they are forewarned you will be arriving with this complication.

Of course if the mother is crowning, and you are seeing the buttocks instead of a head, it is likely birth is imminent. If you can deliver on your stretcher, rather than in some back bedroom upstairs with your equipment spread out all over, it will make it a lot easier to pick up and head out for the ED. The steps for a breech delivery are identified in **Table 11-5**. If you suspect that the mother or fetus is in distress, the only drug for consideration would be supplemental oxygen.

Prolapsed Umbilical Cord

When the patient is examined for crowning, if you note that the umbilical cord is outside of her birth canal (vaginal opening), this can be a serious complication. The procedure for handling the prolapsed cord is described in **Table 11-6**.

Complications

A number of complications can occur that are not considered to be abnormal deliveries (**Table 11-7**).

Table 11-5 Breech Delivery Procedure

1	Support the buttocks or extremities until the back appears.
2	Grasp the infant's iliac wings and apply gentle downward traction. Do not pull on the legs or back as this may cause spinal dislocation or adrenal hemorrhage.
3	Gently swing the infant's body in the direction of least resistance. By swinging anteriorly and posteriorly, both shoulders should deliver posteriorly.
4	Splint the humerus bones with your two fingers and apply gentle traction with your fingers.
5	Gentle, downward compression of the uterus will assist in the head's delivery. Swing the legs upward until the body is in a vertical position. This will permit the delivery of the head.

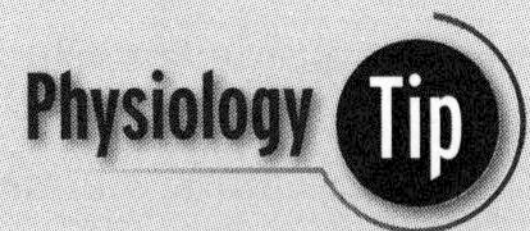

Types of Breech Births

Frank Breech: Buttocks will present first.

Footling Breech: One or both feet will present outside of the birth canal.

Shoulder Breech: The shoulder will present first.

Table 11-6 Prolapsed Cord Procedure

1	Place the mother in a face-up position on your stretcher, with her hips elevated by blankets.
2	Place a gloved hand in the vagina and attempt to hold the infant's head away from the cord.
3	Keep the cord moist, using a sterile dressing and sterile water.
4	Transport as soon as possible and notify the ED of the situation.

If for any reason the fetus was distressed in utero, it may have had its first bowel movement. The fetal bowel contents are mostly a bile-like substance that looks like brownish-green, tarry matter. This is called meconium, and can be problematic if prior to or during the delivery the newborn aspirates the substance. If the infant has evidence of thick meconium staining of the amniotic fluid, the paramedic should be sure to carefully suction the mouth and then the nose with the bulb syringe. If the newborn is completely covered in meconium and you suspect aspiration has occurred in a depressed-appearing newborn, deep suctioning with an appropriate sized ET tube is appropriate to consider.

Another minor complication that can occur with a normal delivery is the amniotic sac not rupturing. In this case, as the newborn's head emerges, you will see that the newborn's head is still in the sac. Simply grasp a piece of the thin sac and strip it away from the infant. If necessary, carefully puncture the sac with your gloved finger or a sterile scalpel or scissor. Be very careful not to cut the infant!

Prenatal Care

Every pregnancy has the potential to develop complications that can place the mother, fetus, or newborn at risk for morbidity or mortality before or after delivery. Prenatal care is essential to discover present or potential risk factors. Regular evaluations, monitoring, screenings, knowledge, and advice are provided during this important time. As a result of prenatal care, and when a pregnancy is classified as high risk, this helps to ensure that the patient receives extra

Table 11-7 Complications of Labor and Delivery

Complication	Description/Management
Meconium staining	The fetus has an intrauterine bowel movement, usually due to some stress, causing a thick, brownish-green staining of the amniotic fluid. The major complication is the potential for aspiration of the substance into the infant's lungs upon birth. Suction will be needed.
Amniotic sac not rupturing	The infant is born with the sac intact. The paramedic will need to carefully break the sac without injuring the newborn.
Postpartum hemorrhage	Heavy bleeding after childbirth due to incomplete removal of the placenta/retained products of conception, or failure of the uterus to contract. Oxygen and fluid administration will be necessary.
Uterine rupture	Tearing of the uterus due to trauma, extended labor, or a weakened section of the uterus from previous scarring. The patient will need rapid transport, oxygen administration, and fluid resuscitation.
Uterine inversion	In this condition, the uterus prolapses and turns inside out after delivery. Because the highly vascular uterine endometrial surface is exposed and uncompressed, severe blood loss and shock result. The patient will need rapid transport, oxygen administration, and fluid resuscitation.
Pulmonary embolism	Results from a blood clot in the lower extremity, limiting pelvic circulation. This can occur during third trimester pregnancy and into the early postpartum phase. Oxygenation and transport are a must with this patient.
Amniotic fluid embolism	Has a high mortality rate but fortunately this is rare. A clot formed of amniotic fluid crosses into maternal circulation during labor, delivery, or the postpartum phase. Oxygenation and transport are a must with this patient.

attention. The most common causes of maternal and infant mortality are:

Maternal mortality

- Motor vehicle collisions
- Embolism
- Complications with anesthesia
- Bleeding
- Infection
- Hypertension

Infant mortality (peri-natal)

- Prematurity
- Congenital problems
- Abruptio placenta
- Multiple pregnancies
- Placenta previa
- **Preeclampsia** and **eclampsia**
- Abnormal presentation

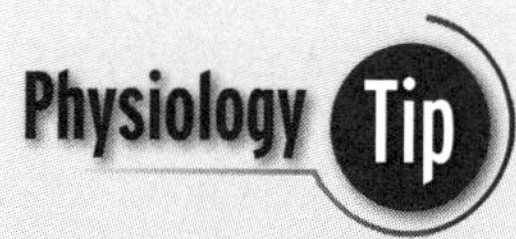

Meconium Staining: What Is Meconium?

The first stool the fetus or infant has is **meconium**. This may occur in utero or postpartum. Meconium is a brownish-green, tarry substance, has little to no odor, and is extremely thick and sticky. Meconium consists of digested cells from the lining of the gastrointestinal (GI) tract, as well as digestion of amniotic fluid and mucus. Fetal meconium occurs in utero due to fetal distress. Any event that causes stress to the mother can cause stress to the infant, but typically it is an event that causes fetal hypoxia. You should be observant for meconium in the amniotic fluid when the bag of waters ruptures and during delivery of the child. Meconium should be rapidly wiped from the mouth and face, and suctioning of the nares and oral pharynx with a bulb syringe, Dee-Lee mucus trap, or meconium aspirator (during intubation) should be performed.

Pregnancy and Hypertension

High blood pressure (hypertension) and pregnancy is a potentially fatal combination. In the prehospital setting, any pregnant patient with a new onset of hypertension (either systolic pressure of 140 mm Hg or above, or a diastolic pressure of 90 mm Hg or above, or an increase of ≥ 30 mm Hg systolic or an increase of ≥ 15 mm Hg diastolic from baseline, even if it does not exceed 140/90 mm Hg) must be evaluated for possible toxemia (which could lead to eclampsia).

The cause of preeclampsia and eclampsia is poorly understood and develops between the 20th week of gestation and 1 week postpartum. Signs and symptoms of preeclampsia include hypertension as described above, edema, headache, vision problems, oliguria (decreased urination), pulmonary edema, **proteinuria** (necessary for the diagnosis), and epigastric pain. A leading complication is abruptio placenta. The preeclamptic mother can develop seizures during her pregnancy; a small percentage may go on to develop eclampsia. Eclampsia is the most serious consequence of hypertension during pregnancy and is usually fatal if left untreated. Signs and symptoms progress from preeclampsia to syncope, seizures, and coma.

When the patient has a history of hypertension prior to becoming pregnant, the condition requires close monitoring. Additional complications that may arise from hypertension during pregnancy include stroke, renal failure, and acute pulmonary edema.

Case Study II Eclampsia

Part 1

Your unit is dispatched to an inner-city, low-income basement apartment for a call for a patient having a seizure. As you are en route, the dispatcher calls back with additional information. It seems the patient is a 17-year-old female who is 8 months pregnant. Your supervisor and the police are also responding since there have been some recent drug activities at the location of the call. When you arrive, the police are already there and give you the signal to enter. The apartment smells of cigarettes and beer. There are full ashtrays and empty beer cans around the living space. The patient is lying on the couch and appears to be unconscious. Two people are in the apartment and they claim to be friends of the patient. They tell you that she has been feeling sick for a couple of days with a headache and an upset stomach and explain that the patient had a sudden loss of consciousness with seizure activity. The initial assessment reveals that the patient's airway is open, with gurgling (see **Table 1**). She is pale, warm, and moist; lung sounds are present with a shallow effort, and the distal pulse is tachycardic and regular. Your partner begins suctioning while you reach for the oxygen tank. The patient is obese and you confirm with her friends that the patient is pregnant. You wonder if the patient has an underlying history of seizures. Perhaps she could have been noncompliant with her medications, due to the pregnancy. All of these questions come to mind. You know that seizure activity during late-term pregnancy is a potentially serious problem indicating eclampsia.

Table 1 Initial Assessment

Initial Assessment	Recording Time: 2 Minutes
General Impression/ Appearance	Looks wiped out, poor general condition, very pale
Mental Status	Moaning (postictal)
Airway	Open with secretions
Breathing	Shallow and rapid
Circulation	Radial pulse at 140 beats/min
Priority/Plan	High due to combination of altered mental status, seizure, and pregnancy

This patient has no apparent new trauma, although there seems to be a number of bruises in different stages of healing. You consider the fact that she could have a severe head injury, given the evidence of bruising on her body. A head injury is not apparent on a physical examination, yet head injuries can produce all of the signs and symptoms that she has.

She is a medical patient who is initially postictal but is slowly beginning to respond. She will need a focused history and physical examination for a responsive medical patient. You will also need to elaborate on the chief complaint of seizures and third trimester pregnancy using the OPQRST acronym.

Question 1: What is the significance of the patient's surroundings?

Question 2: What do you consider to be possible causes of the seizure activity in this patient?

Part 2

As you question the friends, you learn that the patient's name is Gini and she is pregnant, possibly 8 months. The seizure activity lasted 3 to 4 minutes and you confirm that she has no seizure history. She went to Planned Parenthood to get a pregnancy test 6 or 7 months ago and has had no prenatal care since. She is a heavy smoker, drinks alcohol, and does crack cocaine when she can get it. Her friends do not know if she has had any alcohol or drugs today. Your partner obtains vital signs and you begin a focused neurologic examination as part of the focused history and physical examination (see **Table 2**). Gini moans when you stimulate a pain response; her pupils constrict normally when you lift the lids. She is not answering any questions and her extremities are limp. She has urinated. In addition to the bruises noted earlier, the physical examination reveals significant edema of the face, fingers, hands, arms, legs, ankles, and feet.

Table 2 Focused History and Physical Examination

Baseline Vital Signs	Recording Time: 5 Minutes
Skin CTC (color, temperature, condition)	Pale, cool, and clammy
Pulse	140 beats/min and regular
Blood Pressure	156/98 mm Hg
Respirations	24 breaths/min and shallow

Question 3: How do drugs affect the fetus?

Question 4: How does smoking affect the fetus?

Case Study II Continued

Part 3

As part of the SAMPLE history, Gini's friends were also able to tell you that this is her third pregnancy but the last two were abortions (see **Table 3**). Just as they tell you this, Gini begins seizing again. Your partner assesses the airway while you obtain a fingerstick for a blood glucose reading. Your supervisor has brought the stretcher and obtains the report from you. He will talk to medical control while you get Gini on the stretcher. The blood glucose reading is 190 mg/dL and is not the cause of the seizures. A second seizure is very concerning, especially without a period of consciousness in between. You want to get her to the ambulance. This is presenting like a case of eclampsia, a life-threatening condition for the mother and fetus. On the way out, one of the officers hands you two metered-dose inhalers with Gini's name on them.

Table 3 SAMPLE History

SAMPLE History	Comments
Signs/symptoms	Sick for 2 days with headache and upset stomach; first-time seizure activity, significant peripheral edema and hypertension
Allergies	Unknown
Medications	Bronchodilators
Pertinent past medical history	Asthma, evidence of prior trauma, two abortions, no prenatal care, smoker, alcohol and drug use
Last oral intake	Unknown
Events leading up to the incident	High-risk pregnancy with multiple risk factors

Treatment Plan

1. The ABCs are the priority, as with any patient. In treating preeclampsia or eclampsia, the goal is to sustain the mother's life and health and the fetus will respond accordingly.
2. Because the cause of the seizure is unknown, the focus is to end the seizures and obtain some control over the blood pressure. In this specific case, the drug of choice is most likely going to be magnesium sulfate. You know that magnesium sulfate relaxes smooth muscle contractions without producing harmful CNS depression in the mother or fetus. It also helps to control hypertension. You consider other antiseizure options such as IV benzodiazepines.
3. This is an extremely high-risk situation that demands emergency attention on scene, en route, and upon arrival at the hospital. Because hypertension is a factor, you will consult with medical control, who may consider metoprolol tartrate [Lopressor] 5 mg slow IV given over 2 minutes at 2-minute intervals (until heart rate < 60 beats/min or blood pressure is adequately controlled).

Medication options for seizing or status epilepticus during pregnancy include:

- Magnesium sulfate: 1 to 4 g IV/IO over 3 minutes, followed by a 2 g/h IV drip (maximum of 30–40 g/day) (see **Table 4**).
- Diazepam [Valium]: 5 to 10 mg IV every 10 to 15 minutes as necessary (see **Table 5**).
- Midazolam [Versed]: 2.0 to 2.5 mg slow IV over 2 to 3 minutes (see **Table 6**).
- Because hypertension is a factor, you will consult with medical control, who may consider metoprolol tartrate [Lopressor] (see **Table 7**).

Question 5: How does alcohol affect the fetus?

Question 6: What is another possible cause for the seizure activity, hypertension, recent headache, and upset stomach?

Table 4 Magnesium Sulfate

Do you know?	Comments
Right drug? Generic name: [**Magnesium sulfate**]	This drug is an electrolyte that reduces the striated muscle contractions and blocks peripheral neuromuscular transmission by reducing acetylcholine release at the myoneural junction. It manages seizures in pregnancy (eclampsia) and causes uterine relaxation.
Right patient?	Antepartum (prior to delivery) and 1 week postpartum (after delivery) seizures that do not stop after administering the first-line antiseizure medications (ie, diazepam [Valium] or phenobarbital [Luminal]). *continues*

Case Study II Continued

Table 4 Magnesium Sulfate (*Continued*)

Do you know?	Comments
Right dose?	Adult dose for seizure associated with pregnancy is 1 to 4 grams over 3 minutes (maximum daily dose of 30–40 g/day).
Right route?	IV or IO.
Right time?	Confirmed or suspected eclampsia; or after other antiseizure medications have proven ineffective in the seizing pregnant patient.
Right documentation?	Document the administration of the medication as well as the ongoing assessent findings, including lung sounds, on the patient care report.
Expected action	Given for seizures of eclampsia, torsades de pointes, hypomagnesemia,or pulseless ventricular fibrillation or ventricular tachycardia. Can also be used for bronchodilation after beta agonists and anticholinergics have been used.
Side effects	May cause CNS depression, facial flushing, diaphoresis, depressed reflexes, circulatory collapse, or hypotension.
Contraindications	Heart blocks and myocardial damage.
Precautions	Use with caution in patients with renal failure. Not recommended to be given within 2 hours of emergency childbirth. IV calcium chloride or calcium gluconate should be available as an antagonist if needed.
Pharmacokinetics	Onset: immediate IV/IO, IM 3–4 hours; duration: 30 minutes IV/IO, 3–4 hours IM; excreted in urine.

Table 5 Diazepam

Do you know?	Comments
Right drug? Generic name: [**Diazepam**] Trade name: [Diastat, Valium]	This drug is a benzodiazepine. It is used to treat anxiety and convulsive disorders.
Right patient?	Status epilepticus.
Right dose?	5 to 10 mg IV every 10 to 15 minutes as needed.
Right route?	IV.
Right time?	Seizing patient after airway and ventilation are managed and contraindications have been considered.
Right documentation?	Always document how and when the drug was administered as well as the patient's response to the medication on your patient care report.
Expected action	Relief of seizure activity.
Side effects	Potentiates antihypertensive effects of thiazides and other diuretics.
Contraindications	Known sensitivity, narrow-angle glaucoma.
Precautions	May worsen seizure activity.
Pharmacokinetics	Onset: rapid IV, rapid PR, 15–30 minutes IM; peak effect: 15 minutes IV, 30–90 minutes IM; metabolized in the liver and excreted in urine.

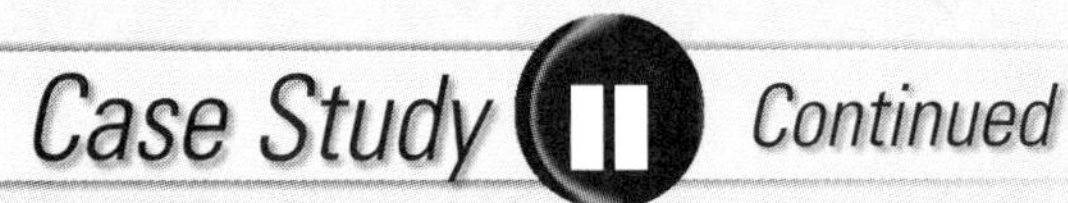

Table 6 Midazolam

Do you know?	Comments
Right drug? Generic name: [**Midazolam**] Trade name: [Versed]	This drug is a short-acting benzodiazepine CNS depressant. Anxiolytic and sedative properties similar to other benzodiazepines, memory impairment.
Right patient?	Indicated in a patient in need of sedation, anxiolytic prior to ET or nasotracheal intubation; as an adjunct for procedural sedation.
Right dose?	Adult dose is 2.0 to 2.5 mg slow IV over 2 to 3 minutes. May be repeated to a total maximum of 0.1 mg/kg.
Right route?	IV slow over 2 to 3 minutes.
Right time?	Can be given for chemical restraint in concert with haloperidol [Haldol]. (Not an issue in this case.)
Right documentation?	Always document how and when the drug was administered as well as the patient's response to the medication on your patient care report.
Expected action	Sedation and anxiolytic reaction similar to other benzodiazepines.
Side effects	Hiccough, cough, oversedation, nausea, vomiting, injection site pain, headache, blurred vision, hypotension, respiratory depression, and arrest.
Contraindications	Glaucoma, shock, coma, alcohol intoxication, overdose, depressed vital signs, concomitant use with other CNS depressants, barbiturates, alcohol, narcotics.
Precautions	Should not be used in patients who have taken a CNS depressant.
Pharmacokinetics	Onset: 1–3 minutes IV and dose-dependent; peak effect: variable 15 minutes; duration: 2–6 hours dose-dependent; metabolized in the liver and excreted in urine.

Table 7 Metoprolol Tartrate

Do you know?	Comments
Right drug? Generic name: [**Metoprolol Tartrate**] Trade name: [Lopressor]	This is a beta-adrenergic receptor blocking agent.
Right patient?	This drug is used to treat hypertension, angina, and acute myocardial infarction (MI) when the patient is stable.
Right dose?	Typically three IV injections of 5 mg each given over 2 minutes at 2-minute intervals.
Right route?	IV bolus.
Right time?	After cardiothoracic assessment and contraindications have been considered.
Right documentation?	Always document how and when the drug was administered as well as the patient's response to the medication on your patient care report.
Expected action	Decreases cardiac work load; slows heart rate and lowers blood pressure.
Side effects	For suspected MI, side effects include: CNS symptoms (tiredness, vertigo, sleep disturbances, hallucinations, headache, dizziness, visual disturbances, and confusion), respiratory symptoms (dyspnea), GI symptoms (nausea and abdominal pain), and dermatologic symptoms (rash and worsened psoriasis).
Contraindications	Heart rates less than 45 beats/min, second- and third-degree heart block, and systolic blood pressure of less than 100 mm Hg. Moderate to severe heart failure.
Precautions	Use with caution in patients with hepatic dysfunction, advanced chronic obstructive pulmonary disease (COPD), or reactive airway disease.
Pharmacokinetics	Onset: 1–5 minutes; peak effect: 90 minutes; metabolized in the liver and excreted in urine.

Case Study II Continued

Part 4

In the ambulance, the three of you work fast to manage the airway, attach the monitor, and start two IVs. Medical control has given an order for a magnesium sulfate bolus to be followed up with a drip. A nasal airway has been inserted and the patient is being ventilated with a bag-mask device. Suction is close at hand and seizure activity is persisting. Vital signs are reassessed after the first bolus, and the infusion is prepared and set in place (see **Table 8**). Transport time is 10 to 15 minutes so there will be time to reassess the patient once the infusion is up and running.

Question 7: Why is magnesium sulfate the drug of choice for eclampsia?

Question 8: What complications is this fetus at risk for during and after birth?

Table 8 Reassessment and Ongoing Assessment of the Patient

Serial Vital Signs and Relevant Data	Recording Time: 15 Minutes
Skin CTC	Warm, pale, and moist
Pulse	136 beats/min, regular
Blood Pressure	160/110 mm Hg
Respirations	Shallow, but assisted by bag-mask device
Mental status/LOC	Unresponsive
ECG	Sinus tachycardia
SpO_2	96%
Lung sounds	Clear bilaterally
Other (ie blood glucose, core body temperature)	190 mg/dL

Part 5

Upon arrival at the ED, the seizure activity has stopped, but Gini remains unresponsive. En route, the decision to intubate was made. Her SpO_2 is 100%, $EtCO_2$ is 42 mm Hg, and she remains tachycardic and hypertensive. There has been no movement from the fetus during the entire transport. There were several factors recognized for Gini having a high-risk pregnancy—prior miscarriages (abortions), smoking, alcohol and substance abuse, possible traumatic injury, and no prenatal care. Her signs and symptoms (seizures, hypertension, edema, headache, and GI distress) are consistent with those of eclampsia. Hypertension during pregnancy is dangerous for the mother and the fetus. New-onset hypertension during pregnancy must be evaluated for a specific cause and to rule out preeclampsia. After managing the ABCs, the goal is to sustain the mother's life and health as the principal means for ensuring a positive fetal outcome. Magnesium sulfate is the drug of choice for the treatment of eclampsia and was used in Gini's case. If the fetus survives, there is a high risk of complications, including low birth weight, withdrawal symptoms, respiratory depression, fetal alcohol syndrome, mental retardation, CNS deformities, genitourinary deformities, skeletal defects, behavioral disturbances, and learning deficiencies.

Predisposition to Eclampsia or Preeclampsia

Women who have a demonstrated prenatal history of fluid retention, excessive weight gain, and elevated blood pressure have an increased risk of hypertension in their pregnancies. Management of the mother is the highest priority. Providing oxygen and controlling seizure activity should take place simultaneously. By managing the mother, you reduce the stress that the fetus is having. Magnesium sulfate or a benzodiazepine should be used to manage the eclamptic patient. Magnesium sulfate is typically used as a first-line management for seizures.

Trauma in Pregnancy

The leading cause of maternal mortality due to trauma is motor vehicle crashes. Other major causes include falls and assaults. Trauma to the abdomen may produce premature labor, spontaneous abortion, abruptio placenta, uterine rupture, and fetal death. Caring for the pregnant trauma patient requires extra attention. Placing the patient on a backboard puts the patient at risk for supine hypotension syndrome (weight of the fetus compresses the inferior vena cava, preventing blood return to the heart and causing hypotension due to loss of effective preload). Tilting the board 15° to the left shifts the weight of the fetus off the vena cava and alleviates this complication (**Figure 11-4▼**).

Additionally, the airway may become compromised because the pregnant patient is prone to gastroesophageal reflux, with the attendant risk of emesis and aspiration. Careful monitoring of the airway and breathing with suction close at hand can reduce this risk.

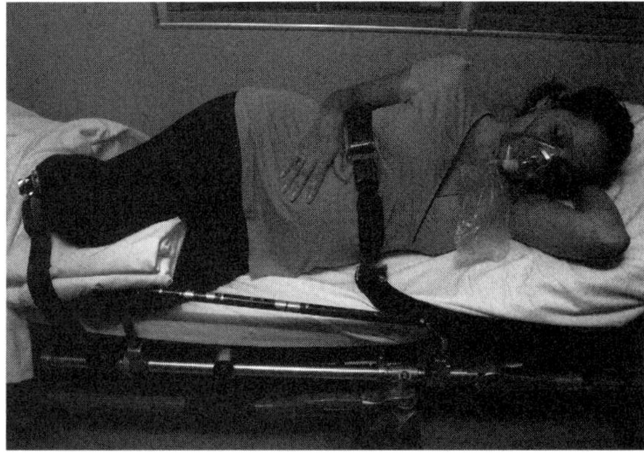

Figure 11-4 Transport a pregnant patient on her left side to allow for sufficient circulation through the vena cava.

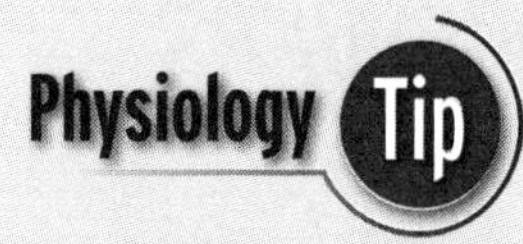

Preeclampsia: A hypertensive disorder that occurs in approximately 8% of all pregnancies. This is characterized by hypertension, first time pregnancies, pregnancies in women older than 40 years of age, renal disease, and diabetes. Manifesting after the 20th week of gestation, symptoms include headache, unusual weight gain, agitation, swelling in the hands and feet, onset of hypertension, and protein in the urine. You cannot check for protein in the urine, so instead ask the patient if her urine has a heavier or more concentrated smell than normal, almost like the first urine of the day. Urine that has elevated protein tends to be darker in color and have a stronger odor. Blood pressure in the preeclamptic patient may be 160 to 180 mm Hg systolic and >105 mm Hg diastolic. These patients are at high risk for miscarriages, fetal retardation, and seizures.

Eclampsia: Occurs when the preeclamptic patient has a seizure.

Both conditions have been known to occur as long as 6 months postpartum, especially if the mother is nursing.

Remember that lack of adequate prenatal care and/or use of alcohol, drugs, and tobacco products markedly increase the risk for pregnancy- and delivery-related complications. During the initial interview, be sure to ask "When was your last prenatal visit?" and "Have there been any issues so far with this pregnancy that we should know about?" The answers to both these questions usually furnish the rescuer with the insight needed to take an extra few seconds to mentally and physically prepare for a potentially catastrophic delivery or associated peripartum event.

Case Study ANSWERS

Case Study I Normal Childbirth

Question 1: What is the significance of learning that Betsy has been going for prenatal care?

Answer 1: It means that both she and the fetus have been getting regular evaluations and advice. The obstetrics team has been monitoring weight gain, vital signs, and screening labs, and helping to prepare her for labor and the delivery. They have also advised her to stop engaging in any activities that may be harmful to the developing child.

Question 2: If this was Betsy's first pregnancy, how long would labor be expected to take?

Answer 2: It is not uncommon for the average first stage of labor, dilation, and effacement of the cervix to take between 8 and 12 hours. For the first pregnancy, it is expected the woman will be on the higher end of this average (ie, 12 to 24 hours).

Question 3: What is the significance of the urge to move her bowels?

Answer 3: It means that the fetus has moved down into the birth canal, with the head pushing back on the rectum, and is therefore likely to be delivered very soon. When the pains are at 1- to 2-minute intervals lasting 45 to 60 seconds, birth is considered imminent.

Question 4: How do you count the labor pains?

Answer 4: Count the time from the start of the strong contraction to the end of the contraction or cramps. Then count the interval length between the end of one labor pain and the start of the next labor pain.

Question 5: Why is it so important to suction the infant, even before delivery is complete?

Answer 5: The delivery may involve bleeding and certainly plenty of amniotic fluid and secretions. The infant should be suctioned right away and resuctioned at a later point to avoid aspiration of the secretions as it takes its first breaths.

Question 6: Why are the umbilical cord clamps placed so far from the infant?

Answer 6: As EMT-Basics, we were all taught to place the first clamp about 8″ to 9″ from the infant and 6″ to 7″ away from the mother. The cord is cut between the two clamps. The reason why they are so far from the infant is to allow plenty of room to place a third clamp in the event that after the cord is clamped, the cord continues to bleed. This will all be cleaned up in the hospital over the next day and ultimately the stub of the cord will fall off.

Question 7: If Betsy's placenta was not delivered within a few minutes, is that a problem?

Answer 7: Not really. Some women take longer to deliver the placenta. Notify the ED en route if it takes more than 20 minutes or the patient continues to bleed postpartum.

Question 8: If there is excessive bleeding as Betsy's placenta is being delivered, what treatment strategies are available to you in the field?

Answer 8: If the patient has excessive postpartum bleeding, there are not a lot of treatment options. First treat Betsy for shock, raising her legs, keeping her warm, and administering supplemental oxygen (switch that nasal cannula to a nonrebreathing mask). Run the IV wide open and check serial vital signs. Expeditiously move to the hospital and notify the ED of the patient's change in condition so they can be prepared for a patient who could be bleeding out. Ask the mother to attempt to nurse her child. This helps stimulate release of the body's own oxytocin. Remember to vigorously apply external uterine massage, as if you were kneading bread dough or were dealing with a hunk of clay. Consult with medical control about administering IV oxytocin [Pitocin] to increase the strength of the uterine contractions, which could help control excessive bleeding.

Case Study II Eclampsia

Question 1: What is the significance of the patient's surroundings?

Answer 1: Cigarettes, alcohol, and the recent history of drug activity in the area are all teratogens. If this activity is routine, the patient is a high-risk pregnancy.

Question 2: What do you consider to be possible causes of the seizure activity in this patient?

Answer 2: She may have an underlying history of seizures and has been noncompliant with her medications because of a variety of factors, including the pregnancy. She may also have suffered a severe head injury given the evidence of bruising on her body. First and foremost, you must be concerned with the possibility of eclampsia.

Case Study ANSWERS

Question 3: How do drugs affect the fetus?

Answer 3: Drugs taken by the mother during pregnancy can cross the placental barrier and adversely affect the development of the fetus by producing developmental deformities, physical dependency, and/or toxic or lethal effects.

Question 4: How does smoking affect the fetus?

Answer 4: Carbon monoxide avidly binds to fetal hemoglobin and causes both hypoxic and toxic effects, while nicotine causes uteroplacental vasoconstriction that produces problems in bringing the pregnancy to term. Maternal smoking adversely affects the fetus and has been demonstrated to cause lower birth weights, congenital heart defects, and orofacial clefts. Maternal smoking is also associated with SIDS, deficits in physical growth, and problems with intellectual development and behavior.

Question 5: How does alcohol affect the fetus?

Answer 5: The consumption of alcohol in any amount during pregnancy has the potential to affect the developing fetus. The most serious consequences of maternal alcohol use are mental retardation, cardiovascular defects, and death.

Question 6: What is another possible cause for the seizure activity, hypertension, recent headache, and upset stomach?

Answer 6: Trauma. Gini has multiple bruises at various stages of healing. She could have a head injury that is not apparent on the physical examination. Head injuries can produce all the signs and symptoms that Gini has.

Question 7: Why is magnesium sulfate the drug of choice for eclampsia?

Answer 7: Magnesium sulfate relaxes smooth muscle contractions without producing harmful CNS depression in the mother or fetus. It also helps to control hypertension.

Question 8: What complications is this fetus at risk for during and after birth?

Answer 8: There were several factors recognized for Gini having a high-risk pregnancy—prior miscarriages (abortions), smoking, alcohol and substance abuse, possible traumatic injury, and no prenatal care. If the fetus survives, there is a high risk of complications, including low birth weight, withdrawal symptoms, respiratory depression, fetal alcohol syndrome, mental retardation, CNS deformities, genitourinary deformities, skeletal defects, behavioral disturbances, and learning deficiencies.

Medication Review

Diazepam (Valium)

Indications Acute anxiety states, acute alcohol withdrawal (delirium tremens), muscle relaxant, seizure activity, agitation. Analgesia for medical procedures (fracture reduction, cardioversion).

Contraindications Hypersensitivity, glaucoma, coma, shock, substance abuse, head injury.

Dosage and administration Seizure activity: Adult: 5–10 mg IV every 10–15 minutes as necessary (5 mg over 5 min) (maximum dose, 30 mg). Seizure activity: Pediatric: 0.2–0.5 mg slowly every 2–5 minutes up to 5 mg (maximum dose, 10 mg/kg). Rectal diazepam: 0.5 mg/kg via rectal catheter and flush with 2–3 mL air after administration. Sedation for cardioversion: 5–15 mg IV over 5–10 minutes prior to cardioversion.

Magnesium Sulfate

Indications Seizures of eclampsia (toxemia of pregnancy), torsade de pointes, hypomagnesemia, Class IIa agent for V-fib /pulseless V-tach that is refractory to lidocaine.

Contraindications Heart blocks, myocardial damage.

Dosage and administration Adult: Seizure activity associated with pregnancy: 1–4 g IV/IO over 3 minutes; maximum dose of 30–40 g/day. Cardiac arrest due to hypomagnesemia or torsade de pointes: 1–2 g (2–4 mL of a 50% solution) diluted in 10 mL of D_5W IV/IO over 5–20 minutes. Torsade de pointes with a pulse or AMI with hypomagnesemia: Loading dose of 1–2 g mixed in 50–100 mL D_5W over 5–60 minutes IV. Follow with 0.5–1 g/hr IV (titrate to control torsade de pointes). Pediatric: IV/IO infusion: 25–50 mg/kg (maximum dose: 2 g) over 10–20 minutes; faster for torsade de pointes. For asthma: 25–50 mg/kg (maximum dose: 2 g) over 10–20 minutes.

Metoprolol Tartrate (Lopressor)

Indications Suspected ACS provided heart rate is > 80 and systolic BP is > 120 mm Hg.

Patients may be taking the tablet form for hypertension or angina. The usual tablet initial dose is 100 mg and effective dose is between 100 and 400 mg daily. Has also been used for ventricular arrhythmias and migraine headaches. Paramedic protocols are usually for the IV dose of the drug.

Contraindications In the context of a suspected MI, the drug is contraindicated in patients with a heart rate < 45 beats/min; second- and third-degree heart block; significant first-degree heart block (P-R interval ≥ 0.24 sec); systolic blood pressure < 100 mm Hg; or moderate-to-severe cardiac failure. Hypersensitivity to the drug, related derivatives, or other beta-blockers (cross sensitivity between beta-blockers can occur).

Dosage and administration Adult: 5 mg slow IV bolus, may be repeated every 2 minutes up to maximum of 15 mg, Pediatric: Not recommended.

Medication Review

Midazolam (Versed)

Indications Sedation, anxiolytic prior to endotracheal or nasotracheal intubation; administer for conscious sedation.

Contraindications Glaucoma, shock, coma, alcohol intoxication, overdose, depressed vital signs, concomitant use with other CNS depressants, barbiturates, alcohol, narcotics.

Dosage and administration Adult: 2.0–2.5 mg slow IV over 2–3 minutes; may be repeated to total maximum: 0.1 mg/kg. Pediatric: Not recommended.

Ondansetron Hydrochloride (Zofran)

Indications For the prevention or control of nausea or vomiting. Also used in the hospital setting for patients undergoing chemotherapy or surgical procedures.

Contraindications Known allergy to this medicine or other 5-HT3 receptor antagonists.

Dosage and administration Adult: 4 mg IV or IM (may repeat in 10 minutes). Pediatric: 0.1 mg/kg IV or IM.

Oxygen

Indications Confirmed or expected hypoxemia, ischemic chest pain, respiratory insufficiency, prophylactically during air transport, confirmed or suspected carbon monoxide poisoning, all other causes of decreased tissue oxygenation, decreased level of consciousness.

Contraindications Certain patients with COPD or emphysema who will not tolerate oxygen concentrations over 35%, hyperventilation. Oxygen should never be withheld from a patient who needs it, however. Be prepared to assist with ventilations in a patient with COPD who requires high oxygen concentrations as apnea may result.

Dosage and administration Adult: Cardiac arrest and carbon monoxide poisoning: 100%. Hypoxemia: 10–15 L/min via nonrebreathing mask. COPD: 1–6 L/min via nasal cannula or 28%–35% Venturi mask. Be prepared to provide ventilatory support if higher concentrations of oxygen needed. Pediatric: Same as for adult with exception of premature infant.

Oxytocin (Pitocin)

Indications Postpartum hemorrhage after infant and placental delivery.

Contraindications Presence of second fetus, unfavorable fetal position, hypersensitivity.

Dosage and administration IM administration: 3–10 units after delivery of placenta. IV administration: Mix 10–40 units in 1,000 mL of a nonhydrating diluent: Infused at 20–40 milliunits/min, titrated to severity of bleeding and uterine response.

Promethazine Hydrochloride (Phenergan)

Indications Nausea, vomiting, motion sickness; sedation for patients in labor; potentiation of analgesic effects of narcotics.

Contraindications Hypersensitivity, coma, CNS-depressed patients from alcohol, barbiturates, narcotics, Reye's syndrome.

How supplied 25 and 50 mg/mL in 1-mL ampules and Tubex syringes.

Dosage and administration Adult: 12.5–25 mg IV, deep IM, PO, rectally. Pediatric: (older than 2 years old) 0.25–0.5 mg/kg dose IM.

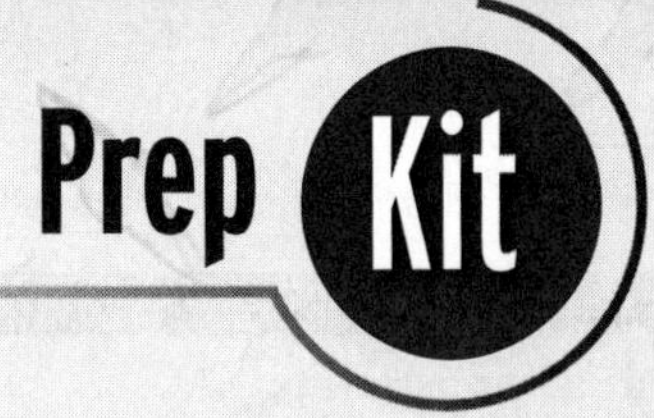

Chapter Summary

- There are three stages of labor.
- Assessment of the obstetrical patient focuses around determining the patient's significant history, if birth is imminent, and examining for crowning when necessary.
- Since 1975, the FDA required that drug labeling include a subsection on a drug's ability to cause birth defects and other effects on reproduction and pregnancy.
- Prochlorperazine [Compazine] is currently the most commonly prescribed medication in the United States for the treatment of nausea and vomiting in pregnancy.
- Drugs used during labor and delivery must be given carefully to avoid toxicity to the fetus.
- Drugs taken by the mother during pregnancy can adversely affect the development of the fetus by producing developmental deformities, physical dependency, and/or toxic or lethal effects.
- Alcohol is the most common cause of drug-induced teratogenesis.
- Smoking reduces the supply of oxygenated blood to the developing fetus.
- There are no pharmacologic remedies for abnormal presentations such as a breech presentation.
- Prenatal care is essential to discover current and potential risk factors.
- High blood pressure (hypertension) and pregnancy is a potentially fatal combination due to the risk of the patient developing eclampsia.
- Magnesium sulfate or a benzodiazepine should be used to manage the eclamptic patient.
- The leading cause of maternal mortality due to trauma is motor vehicle crashes.

Vital Vocabulary

Abruptio placenta A premature separation of the placenta from the wall of the uterus.

Eclampsia The most serious consequence of hypertension during pregnancy, which can be fatal to both mother and child if left untreated. Signs and symptoms are the same as preeclampsia; however, mental status changes including seizures, syncope, or coma occur with eclampsia.

First stage of labor The stage of labor that begins with the onset of regular labor pains, crampy abdominal pains during which the uterus contracts and the cervix effaces.

Gravida The number of all pregnancies a woman has had, including those not necessarily carried to term.

Hyperemesis gravidarum A condition of persistent nausea and vomiting during pregnancy.

Hypoxia A lack of oxygen to the body's cells or tissue.

Ketonuria An excess of ketone bodies in the urine.

Meconium An intrauterine bowel movement by a distressed fetus. The bowel's contents are mostly a bile-like matter that looks like a brownish-green tarry substance.

Parity The number of live births a woman has had.

Placenta previa A condition in which the placenta develops over and covers the cervix.

Preeclampsia Pregnancy-induced hypertension (PIH) in association with various signs and symptoms, including diffuse edema, headache, vision problems, oliguria (decreased urination), and abdominal pains. Often associated with abruptio placenta.

Proteinuria An excess of serum proteins in the urine, as in renal disease or after strenuous exercise.

Second stage of labor The stage of labor in which the baby's head enters the birth canal, during which contractions become more intense and more frequent.

Teratogen Any substance that harms normal cellular embryonic or fetal development.

Third stage of labor The stage of labor in which the placenta is expelled.

Uteroplacental vasoconstriction The constriction of the vessels that provide the circulation from the placenta to the uterus. This has been shown to be caused by drugs such as nicotine and may be dangerous to the fetus.

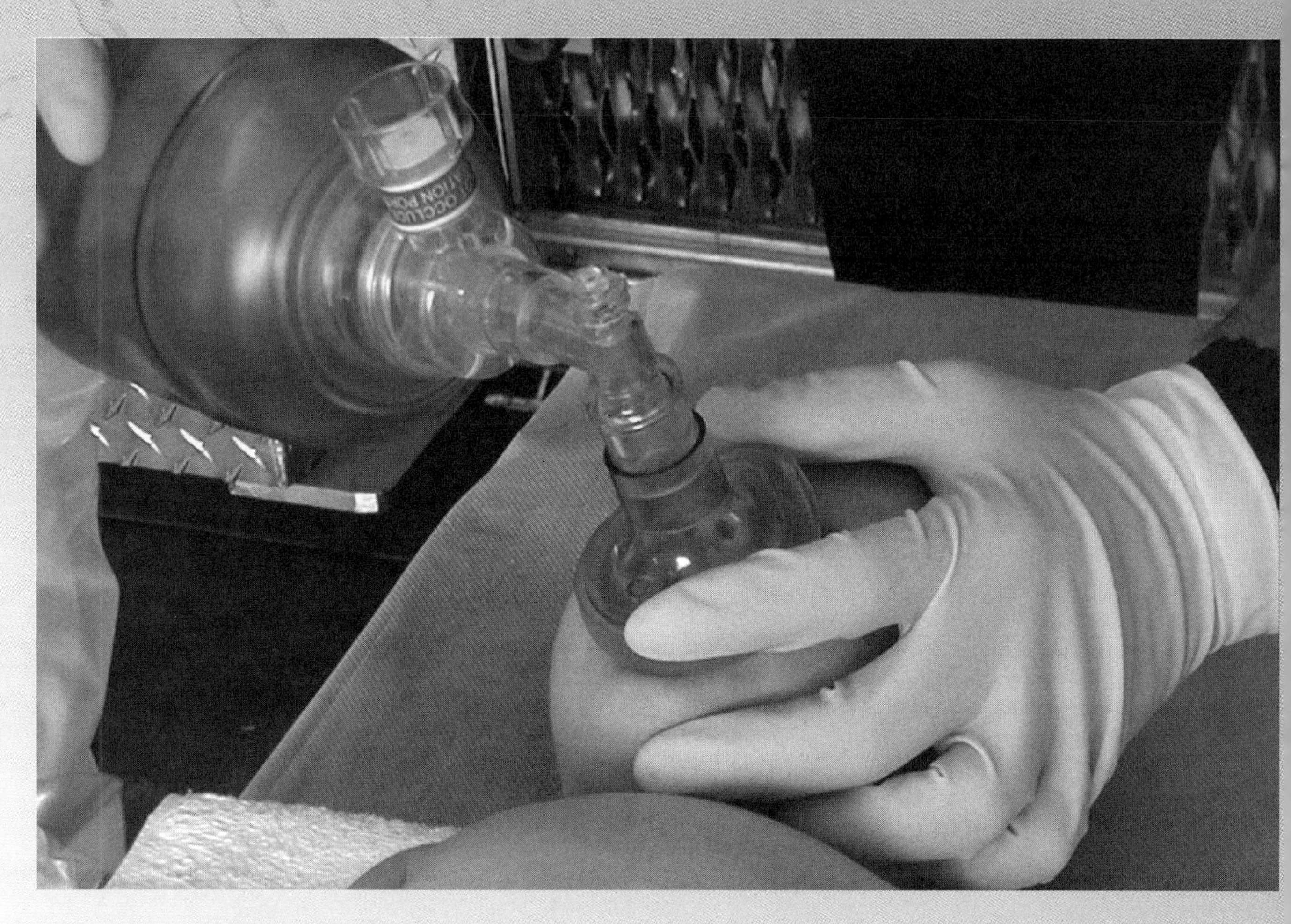

Neonatal Emergencies 12

Objectives

Cognitive

6-1.23 Discuss the routes of medication administration for a newborn. (pages 351–352)

6-1.31 Discuss the effects maternal narcotic usage has on the newborn. (pages 344–350, 352)

6-1.32 Determine the appropriate treatment for the newborn with narcotic depression. (pages 351–352)

6-1.47 Discuss the management/treatment plan for bradycardia in the neonate. (page 352)

6-1.67 Discuss the management/treatment plan for hypothermia in the neonate. (pages 344–350, 352)

6-1.71 Discuss the management/treatment plan for hypoglycemia in the neonate. (page 352)

6-1.87 Discuss the management/treatment plan for cardiac arrest in the neonate. (pages 344–352)

Affective

None

Psychomotor

None

Additional Objectives

1-1 Distinguish between a neonate and a newborn. (page 344)

1-2 Discuss the following medications used in the prehospital setting for neonatal patients: epinephrine [Adrenalin], naloxone hydrochloride [Narcan], 10% dextrose in water ($D_{10}W$), and sodium bicarbonate. (pages 347–349)

1-3 Discuss the use of the APGAR Score. (page 345)

Resuscitation Age Groups

Approach and management of the child is often specific to the age group that the child fits into. The **newborn** refers to an infant within the first few hours after birth. A **neonate** refers to an infant within the first month after birth. Infants, discussed in chapter 13, Pediatric Emergencies, are persons who are from 1 month to 1 year of age.

As you know, pediatric care is even more complex than determining the resuscitation "age groups." Significant anatomic, physiologic, and emotional differences exist between each age group. Pathophysiology also differs as the child grows. Age group descriptions commonly used include:

- Neonatal period—the first month of life
- Infancy—the rest of the first year
- Toddler—ages 1 to 3
- Preschool—ages 3 to 6
- School-age—ages 6 to 12
- Adolescence—ages 13 to 18

In the last 25 years, infant mortality has decreased by nearly half. This fact is credited to a decrease in Sudden Infant Death Syndrome and advances in the treatment of the smallest and sickest babies. As a result, more **premature** and low birth weight babies are surviving. Several factors have been associated with these babies, and as a result, can help to predict when a high-risk birth may occur. These factors include:

- Premature labor
- Multiple fetuses
- Gestational diabetes
- Hypertension syndromes
- Third trimester bleeding
- Maternal smoking
- Maternal use of alcohol and drugs
- Maternal hormonal imbalances
- Inadequate or no prenatal care
- Preexisting medical conditions
- Mother's age is younger than 16 years or older than 35

Assessment of the pediatric patient involves a "from-the-doorway" view of the patient. The Pediatric Assessment Triangle was developed to remind you of the essential elements of appearance, work of breathing, and circulation to the skin that should be observed as you are making your initial approach to the child (**Figure 12-1** ▼).

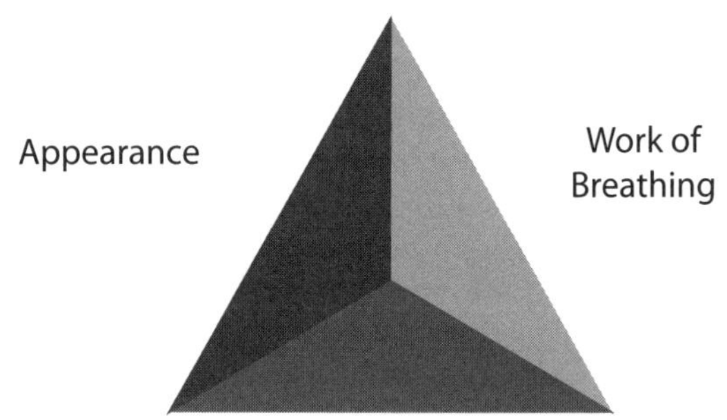

Figure 12-1 The Pediatric Assessment Triangle.

Case Study 1 Prematurity and Hypothermia

Part 1

You have been assigned to a call for the birth of a child at the county correctional facility. Getting into the facility takes time as you have to wait to be let in and then wait for an escort to take you to the infirmary. You receive no further dispatch information on the way to the facility. The guards escort you down to the infirmary in a hurry. One of the inmates has delivered prematurely while on the commode. The baby came out and fell into the toilet bowl. One of the infirmary staff had retrieved the baby and washed it off. When you get to the infirmary you can see a blue premature baby. As you prepare for the initial assessment, you recall that a premature neonate is born before 37 weeks gestation and weighs less than 5.5 lb (2,500 g) (see **Table 1**). The newborn child is lying in a towel, his eyes are closed, and the only movement is a slow chest rise with shallow breathing that is noticeably slow. The cord was clamped and cut so you check to see if there is any bleeding from the stump and there is not. The pulse can be felt at the stump and it has a rate of 50 beats/min.

You rapidly dry the baby and begin ventilations. After 30 seconds, the heart rate is still around 50 beats/min so you begin CPR. The mother's voice can be heard in another room, and she is upset and crying. Your partner calls for another ambulance to transport the mother to the hospital and then turns

Case Study 1 Continued

back to help you. He opens the pediatric bag and pulls out the pediatric resuscitation tape and other necessary items. It has been at least 10 minutes since the baby was born. No APGAR score has been obtained so you will do one now (see **Table 2**).

Table 1 Initial Assessment

Initial Assessment	Recording Time: 1 Minute
General Impression/ Appearance	Poor, premature delivery, infant in near arrest
Mental Status	Unresponsive
Airway	Open manually
Breathing	Shallow and slow
Circulation	Inadequate
Priority/Plan	High

Based on the information provided at this point, it seems that the resuscitation will be a medical resuscitation and there is no apparent trauma involved. This patient is a high priority and will need to be closely attended to as well as rapidly transported.

Question 1: How is a premature infant defined in terms of weight?

Question 2: How can resuscitation medication doses for infants and young children best be determined in the field setting?

Table 2 The Apgar Score

		Points	10 minute
A	**Appearance (skin color)**		
	Blue or pale extremities	0	0
	Pink trunk and blue extremities	1	
	Completely pink	2	
P	**Pulse**		
	Absent	0	
	< 100	1	1
	> 100	2	
G	**Grimace (irritability)**		
	No response	0	0
	Grimace or whimpers	1	
	Actively cries	2	
A	**Activity (muscle tone)**		
	Flaccid, limp	0	0
	Some flexion of extremities	1	
	Active extremity motion	2	
R	**Respiratory Effort**		
	Absent	0	
	Slow and irregular	1	
	Strong cry	2	1
	TOTAL SCORE		**2**

Part 2

The staff and guards in the infirmary are nervously excited as this type of incident has never happened in this facility. As you prepare for the focused history and physical examination, the nurse in charge tells you that the mother was at 22 weeks gestation with her fourth child (see **Table 3**). She had cramps for the last 10 hours with some vaginal bleeding before delivering in the toilet. She has been incarcerated for 2 weeks, is

Table 3 Focused History and Physical Examination

Baseline Vital Signs	Recording Time: 2 Minutes
Skin CTC (color, temperature, condition)	Blue and cool
Pulse	50 beats/min umbilical
Blood Pressure	Not obtained
Respirations	Assisted
APGAR	0-1-0-0-1 = 2

Case Study I Continued

a smoker, and is asthmatic. She has taken no medications that they know of since being incarcerated.

The baby is premature and will have poorly developed lungs and respiratory muscles. Resuscitation is going to be directed at airway management, ventilation, chest compressions, and providing warmth. He is at risk for developing several significant complications including hypoxia, hypothermia, hypoglycemia, and hypovolemia. Hypoxia causes the heart rate to drop and the adequacy of respirations is determined by the heart rate. This baby's heart rate indicates he is very hypoxic. You know that newborns must be kept warm because they lose heat rapidly as their body surface area is larger in relation to their weight, they have small amounts of subcutaneous fat to keep them warm, and their thermoregulatory systems are too immature to produce body heat, thus heat loss occurs faster.

This baby was dropped into toilet water and washed off with water so the chances of hypothermia are high. You know that once a newborn is cold, the resuscitation is less likely to be successful. Newborns have higher glucose needs than infants and older children. At birth, glucose reserves are in short supply. They can become hypoglycemic quickly following birth so the glucose should be assessed at some point during the resuscitation.

Question 3: Why should this infant be assessed for hypothermia?

Question 4: Why are premature babies, newborns, neonates, and infants poor at thermoregulation?

Part 3

The second ambulance is on the way and the nurse reports that the mother is stable. You consider the needs of the baby and make the decision to continue CPR and begin moving out to the ambulance. Once in the ambulance, the heater is turned up and the baby is reassessed. A SAMPLE history is obtained (see **Table 4**). The baby appears to weigh no more than 1 kilogram, and his core is not blue anymore but his extremities are. The pulse is still less than 60 beats/min so you continue CPR while your partner attaches electrodes, pulse oximetry, and opens the pediatric advanced airway kit. Plastic wrap is fashioned as a cap and placed on top of the baby's head to keep in the warmth. The second ambulance has arrived with a third person who will drive your ambulance. She jumps in and you give her the okay to begin transport.

Table 4 SAMPLE History

SAMPLE History	Comments
Signs/symptoms	Premature delivery at 22 weeks gestation
Allergies	Unknown
Medications	None
Pertinent past medical history	Mother is a smoker, unknown maternal use of drugs, asthma
Last oral intake	None
Events leading up to the incident	High risk pregnancy

Treatment Plan

The treatment plan is to follow the neonatal resuscitation algorithm for this premature infant.

1. Provide warmth.
2. Position, clear airway as necessary.
3. Dry, stimulate, reposition.
4. Evaluate respirations, heart rate, and color. The heart rate is < 60 beats/min.
5. Provide positive pressure ventilation and administer chest compressions. If the respiratory effort and pulse rate do not improve, you will consider causes (narcotic overdose, hypoxia, hypothermia, hypovolemia, acidosis etc.) and may continue with the following: Administer epinephrine [Adrenalin] and/or consider fluid infusion (see **Table 5**). An IV, IO, or umbilical vein is the preferred route for vascular access. Fluid volume expanders such as normal saline or lactated ringers are used in most EMS systems (see **Table 6**). Other fluid volume expanders such as plasma protein fraction [Plasmanate] or dextran are not universally used and will always be a function of local medical protocols and the patient's condition.

When a patient is in cardiac arrest and the rhythm is asystole or PEA, consider the "H's and T's" (hypovolemia, hypoxia, hydrogen ion, hypo-/hyperkalemia, hypoglycemia, hypothermia, toxins, tamponade, tension pneumothorax, thrombosis, trauma). For the neonatal patient, this will involve consulting with medical control about considering dextrose for the

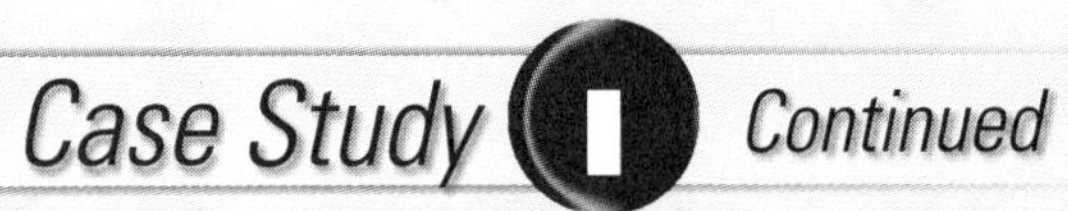

Table 5 Epinephrine

Do you know?	Comments
Right drug? Generic name: [**Epinephrine**] Trade name: [Adrenalin]	This drug is a sympathomimetic. It has the property (vasopressor) to cause contraction of smooth muscle of arteries and arterioles. In a cardiac arrest, a vasopressor is administered every 3–5 minutes. Epinephrine is the drug of choice in cardiac arrest as well as severe allergic reaction and asthma. It can also be effective in symptomatic bradycardia as an alternative to dopamine [Intropin], and severe hypotension that is secondary to bradycardia and not responsive to atropine or transcutaneous pacing.
Right patient?	The vasopressor of choice for the pulseless arrest patient.
Right dose?	0.01 mg/kg of the 1:10,000 solution.
Right route?	Epinephrine is administered by the IV or IO route. Also acceptable by the umbilical vein in an infant this small. It is possible to administer by the ET route but its effectiveness is questionable at best.
Right time?	Every 3–5 minutes of the cardiac arrest.
Right documentation?	Dose, route, time administered, and reassessment should be clearly documented on your patient care report.
Expected action	This drug is a direct-acting alpha- and beta-agonist. The alpha effect is vasoconstriction and Beta-1 is positive inotropic, chronotropic, and dromotropic effects. The Beta-2 effects, which are not immediately relevant to the cardiac arrest patient, are bronchial smooth muscle relaxation and dilation of the skeletal vasculature.
Side effects	Can cause hypertension, tachycardia, arrhythmias, pulmonary edema, anxiety, restlessness, agitation, nausea, headache, and angina.
Contraindications	Hypertension, hypothermia, pulmonary edema, myocardial ischemia, and hypovolemic shock.
Precautions	Epinephrine can potentiate other sympathomimetics. It can be deactivated by alkaline solutions (ie, sodium bicarbonate). Use of MAOIs may potentiate effects and beta-blockers may blunt its effects.
Pharmacokinetics	Onset: immediate; peak effect: minutes; duration: several minutes. Metabolism takes place in the liver.

Table 6 Volume Expanders

Do you know?	Comments
Right drug? [**Volume Expanders**] Generic name(s): [**Normal Saline**] or [**Lactated Ringer's Solution**]	Volume expanders should be administered when clinical signs of hypovolemia (pallor, weak pulses, and delayed capillary refill) are present with an adequate heart rate or high quality chest compressions.
Right patient?	Newborn with significant intravascular volume depletion.
Right dose?	10 mL/kg over 5–10 minutes; multiple doses may be administered when the patient remains hypovolemic.
Right route?	IV or IO.
Right time?	After vascular access has been established and signs of hypovolemia persist with an adequate heart rate or high quality chest compressions.
Right documentation?	Dose(s), route, time administered, and reassessment should be clearly documented on the patient care report.
Expected action	Relief of hypovolemia.
Side effects	Be cautious about overhydration.
Contraindications	None when hypovolemia is present.
Precautions	Carefully monitor fluid boluses to avoid overhydration.
Pharmacokinetics	The impact of expanding the volume should be immediate. Excess fluid is not easily eliminated and will go through the kidneys and urine.

Case Study I Continued

hypoglycemic patient, sodium bicarbonate for the lengthy cardiac arrest (metabolic acidosis), and naloxone hydrochloride [Narcan] for the neonate who may be overdosed on a narcotic (or born to a narcotic abuser who is high) (see **Table 7**, **Table 8**, and **Table 9**).

Question 5: What are some examples of factors associated with premature birth and low birth weight?

Question 6: When should medications be considered in the resuscitation of a newborn and how should they be administered?

Table 7 10% Dextrose in Water

Do you know?	Comments
Right drug? Generic name: [**10% Dextrose**] Trade name: [$D_{10}W$]	This is a hypertonic carbohydrate solution. Also called glucose or d-glucose.
Right patient?	Depressed neonate with documented low blood glucose. Severe hypoglycemia from any cause.
Right dose?	Typical dose is 0.5 g to 1 g/kg.
Right route?	A good vascular access.
Right time?	As soon as possible after glucose level is determined to be below the normal range.
Right documentation?	The patient care report should state the glucose level, the amount of $D_{10}W$ administered, and the serial vital signs as well as the patient's response to the medication.
Expected action	Relief of hypoglycemic state.
Side effects	None when administered in a good site. Redness or pain may occur at the injection site. If $D_{10}W$ leaks into the surrounding tissue (extravasation), it can cause tissue necrosis.
Contraindications	Previous hypersensitivity to dextrose solution. Diabetic coma while patient is hyperglycemic. Intracranial or intraspinal hemorrhage.
Precautions	Assess the site for signs of extravasation.
Pharmacokinetics	Short-term therapy; duration varies with the severity and cause of hypoglycemia.

Table 8 Sodium Bicarbonate

Do you know?	Comments
Right drug? Generic name: [**Sodium Bicarbonate**] Trade name: [Sodium Bicarbonate]	This drug is an alkalinizing agent, antacid, and electrolyte. It is used to treat acute metabolic acidosis caused by shock, severe dehydration, anoxia, uncontrolled diabetes, renal disease, cardiac arrest, and severe lactic acidosis.
Right patient?	Suspected or known mild or moderate metabolic acidosis due to shock, severe dehydration, anoxia, uncontrolled diabetes, renal disease, cardiac arrest, and severe primary lactic acidosis. Can also be used to treat overdose of aspirin and cyclic-antidepressants.
Right dose?	1 mEq per kg IV bolus (may repeat every 10 minutes at ½ initial dose). Paramedics use the 8.4% solution; (50 mEq in 50 mL) preload syringe. In infants, the 4.2% solution is recommended for intravenous administration at a dose not to exceed 8 mEq/kg/day. Slow administration rates and the 4.2% solution are recommended in neonates to guard against the possibility of producing hypernatremia. If you do not carry the 4.2% solution, the 8.4% solution can be diluted 1:1 with D_5W solution.
Right route?	IV bolus in a secondary line.
Right time?	When bradycardia persists even after adequate oxygenation, ventilation, chest compressions, and fluid bolus.
Right documentation?	Dose, route, time administered, and reassessment should be clearly documented on the patient care report.

continues

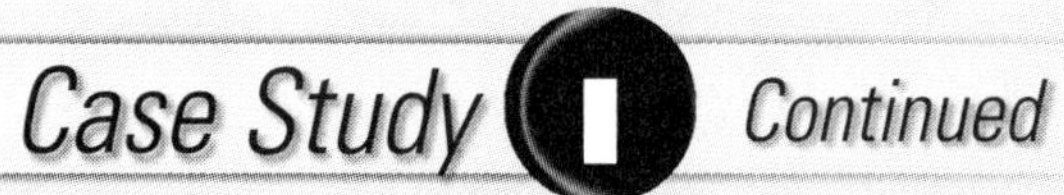

Table 8 Sodium Bicarbonate (*Continued*)

Do you know?	Comments
Expected action	Relief of metabolic acidosis.
Side effects	Hypernatremia, alkalosis, tetany, and fluid overload.
Contraindications	Metabolic and respiratory alkalosis, hypertension, convulsions, and CHF.
Precautions	Administer slow IV push especially in preemies to avoid causing a rapid change in pH that can produce cerebral bleeding. Do not mix in the same IV line as calcium chloride without first flushing the line or the drugs may precipitate.
Pharmacokinetics	Duration of action: Onset is seconds; peak effect is 1–2 minutes; duration is 10 minutes. Metabolized in the kidneys and through respiration. Rapidly metabolized to carbonic acid that rapidly dissociates into water and carbon dioxide. The carbon dioxide is excreted via the lungs.

Table 9 Naloxone Hydrochloride

Do you know?	Comments
Right drug? Generic name: [**Naloxone Hydrochloride**] Trade name: [Narcan]	This drug is a narcotic antagonist. When the paramedic suspects that the patient's respiratory depression is due to an overdose of a narcotic or opiate, such as morphine or heroin, or methadone, the drug of choice to reverse the effects of the narcotic or opiate is naloxone hydrochloride [Narcan].
Right patient?	Babies with depressed respirations induced by narcotics or opiates taken by the mother within 4 hours of delivery.
Right dose?	The dose is 0.1 mg/kg; maximum dose of 0.8 mg.
Right route?	Can be given by IV, IM, SC, or ET (diluted) routes although the ET route is the least effective and not generally recommended if other routes are available.
Right time?	If the baby has respiratory depression, assist the ventilations with a bag-mask device while properly positioning the airway.
Right documentation?	Always document how and when the drug was administered as well as the patient's response to the medication on your patient care report.
Expected action	Antagonistic to narcotic or opiate medications. Expect it to reverse the effect of the overdose. Small doses should improve the patient's ventilations.
Side effects	Nausea, upset stomach, drowsiness, and other signs and symptoms of opiate withdrawal can occur. More serious side effects include: vomiting, diaphoresis, tremors, seizures, rapid and pounding irregular pulse.
Contraindications	Use with caution in narcotic-dependent patients; use with caution in neonates of narcotic-addicted mothers.
Precautions	Give rapidly to reverse drug-induced effects of respiratory depression.
Pharmacokinetics	Onset: within 2 minutes; peak effect: variable; duration: 30–60 minutes, metabolized in the liver and excreted in urine.

Part 4

The back of the ambulance is hot now! En route your partner attempts to place an ET tube. The placement was good, and it has been confirmed with capnography. Keeping the tube in place will be challenging due to compressions and the rough ride, so it should be reassessed frequently. The ventilation method, utilizing the appropriate-sized bag-mask device, is effective and produces adequate chest rise. Warm packs are placed in the towel surrounding the baby. IO access is considered because the baby is not responding well and fluids and medications may be necessary. In this

Case Study I Continued

case, the decision is made to use the umbilical vein since it is easily accessible and there is not a lot of bone to puncture in this premature infant. You reassess the baby prior to giving a call to the hospital (see **Table 10**).

Question 7: When a newborn is initially depressed, when should chest compressions be started?

Question 8: What are the two most common drugs used in neonatal resuscitation?

Table 10 Reassessment and Ongoing Assessment of the Patient

Serial Vital Signs and Relevant Data	Recording Time: 10 Minutes
Skin CTC	Core pink, extremities blue
Pulse	80 beats/min
Blood Pressure	Not obtained
Respirations	Assisted with bag-mask device
Mental Status	Unresponsive, flaccid
ECG	Sinus bradycardia
SpO_2	94%
Lung Sounds	Clear with good chest rise
Other (ie, glucose, core body temperature)	Not obtained

Part 5

En route to the hospital the baby's heart rate increased to 80 beats/min so chest compressions were stopped and ventilations continued. Medical control was contacted and notified of the resuscitation and no additional orders were provided. At the ED a team is waiting in room #6 with an incubator and respiratory therapy.

Newborns who are depressed at birth require immediate attention. The neonatal resuscitation algorithm is used to help the health care provider focus on interventions and assessment, and to recognize the need to progress to the next level of resuscitation delineated in 30-second intervals. Resuscitation is centered on airway management, ventilation, chest compressions, and providing warmth. Intubation, vascular access, and drugs are only considered after effective oxygenation, ventilation, and chest compressions do not improve the condition.

A premature neonate is born before 37 weeks gestation and weighs less than 5.5 lb (2,500 g). Premature babies have poorly developed lungs and respiratory muscles and are at risk for developing several complications including: hypoxia, hypothermia, hypoglycemia, and hypovolemia. In this case, the baby was delivered at 22 weeks gestation into cold water and was found blue, with depressed respirations and a slow pulse resulting in a low APGAR score. After drying the baby, ventilations were provided for 30 seconds which did not increase the heart rate so chest compressions were started. Warmth was provided, intubation performed, and vascular access was obtained via the IO route. The decision to ventilate by bag-mask to ET tube was appropriate but the paramedic does recognize that the tube placement may be difficult to maintain. Constantly monitoring the tube position is a good decision for this baby because of the need to do chest compressions and the rough transport. The common causes of neonatal depression (narcotic overdose, hypoxia, hypothermia, hypovolemia, acidosis, etc.) were considered as well as the treatment options for each. Overall, prematurity and hypothermia are the most obvious causes of depression in this case. Both are conditions that are very dangerous for the newborn and can result in hypoglycemia and metabolic acidosis, and can be fatal. En route to the hospital, the heart rate increased enough to stop compressions, although ventilations were continued.

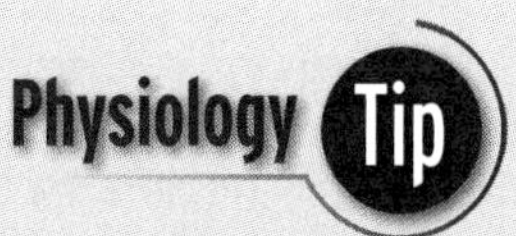

The two most common drugs used in neonatal resuscitation are epinephrine [Adrenalin] and naloxone hydrochloride [Narcan].

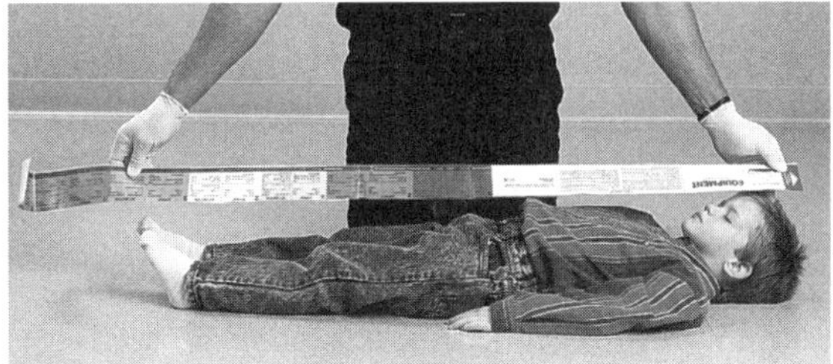

Figure 12-2 Length-based resuscitation tape.

Neonatal Resuscitation

A very stressful event in the care of the neonate is the need for resuscitation. Most paramedics have very little experience with resuscitations in patients this young and small. It is always helpful to have reference charts or resources available to refer to. An excellent tool designed to help guide you through the resuscitation of the newborn is the Neonatal Resuscitation Algorithm (see page 40.11 of Nancy Caroline's *Emergency Care in the Streets, Sixth Edition*). Another useful tool is the length-based resuscitation tape (**Figure 12-2**▲). The tape allows you to estimate a child's weight and identify the correct size for equipment and medication doses.

This tool is designed to move you through the resuscitation quickly and it emphasizes the strategies that should be applied to the newborn in distress with time frames of 30 seconds. It is clear that the initial strategies are high-quality assessment and basic life support procedures and not endotracheal intubation or the administration of medications. The key is to follow the algorithm, take the management steps, reassess, and then move on to the next steps quickly.

Medication Administration in Neonatal Resuscitation

Medication administration in neonatal resuscitation is one of the last treatment options and should only be considered after the airway, ventilation, and circulation components have been managed appropriately. Epinephrine [Adrenalin] and naloxone hydrochloride [Narcan] are the two most common drugs administered to newborns following birth. Epinephrine [Adrenalin] is a first-line vasopressor used in resuscitation and naloxone hydrochloride [Narcan], although not specifically spelled out in the resuscitation algorithm, is used in cases where the neonate was either accidentally overdosed on a narcotic or born to a narcotic abuser.

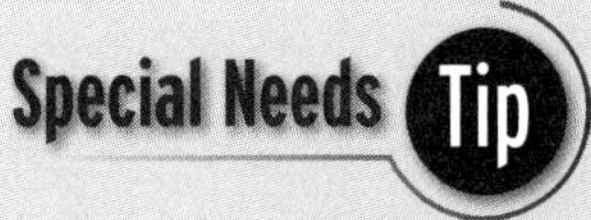

A good rule of thumb when managing newborns is to keep them warm, pink, and sweet. Aggressive warming causes stimulation and improves perfusion and breathing; blow-by oxygen will help "pink" them up; and newborns tend to use glucose very fast, especially when stressed. Airway management should be progressive from least aggressive to most invasive. Start with blow-by oxygen, then progress to oxygen by mask, then try assisting ventilations with a bag-mask device, and finally consider intubation. If you feel the newborn may require more aggressive oxygen therapy, then hook up the neonate bag-mask device to oxygen and use that to provide blow-by, then mask, and then assisted ventilations. The bag-mask is the one device used in the NICU to support ventilation in this sequential manner. It also reduces the stress of having to move from one device to another during an extremely stressful situation. Keeping it simple can help you manage the newborn quickly and efficiently.

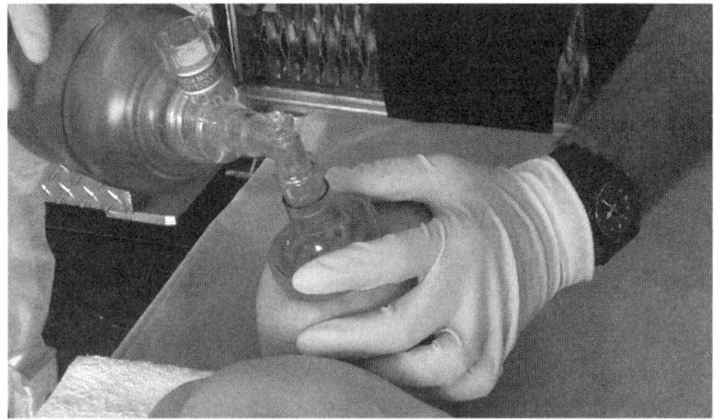

Figure 12-3 Bag-mask ventilation of the newborn.

Intubation

In most situations, the airway of the neonate can be managed with manual maneuvers and ventilation accomplished with a bag-mask device (**Figure 12-3**▲).

Intubation of the trachea is not a difficult procedure but most paramedics have very little field practice with the technique in young patients. If a neonate does need to be intubated, use the person most experienced in intubation and be very careful to assess the placement using numerous methods including capnography.

In the prehospital setting, uncuffed tubes are typically used to intubate neonates and children younger than 8 years old. When properly sized and placed, the uncuffed tube tip rests in the trachea at the subglottic narrowing distal to the vocal cords. This configuration works well to minimize inadvertent gastric distension while not risking pressure necrosis of the fragile tracheal lining that can accompany tube cuff inflation.

Complications of Intubation

The process of ventilating the neonate either by mask or tube is potentially complicated by some degree of gastric insufflation and distention. Gastric distention in a child can compromise mechanical ventilation because the abdominal organs tend to push up against the diaphragm, making it difficult for the lungs to subsequently expand properly. To avoid or relieve gastric distention, an orogastric tube is commonly placed along with or shortly after intubation. This should be done with extreme caution in the case of an extremely premature delivery.

The most common complication of intubation is a misplaced tube. The tube may be initially misplaced or it may slip out of place with patient or rescuer movement. There is a slightly increased tendency for slippage to occur with uncuffed tubes. Barotrauma, pneumothorax, and compromised venous return to the heart are additional serious complications that may occur with endotracheal intubation or overzealous use of positive pressure mechanical ventilation.

Bradycardia: An Ominous Sign in Neonates

Hypoxia causes the heart rate to drop (**bradycardia**) and the adequacy of respirations is determined by the heart rate. Bradycardia in a distressed baby is a sign of impending cardiac arrest. Correcting the hypoxia will, in most cases, improve the heart rate and restore adequate circulation. When bradycardia persists despite effective oxygenation and ventilation, and the infant has a pulse rate of less than 60 beats/min, epinephrine 0.1 mg/kg of the 1:10,000 concentration is administered to help stabilize the neonate. This dose may be repeated and followed up with an infusion drip if bradycardia persists.

Medications may be administered through a peripheral IV, umbilical vein, scalp vein, IO, and endotracheal tube (ET). The intraosseous (IO) route has gained popularity in recent years with the advent of modern "bone drills" that can be rapidly employed. IO is a safe, fast, and reliable way to gain vascular access in the prehospital setting and should be considered when IV access is not available quickly (within 90 seconds). The procedure of IO administration is discussed in chapter 1. Medication administration through the ET is the least reliable and is unpredictable; therefore, it should be the last choice.

Hypothermia

All neonates are at risk for hypothermia due to the large surface area to the head and the thin muscle layer under their skin. When treating the neonate, make sure that you do not infuse a drug or fluid that is cold as you will rapidly induce hypothermia in the child. When the core body temperature has been measured and reveals a hypothermic patient, warm, not hot, fluids can be one of many methods used to begin to warm up the patient's core. This should be done very slowly and is best done in the ED setting.

Hypoglycemia

Hypoglycemia in infants is a blood glucose level of less than 40 mg/dL. It is necessary to treat this condition because the longer the brain goes without glucose, the more brain cells are likely to die. The patient should be assessed and managed focusing on the ABCs. Take the vital signs as well as the blood glucose reading and oxygen saturation. Provide supplemental oxygen and IV access so that 10% dextrose in water ($D_{10}W$) may be administered to the patient when hypoglycemia is detected and if medical control concurs.

Other Conditions

Acidosis

Sodium bicarbonate may be considered when **acidosis** is known or suspected in the neonate. The dose is 1 mEq per kg IV bolus (may repeat every 10 minutes at ½ initial dose). Paramedics usually carry the 8.4% solution (50 mEq) in 50 mL preload syringe for adult patients. In infants (up to 2 years of age), the 4.2% solution is recommended for intravenous administration at a dose not to exceed 8 mEq/kg/day. Slow administration rates and the 4.2% solution are recommended in neonates to guard against the possibility of producing **hypernatremia**. If you do not carry the 4.2% solution, the 8.4% solution can be diluted 1:1 with 5% dextrose in water (D_5W).

Mothers Treated Acutely with Narcotics

For babies with depressed respirations induced by narcotics or opiates taken by the mother within 4 hours of delivery, naloxone hydrochloride [Narcan] is indicated and the dose is 0.1 mg/kg with a maximum dose of 0.8 mg. Naloxone hydrochloride [Narcan] can be administered by the IO, IV, IM, SC, or ET routes.

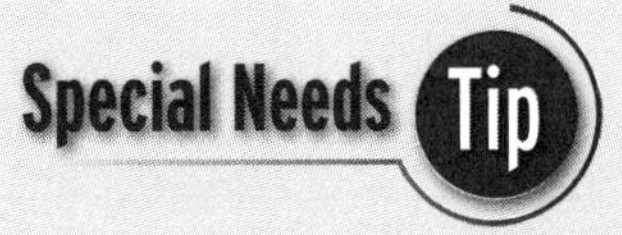

WOW! It is difficult to remember the dose for pediatric medications. Since EMS personnel see fewer critical pediatric patients than adults, it is easy to forget medication doses. There are options for the paramedic. You can create a weight-based dosing chart for all the medications or use a length-weight-based pediatric tape such as the Braselow or a similar product. As soon as you encounter and begin assessing a child, one early question should be, "How much does the child weigh?" If the parents or guardians do not know, or even if they do, simply pull the tape out, and lay it next to the child and leave it there during your management. Even if the child is not acute, frequent and repeated use of the tape will allow you to be less stressed when faced with a critical or urgent pediatric patient.

Physiology Tip

Even though EMS personnel may consider intubating pediatric patients, it is extremely easy to develop tunnel vision and lose focus. One of the most important and easiest things to correct is ventilation. Many rescuers overaggressively ventilate their patient when using a bag-mask device. According to the AHA, ALL HEALTH CARE PROVIDERS need to be cautious and observant when using a bag-mask device and ventilate at the appropriate rate for the patient's age. Ventilating faster will cause respiratory alkalosis (which is more difficult to manage than respiratory acidosis) and gastric distention. Monitor the person performing the ventilations and ensure that he or she is performing them at a rate recommended by the AHA. Remember, it is not about how fast the patient is ventilated, but ensuring delivery of an effective tidal volume.

Not Recommended for Children or the Fetus!

Agents that can cause fetal malformations are referred to as teratogens. Teratogens are discussed in chapter 11. One of the most prominent is the sedative Thalidomide that was used for first trimester morning sickness until it was banned in the 1960s in the USA. Examples of medications or substances that pregnant women should NOT be exposed to and can cause fetal abnormalities include alcohol, coumadin [Warfarin], lead, ACE inhibitors, and certain antibiotics.

There are also a number of medications in your "Adult Drug Formulary" that are not recommended for use with children. **Table 12-1** ▸ is a listing of many of these medications.

Table 12-1 Paramedic Formulary: NOT Recommended for Pediatric Patients

Generic name	Trade name
Digoxin	Lanoxin (not generally used by paramedics in the field)
Diltiazem Hydrochloride	Cardizem
Flumazenil	Romazicon
Glucagon (for calcium channel blocker or beta-blocker OD)	Glucagons
Haloperidol	Haldol
Ketorolac Tromethamine	Toradol IM (not commonly used by paramedics in the field for children)
Labetalol	Normodyne
Metaproterenol 5%	Alupent
Midazolam	Versed
Nalbuphine	Nubain
Nitroglycerin	Nitrostat
Nitro paste	Nitro-Bid Ointment
Streptokinase	Streptase
Tissue Plasminogen Activator	TPA
Vasopressin	Pitressin synthetic

Case Study ANSWERS

Case Study 1 Prematurity and Hypothermia

Question 1: How is a premature infant defined in terms of weight?

Answer 1: A premature infant is born before 37 weeks of gestation and weighs less than 5.5 lb (2,500 g).

Question 2: How can resuscitation medication doses for infants and young children best be determined in the field setting?

Answer 2: First and foremost follow your regional protocols! Many systems use a length-based resuscitation tape system or refer to a weight chart. When in doubt, call Medical Control and discuss with them before administering the wrong dose.

Question 3: Why should this infant be assessed for hypothermia?

Answer 3: This baby was dropped into toilet water and washed off with water so the chances of it being hypothermic to start are high. Once a newborn is cold, the resuscitation becomes much more difficult.

Question 4: Why are premature babies, newborns, neonates, and infants poor at thermoregulation?

Answer 4: Premature babies, newborns, neonates, and infants must be kept warm because they will lose heat rapidly as their body surface area is larger in relation to their weight. Heat loss occurs faster. They have small amounts of subcutaneous fat to keep them warm and their thermoregulatory systems are too immature to produce body heat. A cold baby becomes depressed and deteriorates leading to respiratory and cardiac arrest.

Question 5: What are some examples of factors associated with premature birth and low birth weight?

Answer 5: Examples of factors associated with premature birth and low birth weight include structural irregularities of the uterus, hormonal imbalance in the mother, third trimester bleeding, premature labor, inadequate or no prenatal care, multiple fetuses, and maternal use of drugs, alcohol, and cigarettes.

Question 6: When should medications be considered in the resuscitation of a newborn and how should they be administered?

Answer 6: Medications are one of the last treatment options and should only be considered after the airway, ventilation, and circulation components have been managed appropriately. A patent vascular access is the preferred method for drug administration and medication doses are weight based.

Question 7: When a newborn is initially depressed, when should chest compressions be started?

Answer 7: Chest compressions should be performed when the heart rate drops to less than 60 beats/min and does not increase after 30 seconds of assisted ventilations.

Question 8: What are the two most common drugs used in neonatal resuscitation?

Answer 8: Epinephrine [Adrenalin] is indicated for symptomatic bradycardia that does not improve with effective oxygenation, ventilation, and chest compressions. Naloxone hydrochloride [Narcan] is indicated when babies have depressed respirations induced by narcotics or opiates taken by the mother within 4 hours of delivery.

Medication Review

10% Dextrose in Water ($D_{10}W$)

Indications Hypoglycemia, altered level of consciousness, coma of unknown etiology, seizure of unknown etiology, status epilepticus.

Contraindications Intracranial hemorrhage.

Dosage and administration Pediatric: 0.5–1 g/kg/dose slow IV; may be repeated as necessary.

Epinephrine (Adrenalin)

Indications Cardiac arrest (V-fib/pulseless V-tach, asystole, PEA), symptomatic bradycardia as an alternative infusion to dopamine, severe hypotension secondary to bradycardia when atropine and transcutaneous pacing are unsuccessful, allergic reactions, anaphylaxis, asthma.

Contraindications Hypertension, hypothermia, pulmonary edema, myocardial ischemia, hypovolemic shock.

Dosage and administration Pediatric: Mild allergic reactions and asthma: 0.01 mg/kg (0.01 mL/kg) of 1:1,000 solution SC (maximum of 0.3 mL). Cardiac arrest: IV/IO dose: 0.01 mg/kg (0.1 mL/kg) of 1:10,000 solution every 3–5 minutes during arrest. All endotracheal (ET) doses: 0.1 mg/kg (0.1 mL/kg) of 1:1,000 solution. Symptomatic bradycardia: IV/IO dose: 0.01 mg/kg (0.1 mL/kg) of 1:10,000 solution. Continuous IV/IO infusion: Begin with rapid infusion, then titrate to response. Typical initial infusion: 0.1–1 µg/min. Higher doses may be effective.

Glucagon

Indications Altered level of consciousness when hypoglycemia is suspected. May be used as inotropic agent in beta-blocker overdose.

Contraindications Hyperglycemia, hypersensitivity.

Dosage and administration Pediatric: Hypoglycemia: 0.5–1 mg IM (for children < 20 kg). Calcium channel blocker or beta-blocker overdose: not recommended.

Naloxone Hydrochloride (Narcan)

Indications Opiate overdose, coma; complete or partial reversal of CNS and respiratory depression induced by opioids; decreased level of consciousness; coma of unknown origin; narcotic agonist for the following: morphine sulfate [Astramorph/PF], heroin, hydromorphone (Dilaudid), methadone, meperidine (Demerol), paregoric, fentanyl citrate (Sublimase), oxycodone (Percodan), codeine, propoxyphene (Darvon); narcotic agonist and antagonist for the following: Butorphanol (Stadol), pentazocine (Talwin), nalbuphine (Nubain).

Contraindications Use with caution in narcotic-dependent patients; use with caution in neonates of narcotic-addicted mothers.

Dosage and administration Pediatric: 0.1 mg/kg/dose IV, IM, SC, ET (diluted); maximum dose of 0.8 mg; if no response in 10 minutes, administer an additional 0.1 mg/kg/dose.

Medication Review

Oxygen

Indications Confirmed or expected hypoxemia, ischemic chest pain, respiratory insufficiency, prophylactically during air transport, confirmed or suspected carbon monoxide poisoning, all other causes of decreased tissue oxygenation, decreased level of consciousness.

Contraindications Certain patients with COPD or emphysema who will not tolerate oxygen concentrations over 35%, hyperventilation. This is not a concern with the neonatal patient. Oxygen should never be withheld from a patient who needs it, however. Be prepared to assist with ventilations in a patient with COPD who requires high concentration, as apnea may result.

Dosage and administration Pediatric: Cardiac arrest and carbon monoxide poisoning: 100%. Hypoxemia: 10–15 L/min via nonrebreathing mask. COPD: 1–6 L/min via nasal cannula or 28%–35% Venturi mask. Be prepared to provide ventilatory support if higher concentrations of oxygen are needed. Be careful not to administer directly into the eyes of a premature infant.

Sodium Bicarbonate

Indications Mild or moderate metabolic acidosis due to shock, severe dehydration, anoxia, uncontrolled diabetes, renal disease, cardiac arrest, and severe primary lactic acidosis. To treat overdose of aspirin and cyclic-antidepressants.

Contraindications Metabolic and respiratory alkalosis, hypertension, convulsions, CHF, and other situations where sodium can be dangerous.

Dosage and administration 1 mEq per kg IV bolus (may repeat every 10 minutes at ½ initial dose).

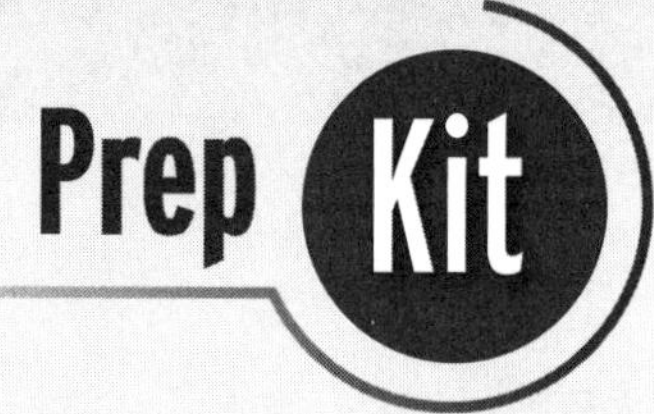

Chapter Summary

- Approach and management of the child is often specific to the age group that the child fits into.
- The pediatric assessment triangle was developed to remind the provider of the essential elements of appearance, work of breathing, and circulation to the skin.
- It is always helpful to have reference charts or resources available to refer to when performing neonatal resuscitation.
- The initial strategies of neonatal resuscitation are high-quality assessment and basic life support procedures.
- Medication administration in neonatal resuscitation is one of the last treatment options. Epinephrine [Adrenalin] and naloxone hydrochloride [Narcan] are the two most common drugs administered to newborns following birth.
- In most situations the airway of the neonate can be managed with manual maneuvers and ventilation accomplished with a bag-mask device. When intubation is needed, uncuffed tubes are typically used to intubate neonates and children younger than 8 years old.
- The most common complication of intubation is a misplaced tube.
- When the core body temperature has been measured and reveals a hypothermic neonate, warm fluids can be one of the methods used to warm up the patient's core.
- Hypoglycemia in infants is a blood glucose level of less than 40 mg/dL.
- Medications or substances that pregnant women should not be exposed to and can cause fetal abnormalities include alcohol, warfarin [Coumadin], lead, ACE inhibitors, and certain antibiotics.
- There are many medications in the adult drug formulary that are not recommended for use with children.

Vital Vocabulary

Acidosis A blood pH of less than 7.35. A pathologic condition resulting from the accumulation of acids in the body.

Bradycardia A slow heart rate, less than 60 beats/min; a pulse rate of less than 100 beats/min in the newborn.

Hypernatremia A blood serum sodium level greater than 148 mEq/L and a serum osmolarity greater than 295 mOsm/kg.

Neonate Infant during the first month after birth.

Newborn Infant within the first few hours after birth.

Premature Born before 37 weeks of gestation and weighs less than 5.5 lb (2,500 g).

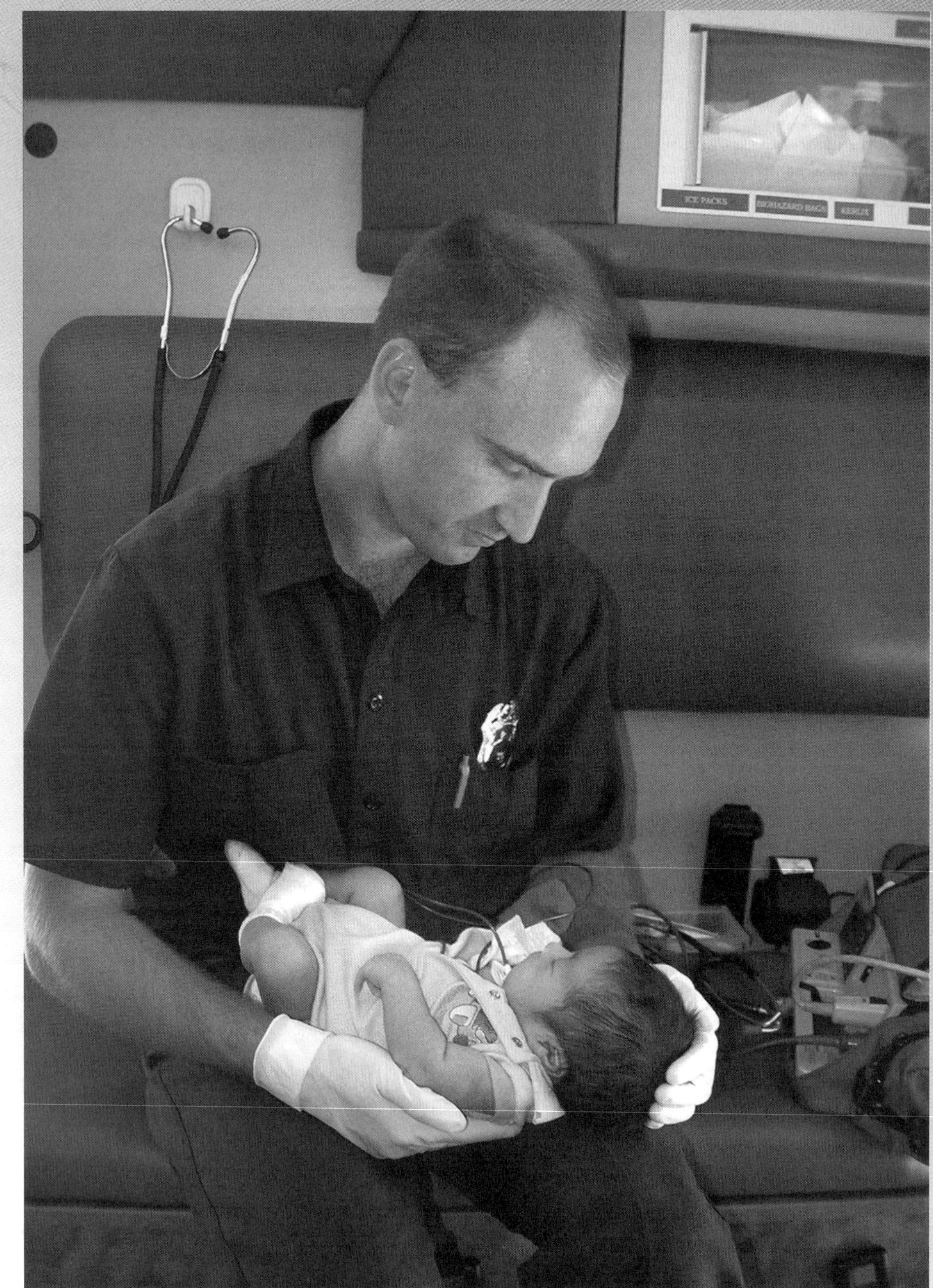
ICE PACKS
BIOHAZARD BAGS
KERLIX

Pediatric Emergencies 13

Objectives

Cognitive

6-2.40 Determine when pain management and sedation are appropriate for infants and children. (pages 383–389)

6-2.50 Discuss the indications, dosage, route of administration and special considerations for medication administration in infants and children. (pages 360–389)

6-2.64 Discuss the management/treatment plan for cardiac arrhythmias in infants and children. (page 383)

Affective

None

Psychomotor

None

Additional Objectives

13-1 List the pediatric doses and routes for medication administration. (pages 360–374)

13-2 Discuss the Wong-Baker FACES Pain Rating Scale and its use in the assessment of pain management. (page 384)

13-3 List medications/substances that can be potentially lethal to the toddler. (pages 381–382)

The Pediatric Patient

Children present unique assessment and management opportunities for the paramedic. They have different physical, emotional, intellectual, and developmental traits as they pass through each age group—from infant to toddler to preschooler to school-age to adolescent. In this chapter, we will touch on some of the assessment and management features that make them unique as well as the specific pharmacologic interventions involving the pediatric patient. In general, there are not a lot of adult medications that are not used in children, although the doses are usually weight-based in children rather than a specific dose, as may be the case with an adult. Specifically, we will cover the following areas in this chapter: pediatric dosing, respiratory emergencies, toxicologic emergencies, arrhythmias and medical emergencies, trauma, burns, and pain management.

Pediatric Doses

Virtually all, but especially pediatric medication doses, are weight-based. It is important to have some grasp of the weight of the child prior to giving medications. In the hospital setting, when a child is being managed over a period of days to weeks, a chart of the doses based on the child's weight should be clearly posted at the bedside. This way, during critical moments the health care providers are not pressured to do the math. In the prehospital setting, where we often have less in the way of provider assistance and much more pressure exerted upon us by numerous factors, it is extremely helpful to use a tool such as the length-based resuscitation tape (**Figure 13-1** ▲).

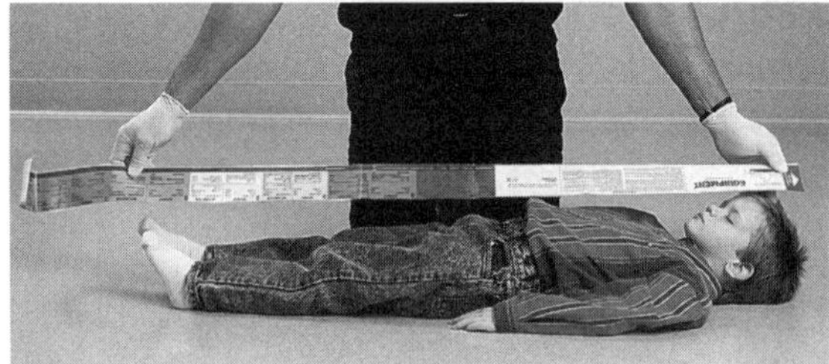

Figure 13-1 Length-based resuscitation tape.

1. Measure the child's length, from head to heel, with the tape (with the red portion at the head).
2. Note the weight in kilograms that corresponds to the child's measured length at the heel.
3. If the child is longer than the tape, use adult equipment and medication doses.
4. From the tape, identify appropriate equipment sizes.
5. From the tape, identify appropriate medication doses.

If you do not have a length-based resuscitation tape available, use a chart in the pediatric kit or refer to a pocket reference for the weight calculations. Always know where that item is located in your unit before starting your shift.

The following **Tables 13-1a/b** ▼ may provide a useful starting point:

Table 13-1a Pediatric Doses (Part I, 4.4–35.2 lb)

Drug	Dose	lb	kg	Administer
Activated charcoal	1–2 g/kg	4.4	2	2–4 g
		6.6	3	3–6 g
		8.8	4	4–8 g
		11	5	5–10 g
		13.2	6	6–12 g
		15.4	7	7–14 g
		17.6	8	8–16 g
		19.8	9	9–18 g
		22	10	10–20 g
		24.2	11	11–22 g
		26.4	12	12–24 g
		28.6	13	13–26 g
		30.8	14	14–28 g
		33	15	15–30 g
		35.2	16	16–32 g
Adenosine [Adenocard] or morphine sulfate [Astramorph/PF]	0.1–0.2 mg/kg	4.4	2	0.2–0.4 mg
		6.6	3	0.3–0.6 mg
		8.8	4	0.4–0.8 mg
		11	5	0.5–1 mg
		13.2	6	0.6–1.2 mg
		15.4	7	0.7–1.4 mg

continues

Table 13-1a Pediatric Doses (Part I) (*Continued*)

Drug	Dose	lb	kg	Administer
		17.6	8	0.8–1.6 mg
		19.8	9	0.9–1.8 mg
		22	10	1–2 mg
		24.2	11	1.1–2.2 mg
		26.4	12	1.2–2.4 mg
		28.6	13	1.3–2.6 mg
		30.8	14	1.4–2.8 mg
		33	15	1.5–3 mg
		35.2	16	1.6–3.2 mg
Albuterol* [Proventil, Ventolin]	0.05–0.15 mg/kg (dilute in 2 mL 0.9% normal saline)	4.4	2	0.1–0.3 mg
		6.6	3	0.15–0.45 mg
		8.8	4	0.2–0.6 mg
		11	5	0.25–0.75 mg
		13.2	6	0.3–0.9 mg
*NOTE: For children ages 2 to 12 the recommended albuterol solution is 0.083%. This strength is not recommended for children less than 15 kg. For adults and children over the age of 12, the albuterol solution used is the 0.5% solution. Most EMS systems simply administer the same dose to adults and children of 2.5 mg (0.5 mL added to 2 mL or normal saline).		15.4	7	0.35–1.05 mg
		17.6	8	0.4–1.2 mg
		19.8	9	0.45–1.35 mg
		22	10	0.5–1.5 mg
		24.2	11	0.55–1.65 mg
		26.4	12	0.6–1.8 mg
		28.6	13	0.65–1.95 mg
		30.8	14	0.7–2.1 mg
		33	15	0.75–2.25 mg
		35.2	16	0.8–2.4 mg
Amiodarone [Cordarone, Pacerone] or phenytoin [Dilantin] (for arrhythmias)	5 mg/kg	4.4	2	10 mg
		6.6	3	15 mg
		8.8	4	20 mg
		11	5	25 mg
		13.2	6	30 mg
		15.4	7	35 mg
		17.6	8	40 mg
		19.8	9	45 mg
		22	10	50 mg
		24.2	11	55 mg
		26.4	12	60 mg
		28.6	13	65 mg
		30.8	14	70 mg
		33	15	75 mg
		35.2	16	80 mg
Atropine sulfate	0.02 mg/kg (0.1 mg minimum)	4.4	2	0.1 mg (min dose)
		6.6	3	0.1 mg (min dose)
		8.8	4	0.1 mg (min dose)
		11	5	0.1 mg
		13.2	6	0.12 mg
		15.4	7	0.14 mg
		17.6	8	0.16 mg
		19.8	9	0.18 mg
		22	10	0.2 mg
		24.2	11	0.22 mg
		26.6	12	0.24 mg
		28.6	13	0.26 mg
		30.8	14	0.28 mg
		33	15	0.30 mg
		35.2	16	0.32 mg

continues

Table 13-1a Pediatric Doses (Part I) (*Continued*)

Drug	Dose	lb	kg	Administer
Calcium chloride	20 mg/kg	4.4	2	40 mg
		6.6	3	60 mg
		8.8	4	80 mg
		11	5	100 mg
		13.2	6	120 mg
		15.4	7	140 mg
		17.6	8	160 mg
		19.8	9	180 mg
		22	10	200 mg
		24.2	11	220 mg
		26.4	12	240 mg
		28.6	13	260 mg
		30.8	14	280 mg
		33	15	300 mg
		35.2	16	320 mg
Dextrose	0.5–1 g/kg	4.4	2	1–2 g
		6.6	3	1.5–3 g
		8.8	4	2–4 g
		11	5	2.5–5 g
		13.2	6	3–6 g
		15.4	7	3.5–7 g
		17.6	8	4–8 g
		19.8	9	4.5–9 g
		22	10	5–10 g
		24.2	11	5.5–11 g
		26.4	12	6–12 g
		28.6	13	6.5–13 g
		30.8	14	7–14 g
		33	15	7.5–15 g
		35.2	16	8–16 g
Diazepam [Valium]	0.2–0.5 mg/kg (higher dose for rectal)	4.4	2	0.4–1 mg
		6.6	3	0.6–1.5 mg
		8.8	4	0.8–2 mg
		11	5	1–2.5 mg
		13.2	6	1.2–3 mg
		15.4	7	1.4–3.5 mg
		17.6	8	1.6–4 mg
		19.8	9	1.8–4.5 mg
		22	10	2–5 mg
		24.2	11	2.2–5.5 mg
		26.4	12	2.4–6 mg
		28.6	13	2.6–6.5 mg
		30.8	14	2.8–7 mg
		33	15	3–7.5 mg
		35.2	16	3.2–8 mg
Diphenhydramine [Benadryl], meperidine hydrocholoride [Demerol], or methylprednisolone sodium succinate [Solu–Medrol] (for asthma)	1–2 mg/kg	4.4	2	2–4 mg
		6.6	3	3–6 mg
		8.8	4	4–8 mg
		11	5	5–10 mg
		13.2	6	6–12 mg
		15.4	7	7–14 mg
		17.6	8	8–16 mg
		19.8	9	9–18 mg
		22	10	10–20 mg
		24.4	11	11–22 mg

continues

Table 13-1a Pediatric Doses (Part I) (*Continued*)

Drug	Dose	lb	kg	Administer
		26.4	12	12–24 mg
		28.6	13	13–26 mg
		30.8	14	14–28 mg
		33	15	15–30 mg
		35.2	16	16–32 mg
Dobutamine [Dobutrex] or dopamine [Intropin]	2–20 μg/kg/min	4.4	2	4–40 μg/min
		6.6	3	6–60 μg/min
		8.8	4	8–80 μg/min
		11	5	10–100 μg/min
		13.2	6	12–120 μg/min
		15.4	7	14–140 μg/min
		17.6	8	16–160 μg/min
		19.8	9	18–180 μg/min
		22	10	20–200 μg/min
		24.2	11	22–220 μg/min
		26.4	12	24–240 μg/min
		28.6	13	26–260 μg/min
		30.8	14	28–280 μg/min
		33	15	30–300 μg/min
		35.2	16	32–320 μg/min
Epinephrine [Adrenalin]	0.01 mg/kg of 1:1,000 solution SC for mild allergic reaction or asthma (max 0.3 mL); 0.01 mg/kg of 1:10,000 solution for cardiac arrest or bradycardia	4.4	2	0.02 mg
		6.6	3	0.03 mg
		8.8	4	0.04 mg
		11	5	0.05 mg
		13.2	6	0.06 mg
		15.4	7	0.07 mg
		17.6	8	0.08 mg
		19.8	9	0.09 mg
		22	10	0.1 mg
		24.2	11	0.11 mg
		26.4	12	0.12 mg
		28.6	13	0.13 mg
		30.8	14	0.14 mg
		33	15	0.15 mg
		35.2	16	0.16 mg
Furosemide [Lasix] and lidocaine hydrochloride [Xylocaine]	1 mg/kg (for lidocaine hydrochloride [Xylocaine], max of 100 mg)	4.4	2	2 mg
		6.6	3	3 mg
		8.8	4	4 mg
		11	5	5 mg
		13.2	6	6 mg
		15.4	7	7 mg
		17.6	8	8 mg
		19.8	9	9 mg
		22	10	10 mg
		24.2	11	11 mg
		26.4	12	12 mg
		28.6	13	13 mg
		30.8	14	14 mg
		33	15	15 mg
		35.2	16	16 mg
Hydroxyzine hydrochloride [Atarax, Vistaril]	0.5–1 mg/kg IM	4.4	2	1–2 mg
		6.6	3	1.5–3 mg
		8.8	4	2–4 mg

continues

Table 13-1a Pediatric Doses (Part I) (*Continued*)

Drug	Dose	lb	kg	Administer
		11	5	2.5–5 mg
		13.2	6	3–6 mg
		15.4	7	3.5–7 mg
		17.6	8	4–8 mg
		19.8	9	4.5–9 mg
		22	10	5–10 mg
		24.2	11	5.5–11 mg
		26.4	12	6–12 mg
		28.6	13	6.5–13 mg
		30.8	14	7–14 mg
		33	15	7.5–15 mg
		35.2	16	8–16 mg
Isoetharine [Bronchosol, Bronkometer]	0.01 mL/kg (dilute in 3 mL saline and nebulize) (max 0.5 mL)	4.4	2	0.02 mL
		6.6	3	0.03 mL
		8.8	4	0.04 mL
		11	5	0.05 mL
		13.2	6	0.06 mL
		15.4	7	0.07 mL
		17.6	8	0.08 mL
		19.8	9	0.09 mL
		22	10	0.1 mL
		24.2	11	0.11 mL
		26.4	12	0.12 mL
		28.6	13	0.13 mL
		30.8	14	0.14 mL
		33	15	0.15 mL
		35.2	16	0.16 mL
Lorazepam [Ativan]	0.05–0.20 mg/kg (slow IV/IO) (max dose 0.2 mg/kg)	4.4	2	0.1–0.4 mg
		6.6	3	0.15–0.6 mg
		8.8	4	0.2–0.8 mg
		11	5	0.25–1 mg
		13.2	6	0.3–1.2 mg
		15.4	7	0.35–1.4 mg
		17.6	8	0.4–1.6 mg
		19.8	9	0.45–1.8 mg
		22	10	0.5–2 mg
		24.2	11	0.55–2.2 mg
		26.4	12	0.6–2.4 mg
		28.6	13	0.65–2.6 mg
		30.8	14	0.7–2.8 mg
		33	15	0.75–3 mg
		35.2	16	0.8–3.2 mg
Magnesium sulfate	25–50 mg/kg (infusion over 10–20 minutes) (max dose 2 g)	4.4	2	50–100 mg
		6.6	3	75–150 mg
		8.8	4	100–200 mg
		11	5	125–250 mg
		13.2	6	150–300 mg
		15.4	7	175–350 mg
		17.6	8	200–400 mg
		19.8	9	225–450 mg
		22	10	250–500 mg
		24.2	11	275–550 mg
		26.4	12	300–600 mg

continues

Table 13-1a Pediatric Doses (Part I) (*Continued*)

Drug	Dose	lb	kg	Administer
		28.6	13	325–650 mg
		30.8	14	350–700 mg
		33	15	375–750 mg
		35.2	16	400–800 mg
Methylprednisolone sodium succinate [Solu-Medrol] (usually in ED and not in field setting)	For acute spinal trauma 30 mg/kg IV (over 30 minutes)	4.4	2	60 mg
		6.6	3	90 mg
		8.8	4	120 mg
		11	5	150 mg
		13.6	6	180 mg
		15.4	7	210 mg
		17.6	8	240 mg
		19.8	9	270 mg
		22	10	300 mg
		24.2	11	330 mg
		26.2	12	360 mg
		28.6	13	390 mg
		30.8	14	420 mg
		33	15	450 mg
		35.2	16	480 mg
Naloxone hydrochloride [Narcan] or pancuronium bromide [Pavulon]	0.1 mg/kg (naloxone hydrochloride, max dose of 0.8 mg) (pancuronium, slow IV/IO)	4.4	2	0.2 mg
		6.6	3	0.3 mg
		8.8	4	0.4 mg
		11	5	0.5 mg
		13.2	6	0.6 mg
		15.4	7	0.7 mg
		17.6	8	0.8 mg
		19.8	9	0.9 mg (max 0.8 mg Narcan)
		22	10	1 mg (max 0.8 mg Narcan)
		24.2	11	1.1 mg (max 0.8 mg Narcan)
		26.4	12	1.2 mg (max 0.8 mg Narcan)
		28.6	13	1.3 mg (max 0.8 mg Narcan)
		30.8	14	1.4 mg (max 0.8 mg Narcan)
		33	15	1.5 mg (max 0.8 mg Narcan)
		35.2	16	1.6 mg (max 0.8 mg Narcan)
Norepinephrine bitartrate [Levophed, Levarterenol]	0.1–1.0 μg/min (IV infusion)	4.4	2	0.2–2 μg/min
		6.6	3	0.3–3 μg/min
		8.8	4	0.4–4 μg/min
		11	5	0.5–5 μg/min
		13.2	6	0.6–6 μg/min
		15.4	7	0.7–7 μg/min
		17.6	8	0.8–8 μg/min
		19.8	9	0.9–9 μg/min
		22	10	1–10 μg/min
		24.2	11	1.1–11 μg/min

continues

Table 13-1a Pediatric Doses (Part I) (*Continued*)

Drug	Dose	lb	kg	Administer
		26.4	12	1.2–12 μg/min
		28.6	13	1.3–13 μg/min
		30.8	14	1.4–14 μg/min
		33	15	1.5–15 μg/min
		35.2	16	1.6–16 μg/min
Phenobarbital [Luminal] or phenytoin [Dilantin] (for seizures)	10–20 mg/kg (IV/IO) (phenytoin slow IV)	4.4	2	20–40 mg
		6.6	3	30–60 mg
		8.8	4	40–80 mg
		11	5	50–100 mg
		13.2	6	60–120 mg
		15.4	7	70–140 mg
		17.6	8	80–160 mg
		19.8	9	90–180 mg
		22	10	100–200 mg
		24.2	11	110–220 mg
		26.4	12	120–240 mg
		28.6	13	130–260 mg
		30.8	14	140–280 mg
		33	15	150–300 mg
		35.2	16	160–320 mg
Pralidoxime chloride [2-PAM chloride, Protopam]	20–40 mg/kg (IV over 15–30 minutes)	4.4	2	40–80 mg
		6.6	3	60–120 mg
		8.8	4	80–160 mg
		11	5	100–200 mg
		13.2	6	120–240 mg
		15.4	7	140–280 mg
		17.6	8	160–320 mg
		19.8	9	180–360 mg
		22	10	200–400 mg
		24.2	11	220–440 mg
		26.4	12	240–480 mg
		28.6	13	260–520 mg
		30.8	14	280–560 mg
		33	15	300–600 mg
		35.2	16	320–640 mg
Procainamide hydrochloride [Procanbid, Pronestyl]	15 mg/kg (IV/IO over 30–60 minutes)	4.4	2	30 mg
		6.6	3	45 mg
		8.8	4	60 mg
		11	5	75 mg
		13.2	6	90 mg
		15.4	7	105 mg
		17.6	8	120 mg
		19.8	9	135 mg
		22	10	150 mg
		24.2	11	165 mg
		26.4	12	180 mg
		28.6	13	195 mg
		30.8	14	210 mg
		33	15	225 mg
		35.2	16	240 mg
Promethazine hydrochloride [Phenergan] (over 2 years old)	0.25–0.5 mg/kg IM	4.4	2	Over 2 years old only
		6.6	3	Over 2 years old only

continues

Table 13-1a Pediatric Doses (Part I) (*Continued*)

Drug	Dose	lb	kg	Administer
		8.8	4	Over 2 years old only
		11	5	1.25–2.5 mg (if over 2 years old)
		13.2	6	1.5–3 mg
		15.4	7	1.75–3.5 mg
		17.6	8	2–4 mg
		19.8	9	2.25–4.5 mg
		22	10	2.5–5 mg
		24.2	11	2.75–5.5 mg
		26.4	12	3–6 mg
		28.6	13	3.25–6.5 mg
		30.8	14	3.5–7 mg
		33	15	3.75–7.5 mg
		35.2	16	4–8 mg
Propranolol hydrochloride [Inderal]	0.01–0.05 mg/kg (slow IV, max dose 3 mg)	4.4	2	0.02–0.1 mg
		6.6	3	0.03–0.15 mg
		8.8	4	0.04–0.2 mg
		11	5	0.05–0.25 mg
		13.2	6	0.06–0.3 mg
		15.4	7	0.07–0.35 mg
		17.6	8	0.08–0.4 mg
		19.8	9	0.09–0.45 mg
		22	10	0.1–0.5 mg
		24.2	11	0.11–0.55 mg
		26.4	12	0.12–0.6 mg
		28.6	13	0.13–0.65 mg
		30.8	14	0.14–0.7 mg
		33	15	0.15–0.75 mg
		35.2	16	0.16–0.8 mg
Succinylcholine chloride [Anectine, Quelicin]	1–1.5 mg/kg (IV/IO)	4.4	2	2–3 mg
		6.6	3	3–4.5 mg
		8.8	4	4–6 mg
		11	5	5–7.5 mg
		13.2	6	6–9 mg
		15.4	7	7–10.5 mg
		17.6	8	8–12 mg
		19.8	9	9–13.5 mg
		22	10	10–15 mg
		24.2	11	11–16.5 mg
		26.4	12	12–18 mg
		28.6	13	13–19.5 mg
		30.8	14	14–21 mg
		33	15	15–22.5 mg
		35.2	16	16–24 mg
Vecuronium bromide [Norcuron]	0.1 mg/kg (IV/IO initial dose)	4.4	2	0.2 mg
		6.6	3	0.3 mg
		8.8	4	0.4 mg
		11	5	0.5 mg
		13.2	6	0.6 mg
		15.4	7	0.7 mg
		17.6	8	0.8 mg
		19.8	9	0.9 mg

continues

Table 13-1a Pediatric Doses (Part I) (*Continued*)

Drug	Dose	lb	kg	Administer
		22	10	1 mg
		24.2	11	1.1 mg
		26.4	12	1.2 mg
		28.6	13	1.3 mg
		30.8	14	1.4 mg
		33	15	1.5 mg
		35.2	16	1.6 mg

NOTES ON TABLE:

1. Metaproterenol [Alupent] 5% inhalation solution is given to children ages 6 to 12 years at a dose of 0.1 to 0.2 mL diluted in 3 mL saline.
2. Terbutaline (not for patients younger than 12 years of age) 0.01 mg/kg (SC every 15–20 minutes with max dose of 0.25 mg)
3. Thiamine 10 to 25 mg (pediatric dose)
4. Verapamil [Isoptin] (not for patients younger than 12 years of age) 0.1 to 0.2 mg/kg (IV/IO over 2 minutes)
5. Glucagon 0.5 to 1 mg IM (children < 20 kg)

Table 13-1b Pediatric Doses (Part II, 39.6–88 lb)

Drug	Dose	lb	kg	Administer
Activated charcoal	1–2 g/kg	39.6	18	18–36 g
		44	20	20–40 g
		48.4	22	22–44 g
		52.8	24	24–48 g
		57.2	26	26–52 g
		61.6	28	28–56 g
		66	30	30–60 g
		70.4	32	32–64 g
		74.8	34	34–68 g
		79.2	36	36–72 g
		83.6	38	38–76 g
		88	40	40–80 g
Adenosine [Adenocard] or morphine sulfate [Astramorph/PF]	0.1–0.2 mg/kg	39.6	18	1.8–3.6 mg
		44	20	2–4 mg
		48.4	22	2.2–4.4 mg
		52.8	24	2.4–4.8 mg
		57.2	26	2.6–5.2 mg
		61.6	28	2.8–5.6 mg
		66	30	3–6 mg
		70.4	32	3.2–6.4 mg
		74.8	34	3.4–6.8 mg
		79.2	36	3.6–7.2 mg
		83.6	38	3.8–7.6 mg
		88	40	4–8 mg
Albuterol* [Proventil, Ventolin]	0.05–0.15 mg/kg (dilute in 2 mL of 0.9% normal saline)	39.6	18	0.9–2.7 mg
		44	20	1–3 mg
*NOTE: For children ages 2 to 12 the recommended albuterol solution is 0.083%. This strength is not recommended for children less than 15 kg. For adults and children over the age of 12, the albuterol solution used is the 0.5% solution. Most EMS		52.8	24	1.2–3.6 mg
		57.2	26	1.3–3.9 mg
		61.6	28	1.4–4.2 mg
		66	30	1.5–4.5 mg
		70.4	32	1.6–4.8 mg
		74.8	34	1.7–5.1 mg

continues

Table 13-1b Pediatric Doses (Part II) (*Continued*)

Drug	Dose	lb	kg	Administer
systems simply administer the same dose to adults and children of 2.5 mg (0.5 mL added to 2 mL or normal saline)		79.2	36	1.8–5.4 mg
		83.6	38	1.9–5.7 mg
		88	40	2–6 mg
Amiodarone [Cordarone, Pacerone] or phenytoin [Dilantin] (for arrhythmias)	5 mg/kg (for phenytoin administer slow IV with max dose of 1 g)	39.6	18	90 mg
		44	20	100 mg
		48.4	22	110 mg
		52.8	24	120 mg
		57.2	26	130 mg
		61.6	28	140 mg
		66	30	150 mg
		70.4	32	160 mg
		74.8	34	170 mg
		79.2	36	180 mg
		83.6	38	190 mg
		88	40	200 mg
Atropine sulfate	0.02 mg/kg (0.1 mg minimum)	39.6	18	0.36 mg
		44	20	0.4 mg
		48.4	22	0.44 mg
		52.8	24	0.48 mg
		57.2	26	0.52 mg
		61.6	28	0.56 mg
		66	30	0.6 mg
		70.4	32	0.64 mg
		74.8	34	0.68 mg
		79.2	36	0.72 mg
		83.6	38	0.76 mg
		88	40	0.8 mg
Calcium chloride	20 mg/kg	39.6	18	360 mg
		44	20	400 mg
		48.4	22	440 mg
		52.8	24	480 mg
		57.2	26	520 mg
		61.6	28	560 mg
		66	30	600 mg
		70.4	32	640 mg
		74.8	34	680 mg
		79.2	36	720 mg
		83.6	38	760 mg
		88	40	800 mg
Dextrose	0.5–1 g/kg	39.6	18	9–18 g
		44	20	10–20 g
		48.4	22	11–22 g
		52.8	24	12–24 g
		57.2	26	13–26 g
		61.6	28	14–28 g
		66	30	15–30 g
		70.4	32	16–32 g
		74.8	34	17–34 g
		79.2	36	18–36 g
		83.6	38	19–38 g
		88	40	20–40 g

continues

Table 13-1b Pediatric Doses (Part II) (*Continued*)

Drug	Dose	lb	kg	Administer
Diazepam [Valium]	0.2–0.5 mg/kg (higher dose for rectal)	39.6	18	3.6–9 mg
		44	20	4–10 mg
		48.4	22	4.4–11 mg
		52.8	24	4.8–12 mg
		57.2	26	5.2–13 mg
		61.6	28	5.6–14 mg
		66	30	6–15 mg
		70.4	32	6.4–16 mg
		74.2	34	6.8–17 mg
		79.2	36	7.2–18 mg
		83.6	38	7.6–19 mg
		88	40	8–20 mg
Diphenhydramine [Benadryl], meperidine hydrochloride [Demerol], or methylprednisolone sodium succinate [Solu-Medrol] (for asthma)	1–2 mg/kg	39.6	18	18–36 mg
		44	20	20–40 mg
		48.4	22	22–44 mg
		52.8	24	24–48 mg
		57.2	26	26–52 mg
		61.6	28	28–56 mg
		66	30	30–60 mg
		70.4	32	32–64 mg
		74.8	34	34–68 mg
		79.2	36	36–72 mg
		83.6	38	38–76 mg
		88	40	40–80 mg
Dobutamine [Dobutrex] or dopamine [Intropin]	2–20 μg/kg/min	39.6	18	36–360 μg/min
		44	20	40–400 μg/min
		48.4	22	44–440 μg/min
		52.8	24	48–480 μg/min
		57.2	26	52–520 μg/min
		61.6	28	56–560 μg/min
		66	30	60–600 μg/min
		70.4	32	64–640 μg/min
		74.8	34	68–680 μg/min
		79.2	36	72–720 μg/min
		83.6	38	76–760 μg/min
		88	40	80–800 μg/min
Epinephrine [Adrenalin]	0.01 mg/kg of 1:1,000 solution SC for mild allergic reaction or asthma (max 0.3 mL); 0.01 mg/kg of 1:10,000 solution for cardiac arrest or bradycardia	39.6	18	0.18 mg
		44	20	0.2 mg
		48.4	22	0.22 mg
		52.8	24	0.24 mg
		57.2	26	0.26 mg
		61.6	28	0.28 mg
		66	30	0.3 mg
		70.4	32	0.32 mg
		74.8	34	0.34 mg
		79.2	36	0.36 mg
		83.6	38	0.38 mg
		88	40	0.4 mg
Furosemide [Lasix] and lidocaine hydrochloride [Xylocaine]	1 mg/kg (for lidocaine hydrochloride [Xylocaine], max of 100 mg)	39.6	18	18 mg
		44	20	20 mg
		48.4	22	22 mg
		52.8	24	24 mg
		57.2	26	26 mg

continues

Table 13-1b Pediatric Doses (Part II) (*Continued*)

Drug	Dose	lb	kg	Administer
		61.6	28	28 mg
		66	30	30 mg
		70.4	32	32 mg
		74.8	34	34 mg
		79.2	36	36 mg
		83.6	38	38 mg
		88	40	40 mg
Hydroxyzine hydrochloride [Atarax, Vistaril]	0.5–1 mg/kg IM	39.6	18	9–18 mg
		44	20	10–20 mg
		48.4	22	11–22 mg
		52.8	24	12–24 mg
		57.2	26	13–26 mg
		61.6	28	14–28 mg
		66	30	15–30 mg
		70.4	32	16–32 mg
		74.8	34	17–34 mg
		79.2	36	18–36 mg
		83.6	38	19–38 mg
		88	40	20–40 mg
Isoetharine [Bronchosol, Bronkometer]	0.01 mL/kg (dilute in 3 mL normal saline and nebulize) (max 0.5 mL)	39.6	18	0.18 mL
		44	20	0.2 mL
		48.4	22	0.22 mL
		52.8	24	0.24 mL
		57.2	26	0.26 mL
		61.6	28	0.28 mL
		66	30	0.3 mL
		70.4	32	0.32 mL
		74.8	34	0.34 mL
		79.2	36	0.36 mL
		83.6	38	0.38 mL
		88	40	0.4 mL
Lorazepam [Ativan]	0.05–0.20 mg/kg (slow IV/IO) (max dose 0.2 mg/kg)	39.6	18	0.9–3.6 mg
		44	20	1–4 mg
		48.4	22	1.1–4.4 mg
		52.8	24	1.2–4.8 mg
		57.2	26	1.3–5.2 mg
		61.6	28	1.4–5.6 mg
		66	30	1.5–6 mg
		70.4	32	1.6–6.4 mg
		74.8	34	1.7–6.8 mg
		79.2	36	1.8–7.2 mg
		83.6	38	1.9–7.6 mg
		88	40	2–8 mg
Magnesium sulfate	25–50 mg/kg (infusion over 10–20 minutes) (max dose 2 g)	39.6	18	450–900 mg
		44	20	500–1,000 mg
		48.4	22	550–1,100 mg
		52.8	24	600–1,200 mg
		57.2	26	650–1,300 mg
		61.6	28	700–1,400 mg
		66	30	750–1,500 mg
		70.4	32	800–1,600 mg

continues

Table 13-1b Pediatric Doses (Part II) (*Continued*)

Drug	Dose	lb	kg	Administer
		74.8	34	850–1,700 mg
		79.2	36	900–1,800 mg
		83.6	38	950–1,900 mg
		88	40	1–2 g
Methylprednisolone sodium succinate [Solu-Medrol] (usually in the ED setting although some regions do administer in the field)	For acute spinal trauma 30 mg/kg IV (over 30 minutes)	39.6	18	540 mg
		44	20	600 mg
		48.4	22	660 mg
		52.8	24	720 mg
		57.2	26	780 mg
		61.6	28	840 mg
		66	30	900 mg
		70.4	32	960 mg
		74.8	34	1.02 g
		79.2	36	1.08 g
		83.6	38	1.14 g
		88	40	1.2 g
Naloxone hydrochloride [Narcan] or pancuronium bromide [Pavulon]	0.1 mg/kg (naloxone hydrochloride max dose of 0.8 mg) (pancuronium, slow IV/IO)	39.6	18	1.8 mg (Narcan max dose 0.8mg)
		44	20	2 mg
		48.4	22	2.2 mg
		52.8	24	2.4 mg
		57.2	26	2.6 mg
		61.6	28	2.8 mg
		66	30	3 mg
		70.4	32	3.2 mg
		74.8	34	3.4 mg
		79.2	36	3.6 mg
		83.6	38	3.8 mg
		88	40	4 mg
Norepinephrine bitartrate [Levophed, Levarterenol]	0.1–1.0 µg/min (IV infusion)	39.6	18	1.8–18 µg/min
		44	20	2–20 µg/min
		48.4	22	2.2–22 µg/min
		52.8	24	2.4–24 µg/min
		57.2	26	2.6–26 µg/min
		61.6	28	2.8–28 µg/min
		66	30	3–30 µg/min
		70.4	32	3.2–32 µg/min
		74.8	34	3.4–34 µg/min
		79.2	36	3.6–36 µg/min
		83.6	38	3.8–38 µg/min
		88	40	4–40 µg/min
Phenobarbital [Luminal] or phenytoin [Dilantin] (for seizures)	10–20 mg/kg (IV/IO) (phenytoin slow IV)	39.6	18	180–360 mg
		44	20	200–400 mg
		48.4	22	220–440 mg
		52.8	24	240–480 mg
		57.2	26	260–520 mg

continues

Table 13-1b Pediatric Doses (Part II) (*Continued*)

Drug	Dose	lb	kg	Administer
		61.6	28	280–560 mg
		66	30	300–600 mg
		70.4	32	320–640 mg
		74.8	34	340–680 mg
		79.2	36	360–720 mg
		83.6	38	380–760 mg
		88	40	400–800 mg
Pralidoxime chloride [2-PAM chloride, Protopam]	20–40 mg/kg (IV over 15–30 minutes)	39.6	18	360–720 mg
		44	20	400–800 mg
		48.4	22	440–880 mg
		52.8	24	480–960 mg
		57.2	26	520–1,040 mg
		61.6	28	560–1,120 mg
		66	30	600–1,200 mg
		70.4	32	640–1,280 mg
		74.8	34	680–1,360 mg
		79.2	36	720–1,440 mg
		83.6	38	760–1,520 mg
		88	40	800–1,600 mg
Procainamide hydrochloride [Procanbid, Pronestyl]	15 mg/kg (IV/IO over 30–60 minutes)	39.6	18	270 mg
		44	20	300 mg
		48.4	22	330 mg
		52.8	24	360 mg
		57.2	26	390 mg
		61.6	28	420 mg
		66	30	450 mg
		70.4	32	480 mg
		74.8	34	510 mg
		79.2	36	540 mg
		83.6	38	570 mg
		88	40	600 mg
Promethazine hydrochlodride [Phenergan] (over 2 years old)	0.25–0.5 mg/kg IM	39.6	18	4.5–9 mg
		44	20	5–10 mg
		48.4	22	5.5–11 mg
		52.8	24	6–12 mg
		57.2	26	6.5–13 mg
		61.6	28	7–14 mg
		66	30	7.5–15 mg
		70.4	32	8–16 mg
		74.8	34	8.5–17 mg
		79.2	36	9–18 mg
		83.6	38	9.5–19 mg
		88	40	10–20 mg

continues

Table 13-1b Pediatric Doses (Part II) (*Continued*)

Drug	Dose	lb	kg	Administer
Propranolol hydrochloride [Inderal]	0.01–0.05 mg/kg (slow IV, max dose 3 mg)	39.6	18	0.18–0.9 mg
		44	20	0.20–1 mg
		48.4	22	0.22–1.1 mg
		52.8	24	0.24–1.2 mg
		57.2	26	0.26–1.3 mg
		61.6	28	0.28–1.4 mg
		66	30	0.30–1.5 mg
		70.4	32	0.32–1.6 mg
		74.8	34	0.34–1.7 mg
		79.2	36	0.36–1.8 mg
		83.6	38	0.38–1.9 mg
		88	40	0.40–2 mg
Succinylcholine chloride [Anectine, Quelicin]	1–1.5 mg/kg (IV/IO)	39.6	18	18–27 mg
		44	20	20–30 mg
		48.4	22	22–33 mg
		52.8	24	24–36 mg
		57.2	26	26–39 mg
		61.6	28	28–42 mg
		66	30	30–45 mg
		70.4	32	32–48 mg
		74.8	34	34–51 mg
		79.2	36	36–54 mg
		83.6	38	38–57 mg
		88	40	40–60 mg
Vecuronium bromide [Norcuron]	0.1 mg/kg (IV/IO initial dose)	39.6	18	1.8 mg
		44	20	2 mg
		48.4	22	2.2 mg
		52.8	24	2.4 mg
		57.2	26	2.6 mg
		61.6	28	2.8 mg
		66	30	3 mg
		70.4	32	3.2 mg
		74.8	34	3.4 mg
		79.2	36	3.6 mg
		83.6	38	3.8 mg
		88	40	4 mg

Respiratory Emergencies

Respiratory emergencies are one of the most common pediatric medical complaints. The pediatric airway is smaller in proportion to that of an adult and the airway anatomy predisposes children to developing obstructions. These obstructions can come from foreign objects getting lodged in the upper airways, secretions in the lower airways, bronchoconstriction, swelling, or any combination. Signs and symptoms of respiratory failure are outlined in **Table 13-2 ▸**. Asthma, bronchiolitis,

Table 13-2 Signs of Respiratory Failure

Assess	Sign
Mental status	Agitation, restlessness, confusion, lethargy (VPU of AVPU)
Skin color	Cyanosis, pallor
Respiratory rate	Tachypnea → bradypnea → apnea
Respiratory effort	Severe retractions, nasal flaring, grunting, paradoxical abdominal motion, tripod positioning
Auscultation	Stridor, wheezing, rales, or diminished air movement
Blood oxygen saturation	< 90% with supplemental oxygen
Pulse rate	Tachycardia, bradycardia, or cardiac arrest

Table 13-3 Common Pediatric Respiratory Conditions

Condition	Description	Typical Treatment
Asthma	Most common respiratory condition. Lower airway emergency. Constriction of the lower airways with mucus production. Often associated with a history of environmental allergy and/or bronchospasm. Many children grow out of this disease as the airway gets larger.	Supplemental oxygen; bronchodilators may be delivered by nebulizer or metered-dose inhaler. 2.5 mg albuterol [Proventil] premixed with 2 mL of normal saline (for severe distress in the adolescent, as it is not commonly used with younger children, consider 5 mg albuterol [Proventil]). Albuterol and inhaled ipratropium bromide [Atrovent] together may also be effective. Levalbuterol [Xopenex] has fewer side effects than albuterol. For severe distress or diminished air movement, epinephrine [Adrenalin] SC or IM may be required (0.01 mg/kg of 1:1,000). A smooth muscle relaxer (ie, magnesium sulfate) and an anti-inflammatory corticosteroid (ie, methylprednisolone sodium succinate) may also be considered.
Bronchiolitis	Lower airway emergency. Viral infection in the bronchioles causing inflammation. Associated with infections in the upper airways. Predominantly affects infants and young toddlers.	Position the child comfortably. Provide supplemental oxygen. Use of bronchodilators (ie, inhaled albuterol [Proventil], or nebulized racemic epinephrine [Micronefrin]), 0.5 mL of a 2.25% solution for inhalation may be given for moderate to severe respiratory distress.
Croup	Upper airway emergency. Viral infection affecting the upper airways producing subglottic swelling of the soft tissues.	Keep child calm; nebulized epinephrine (racemic: 0.5 mL mixed in 3 mL of normal saline. L-epinephrine: 0.25 to 0.5 mg/kg of the 1:1,000 solution, can be diluted with normal saline to bring volume to 3 mL). May need to assist ventilations with a bag-mask device.
Epiglottitis and Bacterial Infections	Upper airway emergency. Viral or bacterial infection affecting the epiglottis. It is potentially lethal, producing swelling of the epiglottis.	Keep child calm, provide supplemental oxygen if tolerable. Expeditious transport to a capable center with early notification to the receiving facility.
Anaphylaxis	Upper airway emergency. A potentially life-threatening allergic reaction triggered by exposure to an antigen. Nuts, shellfish, eggs, milk, and bee stings are common causes of anaphylaxis in children.	Epinephrine [Adrenalin] via SC or IM; 0.01 mg/kg of the 1:1,000 solution to a maximum dose of 0.3 mg. Include supplemental oxygen, diphenhydramine [Benadryl] for its antihistamine effect, and fluid resuscitation for shock.

croup, epiglottitis, and anaphylaxis are common causes of respiratory emergencies in children. **Table 13-3▲** contains a description of the common respiratory conditions and how they are managed. The normal respiratory rates of children are listed in **Table 13-4▶**.

The asthma triad shows the primary components of asthma and the corresponding treatments for each (**Figure 13-2▶**). The treatments are described in more detail in the following sections.

Table 13-4 Normal Respiratory Rates by Age

Age	Respiratory Rate (breaths/min)
Infant	25–50
Toddler	20–30
Preschool-age child	20–25
School-age child	15–20
Adolescent	12–16

Special Needs Tip

Good ventilations are sometimes noisy. When you evaluate breath sounds you may hear wheezing, either loud or diminished. You may also encounter absent breath sounds even though the child is breathing. Opting to give a bronchodilator is prudent in these cases. You can anticipate an improvement of the breath sounds. However, sometimes the breath sounds may become very noisy, indicating turbulence in the air passages. If this occurs, DO NOT PANIC! Recall that quiet or silent breathing in the patient with respiratory distress is not a good sign; it is indicative of significant bronchoconstriction or obstruction. If the breath sounds become noisier, it is usually a sign that more air is passing through the respiratory tree. Increased turbulence due to increased air movement is a positive sign, especially in the patient that had little to no air movement initially. Continue your therapy, and continue reassessing breath sounds. Be observant for exhaustion associated with exacerbation of respiratory distress.

When a child in respiratory distress is grunting, this is a "red flag" that the child is in severe distress and must be given close attention and care. The sound is usually associated with the closing of the glottic opening at the end of the exhalation to maintain back pressure in the alveoli to help to avoid their collapse (atelectisis). It requires great effort on the part of the patient to provide positive end-expiratory pressure (PEEP), and this effort can be exhausting over time. Children in respiratory distress due to lower airway disease do not get better on their own. If a child is wheezing and in distress and he or she begins to quiet down prior to administration of a bronchodilator, this is most likely due to decreased air movement as a result of tiring, which can be deadly.

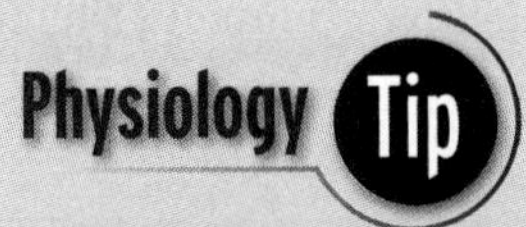

Management of patients in respiratory distress should consist of three components: bronchodilation, fluid replacement, and the treatment of inflammation.

Bronchodilators

Bronchodilation is accomplished by providing the patient with a bronchodilator medication. Some inhaled bronchodilatory medications are much better for overall patient care. Frequently, patients in respiratory distress will have an elevated heart rate. Bronchodilators such as Albuterol [Proventil], a sympathomimetic, and ipratropium bromide [Atrovent], a parasympatholytic, do an excellent job dilating the bronchi but have a side effect of elevating the heart rate. Medications such as levalbuterol [Xopenex] have the same desired effect on the bronchi but with less of an effect on the heart rate. Another thing to determine is whether your patient has been using his or her personal inhaler frequently (typically albuterol [Proventil] or ipratropium bromide [Atrovent]). A nebulized dose of the same medication may not have the desired effect. Many paramedic systems only use the albuterol [Proventil] mix with ipratropium bromide [Atrovent] with older children (adolescents) because the research on smaller children is not supportive at this time. Switching to a different medication may provide a much better outcome for the patient. If a different medication is not available, you may wish to consider an infusion of magnesium sulfate.

Magnesium sulfate is a potent, smooth-muscle relaxant that is extremely effective at dilating the air passages of patients in severe respiratory distress. The pediatric dose is 25 to 50 mg/kg IV drip, administered over 10 to 20 minutes. This is usually accomplished by mixing 1 g of the medication in 100 mL of 0.9% normal saline, which will produce a 10 mg/1 mL mixture (ie, a 20-kg child would get 20 × 25 = 500 mg or half the bag [50 mL] over the 10 to 20 minutes).

Airway edema
Treat with corticosteroids

Increased mucous production
Treat with water and expectorants

Bronchospasm
Treat with bronchodilator

Figure 13-2 The asthma triad demonstrates the three primary components of asthma, and the corresponding treatments for each component.

Epinephrine [Adrenalin]

Epinephrine [Adrenalin] 1:1,000 has fallen out of favor with most pulmonologists because of its severe effects on the heart, which could precipitate myocardial ischemia or worse, an infarction, even in a child. Furthermore, epinephrine [Adrenalin] 1:1,000 is more effective at dilating the upper airway than the lower airways where most airway disease manifests. Still recommended for cases of moderate to severe anaphylaxis, epinephrine [Adrenalin] is administered to those children at a dose of 0.1 mL/kg, (0.1 mL/kg).

Fluid Replacement Therapy

Fluid replacement should be part of the management plan. Patients in respiratory distress breathe faster and dry out their respiratory mucosal membranes faster than healthy individuals would. Approximately 10% of water is lost during normal ventilation. The patient who is breathing faster will lose water faster, thereby more quickly drying out the respiratory tree and respiratory secretions. Patients should be given a fluid bolus of 10 to 20 mL/kg of 0.9% normal saline to rehydrate the respiratory tree and aid in moistening concretions.

Corticosteroids

When bronchoconstriction occurs, inflammation of the airway begins. This process is slow and may take several hours to fully develop. Cases of prolonged bronchoconstriction that have remained refractory to bronchodilators are due to significant inflammation of the respiratory tree. This is commonly referred to as a "rebound effect." The only medications that may be able to break this are corticosteroids such as methylprednisolone sodium succinate [Solu-Medrol] or dexamethasone sodium phosphate [Decadron]. These medications work over several hours, slowing down and limiting the extent of the inflammation. So it is crucial that these medications be given early during the management of acute respiratory distress.

Continuous Positive Airway Pressure (CPAP)

A relatively new method of managing patients suffering from acute respiratory distress in the prehospital setting includes the use of continuous positive airway pressure (CPAP). CPAP is used to force enriched oxygen into the alveolar tissue. When combined with a nebulized bronchodilator, it will not only dilate the most distal respiratory tissues, but also improve the hypoxia.

Case Study 1 Respiratory Emergency

Part 1

Your unit has been dispatched to a middle school where a 12-year-old child is having difficulty breathing during gym class. You are instructed to report to the nurse's office and you understand that the child's parent has already been called. On arrival the scene is safe and you and your partner load equipment onto the stretcher and enter the school. A hall monitor leads you to the office. As you enter, you can hear the child's wheezing. The patient, Tommy Jones, was playing dodge ball and seemed to be having an asthma attack. The nurse has checked the boy's records, and found that he is on a number of medications for his asthma. She said that his mother is already en route and should be there in about 5 to 10 minutes.

Seeing that Tommy is in obvious distress, you introduce yourself and begin the initial assessment while your partner sets up a nonrebreathing mask (see **Table 1**). Tommy is scared, in the tripod position, and in obvious distress, yet still able to answer your questions and follow instructions.

Due to the lack of any trauma and the chief complaint of respiratory distress, you will need to do a focused history and physical examination on a responsive medical patient after completing your initial assessment.

Table 1 Initial Assessment

Initial Assessment	Recording Time: 2 Minutes
General Impression/ Appearance	Young conscious male in distress
Mental Status	Alert (oriented to person, place, and day); speaking in short choppy sentences
Airway	Open but partial lower obstruction
Breathing	Rapid, noisy (expiratory wheezes), and labored
Circulation	Rapid radial pulse
Priority/Plan	High due to respiratory distress

Question 1: If the child has a life threat, can you treat him if the school nurse is present?

Question 2: Would it be likely that the child may have already self-administered his prescribed inhaler prior to your arrival?

Case Study I Continued

Part 2

With a chief complaint of breathing difficulty, you proceed to ask the OPQRST questions to elaborate on the chief complaint. Meanwhile, your partner gets a set of baseline vital signs. You decide to switch the nonrebreathing mask to a nebulizer treatment after listening to Tommy's lung sounds. He now seems to have both inspiratory and expiratory wheezing. The rest of your assessment, after completing the initial assessment, will include the focused history and physical examination of a responsive medical patient (see **Table 2**). Tommy is able to answer many of your questions, although he is speaking only a few words at a time and you are concerned because he seems to be getting worse.

Table 2 Focused History and Physical Examination

Baseline Vital Signs	Recording Time: 5 Minutes
Skin CTC (color, temperature, condition)	Pale, cool, and dry
Pulse	128 beats/min and regular
Blood Pressure	84/68 mm Hg
Respirations	26 breaths/min and labored

Question 3: What would you expect to see as a normal pulse rate for a school-aged child?

Question 4: What would you expect to see as a normal respiratory rate for a school-aged child?

Part 3

You begin to ask Tommy a few questions about his medical history as his mother arrives at the school. She is calm and collected and it is obvious that she has been in this situation before. She immediately asks him "How tight is your chest?" "When did this start?" And, of course, "Why were you playing dodge ball?" Tommy continues to wheeze but you sense he is not increasing in his anxiety level due to his mother's line of questioning. He seems rather comforted that she is now on the scene.

You begin to talk with Mrs. Jones about Tommy's SAMPLE history (see **Table 3**).

Table 3 SAMPLE History

SAMPLE History	Comments
Signs/symptoms	Nasal flaring, use of accessory muscles, and an overall tired look
Allergies	There is a long list of allergens, mostly due to environmental substances.
Medications	Budesonide [Pulmicort], and albuterol [Proventil]
Pertinent past medical history	Has had asthma since he was about 2 years old. It is worse in the springtime and fall. Sometimes also made worse by exercise, thus the "no dodge ball rule."
Last oral intake	Breakfast about 3 hours ago
Events leading up to the incident	A little short of breath all day, respiratory distress increased during exercise at school

Treatment Plan

1. Ensure the ABCs are maintained.
2. Obtain baseline vital signs and lung sounds.
3. Provide airway management with supplemental oxygen by nonrebreathing mask.
4. Administer albuterol [Proventil] 2.5 mg (0.5 mL) in 2 mL normal saline via nebulizer (see **Table 4**). This dose can be repeated up to three times as needed.
5. Monitor the ECG for cardiac irritability.
6. Reassess the patient's lung sounds. Since the condition is severe, and if the nebulizer is not successful, you should consider the following medications:
   a. Epinephrine [Adrenalin] 1:1,000 dose 0.01 mg/kg SC (max dose of 0.5 mg) (see **Table 5**).
   b. If the patient is not improving, obtain vascular access and consider IV fluids and methylprednisolone sodium succinate [Solu-Medrol] 1 mg/kg IV (see **Table 6**).
   c. Can also administer epinephrine [Adrenalin] 1:1,000 dose 0.3 mg mixed with 3 mL of normal saline via nebulizer.
   d. Consider the need for treatment of refractory bronchospasms with a methylxanthine [Aminophylline, Somophyllin] or smooth muscle calcium antagonist (magnesium sulfate).
7. Reassess and transport to the ED (if not already doing so at this point).

Case Study 1 Continued

In some EMS systems and with older children (ie, adolescents), paramedics are trained to only use an albuterol [Proventil] and ipratropium bromide [Atrovent] mix as is done commonly with adults (see Chapter 3). The research on smaller children is not supportive at this time.

Table 4 Albuterol

Do you know?	Comments
Right drug? Generic name: [**Albuterol**] Trade name: [Proventil, Ventolin]	Used to treat wheezing, cough, and dyspnea from reactive airways. Often patients may have already-self-administered by a metered-dose inhaler (MDI), most effectively used with a spacer device. This is one of the typical drugs that EMT-Basics are trained to assist the patient with (provided the medication is prescribed to the patient). In some regions, the Basic-level ambulances actually carry MDIs or nebulizers.
Right patient?	The patient with reactive airway disease who has bronchoconstriction.
Right dose?	A spray from an MDI canister delivers approximately 90 µg per actuation. Each canister contains 17 g and is designed to administer up to 200 doses. When given by paramedics in the field, the MDI is usually not used. The administration method in the field by paramedics is via nebulizer. For adults and children ages 2 to 12, the recommended dose of albuterol solution 0.083 percent is one vial (2.5 mg) three to four times daily using a nebulizer. This strength of albuterol is not recommended for children that weigh less than 15 kg (about seven pounds). For adults and children age 12 and over, the recommended dose of albuterol solution 0.5 percent is 2.5 mg three to four times daily using a nebulizer. Thus, this is why most EMS systems administer the same dose of 2.5 mg (0.5 mL) added to 2 mL of normal saline to adults and pediatrics.
Right route?	Given as an MDI, as a nebulizer treatment, or may be ventilated into the patient using a bag-mask device.
Right time?	Typically the first-line agent in asthma. While the patient is still able to breathe and hold his/her breath.
Right documentation?	Document the administration of the medication as well as the ongoing assessment findings, including lung sounds, on the patient care report.
Expected action	Bronchodilation and ease of breathing with less wheezing and improved airflow and gas exchange.
Side effects	Although there are many potential side effects, these are almost all minimal and very well tolerated by patients. They may include: tremulousness, anxiety, nausea, vomiting, cough, throat irritation, difficulty swallowing, and hoarseness. Palpitations and tachycardia may indicate a serious adrenergic response in the heart.
Contraindications	Known prior hypersensitivity reactions to albuterol. Tachycardia arrhythmias, especially those caused by digitalis. Synergistic with other sympathomimetics.
Precautions	Shallow respirations may prevent drug delivery when an MDI is used. Always shake the MDI before administration.
Pharmacokinetics	Onset: 5–15 minutes; peak effect: 30 minutes to 2 hours; duration: 3–4 hours.

Table 5 Epinephrine Hydrochloride

Do you know?	Comments
Right drug? Generic name: [**Epinephrine Hydrochloride**] 1:10,000 or 1:1,000 Trade name: [Adrenalin Chloride]	Sympathomimetic drug that is a direct-acting alpha and beta agonist. In asthma, the drug is given for its beta-2 stimulation. It also has alpha and beta-1 effects that are discussed in Chapter 1.
Right patient?	Used for the patient experiencing a severe allergic reaction or asthma attack.
Right dose?	In a mild allergic reaction or asthma, the patient is given 0.01 mg/kg up to 0.3 mg SC of the 1:1,000 solution. In a severe reaction, 0.01 mg/kg up to 0.3 mg epinephrine hydrochloride [Adrenalin chloride] 1:10,000 via IV/IO route. EpiPen auto-injectors are all 1:1,000 concentration, 0.15 or 0.3 mg administered IM.

continues

Case Study I Continued

Table 5 Epinephrine Hydrochloride (*Continued*)

Do you know?	Comments
Right route?	Given by the SC injection. If the patient is severe it can be given by the IV route, but the concentration used is the 1:10,000. For a severe allergic reaction or anaphylaxis, it is given by the IM route with the use of an EpiPen auto-injector. (EpiPens are all 1:1,000 concentration, 0.15 or 0.3 mg, IM auto-injected only.)
Right time?	1:1,000 is rarely used in cases of a severe refractory asthma attack. If the asthma is severe, the patient can be given 0.01 mg/kg up to 0.3 mg epinephrine hydrochloride [Adrenalin chloride] 1:10,000 via IV/IO route.
Right documentation?	Document the administration of the medication as well as the ongoing assessment findings, including vital signs, 12-lead ECG tracings, and lung sounds, on the patient care report.
Expected action	Immediate action of bronchial smooth muscle relaxation and dilation of the skeletal vasculature.
Side effects	Hypertension, tachycardias, arrhythmias, anxiety, restlessness, psychomotor agitation, nausea, headache, angina, and myocardial infarction. It may increase the myocardial oxygen demand. It potentiates other sympathomimetics and is deactivated by alkaline solutions.
Contraindications	Hypertension, hypothermia, pulmonary edema, acute coronary syndrome, and hypovolemic shock.
Precautions	Use with caution in diabetes mellitus, tuberculosis, long-standing asthma, elevated heart rates. SC route is ineffective in poor perfusion states (ie, delayed capillary refill).
Pharmacokinetics	Onset: immediate IV, 5–15 minutes SC/IM; peak effect: 5–30 minutes; duration 1–3 hours. Metabolism takes place in both liver and other tissues by monoamine oxidase (MAO) and catechol-O-methyltransferase (COMT) to inactive metabolites.

Table 6 Methylprednisolone Sodium Succinate

Do you know?	Comments
Right drug? Generic name: [**Methylprednisolone Sodium Succinate**] Trade name: [Solu-Medrol]	A potent anti-inflammatory glucocorticoid, it is a synthetic corticosteroid that suppresses inflammation. It also potentiates vascular smooth muscle relaxation by beta-adrenergic agonism.
Right patient?	Used with the acute spinal cord trauma patient, anaphylaxis, and as a bronchodilator for unresponsive acute asthmatics.
Right dose?	For asthma, children should receive 1–2 mg/kg IV.
Right route?	Given by the IV route.
Right time?	Administered to the asthmatic who is not responsive to other therapy.
Right documentation?	Document the administration of the medication as well as the ongoing assessment findings, including lung sounds, on the patient care report.
Expected action	Used as a bronchodilator for asthma. Also can be used for anaphylaxis.
Side effects	May cause headache, hypertension, sodium and water retention, congestive heart failure, hypokalemia, alkalosis, peptic ulcer disease, nausea or vomiting.
Contraindications	Virtually none in the setting of single-dose prehospital administration. Some sources do not recommend use for premature infants and patients with fungal infections.
Precautions	Use with caution in patients with gastrointestinal bleeding. The drug can interact by blunting the effects of insulin and hypoglycemic agents. Potassium-depleting agents may exacerbate hypokalemic effects.
Pharmacokinetics	Onset: 1–2 hours; peak effect: variable; duration of action: 8–24 hours.

Case Study I Continued

Question 5: If prior to administering a bronchodilator the child begins to get a quieter chest, what does this indicate?

Question 6: When should you start an IV on a pediatric patient in respiratory distress?

Part 4

After administering the nebulizer treatment twice, you note that Tommy starts to look like he is in less distress en route to the ED. He is able to talk in full sentences and that mottled grey coloring is turning to a normal color. He is having a conversation with his mother as you load the stretcher into the back of the ambulance. Next you will get another set of vital signs and listen to his lungs one more time. This is the reassessment stage (see **Table 7**). En route, you will give the ED a quick report on his condition and the fact that the medication was helpful.

Question 7: Why does the prevalence of asthma decrease as children get older?

Question 8: If a child in respiratory distress was grunting, what does that indicate?

Table 7 Reassessment and Ongoing Assessment of the Patient

Serial Vital Signs and Relevant Data	Recording Time: 10 Minutes
Skin CTC	Normal color and temperature, dry
Pulse	120 beats/min regular and strong
Blood Pressure	80/64 mm Hg
Respirations	22 breaths/min and shallow
Mental status	Alert (oriented to person, place, and day)
ECG	Sinus tachycardia with no ectopy
SpO_2	95% with supplemental oxygen
Lung sounds	Expiratory wheezing (less than previously) yet flow is getting better
Other (ie, glucose, core body temperature)	Seems to be less work of breathing

Part 5

The ride to the ED is basically uneventful. Tommy is looking much better so all the therapy you provided was helpful. You have a nice conversation with his mother and he chimes in occasionally.

Fortunately, this call had a good outcome. Not all asthmatics are as fortunate as Tommy, as asthma is a very serious disease that can be life-threatening at times.

Beware When Suctioning a Child

Stimulation of the **tenth cranial nerve** (vagus nerve) can cause the heart rate to slow down. Younger children are especially susceptible to vagal stimuli and have been known to have their heart rates plummet when a rescuer inadvertently stimulated the vagus for too long a period of time. Vagal stimulation occurs via a variety of mechanisms, including pressure on the eyeballs, irritation to the back of the throat that would potentially cause gagging or retching, pressure over the anterior neck and carotid bodies, ice to the front of the face, and bearing down as in trying to move the bowels. All of this is important to know when you need to manage the airway with pharyngeal suction or airway placement, or when placing an endotracheal tube (**Figure 13-3** ▸).

Children in need of these interventions should be placed on a cardiac monitor and watched for evidence of vagal stimulation and bradycardia.

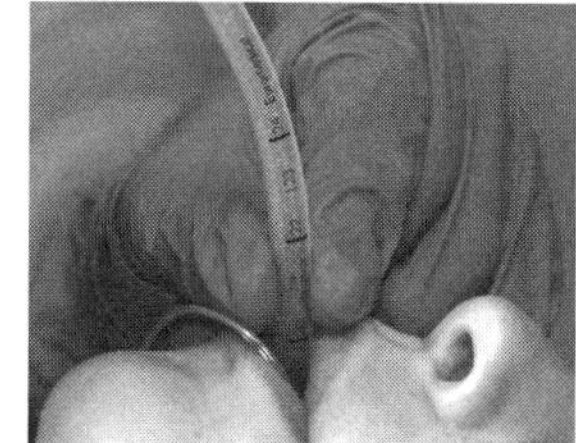

Figure 13-3 Endotracheal tube placement.

Toxicology Emergencies

One of the problems that occurs in pediatric patients, particularly the toddler and preschool age groups, is poisoning. As discussed in Chapter 9, poisoning occurs by four major routes: ingestion, inhalation, injection, and absorption through the skin. Toddlers and

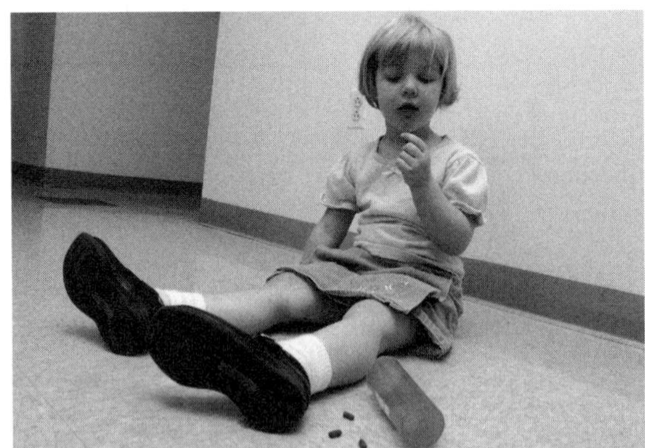

Figure 13-4 Children will put many things into their mouths, including dangerous medications.

preschool children tend to explore all things, whether or not they are familiar with them (**Figure 13-4**▲).

This includes food containers. To avoid poisoning, never transfer dangerous substances into food product containers (eg, paint thinner stored in an old milk container) as children are likely to drink from the container.

The products stored under the sink (ie, cleaners, alcohol, and petroleum-based products) are a common problem. They may come packaged in visually appealing containers, often with a pleasing scent attached to them (**Figure 13-5**▸).

Often a preventable situation, small children are likely to become poisoned by ingestion of toxic substances they come in contact with when unsupervised by an adult. Fortunately, the poison control centers tell us that most of these incidents are not fatal poisonings. All hazardous substances should be kept in the proper containers and out of reach of children.

Poisonous plants found around the home can include: angel's trumpet (Datura meteloides), azalea (Rhododendron), Jerusalem cherry (Solanum pseudocapsicum), and Jimsonweed (Datura stramonium). Other examples of potentially lethal ingestions and their common uses are shown in **Table 13-5**▼.

Older children (ie, school-aged children and adolescents) have been injured by intentional exposure to inhalants (ie, huffing) and overdose of recreational or prescription drugs. The common drugs used by these two age groups would include: alcohol, nicotine, marijuana, LSD, PCP, hashish, central nervous system stimulants (ie, cocaine, crack, and amphetamines), CNS depressants (ie, barbiturates), and hydrocarbons and fluorocarbons (ie, kerosene, naphtha, glue, chloroform, and aerosol products).

With the exception of food poisoning, poisonings usually involve substances that were not typically intended for human consumption and overdoses usually involve substances (most frequently medicines) that were designed for human consumption but have been taken, either accidentally or purposefully, in excess.

The management of a toxicologic emergency includes attention to the ABCs, decontamination, and a possible antidote (**Table 13-6**▸). The dose depends on the weight of the child.

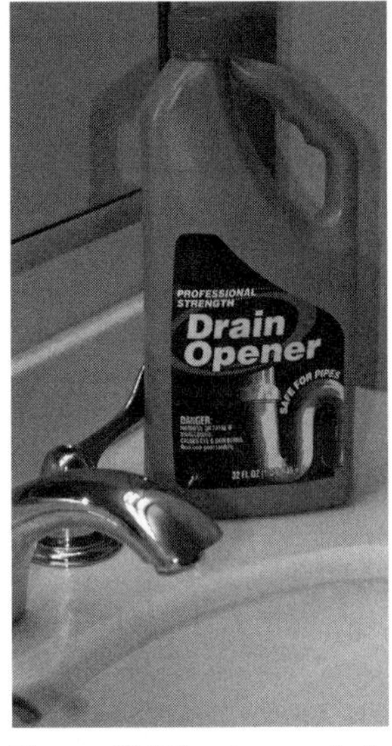

Figure 13-5 Cleaning products and other harmful agents should be stored out of the reach of children.

Table 13-5 Examples of Potentially Lethal Toddler Ingestion

Medicine	Source/Use	Lethal Dose
Camphor	Ketone derived from a tree or produced synthetically; counterirritant for infections and in the treatment of pain and itching	One teaspoon of oil
Chloroquine	Synthetic substance; used to control malaria attacks	One 500-mg tablet
Clonidine	Synthetic substance; used in the treatment of high blood pressure	One 0.3-mg tablet
Glyburide	Hypoglycemic substance; used in the treatment of diabetes mellitus	Two 5-mg tablets
Imipramine	Tricyclic antidepressant; used for the symptomatic relief of depression	One 150-mg tablet
Lindane	Agricultural pesticide; also used in the treatment of scabies and lice	Two teaspoons of 1% lotion
Diphenoxylate/atropine	Hydrochloride; used in the treatment of diarrhea	Two 2.5-mg tablets
Propranolol [Inderal]	Beta-blocker; used in the treatment of arrhythmias, hypertension, and angina pectoris	One or two 160-mg tablets
Theophylline	Extracted from tea leaves or produced synthetically; a poisonous alkaloid; used as a diuretic, in the treatment of certain heart conditions, and bronchial spasms	One 500-mg tablet
Verapamil [Isoptin]	Calcium blocker; used in the treatment of angina and certain arrhythmias	One or two 240-mg tablets

Table 13-6 Common Antidotes

Poison	Antidote
Carbon monoxide	Oxygen
Organophosphate	Atropine/pralidoxime
Tricyclic antidepressants	Sodium bicarbonate
Opiates	Naloxone hydrochloride
Beta-blockers	Glucagon
Calcium channel blockers	Calcium chloride
Benzodiazepine	Flumazenil

Cardiovascular Emergencies

Cardiovascular emergencies rarely occur in children. There are some children who are born with congenital heart or valve defects, but this is rare. Whenever a young child has a syncopal episode, consider a cardiovascular event. Most states are moving to requiring that AEDs and trainers certified in CPR should be available at all school sporting events.

Arrhythmias

Hypoxia is the leading cause of cardiac arrhythmias in children. Arrhythmias that produce acute emergencies in children include **tachycardia**, **bradycardia**, and absent (pulseless). **Sinus tachycardia (ST)** is a reactive arrhythmia, and is the most common arrhythmia found in children. ST is a sinus rhythm with a heart rate greater than 100 beats/min. ST is typically a sign of some other underlying problem or it may be due to fever, pain, or anxiety. The treatment is to correct the condition producing the fast heart rate (ie, fever, infection, pain, dehydration, and intrinsic tachycardias). **Supraventricular tachycardia (SVT)** can also occur in children; the treatment is similar to adults, and includes the use of adenosine [Adenocard] and cardioversion. The normal pulse rates for children are listed in **Table 13-7 ▸**. The rates for distinguishing tachycardias in children are shown in **Table 13-8 ▸**.

As discussed previously, children do not tolerate bradycardias well and the presence of slow heart rates should alert the rescuer to the potential for an impending catastrophe. Bradycardias in the very young have a tendency to deteriorate to cardiac arrest. Hypoxia is the primary cause of bradycardia, so treatment should be focused on optimizing oxygenation and ventilation (**Figure 13-6 ▸**).

If bradycardia persists, treatment is similar to adults and can include the use of epinephrine [Adrenalin], atropine sulfate, and transcutaneous pacing in either the prehospital or in-hospital settings.

Medical Emergencies

Aside from the respiratory medical emergencies we have already discussed that are very common in children, other medical emergencies occur that can involve paramedic assessment and management in the field. Seizure is another common complaint in children for which you may need to intervene with a drug. Remember, all emergencies in children involve a very focused assessment and field management of the ABCs, or for that matter, as many pediatricians might say: airway, airway, and airway!

Table 13-7 Normal Pediatric Pulse Rates

Age	Pulse Rate (beats/min)
Infant	100–160
Toddler	90–150
Preschool-age child	80–140
School-age child	70–120
Adolescent	60–100

Table 13-8 Distinguishing ST from SVT in Children

	Pulse Rate	Treatment
ST	< 220 beats/min (infant) < 180 beats/min (child)	Fluids, oxygen, splinting, analgesia, or sedation
SVT	> 220 beats/min (infant) > 180 beats/min (child)	Vagal maneuvers (ice to face), adenosine [Adenocard], synchronized electrical cardioversion

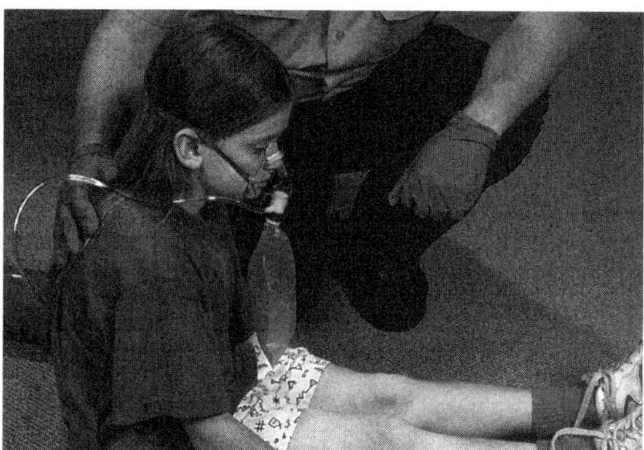

Figure 13-6 A pediatric nonrebreathing mask is an appropriate choice to deliver oxygen to children who can tolerate the mask.

Febrile Seizure

Febrile seizures are a frequent cause for an EMS call and occur in about 25% of young children. A febrile seizure is associated with a rapid rise, or change, in body temperature, usually above 102°F (39°C), and occurs in children between the ages of 6 months and 6 years, with the highest frequency in the ages between 6 months and 3 years. In most cases, the seizure is generalized and brief, followed by a short

Table 13-9 Normal Blood Pressure for Age

Age	Minimal Systolic Blood Pressure (mm Hg)
Infant	> 60
Toddler	> 70
Preschool-age child	> 75
School-age child	> 80
Adolescent	> 90

postictal period. With any seizure, assess for hypoxia and hypoglycemia as the possible cause prior to treating for any other causes.

Febrile seizures have no lasting neurologic effect, but the child must be evaluated by a physician to make this determination and be observed for another breakthrough seizure. Treatment is supportive for the airway, and includes removing excess clothing to begin cooling. The parent may have already considered the administration of acetaminophen to reduce the fever. Rarely, the seizure may be prolonged or a second seizure may occur. In these cases, oxygen and an anticonvulsant are administered. First-line medications include benzodiazepines (diazepam [Valium], midazolam [Versed], or lorazepam [Ativan]). These may be administered IV, IM, or via the rectal route. Second-line medications include phenobarbital [Luminal], phenytoin [Dilantin], and fosphenytoin [Cerebyx]. Benzodiazepines and phenobarbital [Luminal] can cause respiratory depression; therefore, use of these medications requires extra attention to airway and ventilation management. Phenobarbital [Luminal] and phenytoin [Dilantin] may cause hypotension. Monitor blood pressure closely with these two drugs. Normal blood pressure for children is outlined in **Table 13-9▲**.

Trauma

Trauma is the young person's disease, and many children are taken from their families suddenly due to tragic accidents. Your field assessment and management should focus on determining and managing life threats to the ABCs as well as rapidly transporting the child to a facility prepared to deal with the injuries that were sustained. With respect to medications, oxygen therapy, fluid administration, and occasionally pain management are the focus of prehospital treatment.

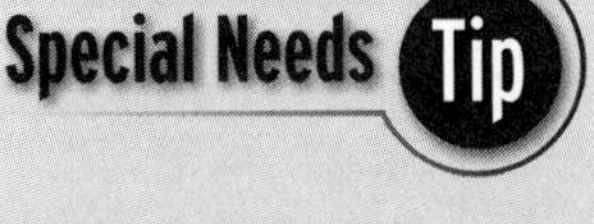

Epiphyseal plate or growth plate injuries occur in children and adolescents. The **epiphyseal plate** is the area of growing tissue near the end of the long bones and determines the future length and shape of the mature bone. It is also the weakest area of the growing skeleton.

Complications that occur are related to the severity of the injury. The most common complication of a growth plate fracture is growth arrest (stunted growth). The affected bone stops growing at the affected growth plate, resulting in a limb-length inequality as compared to the contralateral (opposite) unaffected limb. When only part of the growth plate is injured, growth may be asymmetrical and the limb may grow abnormally. When the injury is open, there is a risk of infection that could also injure the growth plate. Injuries to these areas can occur acutely with trauma (ie, falls, sports injuries, inappropriate IO placement, and child abuse) and chronically with overuse as seen with repetitive movement in athletes, radiation therapy, and certain neurologic and musculoskeletal disorders. Signs and symptoms include severe joint pain, deformities, reduced range of motion, reduced play, or inability to play.

Pain Management

Assessment of the quantity of pain in a child is subjective and best done with a reasonable yardstick that can be used to measure the child's present pain to his or her pain at a point in the near future, especially after an intervention has been tried. The Wong-Baker FACES pain rating scale is particularly useful with children. The scale uses a series of faces as shown in **Figure 13-7▼**.

Many articles have been published on the management of patients' pain by hospital providers. The common thread is that hospital providers fail to manage pain quickly and effectively. It is safe to say that prehospital providers probably have similar statistics. Many agencies across the nation have begun aggres-

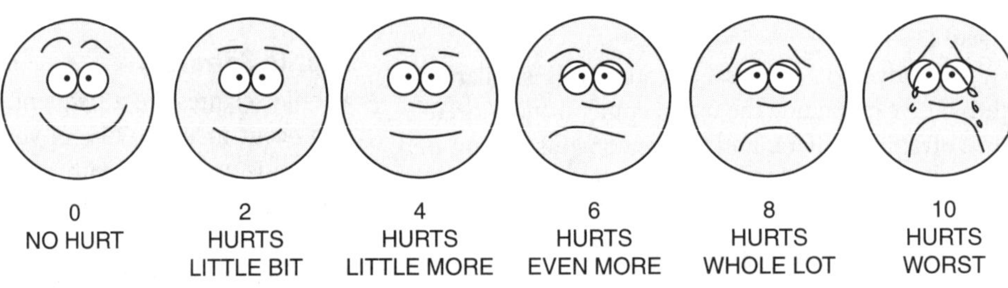

Figure 13-7 The Wong-Baker FACES Pain Rating Scale. From Hockenberry MJ, Wilson D, Wikelstein ML: *Wong's Essentials of Pediatric Nursing*, ed. 7, St. Louis, 2005, p. 1259. Used with permission. Copyright, Mosby.

sively managing patients' pain. Pain management should be a progressive process. First, evaluate the patient's pain using the Wong-Baker scale or a similar pain management tool. Second, ensure that you have a comprehensive set of vital signs. Pain management in many instances should be done on scene with the patient. The goal is not to relieve the pain, but make it tolerable, in other words "take the edge off." Pain management can begin with nitrous oxide [Nitronox], and progress to narcotics of either morphine sulfate [Astramorph/PF], fentanyl citrate [Sublimase], butorphanol tartrate [Stadol], nalbuphine hydrochloride [Nubain], or ketorolac tromethamine [Toradal]. Some agencies even recommend dosing with a benzodiazepine such as midazolam [Versed] or diazepam [Valium] to relieve muscle spasms and to potentiate the narcotics. Frequent vital sign assessment should be performed as well as repeated for the patient's response to the therapy. Consider redosing the patient prior to arrival at the ED if it is anticipated that the patient may have a prolonged wait. Most services even allow for continued pain management in the ED, until the patient has been released to ED staff. Caution should be exercised if the patient has intoxicating substances in his or her system.

Case Study II Pain Management

Part 1

Your unit has been dispatched to the Olympian Gymnastics Training Center, a large gymnastics school on the outskirts of town. An ambulance is already on the scene with a 12-year-old girl who fell during a gymnastics routine on the uneven bars. You are told the bars are twice as high as her height. The EMT-Basics are calling you because she has the most severely angulated forearm they have ever seen and they do not carry pain relievers (analgesics) on their unit.

As you pull up in front of the location, you are ushered inside where a small crowd is gathered around the young athlete. It is obvious by the look on her face that she is holding back the tears while an EMT-B is attempting to support her right arm. As you are given an arrival report, it is clear that the initial assessment has been completed and she has no life threats (see **Table 1**). Her mother is nearby, on her cell phone, as is her trainer, who tells you someone was sent to go get some ice. The patient's name is Elizabeth but she says, "Call me Liz."

Apparently, Liz fell off the bars and her entire body weight landed on her outstretched arm, fracturing it in several places. Because the mechanism of injury (MOI) is significant due to the height of the fall, she will get a rapid trauma examination to make sure there are no other injuries present. Since there is no pulse in the injured arm, you know that the fracture may have injured the nervous or vascular supply to the extremity. You also assign someone to hold cervical spine immobilization. Aside from its main purpose of immobilizing the patient, this will help to distract Liz from her pulseless, angulated arm as you finish up your examination.

Table 1 Initial Assessment

Initial Assessment	Recording Time: 2 Minutes
General Impression/ Appearance	Pale, conscious, and nervous-looking
Mental Status	Alert (oriented to person, place, and day)
Airway	Open and clear
Breathing	Rapid and shallow
Circulation	Weak, rapid pulse in the uninjured arm (radial). Lack of pulse in the injured extremity.
Priority/Plan	High due to pain and questionable pulse in the injured extremity

Question 1: Why would you consider this mechanism of injury significant?

Question 2: What is the significance of the lack of a distal pulse in the extremity?

Case Study II Continued

Part 2

As your partner assists the EMT-Basics in positioning a splint for the extremity, you begin to ask Liz and her mother a number of questions. She is sitting on a mat, and one of the EMT-Basics has been holding her head and neck still. Apparently, she came down on the arm and rolled on the mat. She does not have any pain in the head, neck, or chest. Her right shoulder is sore, but there does not appear to be an injury present. On a scale of 1 to 10, Liz states that she would give the pain an 8.

As you complete your rapid trauma examination, it is decided that the cervical collar is still appropriate due to the single extremely painful injury to the arm. Once the arm is splinted and cold has been applied, she will be placed in a supine position, due to the MOI, on a long back board. Your partner gets a set of baseline vital signs as part of the focused history and physical examination (see **Table 2**).

Table 2 Focused History and Physical Examination

Baseline Vital Signs	Recording Time: 5 Minutes
Skin CTC (color, temperature, condition)	Pale, cool, and clammy
Pulse	120 beats/min and regular
Blood Pressure	88/60 mm Hg
Respirations	22 breaths/min and shallow

Question 3: Why is it appropriate to immobilize this patient's spine?

Question 4: What would you expect to see as a normal blood pressure for a school-aged child?

Part 3

After the splint is applied and Liz is immobilized, you start an IV and contact medical control for permission to administer a dose of morphine sulfate [Astramorph/PF] to help take the edge off the pain. Within a few minutes of starting the pain reliever, Liz is beginning to talk more about the routines she was doing when the accident occurred. When asked, she states that the pain is now about a 4 on a scale of 1 to 10 and denies any nausea. You reassess the extremity; there is a faint distal pulse and the splint is not too tight.

You are able to obtain the SAMPLE history information from her mother (see **Table 3**).

Table 3 SAMPLE History

SAMPLE History	Comments
Signs/symptoms	Poor distal pulse in injured arm, severe pain, and a severely angulated fracture with multiple breaks
Allergies	Penicillin
Medications	Multiple vitamins and supplements
Pertinent past medical history	Old fractured left shoulder, concussion about 3 years ago, borderline underweight (possible eating disorder)
Last oral intake	Breakfast about 4 hours ago
Events leading up to the incident	Practicing gymnastics routine on the uneven bars for a meet in 2 days

Treatment Plan

1. Assess and maintain the ABCs.
2. Assess the injured extremity, determining distal pulses and motor and sensory function (PMS).
3. Splint the extremity, apply cold throughout transport, and immobilize the neck and back. Continued use of the ice will be effective in decreasing swelling, which will help reduce pain and the length of the recovery time.
4. Administer supplemental oxygen with a nonrebreathing mask.
5. Monitor the ECG.
6. Obtain IV access.
7. Consult with medical control concerning morphine sulfate [Astramorph/PF] or fentanyl citrate [Sublimase] for the pain (see **Table 4** and **Table 5**).

   The dose for morphine sulfate [Astramorph/PF] would be 0.1–0.2 mg/kg (estimated 80-lb or 36-kg patient would be 3.6–7.2 mg) IV and the dose for fentanyl citrate [Sublimase] would be 1.7–3.3 µg/kg IM, IVP, or IO. The adult dose, which is administered to people older than age 12 years, is 25 to 100 µg (0.5–1 µg/kg) and may also be administered by the atomized intranasal route. Keep naloxone hydrochloride [Narcan] handy in case it is needed.
8. Reassess and monitor for respiratory depression and nausea.
9. Consider an antiemetic (ie, ondansetron hydrochloride [Zofran]) as needed (and used in your EMS system) (see **Table 6**).

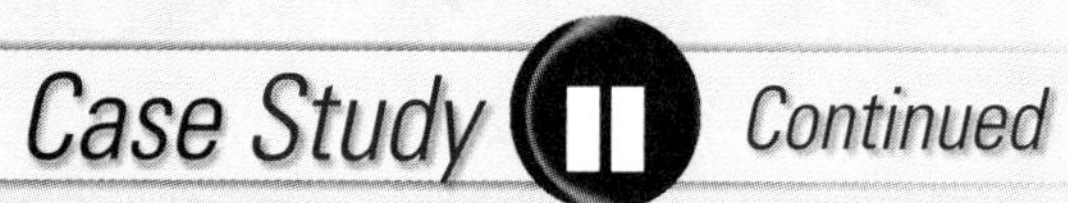

Table 4 **Morphine Sulfate**

Do you know?	Comments
Right drug? Generic name: [**Morphine Sulfate**] Trade name: [Astramorph/PF]	This is a narcotic analgesic. It can be used for pain relief and sedation (although there are better agents used in many EMS systems).
Right patient?	In this situation, the medication is being administered to relieve pain.
Right dose?	0.1–0.2 mg/kg.
Right route?	IV, IO, IM, SC.
Right time?	After assessment including vital signs.
Right documentation?	Document the administration of the medication as well as the ongoing assessment findings, including lung sounds, on the patient care report.
Expected action	Relief of pain.
Side effects	Hypoventilation and/or hypovolemia.
Contraindications	Known allergy, mental status changes, hypotension.
Precautions	Use with caution for asthma. Monitor respiratory effort and blood pressure carefully (have naloxone hydrochloride [Narcan] available). Watch for oversedation or respiratory depression. This patient is light for her age.
Pharmacokinetics	Onset: immediate; peak effect: 20 minutes; duration of action: 2–7 hours; metabolized in the liver and excreted in urine.

Table 5 **Fentanyl Citrate**

Do you know?	Comments
Right drug? Generic name: [**Fentanyl Citrate**] Trade name: [Sublimase]	This drug is a narcotic analgesic (schedule II narcotic). It is used to treat severe pain and is used with anesthesia. It has actions similar to morphine sulfate [Astramorph/PF] and meperidine hydrochloride [Demerol].
Right patient?	Relief of severe pain.
Right dose?	For a child from 2–12 years old, the dose is 1.7–3.3 µg/kg. The adult dose is 25–100 µg (0.5–1 µg/kg).
Right route?	IM, IVP, IO, or atomized intranasal (adult route).
Right time?	After assessment and contraindications for use have been considered.
Right documentation?	Always document how and when the drug was administered as well as the patient's response to the medication on your patient care report.
Expected action	Relief of pain.
Side effects	Skeletal and thoracic muscle rigidity, bradycardia, seizures, and diaphoresis.
Contraindications	Myasthenia gravis, children younger than 2 years old.
Precautions	May cause life-threatening hypoventilation. Should have naloxone hydrochloride [Narcan] readily available.
Pharmacokinetics	Onset: immediate IV, 7–15 minutes IM; peak effect: 3–5 minutes IV, 30 minutes IM; duration: 30–60 minutes IV, 1–2 hours IM; metabolized in the liver and excreted in urine.

Case Study II Continued

Table 6 Ondansetron Hydrochloride

Do you know?	Comments
Right drug? Generic name: [**Ondansetron Hydrochloride**] Trade name: [Zofran]	This drug is an antiemetic. It is used to relieve or prevent nausea and vomiting in a variety of situations.
Right patient?	Nausea with pain and with the use of a narcotic.
Right dose?	0.1 mg/kg; may be repeated; follow local protocol.
Right route?	IM or IV.
Right time?	Adjunct treatment with narcotics in pain management.
Right documentation?	Document the administration of the medication as well as the ongoing assessment findings, including lung sounds, on the patient care report.
Expected action	Relief of nausea.
Side effects	Seizures, tachycardia, bradycardia, headache, sedation, chest pain, bronchospasm, wheezing, acute dystonic reactions, blurred vision, hypokalemia, fever, skin rash, and hives.
Contraindications	Known allergy to this medication or other 5-HT3 receptor agonists.
Precautions	May worsen preexisting symptoms.
Pharmacokinetics	Onset: 30 minutes; peak effect: 2 hours; duration of action: 3–6 hours; metabolized in the liver, excreted in urine.

Question 5: With multiple fractures in the extremity, what is the prehospital management likely to involve?

Question 6: What is the most serious side effect of morphine sulfate [Astramorph/PF] in this case?

Part 4

As you load Liz and her mother into the ambulance, you begin to learn all about the gymnastic routines that Liz competes in. She had been practicing for a meet that is to occur in the next 2 days. As you reassess her vital signs, you decide it is best to let her talk since it has a calming effect and has taken her mind off of the pain (see **Table 7**). Her mother describes some of the finer points of the scoring for the uneven bars routines and you learn that Liz has been competing for the past 7 years!

The morphine sulfate [Astramorph/PF] has been helpful and there certainly are no harmful side effects to be concerned about.

Question 7: With an SpO_2 of 98%, and if Liz is uncomfortable with the nonrebreathing mask, can you remove it?

Question 8: What is the value of continuing to keep the extremity cold?

Table 7 Reassessment and Ongoing Assessment of the Patient

Serial Vital Signs and Relevant Data	Recording Time: 15 Minutes
Skin CTC	Normal, warm, dry
Pulse	100 beats/min and regular
Blood pressure	94 mm Hg/palpation
Respirations	20 breaths/min and normal
Mental status	Alert (oriented to person, place, and day)
ECG	Normal sinus rhythm
SpO_2	98% on nonrebreathing mask
Lung sounds	Clear bilaterally
Other (ie, glucose, core body temperature)	Additional cold is applied to the fracture site, distal pulse is still faint but present, she is able to feel you touch her fingers and wiggle her fingers

Case Study II Continued

Part 5

Gymnastics is a very active and competitive sport. It requires intense concentration and plenty of practice to excel. Liz is a very competitive young lady who has been injured before and was injured again today. It will be a setback for her training but she will be back as soon as her injury and its rehabilitation allow. Aside from the severe pain that she had to endure, she was very lucky to not have injured her shoulder or head during the fall. It was obvious that the pain medication helped to take the edge off and make it much more tolerable for Liz. You learned a lot today about a sport you were not that familiar with as well as the perseverance and strength of a 12-year-old girl.

Burns

Just like adult patients, children also can experience devastating burn trauma. The patients who are at risk for complications of burns are those at the beginning and end of the life cycle. Your assessment and management of burn-injured children will be essential to their survival and dealing with these critical injuries. As far as pharmaceutical interventions, when a child is seriously burned, the focus is on oxygenation, bronchodilation as needed, fluid resuscitation, and pain relief.

Cold packs are great tools to use to relieve pain and reduce soft-tissue swelling. However, ice and chemical cold packs should NEVER be placed directly against the skin, as prolonged exposure to the skin can result in frost nip or frostbite. Ensure that a hand towel or 4 × 4 gauze is placed between the cold pack and the patient's skin.

If an IV site is not readily apparent and the situation does not warrant IV fluid administration or IO, always consider the IM route if medical control agrees.

Case Study ANSWERS

Case Study I Respiratory Emergency

Question 1: If the child has a life threat, can you treat him if the school nurse is present?

Answer 1: In most states, the school nurse can act in the place of the parent if the parent cannot be located. If the child has a life threat or is not conscious, the emergency rule or implied consent should provide adequate coverage. In this case, the parent has been called and will be there in a short amount of time to help you decide on the location to transport the child to as well as authorize treatment.

Question 2: Would it be likely that the child may have already self-administered his prescribed inhaler prior to your arrival?

Answer 2: Not really, because most elementary schools require that the child's medication be kept in the nurse's office and the child must go to the nurse's office to retrieve the medication.

Question 3: What would you expect to see as a normal pulse rate for a school-aged child?

Answer 3: Normal pulse rate for a school-aged child would be in the range of 70 to 120 beats/min. The rest of the ranges are as follows:

Age	Pulse Rate (beats/min)
Infant	100–160
Toddler	90–150
Preschool-aged child	80–140
School-aged child	70–120
Adolescent	60–100

Question 4: What would you expect to see as a normal respiratory rate for a school-aged child?

Answer 4: Normal respiratory rate for a school-aged child would be in the range of 15 to 20 breaths/min. The rest of the ranges are as follows:

Age	Respiratory Rate (breaths/min)
Infant	25–50
Toddler	20–30
Preschool-aged child	20–25
School-aged child	15–20
Adolescent	12–16

Question 5: If prior to administering a bronchodilator the child begins to get a quieter chest, what does this indicate?

Answer 5: Children usually do not just get better on their own. If the chest is getting quieter, it usually means the child is simply no longer moving enough air to cause the wheezing, which could indicate status asthmaticus or imminent respiratory arrest.

Question 6: When should you start an IV on a pediatric patient in respiratory distress?

Answer 6: Don't—if the child gets better with the first nebulizer treatment, the attack was not that severe and the child will not have to endure the pain and discomfort of the IV.

Question 7: Why does the prevalence of asthma decrease as children get older?

Answer 7: Their airways get larger and many children "grow out" of the disease.

Question 8: If a child in respiratory distress was grunting, what does that indicate?

Answer 8: That would be a "red flag" that the child is in severe distress and must be given close attention and care. It is actually the closing of the glottic opening at the end of the exhalation to maintain back pressure in the alveoli and help to avoid their collapse (atelectisis). It is an effort on the part of the patient to provide PEEP, or positive end-expiratory pressure.

Case Study II Pain Management

Question 1: Why would you consider this mechanism of injury significant?

Answer 1: Liz fell from the uneven bars, which is a fall from twice (or more) her own height constituting a significant mechanism of injury (MOI). In addition, due to the severity of the single (at this point) isolated injury, it should be handled as a significant MOI.

Question 2: What is the significance of the lack of a distal pulse in the extremity?

Answer 2: If an injured extremity has no sensation or pulse, it is likely that the fracture may have injured either the nervous or vascular supply to the extremity. These physical findings considerably increase the care priority as the patient could sustain permanent

Case Study ANSWERS

limb-threatening damage to the extremity if it is not treated promptly.

Question 3: Why is it appropriate to immobilize this patient's spine?

Answer 3: The presence of a distracting injury, such as Liz's severely angulated fracture, and a concerning mechanism should motivate the provider to immobilize the spine, as the distractor may prevent the patient from adequately focusing on spinal tenderness when the initial examination is done by the rescuer.

Question 4: What would you expect to see as a normal blood pressure for a school-aged child?

Answer 4: Normal blood pressure for a school-aged child would be in the range of 102–124 mm Hg. (systolic 90 + (child's age in years × 2). The minimal systolic ranges are as follows:

Age	Minimal Systolic Blood Pressure (mm Hg)
Infant	> 70
Toddler	> 80
Preschool-aged child	> 80
School-aged child	> 80
Adolescent	> 90

Question 5: With multiple fractures in the extremity, what is the prehospital management likely to involve?

Answer 5: That depends on the orthopaedic surgeon's approach. Certainly the first, best approach will involve continued care with ice, immobilization, and pain medication. Following radiographic examination, she will end up in a cast, and then may undergo surgical correction of her injury. Because she is a dedicated athlete with a prior history of orthopaedic injury, she most likely already has a close relationship to an orthopaedist that specializes in sports medicine who will ultimately guide her care and recovery. Specifically, the treatment plan consists of:

1. Assess and maintain ABCs.
2. Assess the injured extremity determining distal pulses, motor function, and sensory function (PMS).
3. Splint the extremity, apply cold, and immobilize the neck and back.
4. Administer supplemental oxygen with a nonrebreathing mask.
5. Monitor the ECG.
6. Obtain IV access.
7. Consult with medical control concerning morphine sulfate [Astromorph/PF] or fentanyl citrate [Sublimase] for pain.
8. Reassess and monitor for respiratory depression and nausea.
9. Consider an antiemetic as needed.

Question 6: What is the most serious side effect of morphine sulfate [Astramorph/PF] in this case?

Answer 6: Because she is light in weight for her age, the morphine sulfate [Astramorph/PF] may cause oversedation or respiratory depression if too much is given, or her body does not handle the dose properly.

Question 7: With an SpO_2 of 98%, and if Liz is uncomfortable with the nonrebreathing mask, can you remove it?

Answer 7: Based on the fact that her mental status is alert, her vitals are normal for a child her age, and her SpO_2 is 98%, if she is uncomfortable with the mask it would certainly be appropriate to either remove it or switch to a nasal cannula.

Question 8: What is the value of continuing to keep the extremity cold?

Answer 8: The cold may be effective in decreasing the swelling, which might help reduce the pain.

Medication Review

Activated Charcoal

Indications Most oral poisonings and medication overdoses; can be used after evacuation of poisons.

Contraindications Oral administration to comatose patient; after ingestion of corrosives, caustics, or petroleum distillates (ineffective and may induce vomiting); simultaneous administration with other oral drugs.

Dosage and administration Note: if not in premixed slurry, dilute with 1 part charcoal/4 parts water. Pediatric: 1–2 g/kg PO or via NGT.

Adenosine (Adenocard)

Indications Conversion of PSVT to sinus rhythm. May convert re-entry SVT due to Wolff-Parkinson-White syndrome. Not effective in converting atrial fibrillation/flutter or V-tach.

Contraindications Second- or third-degree block or sick sinus syndrome, atrial flutter/atrial fibrillation, ventricular tachycardia, hypersensitivity to adenosine, poison-induced tachycardia.

Dosage and administration Pediatric: 0.1–0.2 mg/kg rapid IV; maximum single dose, 12 mg.

Albuterol (Proventil, Ventolin)

Indications Treatment of bronchospasm in patients with reversible obstructive airway disease (COPD/asthma). Prevention of exercise-induced bronchospasm.

Contraindications Known prior hypersensitivity reactions to albuterol. Tachycardia arrhythmias, especially those caused by digitalis. Synergistic with other sympathomimetics.

Dosage and administration Pediatric: (between the ages of 2 and 12) administer 2.5 mg (0.5 mL of the 0.083% solution) added to 2 mL of normal saline for inhalation by nebulizer treatment and administer over 10–15 minutes. May repeat every 20 minutes up to three times.

Amiodarone (Cordarone, Pacerone)

Indications Indicates V-fib/pulseless V-tach and unstable V-tach in patients refractory to other therapy. Also persistent SVTs unresponsive to other treatment.

Contraindications Known hypersensitivity, cardiogenic shock, sinus bradycardia, and second- or third-degree AV block (unless a functional pacemaker is available).

Dosage and administration Pediatric: Refractory V-fib/pulseless V-tach: 5 mg/kg IV/IO bolus. Can repeat the 5 mg/kg IV/IO bolus up to a total dose of 15 mg/kg per 24 hours. Maximum single dose is 300 mg. Perfusing supraventricular and ventricular tachycardias: Loading dose of 5 mg/kg IV/IO over 20–60 minutes (maximum single dose of 300 mg). Can repeat to maximum of 15 mg/kg per day.

Amyl Nitrite, Sodium Nitrite, Sodium Thiosulfate (Cyanide Antidote Kit)

Indications Cyanide or hydrocyanic acid poisoning.

Contraindications Not applicable.

Dosage and administration Pediatric: Amyl nitrite: breathe 30 seconds out of every minute. Sodium thiosulfate and sodium nitrite: IV per antidote kit directions.

Atropine Sulfate

Indications Hemodynamically unstable bradycardia, asystole, bradycardic (< 60 beats/min) pulseless electrical activity (PEA), organophosphate poisoning, bronchospastic pulmonary disorders.

Contraindications Tachycardia, hypersensitivity, unstable cardiovascular status in acute hemorrhage and myocardial ischemia, narrow-angle glaucoma.

Dosage and administration Pediatric: 0.02 mg/kg via IV/IO push; may double this dose for second IV/IO dose. Minimum single dose: 0.1 mg. Maximum doses: child single dose: 0.5 mg, child total dose: 1 mg, adolescent single dose: 1 mg, adolescent total dose: 2 mg. Endotracheal administration: 0.03 mg/kg (absorption may be unreliable).

Medication Review

Calcium Chloride

Indications Hypocalcemia, hyperkalemia, magnesium sulfate overdose, calcium channel blocker overdose, adjunctive therapy in treatment of insect bites and stings.

Contraindications Hypercalcemia, V-fib, digitalis toxicity.

Dosage and administration Pediatric: 20 mg/kg (0.2 mL/kg) slow IV/IO push. Maximum 1 g dose; may repeat in 10 minutes.

Dexamethasone Sodium Phosphate (Decadron, Hexadrol)

Indications Anaphylaxis, asthma, croup, elevated intracranial pressure (prevention and treatment), as an adjunct to treatment of shock.

Contraindications Hypersensitivity to product, systemic sepsis, bacterial infection.

Dosage and administration Pediatric: 0.25–1.0 mg/kg/dose IV, IO, IM.

Dextrose

Indications Hypoglycemia, altered level of consciousness, coma of unknown etiology, seizure of unknown etiology, status epilepticus.

Contraindications Intracranial hemorrhage.

Dosage and administration Pediatric: 0.5–1 g/kg/dose slow IV; may be repeated as necessary.

Diazepam (Valium)

Indications Acute anxiety states, acute alcohol withdrawal (delirium tremens), muscle relaxant, seizure activity, agitation. Analgesia for medical procedures (fracture reduction, cardioversion).

Contraindications Hypersensitivity, glaucoma, coma, shock, substance abuse, head injury.

Dosage and administration Pediatric seizure activity: 0.2–0.5 mg slowly every 2–5 minutes up to 5 mg (maximum dose, 10 mg/kg). Rectal diazepam: 0.5 mg/kg via rectal catheter and flush with 2-3 mL air after administration.

Diphenhydramine (Benadryl)

Indications Symptomatic relief of allergies, allergic reactions, anaphylaxis, acute dystonic reactions (phenothiazines). Blood administration reactions; used for motion sickness, hay fever.

Contraindications Asthma, glaucoma, pregnancy, hypertension, narrow-angle glaucoma, infants, patients taking monoamine oxidase inhibitors (MAOIs).

Dosage and administration Pediatric: 1–2 mg/kg IV, IO slowly or IM. If given PO: 5 mg/kg/24 hours.

Dobutamine (Dobutrex)

Indications Cardiogenic shock, CHF, left ventricular dysfunction. Often used in conjunction with other drugs.

Contraindications Tachyarrhythmias, IHSS, severe hypotension.

Dosage and administration Pediatric: 2–20 µg/kg/min titrated to desired effect.

Dopamine (Intropin)

Indications Cardiogenic, septic or spinal shock, hypotension with low cardiac output states, distributive shock.

Contraindications Hypovolemic shock, pheochromocytoma, tachyarrhythmias, V-fib.

Dosage and administration Pediatric: 2–20 µg/kg/min titrated to patient response.

Medication Review

Epinephrine (Adrenalin)

Indications Cardiac arrest (V-fib/pulseless V-tach, asystole, PEA), symptomatic bradycardia as an alternative infusion to dopamine, severe hypotension secondary to bradycardia when atropine and transcutaneous pacing are unsuccessful, allergic reactions, anaphylaxis, asthma.

Contraindications Hypertension, hypothermia, pulmonary edema, myocardial ischemia, hypovolemic shock.

Dosage and administration Pediatric: Mild allergic reactions and asthma: 0.01 mg/kg (0.01 mL/kg) of 1:1,000 solution SC (maximum of 0.3 mL). Cardiac arrest: IV/IO dose: 0.01 mg/kg (0.1 mL/kg) of 1:10,000 solution every 3–5 minutes during arrest. All endotracheal (ET) doses: 0.1 mg/kg (0.1 mL/kg) of 1:1,000 solution. Symptomatic bradycardia: IV/IO dose: 0.01 mg/kg (0.1 mL/kg) of 1:10,000 solution. Continuous IV/IO infusion: Begin with rapid infusion, then titrate to response. Typical initial infusion: 0.1–1 µg/min. Higher doses may be effective.

Epinephrine Racemic (microNefrin, Vaponefrin)

Indications Bronchial asthma, prevention of bronchospasm. Croup, laryngotracheobronchitis, laryngeal edema.

Contraindications Hypertension, underlying cardiovascular disease, epiglottitis.

Dosage and administration Pediatric: Solution: dilute 0.25 mL (0.1%) in 2.5 mL NS (if less than 20 kg); dilute 0.5 mL in 2.5 mL NS (if 20–40 kg); dilute 0.75 mL in 2.5 mL NS (if greater than 40 kg). Administer by aerosolization.

Fentanyl Citrate (Sublimase)

Indications This drug is used to treat severe pain and is used with anesthesia.

Contraindications Myasthenia gravis, children under 2 years old. May cause life-threatening hypoventilation so naloxone hydrochloride [Narcan] should be readily available.

Dosage and administration Pediatric 2–12 years old: 1.7–3.3 µg/kg IM, IO, IVP. Adult dose is 25–100 µg (0.5–1 µg/kg) IM, IO, IVP or atomized intranasal.

Furosemide (Lasix)

Indications CHF, pulmonary edema, hypertensive crisis.

Contraindications Hypovolemia, anuria, hypotension (relative contraindication); hypersensitivity, hepatic coma.

Dosage and administration Pediatric: 1 mg/kg/dose IV, IO.

Glucagon

Indications Altered level of consciousness when hypoglycemia is suspected. May be used as inotropic agent in beta-blocker overdose.

Contraindications Hyperglycemia, hypersensitivity.

Dosage and administration Pediatric: Hypoglycemia: 0.5–1 mg IM (for children < 20 kg).

Hydrocortisone Sodium Succinate (Solu-Cortef)

Indications Shock due to acute adrenocortical insufficiency.

Contraindications None if given as single dose.

Dosage and administration Pediatric: 0.16–1.0 mg/kg slow IV bolus.

Hydroxyzine Hydrochloride (Atarax, Vistaril)

Indications To potentiate the effects of analgesics; to control nausea and vomiting, anxiety reactions, and motion sickness; preoperative and postoperative sedation.

Contraindications Hypersensitivity.

Dosage and administration Pediatric: 0.5–1.0 mg/kg/dose IM.

Medication Review

Ipratropium bromide (Atrovent)

Indications Maintenance treatment of bronchospasm in patients with reversible obstructive airway disease (COPD/asthma). Can be used alone or in combination with other bronchodilators (especially beta-adrenergics).

Contraindications Known prior hypersensitivity reactions to ipratropium bromide. Hypersensitivity to atropine or any anticholinergic derivatives or to soya lecithin or related food products.

Dosage and administration Pediatric: Safety and effectiveness in the pediatric population below the age of 12 have not been established so many paramedic systems do not utilize this drug in the younger children.

Isoetharine (Bronchosol, Bronkometer)

Indications Acute bronchial asthma, bronchospasm (especially in COPD patient).

Contraindications Use with caution in patients with diabetes, hyperthyroidism, cardiovascular and cerebrovascular disease.

Dosage and administration Pediatric: 0.01 mL/kg; maximum dose: 0.5 mL diluted in 3 mL NS and nebulized.

Levalbuterol (Xopenex)

Indications Used to treat or prevent bronchospasm in patients 6 years or older. Relaxes the smooth muscles of the lower airways.

Contraindications Known sensitivity to the drug.

Dosage and administration Adult and pediatric (6 years and older): 1.25 mg in 3 mL administered by the nebulizer route. It is also administered by MDI (2 puffs) to adult patients.

Lidocaine Hydrochloride (Xylocaine)

Indications Alternative to amiodarone in cardiac arrest from V-fib/pulseless V-tach, stable monomorphic V-tach, stable polymorphic V-tach with normal baseline QT interval.

Contraindications Hypersensitivity, second- and third-degree AV blocks in the absence of artificial pacemaker, Stokes-Adams syndrome, prophylactic use in AMI, wide-complex ventricular escape beats with bradycardia.

Dosage and administration Pediatric: IV/IO dose: 1 mg/kg rapid IV/IO push. Maximum dose: 100 mg. Continuous IV/IO infusion: 20–50 μg/kg/min. Administer bolus dose (1 mg/kg) when infusion is initiated if bolus has not been given within previous 15 minutes. Endotracheal (ET) dose: 2–3 mg/kg.

Lorazepam (Ativan)

Indications Initial control of status epilepticus or severe recurrent seizures, severe anxiety, sedation.

Contraindications Acute narrow-angle glaucoma. Coma, shock, or suspected drug abuse.

Dosage and administration Note: When given IV or IO, must dilute with equal volume of sterile water or sterile saline; when given IM, lorazepam is not to be diluted. Pediatric: 0.05–0.20 mg/kg slow IV, IO slowly over 2 minutes or IM; may repeat in 15–20 minutes to maximum dose of 0.2 mg/kg.

Magnesium Sulfate

Indications Seizures of eclampsia (toxemia of pregnancy), torsade de pointes, hypomagnesemia, Class IIa agent for V-fib/pulseless V-tach that is refractory to lidocaine.

Contraindications Heart blocks, myocardial damage.

Dosage and administration Pediatric: IV/IO infusion: 25–50 mg/kg (maximum dose: 2 g) over 10–20 minutes; faster for torsade de pointes. For asthma: 25–50 mg/kg (maximum dose: 2 g) over 10–20 minutes.

Medication Review

Meperidine Hydrochloride (Demerol)

Indications Analgesia for moderate to severe pain.

Contraindications Hypersensitivity to narcotic agents, diarrhea caused by poisoning, patients taking MAOIs, during labor or delivery of a premature infant, undiagnosed abdominal pain or head injury.

Dosage and administration Pediatric: 1–2 mg/kg/dose IV, IO, IM, SC.

Metaproterenol 5% (Alupent)

Indications Bronchial asthma, reversible bronchospasm secondary to bronchitis, COPD.

Contraindications Tachyarrhythmias, hypersensitivity, tachycardias due to digitalis toxicity.

Dosage and administration Pediatric: MDI: not recommended. Inhalation solution 5%: age 6–12 years: 0.1–0.2 mL diluted in 3 mL saline.

Methylprednisolone Sodium Succinate (Solu-Medrol)

Indications Acute spinal cord trauma, anaphylaxis, bronchodilator for unresponsive asthma.

Contraindications Premature infants, systemic fungal infections; use with caution in patients with gastrointestinal bleeding, sepsis, local infection.

Dosage and administration Pediatric: Acute spinal cord trauma: 30 mg/kg IV over 30 minutes; infusion: 5.4 mg/kg/h. Asthma: 1–2 mg/kg/dose IV.

Morphine Sulfate (Astramorph/PF and others)

Indications Severe CHF, pulmonary edema, chest pain associated with acute MI, analgesia for moderate to severe acute and chronic pain (use with caution).

Contraindications Head injury, exacerbated COPD, depressed respiratory drive, hypotension, undiagnosed abdominal pain, decreased level of consciousness, suspected hypovolemia, patients who have taken MAOIs within the past 14 days.

Dosage and administration Pediatric: 0.1–0.2 mg/kg per dose via IV, IO, IM, or SC; maximum dose of 5 mg.

Naloxone Hydrochloride (Narcan)

Indications Opiate overdose, coma; complete or partial reversal of CNS and respiratory depression induced by opioids; decreased level of consciousness; coma of unknown origin; narcotic agonist for the following: morphine, heroin, hydromorphone (Dilaudid), methadone, meperidine (Demerol), paregoric, fentanyl citrate (Sublimase), oxycodone (Percodan), codeine, propoxyphene (Darvon); narcotic agonist and antagonist for the following: Butorphanol (Stadol), pentazocine (Talwin), nalbuphine (Nubain).

Contraindications Use with caution in narcotic-dependent patients; use with caution in neonates of narcotic-addicted mothers.

Dosage and administration Pediatric: 0.1 mg/kg/dose IV, IM, SC, ET (diluted); maximum dose of 0.8 mg; if no response in 10 minutes, administer an additional 0.1 mg/kg/dose.

Nitrous Oxide: Oxygen (50:50) (Nitronox)

Indications Moderate to severe pain, anxiety, apprehension.

Contraindications Impaired level of consciousness, head injury, inability to comply with instructions; decompression sickness (nitrogen narcosis, air embolism, air transport); undiagnosed abdominal pain or marked distention, bowel obstruction; hypotension, shock, COPD (with history/suspicion of carbon dioxide retention); cyanosis; chest trauma with pneumothorax.

Dosage and administration Pediatric: (Note: Invert cylinder several times before use) Instruct the patient to inhale deeply through demand valve and mask or mouthpiece.

Medication Review

Norepinephrine Bitartrate (Levophed, Levarterenol)

Indications Cardiogenic shock, significant hypotensive (< 70 mm Hg) states.

Contraindications Hypotensive patients with hypovolemia, pregnancy (relative contraindication).

Dosage and administration Pediatric: 0.1–1.0 µg/min IV infusion, titrated to patient response.

Ondansetron Hydrochloride (Zofran)

Indications For the prevention or control of nausea or vomiting. Also used in the hospital setting for patients undergoing chemotherapy or surgical procedures.

Contraindications Known allergy to this medicine or other 5-HT3 receptor antagonists.

Dosage and administration Pediatric: 0.1 mg/kg IV or IM.

Oral Glucose (Insta-Glucose)

Indications Conscious patients with suspected hypoglycemia.

Contraindications Decreased level of consciousness, nausea, vomiting.

Dosage and administration Pediatric: Should be sipped slowly by patient until clinical improvement noted.

Oxygen

Indications Confirmed or expected hypoxemia, ischemic chest pain, respiratory insufficiency, prophylactically during air transport, confirmed or suspected carbon monoxide poisoning, all other causes of decreased tissue oxygenation, decreased level of consciousness.

Contraindications Certain patients with COPD or emphysema who will not tolerate oxygen concentrations over 35%, hyperventilation. Oxygen should never be withheld from a patient who needs it, however. Be prepared to assist with ventilations in a patient with COPD who requires high concentration, as apnea may result.

Dosage and administration Pediatric: Cardiac arrest and carbon monoxide poisoning: 100%. Hypoxemia: 10–15 L/min via nonrebreathing mask. COPD: 1–6 L/min via nasal cannula or 28%–35% Venturi mask. Be prepared to provide ventilatory support if higher concentrations of oxygen needed. (Be careful not to deliver directly into the eyes of a premature infant).

Pancuronium Bromide (Pavulon)

Indications Induction or maintenance of paralysis after intubation to assist ventilations.

Contraindications Hypersensitivity, inability to control airway and support ventilations with oxygen and positive pressure, neuromuscular disease (myasthenia gravis), hepatic or renal failure.

Dosage and administration Pediatric: 0.1 mg/kg slow IV, IO.

Medication Review

Phenobarbital (Luminal)

Indications Prevention and treatment of seizure activity; prophylaxis for febrile seizures; anxiety, apprehension; status epilepticus.

Contraindications Patients with porphyria, hypersensitivity, severe liver or respiratory diseases.

Dosage and administration Pediatric: 10–20 mg/kg IV, IO (less than 1 mg/kg/min) or IM; repeat as needed in 20–30 minutes.

Phenytoin (Dilantin)

Indications Prophylaxis and treatment of major motor seizures, digitalis-induced arrhythmias.

Contraindications Hypersensitivity, bradycardia, second- and third-degree heart block.

Dosage and administration Pediatric: Seizures: 10–20 mg/kg slow IV (1–3 mg/kg/min). Arrhythmias: 5 mg/kg slow IV; maximum, 1 g.

Pralidoxime Chloride (2-PAM Chloride, Protopam)

Indications As an antidote in the treatment of poisoning by organophosphate pesticides and chemicals. In the prehospital arena, is used when atropine is or has become ineffective in management of organophosphate poisoning.

Contraindications Use with caution in patients with reduced renal function; patients with myasthenia gravis and organophosphate poisoning.

Dosage and administration Note: If Protopam is to be used, it should be administered almost simultaneously with atropine. Pediatric: 20–40 mg/kg as IV infusion over 15–30 minutes. Doses may be repeated every 1 hour if muscle weakness persists. If IV administration is not feasible, IM or SC injection may be utilized.

Procainamide Hydrochloride (Pronestyl, Procanbid)

Indications Stable monomorphic V-tach with normal QT interval, reentry SVT uncontrolled by vagal maneuvers and adenosine, stable wide-complex tachycardia of unknown origin, atrial fibrillation with rapid ventricular rate in patients with Wolff-Parkinson-White syndrome.

Contraindications Torsade de pointes, second- and third-degree AV block (without functional artificial pacemaker), digitalis toxicity, tricyclic antidepressant overdose.

Dosage and administration Pediatric: Loading dose of 15 mg/kg IV/IO over 30–60 minutes.

Promethazine Hydrochloride (Phenergan)

Indications Nausea, vomiting, motion sickness; sedation for patients in labor; potentiation of analgesic effects of narcotics.

Contraindications Hypersensitivity, coma, CNS-depressed patients from alcohol, barbiturates, narcotics, Reye's syndrome.

Dosage and administration Pediatric: (greater than 2 years old) 0.25–0.5 mg/kg dose IM.

Propranolol Hydrochloride (Inderal)

Indications Hypertension, angina pectoris, V-tach and V-fib refractory to lidocaine; selected supraventricular tachycardias.

Contraindications Sinus bradycardia, second- or third-degree AV block, asthma, CHF, COPD.

Dosage and administration Pediatric: 0.01–0.05 mg/kg/dose slow IV over 10 minutes; maximum, 3 mg.

Medication Review

Sodium Bicarbonate

Indications Mild or moderate metabolic acidosis due to shock, severe dehydration, anoxia, uncontrolled diabetes, renal disease, cardiac arrest, and severe primary lactic acidosis. To treat overdose of aspirin and cyclic-antidepressants.

Contraindications Metabolic and respiratory alkalosis, hypertension, convulsions, CHF, and other situations where sodium can be dangerous.

Dosage and administration 1 mEq per kg IV bolus (may repeat every 10 minutes at ½ initial dose).

Succinylcholine Chloride (Anectine, Quelicin)

Indications To facilitate intubation, to terminate laryngospasm, to promote muscle relaxation, to facilitate electroconvulsive shock therapy.

Contraindications Acute narrow-angle glaucoma, penetrating eye injuries, inability to control airway or support ventilations with oxygen and positive pressure.

Dosage and administration Pediatric: 1–1.5 mg/kg dose rapid IV, IO; repeat once if needed.

Terbutaline Sulfate (Brethine)

Indications Bronchial asthma, reversible bronchospasm associated with exercise, chronic bronchitis, and emphysema.

Contraindications Hypersensitivity, tachyarrhythmias.

Dosage and administration Pediatric: Not recommended for children under 12 years of age; 0.01 mg/kg/dose SC every 15–20 minutes as needed to maximum 0.25 mg dose. 0.03–0.05 mg/kg in 1.25 mL saline for aerosolization every 4 hours.

Thiamine Hydrochloride (Vitamin B-1)

Indications Coma of unknown origin, delirium tremens, beriberi, Wernicke's encephalopathy.

Contraindications None.

Dosage and administration Pediatric: 10–25 mg slow IV or IM.

Vecuronium Bromide (Norcuron)

Indications To facilitate intubation, to terminate laryngospasm, to promote muscle relaxation, to facilitate electroconvulsive shock therapy.

Contraindications Acute narrow-angle glaucoma, penetrating eye injuries, inability to control airway or support ventilations with oxygen and positive pressure, newborns, myasthenia gravis, hepatic or renal failure.

Dosage and administration Pediatric: 0.1 mg/kg IV, IO; maintenance dose within 20–35 minutes: 0.01–0.05 mg/kg IV push.

Medication Review

Verapamil (Calan, Isoptin)

Indications PSVT, PAT, atrial fibrillation and atrial flutter with rapid ventricular response.

Contraindications Wolff-Parkinson-White syndrome, second-degree or third-degree AV block, sick sinus syndrome (unless patient has functioning pacemaker), hypotension, cardiogenic shock, severe CHF, pulmonary edema, patients receiving IV beta-blockers, wide-complex tachycardias, children less than 12 months of age.

Dosage and administration Pediatric: 0.1–0.2 mg/kg/dose IV, IO push over 2 minutes. Repeat dose in 30 minutes if not effective. (Note: not to be used in children less than 12 months of age.)

0.9% Sodium Chloride (Normal Saline)

Indications Heat-related problems (heat exhaustion, heat stroke), freshwater drowning, hypovolemia, diabetic ketoacidosis, keep open IV.

Contraindications The use of 0.9% sodium chloride should not be considered in patients with congestive heart failure as circulatory overload can be easily induced.

Dosage and administration The specific situation being treated will dictate the rate in which normal saline will be administered. In severe heat stroke, diabetic ketoacidosis, and freshwater drowning, it is likely that you will be called on to administer the fluid quite rapidly. In other cases, it is advisable to administer the fluid at a moderate rate (for example, 100 mL/h).

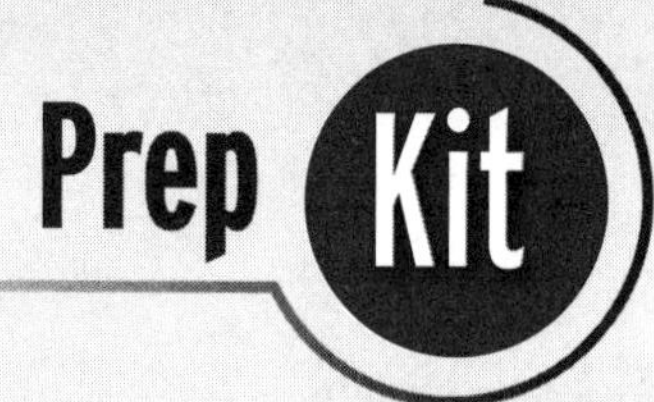

Chapter Summary

- Virtually all, but especially pediatric medication doses, are weight-based.
- The pediatric airway is smaller in proportion to that of an adult and this predisposes children to developing airway obstructions.
- Asthma, bronchiolitis, croup, epiglottitis, and anaphylaxis are common causes of respiratory emergencies in children.
- Bronchodilators such as Albuterol [Proventil], a sympathomimetic, and ipratropium bromide [Atrovent], a parasympatholytic, do an excellent job at dilating the bronchi, but have a side effect of elevating the heart rate. Medications such as levalbuterol [Xopenex] have the same desired effect on the bronchi but with less of an effect on heart rate.
- Epinephrine [Adrenalin] 1:1,000 has fallen out of favor because of its severe effects on the heart, which could precipitate a myocardial ischemia or worse, an infarction, even in a child. Furthermore, epinephrine [Adrenalin] 1:1,000 is more effective at dilating the upper airway rather than the lower airways.
- Fluid replacement should be part of the management plan. Patients in respiratory distress breathe faster and dry out their respiratory mucosal membranes faster than healthy individuals would. Approximately 10% of water is lost during normal ventilation.
- Corticosteroids such as methylprednisolone sodium succinate [Solu-Medrol] or dexamethasone sodium phosphate [Decadron] work over several hours, slowing down and limiting the extent of the inflammation.
- With the exception of food poisoning, poisonings usually involve substances that were not typically intended for human consumption and overdoses usually involve substances (most frequently medicines) that were designed for human consumption but have been taken, either accidentally or purposefully, in excess.
- Hypoxia is the leading cause of cardiac arrhythmias in children.
- The child with a seizure is a common medical complaint in which the paramedic may need to intervene with a drug.
- Trauma is the young person's disease, and many children are taken from their families suddenly due to tragic accidents.
- The Wong-Baker FACES pain rating scale is a particularly useful tool used to measure the level of pain a child is experiencing.

Vital Vocabulary

Bradycardia A slow heart rate, less than 60 beats/min; a pulse rate of less than 100 beats/min in the newborn.

Epiphyseal plate The area of growing tissue near the end of the pediatric long bones that determines the future length and shape of the mature bone. Also called the growth plate.

Sinus tachycardia (ST) A sinus rhythm with a heart rate greater than 100 beats/min.

Supraventricular tachycardia (SVT) An abnormal heart rhythm with a rapid, narrow QRS complex.

Tachycardia A rapid heart rate, more than 100 beats/min.

Tenth cranial nerve The vagus nerve, which runs throughout the body. It is responsible for slowing down the heart rate when stimulated.

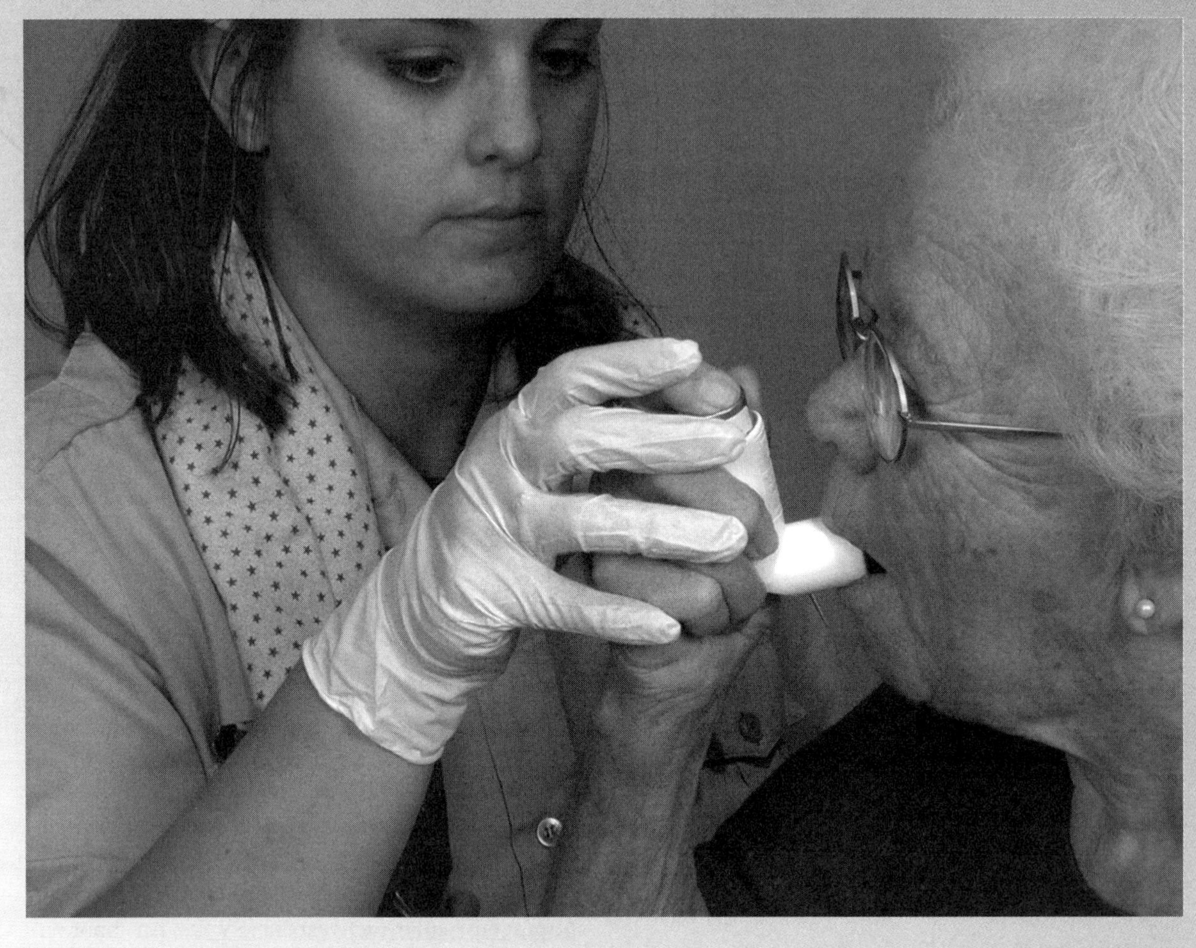

Geriatric Emergencies 14

Objectives

Cognitive

6-3.15 Compare the pharmacokinetics of an elderly patient to that of a young adult. (pages 404–416)

6-3.16 Discuss the impact of polypharmacy and medication non-compliance on patient assessment and management. (pages 406, 408–409)

6-3.17 Discuss drug distribution, metabolism, and excretion in the elderly patient. (pages 409–410)

6-3.18 Discuss medication issues of the elderly including polypharmacy, dosing errors, and increased drug sensitivity. (pages 406, 408–409)

6-3.19 Discuss the use and effects of commonly prescribed drugs for the elderly patient. (page 412)

6-3.25 Develop a treatment and management plan of the elderly patient with pulmonary complaints, including pneumonia, chronic obstructive pulmonary diseases, and pulmonary embolism. (page 418)

6-3.31 Develop a treatment and management plan of the elderly patient with cardiovascular complaints, including myocardial infarction, heart failure, arrhythmias, aneurysm, and hypertension. (page 418)

6-3.37 Develop a treatment and management plan of the elderly patient with complaints related to the nervous system, including cerebral vascular disease, delirium, dementia, Alzheimer's disease, and Parkinson's disease. (page 418)

6-3.43 Develop a treatment and management plan of the elderly patient with endocrine problems, including diabetes and thyroid diseases. (page 418)

6-3.50 Discuss the normal and abnormal changes with age related to toxicology. (pages 404–416)

6-3.51 Discuss the assessment of the elderly patient with complaints related to toxicology. (pages 404–416)

6-3.52 Identify the need for intervention and transport of the patient with toxicological problems. (pages 404–416)

6-3.53 Develop and execute a treatment plan and management of the elderly patient with toxicological problems. (pages 404–416)

6-3.54 Describe the epidemiology in the elderly, including the incidence, morbidity/mortality, risk factors, and prevention strategies for patients with drug toxicity. (pages 404–416)

6-3.55 Compare and contrast the pathophysiology of drug toxicity in the elderly with that of a younger adult. (pages 404–416)

6-3.56 Discuss the assessment findings common in elderly patients with drug toxicity. (pages 404–416)

6-3.61 Discuss the management/considerations when treating an elderly patient with drug and alcohol abuse. (pages 404–416)

Affective

None

Psychomotor

None

Additional Objectives

6-1 Discuss causes of falls in the elderly. (pages 416–417)

6-2 Discuss the management of specific geriatric conditions. (pages 417–423)

Drugs and the Geriatric Population

In this chapter we use the terms elderly and geriatric interchangeably. Because the body works constantly to detoxify and eliminate chemicals such as medications, the effects of most drugs are temporary. As discussed in Chapter 1, the liver is the primary organ for detoxifying and metabolizing most drugs so they can be eliminated through the kidneys. Depending on the drug, the kidneys, lungs, intestinal mucosa, and plasma may also be involved in this process. Some drugs pass through the body partially or almost fully unchanged. Geriatric patients become more susceptible to an adverse response to drug therapy when they develop a decline in liver and kidney functions and cannot eliminate drugs at the same rate as a younger person might. In some cases, potentially heavy medication use might be indicated such as in patients who are terminally ill.

Geriatric Medication Concerns

When a geriatric patient is taking medications, remember that it could be a contributing factor to nearly any health problem. When a problem arises that produces a 9-1-1 call, consider any recent changes in the patient's medication schedules. Look for the starting or stopping of drug administration, changes in dosing, medication non-compliance, and recent changes affecting daily living conditions (ie, limited or loss of mobility, vision problems, loss of financial support, loss of social support, loss of memory, altered mental status, and exacerbation of an existing condition or the development of a new condition).

Geriatric patients often have multiple medical problems for which they may be taking many different medications (**polypharmacy**) (**Figure 14-1** ▸).

These drugs can interact with each other in a negative way, potentiate side effects, or enhance or neutralize one other. Some drugs predispose patients to hypothermia. Some are a blend of medications, creating a risk factor for inadvertent overdose or side effects. Medications may be dispensed with a trade name or a generic name so the patient may have the same drug with different labels. The issues of concern with geriatric medication administration involve polypharmacy, medication non-compliance, potential dosing errors, increased sensitivity, and abuse.

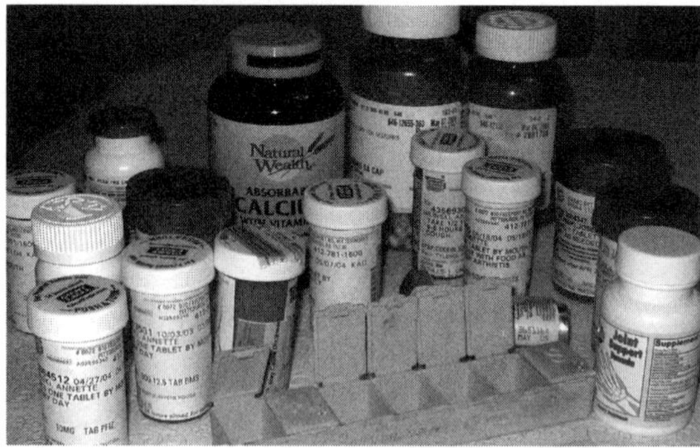

Figure 14-1 Geriatric patients are often prescribed many medications at the same time.

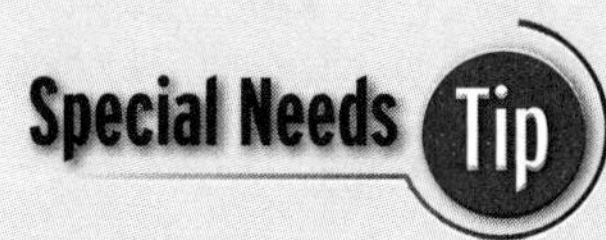

Many geriatric patients take a variety of medications. Often these include analgesics, antihypertensives, and anti-inflammatories. Conditions related to polypharmacy can result in untoward concomitant reactions between these medications. Occasionally the patient will take additional medication to make up for a missed dose, and this must be asked during the history-taking process.

Case Study 1 A Syncopal Episode

Part 1

Your unit has been dispatched to an assisted living center in a quiet community on the east side of town. As you and your partner pull up in front of the Golden Years Community Center, you are met by two elderly women at the curb. They ask you to please come quickly because Mrs. Wilson may have broken her hip.

They tell you that Millie Wilson, their close friend, was playing bingo with the usual group this afternoon when she said she needed to go to the ladies' room. When she did not come back they found her on the floor in the hallway, confused and unable to get up.

You have decided that the scene is safe so you load up the stretcher with equipment and follow the ladies into the building. There is a lot going on inside and it is very noisy. Fortunately it is quieter in the hallway where Mrs. Wilson is.

As you kneel beside the patient you introduce yourself and begin your initial assessment (see **Table 1**). Mrs. Wilson tells you to call her Millie.

The initial assessment does not reveal any immediate life-threats but you decide to maintain manual stabilization of the head and neck because Millie is confused and not sure she remembers passing out. You note that her right leg is shortened and rotated outward. You recall from your medic class that the external rotation is usually a sign of fracture, while internal rotation is dislocation.

Table 1 Initial Assessment

Initial Assessment	Recording Time: 2 Minutes
General Impression/ Appearance	Slightly confused, elderly patient with obviously injured right hip/pelvis
Mental Status	"V" verbally responsive (knows name, and where she is but confused about the day)
Airway	Open and clear
Breathing	Rapid and regular
Circulation	Slow pulse but strong radial pulse, no external bleeding
Priority/Plan	High at this point until more information is obtained

Based on what you have learned so far about Millie, she will need a focused history and physical examination as well as the rapid trauma examination to help narrow down how she ended up on the floor. With a chief complaint of a hip injury and suspected syncope, it will be helpful to elaborate on the chief complaint with the OPQRST questions.

Question 1: What is syncope?

Question 2: What are some of the causes of falls in the geriatric patient?

Part 2

Your partner gets a set of vital signs and applies the ECG electrodes as part of the focused history and physical examination (see **Table 2**). You use the OPQRST questions to elaborate on the chief complaint. Your rapid trauma examination only confirms that Millie has swelling and deformity in the right hip area. She has adequate distal pulses, motor function, and sensation (PMS) in the injured leg. Due to the MOI, you decide to continue to maintain the head/neck immobilization so a rigid cervical collar is applied.

From your interview and conversation with Millie, she is more coherent as compared to when you first introduced yourself. It seems that she was rushing to go to the ladies' room as she wanted to get back to the bingo game. She says that she felt dizzy when she got up from the toilet and as she was rushing back down the hallway she felt like she might pass out. Of course that is all she remembers until she woke up on the floor with a friend calling her name.

Table 2 Focused History and Physical Examination

Baseline Vital Signs	Recording Time: 5 Minutes
Skin CTC (color, temperature, and condition)	Pale, cool, diaphoretic
Pulse	46 beats/min and radial
Blood Pressure	88/64 mm Hg
Respirations	24 breaths/min and regular

Question 3: What is the significance of Millie feeling dizzy when she got up so fast?

Question 4: The fact that Millie woke up on the floor could indicate what to you?

Case Study I Continued

Part 3

The ECG shows a very slow rhythm and you will be looking closer to determine specifically what the cause of the rhythm is. You perform the SAMPLE history (see **Table 3**). From the information obtained during the SAMPLE history, as well as discussion with the patient, it is clear that Millie has a cardiac history and is taking a beta-blocker. It would be appropriate to do a 12-lead ECG because any irregularity in an elderly patient, especially a patient on a beta-blocker, could be masking the symptoms of an acute myocardial infarction (AMI). Millie says that her heart has not been giving her any trouble for the past few months and she does not remember the last time she actually took one of those nitroglycerin pills. It seems that this is not Millie's first dizzy spell as she woke up on the floor in the bathroom about a week ago. This information was obtained by staff at the facility and not volunteered by Millie. It was clear that she did not go to the hospital at that time because she did not say anything to the staff at the time of the incident. They figured it out later that evening.

Table 3 SAMPLE History

SAMPLE History	Comments
Signs/symptoms	Right hip pain and swelling, dizziness, slow heartbeat, denies any chest pain or shortness of breath (SOB)
Allergies	Penicillin, Sumycin (Tetracycline)
Medications	Nitroglycerin, folic acid, quinapril (Accupril), atorvastatin calcium (Lipitor), diazepam (Valium), aspirin, vitamin E, vitamin C, and metoprolol tartrate (Lopressor)
Pertinent past medical history	Cardiac history including angina, an MI in 2005 and another in 2007, an irregular heart rhythm, high cholesterol
Last oral intake	Orange juice and a muffin about an hour ago
Events leading up to the incident	Dizziness and possible syncopal episode. May also have been some seizure activity although there is no prior history.

Treatment Plan

1. Assess and manage the ABCs.
2. Administer supplemental oxygen by nonrebreathing mask.
3. Obtain a 12-lead ECG and interpret the results.
4. Obtain vascular access.
5. Splint and ice the fracture.
6. Check blood glucose (due to altered mental status).
7. Check rhythm. After consulting with medical control, administer atropine sulfate (Atropine) (see **Table 4**).
8. Consult medical control for pain medication such as fentanyl citrate (Sublimise) (see **Table 5**).
9. Manage the arrhythmia.
10. Reassess serial vital signs and alert the receiving facility during transport.

Table 4 Atropine Sulfate

Do you know?	Comments
Right drug? Generic name: [**Atropine Sulfate**] Trade name: [Atropine]	This drug is an anticholinergic agent (parasympathetic blocker). It is used to manage symptomatic bradycardias (ie, hypotension, AMS). It is also used as an antidote for toxicity due to organophosphate nerve agents and cholinergic drugs.
Right patient?	In this case it would be considered for a patient with a hemodynamically unstable bradycardia (< 60 beats/min); also asystole or PEA (although not pertinent to this patient at this point).
Right dose?	For a symptomatic bradycardia 0.5 mg IV push is administered. If the patient goes into cardiac arrest (asystole or PEA), the dose would be 1 mg IV/IO push. May repeat every 3–5 minutes to a maximum of 0.04 mg/kg.
Right route?	IV/IO. Can be administered by ET route which involves 2-3 mg diluted in 10 mL of normal saline (this route has questionable effectiveness).
Right time?	After the patient has received high quality CPR for two cycles and the vasopressor has yet to work in the cardiac arrest situation.
Right documentation?	Dose, route, time administered, and reassessment should be clearly documented on the patient care report. *continues*

Case Study 1 Continued

Table 4 **Atropine Sulfate (*Continued*)**

Do you know?	Comments
Expected action	Parasympatholytic reaction that inhibits the action of acetylcholine at the postganglionic parasympathetic neuroeffector sites. Increased heart rate in life-threatening bradyarrhythmias.
Side effects	Headache, dizziness, palpitations, nausea and vomiting, tachycardia, arrhythmias, anticholinergic effects (blurred vision, dry mouth, urinary retention), paradoxical bradycardia when pushed slowly or at low doses; flushed, hot, dry skin.
Contraindications	Tachycardia, hypersensitivity, unstable cardiovascular status in acute hemorrhage and myocardial ischemia, narrow-angle glaucoma.
Precautions	Potential adverse effects when administered with digoxin (Lanoxin), cholinergics, physostigmine salicylate (Antilirium). Effects enhanced by antihistamines, procainamide (Pronestyl), quinidine (Quinidex), antipsychotics, benzodiazepines, and antidepressants.
Pharmacokinetics	Onset: immediate; peak effect: 1–2 minutes; Duration: 2–6 hours metabolized by the liver, excreted through urine unchanged.

Table 5 **Fentanyl Citrate**

Do you know?	Comments
Right drug? Generic name: [**Fentanyl Citrate**] Trade name: [Sublimase]	This drug is a narcotic analgesic (schedule II narcotic). It is used to treat severe pain and is used individually as an analgesic or in combination with other agents during procedural sedation or anesthesia. It has actions similar to morphine sulfate (Astramorph/PF) and meperidine (Demerol).
Right patient?	Relief of severe pain.
Right dose?	0.5–2 μg/kg IV/IM. Due to the size of the patient it would be best to start dosing on the lower end of the range and consult with medical control.
Right route?	IV/IM.
Right time?	After assessment and contraindications for use have been considered.
Right documentation?	Always document how and when the drug was administered as well as the patient's response to the medication on your patient care report.
Expected action	Pain relief.
Side effects	Skeletal and thoracic muscle rigidity, bradycardia, seizures, and diaphoresis.
Contraindications	Myasthenia gravis.
Precautions	May cause life-threatening hypoventilation.
Pharmacokinetics	Onset: immediate IV, 2–7 minutes IM; peak effect: 30 minutes IM; Duration: 30–60 minutes IV, 1–2 hours IM; metabolized in the liver and excreted in urine.

In Millie's case, the 12-lead does not show any evidence of a new MI or ST-segment elevations. Because syncope can be caused by hypoglycemia, you check her blood glucose. It is within the normal range and sitting up her blood pressure is 90 mm Hg by palpation. Her rhythm is a second-degree type I block and you administer a dose of 0.5 mg IV atropine sulfate [Atropine] per protocol, which proves to be effective in increasing her heart rate to just above 60 beats/min and her mental status to alert. As she becomes alert, she also feels the pain in her right hip more prominently. The fentanyl citrate [Sublimase] will be helpful for the pain and is probably more appropriate than morphine sulfate [Astramorph/PF] in light of her marginal blood pressure.

Question 5: Why is it important to obtain a 12-lead ECG in Millie's case even though she denies chest pain?

Question 6: What is the significance of Millie's past cardiac history?

Case Study I Continued

Part 4

With plenty of help from Millie's friends, you and your partner have carefully immobilized her on the long backboard with plenty of padding to make the ride to the hospital as comfortable as possible. You have also obtained vascular access and administered a dose of fentanyl citrate [Sublimase] to take an edge off the pain.

Millie, it seems, is a big talker and now that her head is clear again she proceeds to tell you about her interesting life before moving to the assisted living center. You listen intently as you continue your reassessment and ongoing assessment of the patient (**Table 6**).

Question 7: Why did you check Millie's blood glucose?

Question 8: If you identified the ECG as a second-degree type II heart block, what would be the primary treatment? You may need to refer to case study IV in Chapter 4, Cardiovascular Emergencies.

Table 6 Reassessment and Ongoing Assessment of the Patient

Serial Vital Signs and Relevant Data	Recording Time: 9 Minutes
Skin CTC	Pale, warm, dry
Pulse	68 beats/min and regular
Blood Pressure	100/70 mm Hg
Respirations	20 breaths/min and regular
Mental Status	"A" alert (oriented to person, place, and day)
ECG	Normal sinus rhythm at this point
SpO_2	98%
Lung Sounds	Clear bilaterally
Other (ie, blood glucose, core temperature)	Blood glucose is 128 mg/dL, good distal pulse in injured extremity, no pedal edema

Part 5

The ride to the ED was an enjoyable one where you reassessed Millie's condition and she was doing well, considering she has a fractured right hip. You called the ED to give them a brief report of her condition and to allow them time to prepare for her. You also had the pleasure of learning all about a wonderful lady who, in her younger days, was a graduate of an Ivy League college, an excellent swimmer and dancer, and was very involved in local politics in her community.

And of course as is the case with many of the patients you have taken out of that home, Millie was extremely grateful for the service you provided in her time of need.

Polypharmacy

Polypharmacy involves the simultaneous use of different medications. It is not uncommon to ask a geriatric patient to produce the medications they are taking only to find they have a shopping bag full of vials. Sometimes patients go to multiple physicians and are able to obtain prescribed medications from each of them. A physician does not always have knowledge of the medications a patient may be taking if prescribed by someone else. This is problematic because some medications have a synergistic effect; others potentiate one another [ie, codeine and alcohol); some cancel each other out; and some are linked to other complications [ie, atorvastatin calcium (Lipitor) and grapefruit juice have been linked to prolonged QT syndrome when used together]. Patients have been known to overdose on nonsteroidal anti-inflammatory drugs (NSAIDs) or aspirin since so many OTC preparations have these substances in them. It is always best to advise the patient that he or she should have a complete written list of the medications he or she is taking. The list should include each drug name, the specific dose and times per day it is administered, and the reason it is administered (as some drugs have multiple indications). This information should be kept in the wallet or purse so it can be shown to the health care providers prior to treatment, or to a new physician prescribing another medication for the patient. The Vial of Life is another option that is used to keep this information in a secure and dry place (**Figure 14-2** ▸).

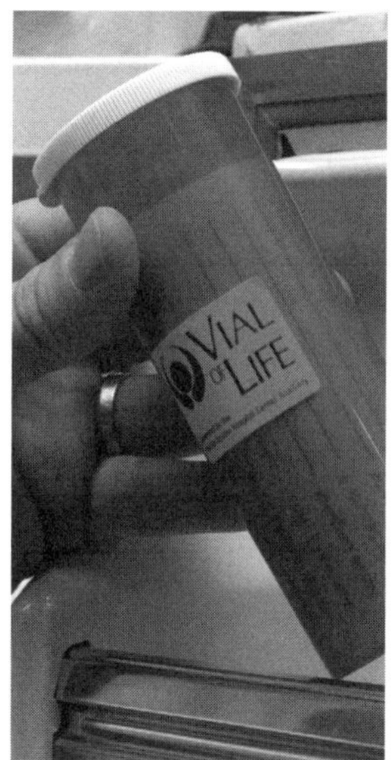

Figure 14-2 Medication containers such as The Vial of Life can be provided to geriatric patients to keep track of medication information.

Medication Non-Compliance

Another major concern with the geriatric patient is medication non-compliance. Some geriatric patients will take it upon themselves to switch back and forth between two medications, rather than taking both medications as a "cost saving" measure. This can be dangerous and in some cases neither of the medications is effective when used inappropriately. When an antibiotic is prescribed, the patient should take the entire prescribed dose. Many geriatric patients stop taking the pills because they feel better one day. For example, when an anticonvulsant is prescribed, a patient cannot skip days because a consistent blood concentration of the medication is imperative. The patient's blood level of the anticonvulsant medication will decrease and he or she is likely to experience a breakthrough seizure. Another example includes corticosteroid use. Patients taking medium to long-term courses of corticosteroids must be gradually weaned off so as to permit the adrenal glands to resume natural cortisol production. A patient cannot abruptly stop using these because eliminating doses too quickly can result in **adrenal crisis** (a life-threatening state caused by insufficient levels of cortisol).

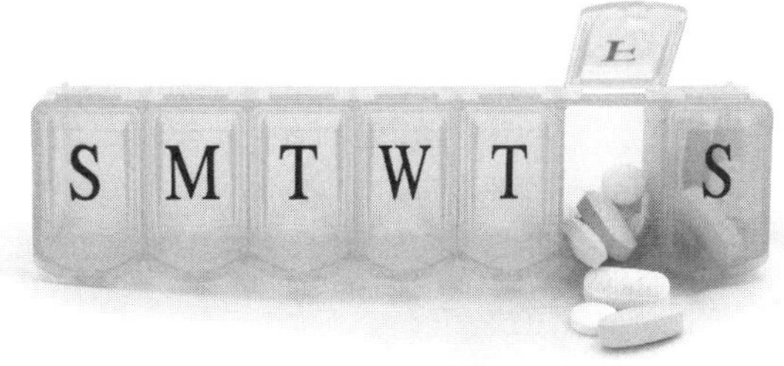

Figure 14-3 7-day containers can be helpful in keeping the patient on his or her daily prescribed medication schedule.

It is not uncommon for the paramedic to find that the geriatric patient has a long list of medications that are supposed to be taken every day.

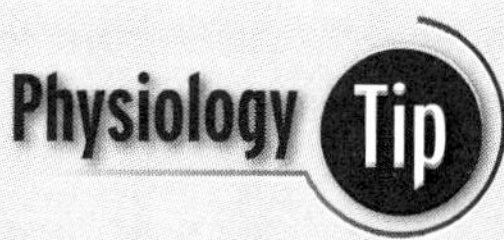

The purpose of pain medication in the prehospital setting is not to completely remove all pain, but to make the pain bearable so the patient is comfortable and able to tolerate the transport to the hospital.

Dosing Errors

The potential for dosing errors is increased in the patient who may suffer from some degree of dementia. A friend or family member should take an active role in helping the geriatric patient separate out the daily medications. Most drug stores have 7-day containers that can be helpful in keeping the patient on his or her daily prescribed medication schedule (**Figure 14-3** ▸). This is particularly useful for the patient who is required to take multiple medications daily.

Drug Sensitivity

Increased drug sensitivity is always a concern in the geriatric patient. The anticoagulant warfarin (Coumadin) is an example of a drug to which the geriatric population is sensitive. Bleeding is the main side effect and may occur from any tissue or organ. Furthermore, this drug increases the risk of bleeding secondary to relatively minor trauma, infection, renal insufficiency, polycythemia vera, vasculitis, and allergic reactions.

Toxicology and the Geriatric Patient

According to the web site www.caregivers.com, America's senior society (older than age 65) consists of only 13% of the population yet it uses 35% of all medications dispensed, and 21% of all hospital admissions are related to adverse medication emergencies, of which 50% are thought to be preventable.

Table 14-1 Drugs Most Commonly Causing Toxic Reactions in Elderly People

Medication	Symptoms
Anti-inflammatory agents (NSAIDs, steroids)	Drowsiness, dizziness, confusion, anxiety, bradypnea, tachypnea, GI bleeding
Antibiotics	GI signs, altered mental status, seizures, coma
Anticholinergics and antihistamines	Urination difficulty, constipation, drowsiness, restlessness, irritability, hypertension
Anticoagulants (warfarin)	Ecchymosis, epistaxis, hematuria, abdominal pain, vomiting, fecal blood
Antiarrhythmics (amiodarone, lidocaine)	Restlessness, hypotension, bradycardia, tachycardia, palpitations, angina
Antidepressants (tricyclics, long-acting selective serotonin reuptake inhibitors)	Confusion, delirium, disorientation, memory impairment
Antihypertensives (diuretics, alpha blockers, beta-blockers; angiotensin-converting enzyme inhibitors)	Hypotension, palpitations, angina, fluid retention, headache
Antipsychotics (phenothiazines, atypicals)	Drowsiness, tachycardia, dizziness, restlessness
Digoxin	Headache, fatigue, malaise, drowsiness, depression
Insulin and oral antidiabetic medications	Hypoglycemia presenting as confusion
Narcotics	Delirium, respiratory depression, apnea, involuntary muscle movements
Sedative-hypnotics (benzodiazepines, barbiturates)	Incoordination, dizziness, disturbances in cognitive function

Patients that have decreased cardiac functions, circulation, or renal and liver functions will have a slower metabolic rate that decreases clearance efficiency and leads to toxic or adverse reactions (**Table 14-1** ▲).

All medications have therapeutic ranges or indexes, but some (ie, warfarin [Coumadin], digoxin [Lanoxin], lidocaine hydrochloride [Xylocaine], and various beta-blockers) have very specific therapeutic ranges and are especially likely to be either ineffective due to slightly low therapeutic blood levels or produce toxicity because of somewhat elevated levels; therefore, geriatric patients must be monitored very closely. Always consider that certain medications are commonly associated with major adverse events in the geriatric patient; examples include: warfarin (Coumadin), heparin, prednisone (Deltasone), furosemide (Lasix), insulin, oxygen, narcotics, NSAIDS, blood pressure medications, medications known to display anticholinergic activity, OTC medications, herbals, and natural home remedies.

Case Study II Sick with the Chills

Part 1

Your unit has been dispatched to a low income housing project where a geriatric person has been feeling ill. The police are already on scene as you pull up in front of building. This is the third time this week you have responded to this location and they still have not fixed the broken elevator. Fortunately, the patient is only on the fourth floor of the 10-story building.

You are met at the doorway by a geriatric gentleman who says his wife has been very sick for the past 2 days. She has been vomiting and has not been able to keep food down. He is afraid she may have pneumonia like she did last winter. The scene is safe so the three of you enter the small apartment. The patient is introduced as Mrs. Alverez. As you walk through the kitchen to the back bedroom, you notice that the oven is on and open which seems strange since there is no smell of cooking.

Your partner decides to question the gentleman who is Mike, her husband of 50 years. In the meantime, your general impression of the patient reveals an ill-looking woman in her 60s who is shivering and sweating with blankets on her. She is sitting up in her bed with a small portable television turned on.

Your initial assessment does not reveal any immediate life-threats to the ABCs (see **Table 1**). Based on the information you have so far and the fact that there is no apparent trauma, you decide this is a responsive medical patient who will need a focused history and physical examination.

Case Study II Continued

Table 1 Initial Assessment

Initial Assessment	Recording Time: 2 Minutes
General Impression/ Appearance	Shivering, diaphoretic, elderly woman
Mental Status	"V" verbal (oriented to person, place, but not the day)
Airway	Open and clear
Breathing	Rapid and shallow
Circulation	Rapid and weak radial pulse
Priority/Plan	High due to the abnormal vital signs. Further information may identify other potential life threats.

Question 1: What could be the reason for the open oven, and does this have an effect on the patient's condition?

Question 2: Why is the patient shivering?

Part 2

According to Mike, Mrs. Alverez has been sick for a few days and is getting worse each day. He says he would not have bothered to call 9-1-1 but she was acting very confused this morning before the ambulance arrived. She has type 2 diabetes. He said her last blood glucose test was a little on the low side. Your partner gets a set of baseline vital signs as you begin to ask the "OPQRST" questions to elaborate on the chief complaint. The plan is to recheck her blood glucose with a finger stick and to ask Mike to gather all of her medications.

You note that the kitchen is warm but the back bedroom is cool. You ask Mike about the heat in the apartment and he says that it has not been working this week. You know with gas there is always a potential for carbon monoxide (CO) poisoning. You turn off the oven and prepare to get moving out of the apartment as soon as possible. It is best to wrap up Mrs. Alverez in a blanket and load her onto the stair chair so you can get her out of the apartment. You can complete the focused history and physical examination as you move toward the ambulance (see **Table 2**). Using the back of your hand, you recognize that the temperature of her skin feels cooler than yours. Just prior to leaving the apartment you get a temperature on Mrs. Alverez and it is a little low at 95.5°F.

Question 3: What factors indicate that you should check the blood glucose on this patient?

Question 4: Why did you check the body temperature on this patient?

Table 2 Focused History and Physical Examination

Baseline Vital Signs	Recording Time: 4 Minutes
Skin CTC (color, temperature, condition)	Pale, warm, and diaphoretic
Pulse	110 beats/min
Blood Pressure	98/68 mm Hg
Respirations	24 breaths/min and shallow

Part 3

She is still shivering so you will try to warm her up with blankets and heat in the ambulance. This may explain why she was a little confused. Of course there may be other explanations for her confusion. Since her blood glucose is borderline (70 mg/dL), you decide to give her some dextrose (Glutose) on a tongue depressor to hold in her mouth against her gums.

Your partner mentions that she could be dehydrated. Her lungs are clear so the pneumonia is not high on the list of suspected conditions. Also a 12-lead ECG will need to be taken because as a geriatric patient, a woman, and a diabetic, she certainly fits the profile for a potential silent MI. Of course, CO poisoning is always a factor because the oven was being used as a source of heat. However, Mike has no symptoms of headache or nausea and he says he has been in the apartment for days. As you begin moving down the stairwell, Mrs. Alverez becomes more talkative, asking if the apartment was locked and if

Case Study II Continued

the oven is turned off. Mike was right on top of both of those things as well as packing a few clothes and bringing along a small bag with her medications. That was fortunate since your focus was to just get her out of the apartment at that point and this will complete your SAMPLE history (see **Table 3**).

As you are exiting the apartment, the fire department arrives. They will be going into the apartment and checking the carbon monoxide levels to see if they are dangerous. You mention to your partner, "It would be nice if we had one of those new CO monitors for cases like this."

Table 3 SAMPLE History

SAMPLE History	Comments
Signs/symptoms	Weak, nausea, vomiting for past few days. An altered level of conciousness today
Allergies	Sulfate drugs, penicillin, novocaine, and tetracycline [Sumycin]
Medications	Furosemide [Lasix], nitroglycerin [Nitrostat], aspirin, glyburide [Diabeta], and vitamins E and C
Pertinent past medical history	Type II diabetic
Last oral intake	Minimal breakfast about 3 hours ago but has not been able to hold down more than tea and dry toast
Events leading up to the incident	Sick for the last few days; getting progressively worse this morning

Treatment Plan

1. Assess and manage the ABCs.
2. Administer supplemental oxygen by nonrebreathing mask.
3. Check blood glucose and treat with dextrose (Glutose) per protocol [ie, if low blood glucose and altered mental status with a good gag reflex consider oral dextrose (Glutose); if altered mental status and questionable gag reflex give either Glucagon (see **Table 4**) or 25 g of dextrose by IV (see **Table 5**)].
4. Obtain vascular access and consider administering IV fluids (as a challenge as long as the lungs are dry). If you think electrolyte imbalance may be a concern, consult with medical control (see **Table 6** and **Table 7**).
5. Obtain an ECG (12-lead would be appropriate) and interpret.
6. Consider the need to manage the arrhythmia (consult with medical control).
7. Reassess serial vital signs and alert ED during transport.

Table 4 Glucagon

Do you know?	Comments
Right drug? Generic name: [**Glucagon**] Trade name: [Glucagon]	This drug is a pancreatic hormone, insulin antagonist. The generic and trade names are the same for this medication. Considered to have a major role in the maintenance of a normal concentration of glucose in the blood. Glucagon is the opposing factor to insulin in keeping glucose within its normal range.
Right patient?	The diabetic patient with a suspected or confirmed low blood glucose level. It has also been used for esophageal strictures with obstruction since it may promote esophageal smooth muscle relaxation. Although not in this case, may be used as an intropic agent in beta-blocker overdose.
Right dose?	0.5 to 1 unit that may be repeated in 7- to 10-minute increments. The drug comes in a container of liquid and a container of dry powder, which needs to be mixed prior to administration.
Right route?	May be administered IM, IV, or SC, and it is likely that family members may have administered the medication to the patient prior to calling EMS.
Right time?	As soon as possible after baseline vital signs since brain cells may be dying without glucose. Family members are usually told to administer the medication while the patient is still conscious.
Right documentation?	The patient care report should state the glucose level, the amount of glucagon administered, the serial vital signs, and the patient's response to the medication. It may not be possible to get a tube of blood prior to administration of the glucagon, since it is often given on a diabetic with poor IV access. In that case, be sure to document an initial finger-stick glucose reading.

continues

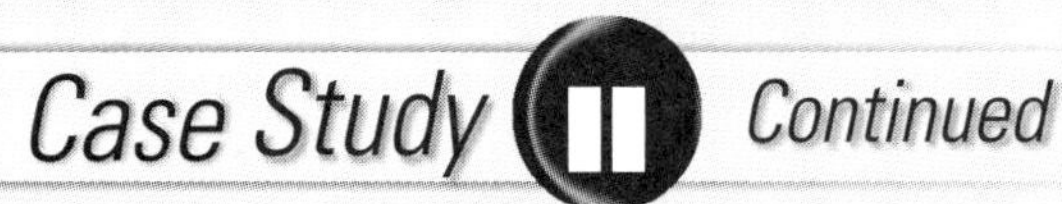

Case Study II Continued

Table 4 Glucagon (*Continued*)

Do you know?	Comments
Expected action	Improvement in the patient's mental status. Increase in blood glucose concentration.
Side effects	Dizziness, light headed, nausea, and vomiting (which are also symptoms of the hypoglycemia) and sometimes urticaria.
Contraindications	A known hypersensitivity to glucagon, hyperglycemia, hypersensitivity.
Precautions	There are none in the prehospital setting.
Pharmacokinetics	Onset: 1 minute; peak effect: 30 minutes; Duration: variable (generally 9–17 minutes); how fast and how effective this drug is will vary on the amount of liver glycogen reserves the patient has.

Table 5 50% Dextrose

Do you know?	Comments
Right drug? Generic name: [**50% Dextrose**] Trade name: [$D_{50}W$]	This is a carbohydrate hypertonic solution. Also called glucose or d-glucose.
Right patient?	Diabetic with a documented low blood glucose. Severe hypoglycemia for any cause (ie, insulin shock, alcoholism).
Right dose?	25 grams IV bolus for the adult patient.
Right route?	A patent large bore IV site.
Right time?	As soon as possible after baseline vital signs since brain cells may be dying without glucose.
Right documentation?	The patient care report should state the glucose level, the amount of $D_{50}W$ administered, and the serial vital signs as well as the patient's response to the medication.
Expected action	The patient's mental status should improve within minutes. Each 100 mL of fluid contains 50 grams of dextrose which delivers 3.4 kcal/g.
Side effects	None provided that the $D_{50}W$ was in a good vein. Redness or pain may occur at the injection site. If the $D_{50}W$ did leak into the surrounding tissue (extravasation) it is so concentrated it can cause local tissue necrosis.
Contraindications	Previous hypersensitivity to dextrose solution. Diabetic coma while patient is hyperglycemic. Intracranial or intraspinal hemorrhage.
Precautions	With patients with suspected stroke check the glucose prior to administering $D_{50}W$. In an ischemic stroke there have been concerns raised that increased blood glucose concentrations may worsen cerebral ischemia and impair recovery.
Pharmacokinetics	Onset: 1 minute; Duration: varies with the severity of hypoglycemia.

Table 6 Sodium Bicarbonate

Do you know?	Comments
Right drug? Generic name: [**Sodium Bicarbonate**] Trade name: [Sodium Bicarbonate]	This drug is an alkalinizing agent, antacid, and electrolyte. It is used to treat tricyclic antidepressant overdose, as well as acute metabolic acidosis caused by shock, severe dehydration, anoxia, uncontrolled diabetes, renal disease, cardiac arrest, and severe lactic acidosis, and as an adjunct in hyperkalemia management.
Right patient?	Tricyclic antidepressant overdose with prolonged QRS duration on ECG.
Right dose?	1 mEq/kg of 8.4% solution.
Right route?	IV bolus in a secondary line.

continues

Case Study II Continued

Table 6 Sodium Bicarbonate (*Continued*)

Do you know?	Comments
Right time?	When bradycardia persists even after adequate oxygenation, ventilation, chest compressions, and fluid bolus.
Right documentation?	Dose, route, time administered, and reassessment should be clearly documented on the patient care report.
Expected action	Relief of metabolic acidosis, narrowing of QRS complex duration.
Side effects	Hypernatremia, alkalosis, tetany, and fluid overload. Be sure to administer slow IV push (especially in premature infants) to avoid causing a rapid change in pH that can produce cerebral bleeding.
Contraindications	Metabolic and respiratory alkalosis, hypertension, convulsions, and CHF.
Precautions	Adverse reactions can include: gastric distention, hypercalcemia, metabolic acidosis; extravasation following IV use may cause tissue sloughing, cellulitis, or necrosis at the site of injection. Do not mix in the same IV line as calcium chloride without first flushing the line or the drugs may precipitate.
Pharmacokinetics	Onset: seconds; peak effect: 1–2 minutes; Duration: 10 minutes. Rapidly metabolized to carbonic acid which rapidly dissociates into water and carbon dioxide. The carbon dioxide is excreted via the lungs.

Table 7 Calcium Chloride

Do you know?	Comments
Right drug? Generic name: [**Calcium Chloride**] Trade name: [Calcium Chloride]	Electrolyte. This drug is used to treat calcium channel blocker (ie, verapamil [Calan, Isoptin]) overdose.
Right patient?	Symptomatic patient from a calcium channel blocker overdose.
Right dose?	500 mg to 1 gram (5-10 mL of a 10% solution) IV/IO push.
Right route?	IVP.
Right time?	When bradycardia persists even after adequate oxygenation, ventilation, chest compressions, and fluid bolus.
Right documentation?	Dose, route, time administered, and reassessment should be clearly documented on the patient care report.
Expected action	Reverse symptoms of calcium channel blocker overdose.
Side effects	Bradycardia, asystole, hypotension, peripheral vasodilation, metallic taste, local necrosis, coronary and cerebral artery spasm, nausea and vomiting.
Contraindications	Hypercalcemia, V-fib, digitalis toxicity.
Precautions	Do not use routinely in cardiac arrest.
Pharmacokinetics	Onset: 5–15 minutes; peak effect: 3–5 minutes; Duration 15–30 minutes but may persist for 4 hours (dose-dependent).

Question 5: Aside from having the fire department test the atmosphere for carbon monoxide, is there any other way to test the patient in the prehospital setting?

Question 6: Why would it be a smart decision to do a 12-lead ECG on this patient?

Case Study II Continued

Part 4

Once outside of the housing complex, the fresh air seems to help perk up Mrs. Alverez. Although it is a cool winter day, the stairwells are hot and you are both dripping wet after carrying her down four flights.

Once in the back of the ambulance, you begin the reassessment by starting an IV and beginning a fluid challenge since her blood pressure is low (90 mm Hg systolic) and her lungs are clear (see **Table 8**). You decide that since she is mentating well at this point it will not be necessary to administer glucagon or 50% Dextrose ($D_{50}W$). Mrs. Alverez is still nauseous so you ask her to hold onto a convenience bag, just in case.

Question 7: Is the sinus tachycardia a problem in Mrs. Alverez?

Question 8: Since Mrs. Alverez's blood glucose is 70 mg/dL, will you need to administer IV dextrose in addition to the oral dextrose [Glutose]?

Table 8 Reassessment and Ongoing Assessment of the Patient

Serial Vital Signs and Relevant Data	Recording Time: 10 Minutes
Skin CTC	Pale, cool, and not as clammy as before
Pulse	108 beats/min at the radial artery
Blood Pressure	100/70 mm Hg
Respirations	22 breaths/min and regular
Mental Status	"A" alert (oriented to person, place, and day)
ECG	Sinus tachycardia. The 12-lead shows no significant ST-segment changes.
SpO_2	97% on nonrebreathing
Lung Sounds	Clear bilaterally
Other (ie, glucose, core temperature)	Glucose is 70 mg/dL and temp is 97°F

Part 5

En route to the hospital you have a nice conversation with the couple. Apparently they have lived in this country for 55 years and have always worked hard for the county. When the county had its cutbacks a few years ago, they were laid off as an early retirement. Unfortunately, having raised six children who have since moved away, they had little savings and the costs of medications, food, and rent were making it very difficult for them to make ends meet. They said they were one of the first families to move into the city housing project, but over the years it has been in disrepair and there is a lot of crime due to the street gangs that moved in nearby. It was interesting to hear of the nicer days in that housing project because for as long as you have been responding there, it has always been a troublesome area.

Just as you arrive at the ED, the fire captain relays that the carbon monoxide levels in the building were elevated but not in a dangerous range. After presenting the patient to the ED physician, he decides he will still follow up with Mrs. Alverez about her diabetes, an intestinal bug that may have caused the initial sickness, as well as watch her body temperature.

Due to the borderline CO levels, the landlord will be forced to fix the heating problem right away. That should be good news for the elderly couple.

Management of Toxicology Emergencies

The treatment and management plan for a geriatric patient with a possible or known adverse medication emergency is to maintain the ABCs, and get a complete list of their prescribed and OTC medications, including changes in dosing, the starting and stopping of a medication, and any known allergies. Attempt to identify the cause and if possible and available, administer an antidote or drug to counter the effects (**Table 14-2** ▸).

Digitalis Toxicity

Digoxin (Lanoxin) is an example of a drug that is very toxic and has a narrow margin of safety between a therapeutic dose and a toxic dose. Serum levels must be evaluated regularly to ensure safe use. The half-life is prolonged in the geriatric patient; therefore, smaller doses may be prescribed. Signs to watch out for with digitalis toxicity are bluish/yellowish tinted vision, a visualized glow or "halo" around objects, generalized GI disturbances, palpitations, confusion, or hallucinations. Additional signs and symptoms of digitalis toxicity include:

- Abdominal pain/distress/bleeding
- Anorexia
- Aphasia
- Arrhythmias

Table 14-2 Management of Drugs Causing Adverse Effects

Drug Causing Adverse Effects	Management
Lidocaine	CNS depression may occur; be alert for respiratory changes. No antidote is used in prehospital care.
Beta-blockers	Provide supportive care and give activated charcoal; consider the use of atropine, epinephrine, and glucagon in symptomatic patient.
Antihypertensives	Provide supportive care. No antidote is used in the prehospital setting to reverse the effects.
Diuretics	Provide supportive care. Consider treatments aimed at restoring volume completion and electrolyte imbalance. No antidote is used in the prehospital setting to reverse the effects.
Digitalis	Provide supportive care. Consider fluid replacement, vasoactive medications such as dopamine, and activated charcoal.
Psychotropics	Provide supportive care. Consider aggressive fluid replacement.
Antidepressants	Provide supportive care. Give fluid therapy for hypotension and sodium bicarbonate.

Table 14-3 Causes of Falls in the Elderly

Cause	Clues to Suggest This Cause
Extrinsic (accidental)	Obvious environmental hazard at the scene, such as poor lighting, scatter rugs, uneven sidewalk, ice or other slippery surface
Intrinsic drop attacks	Sudden fall; patient found on the ground somewhat confused, often temporarily paralyzed and unable to get up; no premonitory symptoms
Postural hypotension	Fall when getting up from a recumbent or sitting position (Check medications the patient is taking, and ask about occult blood loss, such as presence of black stools. Measure blood pressure in recumbent and sitting positions.)
Dizziness or syncope	Marked bradycardia or tachyarrhythmias
Stroke	Other characteristic signs of stroke, such as hemiparesis, hemiplegia, or aphasia
Fracture	Patient felt something snap before falling.

- Bowel necrosis
- Confusion
- Convulsions
- Delirium/hallucinations
- Depression
- Diarrhea
- Epigastric distress
- Fatigue
- Headache
- Hypokalemia
- Hypotension
- Insomnia
- Irritability
- Muscle weakness
- Nausea and vomiting
- Respiratory distress

Falling—A Serious Health Problem

Falling down is a leading cause of injury and death and is a major life threat for geriatric patients. Approximately 30% of people older than age 65 experience a fall each year. The rates of fall-related injuries in the geriatric population rose dramatically in the last decade. The Centers for Disease Control and Prevention (CDC) tells us that the following outcomes are linked to falls in the geriatric patient:

- 20–30% of people who fall suffer moderate to severe injuries (ie, bruises, hip fractures, head trauma). These injuries can make it difficult to get around and limit mobility and independent living as well as increase the risk of early death.
- Falls are the most common cause of traumatic brain injury, accounting for 46% of fatal injuries among geriatric patients.
- Most fractures in geriatric patients are caused by falls, and the most common fractures include those of the spine, hip, forearm, leg, ankle, pelvis, upper arm, and hand.
- In 2000, the direct medical costs of falls in the geriatric patient population totaled $179 million for fatal falls and $19 billion for nonfatal fall injuries.

Common contributing factors include environmental problems, vision problems, cerebrovascular disease, decreased strength, loss of bone mass, and the use of medications (**Table 14-3** ▲).

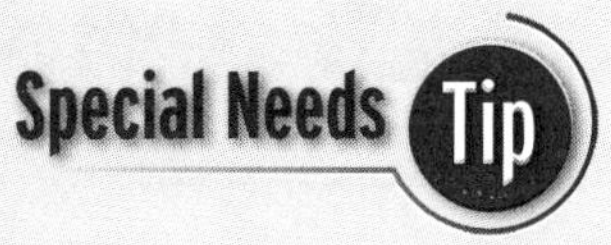

Before you administer medications to a geriatric patient, remember that there are medications that work better than others for this population.

There are certain medications that are associated with falls in the geriatric patient and these medications should be used with caution or, if possible, substituted with another drug (**Table 14-4 ▸**).

According to the American Academy of Orthopaedic Surgeons (AAOS), injuries from falling are the sixth leading cause of death for geriatric patients. Hip fractures are a primary injury associated with these falls. Hip fractures result in medical care costs estimated at $7 billion each year. Only 25% of hip fracture patients will make a full recovery; 40% will require nursing home admission; 50% will be dependent upon a cane or a walker; and 20% will die in 1 year.

Table 14-4 Medications Associated With Falls

Medication	Use
alprazolam [Xanax]	Anti-anxiety medication that causes dizziness
diazepam [Valium]	Anti-anxiety medication that causes dizziness
flurazepam hydrochloride [Dalmane]	Hypnotic medication that causes dizziness
diphenhydramine [Benadryl]	Antihistamine/hypnotic medication that causes blurred vision
digoxin [Lanoxin]	Heart arrhythmia/congestive heart failure medication; toxicity can cause bluish/yellowish tinted vision, a "halo" around objects

Other Concerns With Falling

There are other significant issues regarding falls in geriatric patients. Certainly, cause is always a primary concern. Was the fall due to a trip, slip, or loss of balance? If so, was the patient supposed to be using an assistive device for ambulation and simply failed to do so? Was syncope or pre-syncope an inciting cause? In the cases of geriatric patients who fall and are simply too weak to get up, numerous sources of the problem that may or may not have a link to medication utilization can be identified (ie overdose, underdose, trading off different types of medications to save money, self doctoring by the patient, or medication non-compliance). Cardiovascular and cerebrovascular sources are commonplace, as are septic (urinary tract infection), metabolic (dehydration, electrolyte disorders), and hematologic (anemia, GI bleeding) causes. Injury secondary to the fall is always concerning, and a variety of bone and soft-tissue injuries can result. Regardless of mental status, the case of a geriatric patient who has fallen and struck his or her head while using warfarin [Coumadin] for anticoagulation is a situation that mandates evaluation in the hospital with associated neuroimaging to assess for possible intracranial bleeding.

Management of Specific Conditions

A large number of patients are geriatric patients, and with the baby boomer generation reaching their "golden years," the numbers continue to rise. Here we will address a number of specific conditions found in the geriatric population (**Table 14-5 ▸**).

Table 14-5 Managing Typical Geriatric Conditions

System	Condition	Management
Respiratory System	Pneumonia	ABCs, in-hospital antibiotics, and bed rest.
	Chronic obstructive pulmonary disease (COPD)	Improve oxygenation, administer bronchodilator, corticosteroid for inflammation, and consider CPAP.
	Pulmonary embolism	Continuous oxygen, analgesic as needed for pain, vasopressors for hypotension, antiarrhythmics for arrhythmias, fibrinolytic therapy for massive pulmonary embolism.
Cardiovascular System	Acute coronary syndrome (ACS) including myocardial infarction (MI).	Oxygen, aspirin, nitrates, morphine, beta-blocker, reperfusion strategy.
	Heart failure	Continuous oxygenation, treat for shock, diuretics, ACE inhibitors, digitalis, beta-blockers, and vasopressors for hypotension.
	Arrhythmias	If too slow or too fast or lethal ventricular rhythm, treat the symptomatic patient with electricity or medications (address the etiology).
	Aortic aneurysm	Elective or emergency surgery for graft or excision.
	Hypertension	Antihypertensive drug therapy: diuretic, beta-blockers, calcium channel blockers, ACE inhibitors, angiotensin II receptor blockers, alpha adrenergic blockers, and alpha-beta blockers.
Nervous System	Transient ischemic attack (TIA) or cerebrovascular disease	Antiplatelet or anticoagulation therapy.
	Delirium	May require minimal or no pharmacologic therapy. When behavior or alcohol involvement poses a danger, consider diazepam, lorazepam, haloperidol or droperidol.
	Dementia	Treatment varies widely and is determined by the cause.
	Alzheimer's	Treatment varies widely to slow cognitive decline. Drugs that enhance cholinergic neurotransmission may improve memory at early stages.
	Parkinson's	Dopaminergics, anticholinergics, and Monoamine Oxidase Type B (MAO-B) inhibitor.
Endocrine System	Diabetes	Education in diet and exercise; metabolic control of hyperglycemia while avoiding hypoglycemic episodes that include syncope or fainting.
	Thyroid	Varies depending on the disorder.
	Hyperthyroidism	Iodine, anti-thyroid drugs, beta-blockers, radioactive sodium iodine, surgical treatment.
	Hypothyroidism	Hormone replacement therapy.
	Thyroiditis	High doses of aspirin or NSAIDs.
	Goiter	Thyroid hormone, surgical treatment.

Case Study III Suspected Stroke

Part 1

Your unit has been dispatched to a private residence at 9:00 a.m. on a Sunday. You are met at the doorway by the patient's son who begins to fill you in on what happened. The police are en route but you and your partner decide it is safe to enter the residence.

The son states his name is Tom and his dad's name is Harry Jones. Tom says he heard his dad get up at his usual time, which is 6:00 a.m., but he fell back asleep. When Tom got out of bed he heard the TV on and went to check on him in the family room. Mr. Jones always watches the morning news but today Tom was surprised to see that there were cartoons on. When he called out his name, he stared off into space and was not acknowledging Tom. Mr. Jones was also drooling all over his nice white tee shirt.

As your partner asks Tom to show him the medications Mr. Jones takes, you begin to conduct your initial assessment on Mr. Jones (see **Table 1**).

Case Study III Continued

There is no apparent trauma present so you decide it would be appropriate to do a rapid medical examination. Although he does respond to your verbal commands, he is not able to speak to you at this point. You are able to elaborate on the chief complaint with the answers to a number of the OPQRST questions coming from his son. You and your partner decide that the time for assessment and on scene treatment should be kept to a minimum since it is unclear when he was last seen with normal behavior.

Question 1: What is the significance of the cartoons?

Question 2: What is the significance of the drooling?

Table 1 Initial Assessment

Initial Assessment	Recording Time: 2 Minutes
General Impression/ Appearance	Poor. He is sitting up, confused and drooling
Mental Status	"V" responds to verbal stimuli
Airway	Open but he has a lot of secretions and will need suctioning
Breathing	Rapid and noisy (snoring) due to some apparent partial upper airway obstruction
Circulation	Tachycardic (fast) strong bounding radial pulse
Priority/Plan	High due to altered mental status

Part 2

As your partner returns to the room with a medication list, you learn that Mr. Jones has a history of hypertension, glaucoma, and arthritis, and is currently being treated for arteritis. You begin to ask a few questions of the son to elaborate on the chief complaint of an altered mental status. The examination will be a focused history and physical examination of the neurologic system and will include the Cincinnati Prehospital Stroke Scale (see **Table 2**). Next your partner gets a set of baseline vital signs.

Question 3: What does the Cincinnati Prehospital Stroke Scale involve?

Table 2 Focused History and Physical Examination

Baseline Vital Signs	Recording Time: 2 Minutes
Skin CTC (color, temperature, condition)	Flushed, normal temp, slightly diaphoretic (sweaty)
Pulse	108 beats/min and bounding
Blood Pressure	108/50 mm Hg
Respirations	38 breaths/min and shallow

Question 4: What is the significance of the medical history in this case (ie, hypertension, glaucoma, arthritis, and arteritis)?

Part 3

After suctioning Mr. Jones' mouth, you listen to his lung sounds and they are surprisingly clear. Next you and your partner work to complete the routine tasks for a patient with an altered mental status: administer oxygen to rule out hypoxia, obtain a finger stick to rule out hypoglycemia, perform an ECG, and get a temperature reading. Tom tells you that his dad went to bed early last night with a headache and upset stomach (see **Table 3**). He has no history of stroke, heart attack, or diabetic problems but is being treated for arteritis. He has had a lot of headaches due to the arteritis, and the steroid use has made him feel weak and sometimes depressed.

Mr. Jones appears to be awake but his movements are very slow and he remains nonverbal. He does not give you any help with the Cincinnati Prehospital Stroke Scale. In taking a close look at Mr. Jones' medication bottles you see that the prednisone [Deltasone] he is taking is a high dose of 60 mg a day and the bottle is empty. The date and number of pills listed on the bottle indicate Mr. Jones should have finished this bottle more than 2 weeks ago. You know that corticosteroid use must not be stopped abruptly and ask Tom if there is a refill bottle somewhere. He tells you that his dad may not have refilled the prescription as he tends to be careless with those things. The blood glucose reading is 70 mg/dL, the SpO_2 is 99% with oxygen by nonrebreathing mask, the rhythm is sinus tachycardia, and the temperature is 101.3°F.

Case Study III Continued

Table 3 SAMPLE History

SAMPLE History	Comments
Signs/symptoms	Headache, upset stomach
Allergies	Codeine
Medications	Lisinopril [Zestril], prednisone [Deltasone], and NSAIDs (even though not prescribed nor recommended while taking a steroid)
Pertinent past medical history	Hypertension, glaucoma, arthritis, and is currently being treated for arteritis
Last oral intake	Dinner the night before
Events leading up to the incident	Went to bed not feeling well, acting strange in the morning

High-dose steroids are given occasionally for the most severe cases of inflammatory diseases such as temporal arteritis or rheumatoid arthritis. You know the powerful effects of corticosteroids can result in serious side effects at low or high doses. Patients taking medium- to long-term courses of corticosteroids **must** be gradually weaned off so as to permit the adrenal glands to resume natural cortisol production. Eliminating doses too quickly can result in adrenal crisis (a life-threatening state caused by insufficient levels of cortisol).

Adrenal crisis is also known as Addisonian crisis and acute adrenal insufficiency. Signs and symptoms may include:

- Abdominal pain
- Altered mental status
- Chills and shaking
- Confusion
- Coma
- Darkening of the skin
- Dehydration
- Excessive sweating on face or hands
- Fatigue and weakness
- Fever
- Flank pain
- Joint pain
- Headache
- Hypotension
- Low blood glucose
- Loss of appetite
- Nausea and vomiting
- Slow, sluggish movement
- Skin rash
- Tachycardia
- Tachypnea
- Unintentional weight loss

At this point hypoxia does not appear to be the problem, the blood glucose reading is below the normal range (80–120 mg/dL) [note protocols may differ by region], the temperature is elevated, and the ECG is sinus tachycardia. Mr. Jones' abnormal presentation may have to do with hypoglycemia, infection/sepsis, stroke, adrenal insufficiency, renal insufficiency, or GI bleeding.

Treatment Plan

1. Continued high-flow oxygen.
2. Start an IV and administer 25 grams of dextrose $D_{50}W$ (see **Table 4**).
3. Begin transport.

Table 4 50% Dextrose

Do you know?	Comments
Right drug? Generic name: [**50% Dextrose**] Trade name: [$D_{50}W$]	This is a carbohydrate hypertonic solution. Also called glucose or d-glucose.
Right patient?	Diabetic with altered mental status and documented low blood glucose. Severe hypoglycemia for any cause (ie, insulin shock, alcoholism).
Right dose?	25 grams IV bolus for the adult patient.
Right route?	A patent large bore IV.
Right time?	As soon as possible after baseline vital signs.
Right documentation?	The patient care report should state the glucose level, the amount of $D_{50}W$ administered, and the serial vital signs as well as the patient's response to the medication.
Expected action	The patient's mental status should improve within minutes. Each 100 mL of fluid contains 50 grams of dextrose which delivers 3.4 kcal/g.

continues

Case Study III Continued

Table 4 50% Dextrose (*Continued*)

Do you know?	Comments
Side effects	None provided the $D_{50}W$ was in a good vein. Redness or pain may occur at the injection site. If the $D_{50}W$ did leak into the surrounding tissue (extravasation), it is so concentrated it can cause local tissue necrosis.
Contraindications	Previous hypersensitivity to dextrose solution. Diabetic coma while patient is hyperglycemic. Intracranial or intraspinal hemorrhage.
Precautions	With patients with suspected stroke check the blood glucose prior to administering $D_{50}W$. In an ischemic stroke it has been shown that increased blood glucose concentrations may worsen cerebral ischemic brain damage and impair recovery.
Pharmacokinetics	Onset 1 minute; duration varies with the severity of hypoglycemia.

Question 5: What is a major risk factor for stopping the use of corticosteroids?

Question 6: Can Mr. Jones' low blood glucose be associated with adrenal crisis?

Part 4

After administering $D_{50}W$, Mr. Jones' condition has not changed. A repeat finger-stick reading shows 170 mg/dL (see **Table 5**). As you finish getting him ready and move him out to the ambulance you consider making the call to medical control for further guidance.

Question 7: What are some major side effects of taking NSAIDs?

Question 8: What are the primary organs for detoxifying and metabolizing most drugs?

Table 5 Reassessment and Ongoing Assessment of the Patient

Serial Vital Signs and Relevant Data	Recording Time: 5 Minutes
Skin CTC	Warm, dry, good color
Pulse	Tachycardic (fast) at 124 beats/min
Blood Pressure	102/48 mm Hg
Respirations	34 breaths/min and shallow
Mental Status	Conscious, nonverbal
ECG	Sinus tachycardia
SpO_2	100%
Lung Sounds	Clear
Other (ie glucose, core body temperature)	Glucose 70 mg/dL initial and 170 mg/dL after $D_{50}W$, temperature 101.3°F

Part 5

En route you talked to medical control and for now Mr. Jones will be treated under the stroke protocol. If adrenal insufficiency or crisis was a concern, treatment would include corticosteroids, commonly hydrocortisone [Solu-Cortef]. In this case the priority is attending to the ABCs and expeditious transport to a stroke center.

This case was more complex than others, as is often the way with many elderly patient presentations. There are age-related conditions to consider, possible medication problems, and concurrent disease processes. Mr. Jones presented with altered mental status, modestly decreased blood glucose, elevated temperature, signs of stroke, and concerns of possible medication-related problems. When the administration of oxygen and glucose did not correct or improve his condition, this left a large differential diagnosis and few treatment options in the prehospital setting. Maintaining the ABCs was the priority with Mr. Jones, as well as transport to an appropriate setting.

This is actually a fairly complex case. It might involve a lot of testing in the ED to determine the diagnosis for this patient. You can see how it was handled

Case Study III Continued

in the prehospital phase of care. However, it certainly could turn out to be a number of potential diagnosis pathways in the in-hospital setting (ie, medication reaction/anticholinergic toxicity, stroke, adrenal insufficiency, etc). The bottom line here is that geriatric cases are rarely simple because they have years of medical history and multiple conditions, and the patients are often taking multiple medications. Focus on the ABCs, help support the patient and make him or her comfortable, and do not always expect to solve all medical problems in the prehospital setting!

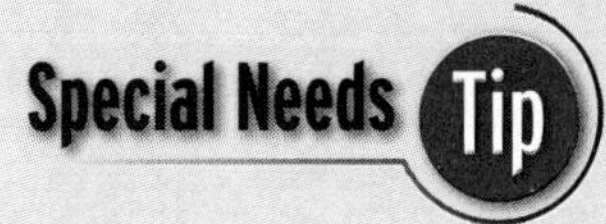

Getting old does not naturally cause conditions related to disease processes.

Chronic Pain

Many geriatric patients experience chronic pain. The pharmacotherapy options for managing chronic pain include the use of **opioid** and **nonopioid** drugs. Nonopioid pain relievers such as NSAIDs and acetaminophen (Tylenol) are effective for treating mild to moderate acute and chronic pain. Opioids such as methadone or morphine can be used alone or in combination with nonopioids to manage severe pain, including cancer pain.

Nonopioid drugs do not produce physical dependence but do have side effects that can cause problems for the geriatric patient. The use of NSAIDs is strongly associated with GI bleeding and over 16,000 Americans die each year secondary to the GI bleeding caused by NSAIDs.

According to the American College of Gastroenterology (ACG) Bleeding Registry, when studied, alcohol is associated with a two-fold risk for GI bleeding and OTC aspirin and NSAIDs were associated with an increase risk for GI bleeding to around two-fold to three-fold. Taking an OTC analgesic and also consuming alcohol increases that risk to around five-fold.

The geriatric population is particularly sensitive to this effect. NSAIDs are known to be somewhat toxic to the kidneys, and should be used with great caution in individuals who have known underlying renal insufficiency. NSAIDs also carry the risk for accidental overdose and toxicity because so many OTC products (ie, cold medicines, muscle creams) contain them as part of the ingredients (**Figure 14-4 ▸**).

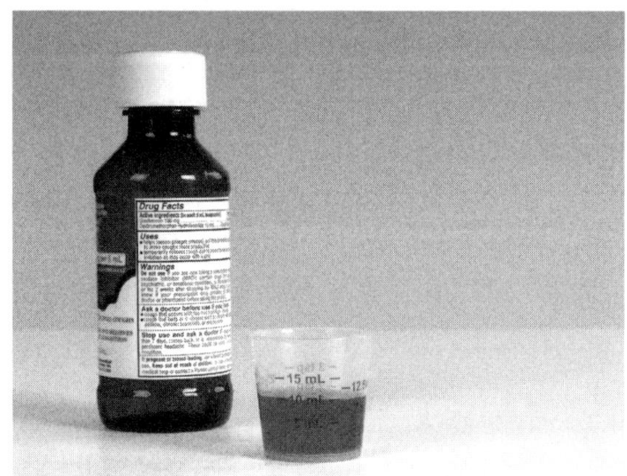

Figure 14-4 Over-the-counter products such as cold medicines contain NSAIDs as part of the ingredients.

Opioids are highly effective for managing severe pain but carry the risk of dependence in the long-term treatment of chronic pain. Side effects include constipation, nausea, hypoventilation, and altered mental status. In addition to being predisposed to side effects, geriatric patients have increased sensitivity to opioids and tend to require smaller doses than younger patients. These drugs should be used with caution in patients with decreased renal and hepatic functions, COPD, **encephalopathy**, and dementia.

When assessing a patient with signs and symptoms of possible opioid overdose or toxicity, examine the patient for transdermal opioid patches (ie, fentanyl citrate [Sublimase] or morphine sulfate [Astramorph/PF]) which may be hidden under clothing. Use gloves when removing these patches and clean the area with water while avoiding contact with your own skin. It is a smart procedure to take the patch with you in a plastic bag, turn it over to a nurse or physician in the ED, and document this on the patient care report. The following is a list of both types of drugs (**Table 14-6 ▸**).

Table 14-6 Nonopioid and Opioid Analgesics

Nonopioid Analgesics	Opioid Analgesics
Acetaminophen (Tylenol)	Fentanyl citrate (Sublimase)—transdermal use for chronic pain
Aspirin	Hydromorphone hydrochloride (Dilaudid)
Diclofenac sodium (Arthrotec)	Levorphanol (Levo Dromoran)—long half-life
Diflunisal (Dolobid)	Methadone (Dolophine)—long half-life
Ibuprofen (Motrin)	Morphine sulfate (Astramorph/PF)—rapid onset
Indomethacin (Indocin)	Oxycodone (Roxicodone)—used for long-term management of chronic pain
Ketoprofen (Orudis)	Oxymorphone (Numorphan)—rapid onset
Mefenamic acid (Ponstel)	Propoxyphene (Darvon)—used to treat mild to moderate pain
Nabumetone (Relafen)	
Naproxen (Naprosyn)	
Oxaprozin (Daypro Alta)	
Piroxicam (Feldene)	
Sulindac (Clinoril)	
Tolmetin sodium (Tolectin)	

Eye Medications

There are several eye problems associated with aging, although they can affect younger adults at any age. They include **presbyopia**, cataracts, glaucoma, retinal disorders, conjunctivitis, **corneal diseases**, eye lid problems, excessively dry or tearing eyes, and **temporal arteritis**. Some of these problems require medications to correct (ie, antibiotic for conjunctivitis and prednisone [Deltasone] for temporal arteritis) or the vision problem can be made worse with medications (ie, the antidepressants amitriptyline [Elavil] and doxepin [Sinequan] can aggravate glaucoma). Be alert for sudden changes in the patient's condition that involves sight as this may be an indication of a much more severe medical emergency.

Sleep Aids

People who live with pain may take analgesics to help them sleep. Additional drugs used as sleep aides include hypnotics, benzodiazepines, antidepressants, and diphenhydramine (Benadryl). As stated earlier, these medications can cause problems for geriatric patients. Some drugs should be avoided completely because of strong anti-cholinergic effects and age-related prolonged half-lives, while others may need the dosage to be lowered.

Temporal Arteritis

Temporal arteritis is the inflammation of the temporal artery and other branches of the external carotid artery system. Inflammation of the medium to large arteries causes thickening of the intimal layer of the vessel with associated narrowing and sometimes occlusion. Arteritis may be localized, multifocal, or widespread. Symptoms are varied and often include severe headache, pain when chewing, tenderness in the temporal area, and visual disturbances. It may be followed by sudden and permanent vision loss. Patients may have preexisting arthritis or carpal tunnel syndrome and have other symptoms including shaking, weight loss, shoulder or hip weakness, and low-grade fever. It may be caused by an impaired immune system. Early treatment with corticosteroids is aimed at reducing vascular inflammation and preventing visual loss.

Case Study ANSWERS

Case Study I A Syncopal Episode

Question 1: What is syncope?

Answer 1: Syncope is fainting or a brief loss of consciousness caused by transiently inadequate blood flow to the brain. It is important to distinguish syncope from near or pre-syncope, and it is often self-correcting as the patient lies in the supine position. Syncope is also easily confused with a seizure so always assess and suspect seizure too. The larger question is to determine what caused the syncope (ie, arrhythmia, ischemic heart disease, dehydration, sepsis, or anemia) and if any injuries sustained as a result of the ensuing fall were from the syncope (ie, head injury, fracture, soft-tissue injury).

Question 2: What are some of the causes of falls in the geriatric patient?

Answer 2: Falls in the elderly are evenly distributed between those resulting from external or extrinsic causes and those resulting from internal or intrinsic causes as shown in Table 14-3.

Question 3: What is the significance of Millie feeling dizzy when she got up so fast?

Answer 3: It could give you a clue to the cause of the fall. Millie may have had orthostatic changes from getting up fast possible due to some internal bleeding. Geriatric patients often do not compensate well for rapid changes in position because their arteries are hardened and lack the flexibility of a younger person's arteries.

Question 4: The fact that Millie woke up on the floor could indicate what to you?

Answer 4: If she did not trip on anything, did she sense a fracture occurring in her leg at the time of the fall? Is it likely that she passed out and found herself on the floor (ie, experienced syncope)?

Question 5: Why is it important to obtain a 12-lead ECG in Millie's case even though she denies chest pain?

Answer 5: Silent or "painless" ischemia events including MI frequently occur, more so in the case of diabetics, women, and geriatric patients.

Question 6: What is the significance of Millie's past cardiac history?

Answer 6: Despite Millie's denial of her recent dizziness, she has a significant cardiac history of angina, an arrhythmia, and two past MIs so there is certainly potential that her syncope is evidence of recurrent cardiac disease.

Question 7: Why did you check Millie's blood glucose?

Answer 7: One of the many causes of syncope and an altered level of conscious can be hypoglycemia. It is also one of the easiest to fix provided you check the patient's blood glucose level.

Question 8: If you identified the ECG as a second-degree type II heart block, what would be the primary treatment?

Answer 8: Heart blocks come in four "flavors:" first-degree, second-degree type 1 and type 2, and third-degree or complete heart block. The first-degree block is typically not treated, second-degree type 1 is when the patient is symptomatic and treated with atropine sulfate [Atropine] and expectant management, whereas second-degree type 2 and complete heart blocks are treated with transcutaneous pacing or dopamine (see case study IV, chapter 4, Cardiovascular Emergencies). If the heart block is associated with chest pain, dyspnea, or ST-segment elevation, consider the potential for AMI and the need for a coronary catheterization lab.

Case Study II Sick with the Chills

Question 1: What could be the reason for the open oven, and does this have an effect on the patient's condition?

Answer 1: In the absence of cooking, it may indicate that the patient is trying to warm the apartment with the heat from the stove. This is a very dangerous thing to do. It was, in this case, a clue that there could be a high level of CO in the atmosphere. Had you suspected CO poisoning initially, the scene assessment would have told us not to enter the premises without the appropriate PPE. In this case you were already inside and made contact with the patient. At this point it is best to wrap her up quickly and get out into the fresh air.

Case Study ANSWERS

Question 2: Why is the patient shivering?

Answer 2: Mrs. Alverez is probably shivering because she is cold and her body is trying to generate heat by moving muscles. It is also possible to shiver when the body's "thermostat" has been reset to high, such as during a fever. Even though the body is actually running a temperature, it senses that the body temperature is low (low as compared to the reset new high) so the body begins to shiver. It is often confusing for a patient to have a high fever and to be shivering. Some medications, such as antipyretics are designed to break the fever and allow the body's thermostat to be reset back to normal. So, you can shiver whether you are cold OR hot.

Question 3: What factors indicate that you should check the blood glucose on this patient?

Answer 3: Mrs. Alverez has a slightly altered mental status as well as type II diabetes and has not been able to hold food down for the last couple of days.

Question 4: Why did you check the body temperature on this patient?

Answer 4: Any patient whose body temperature feels cooler or warmer than yours (back of your hand) should have their temperature taken with an actual thermometer.

Question 5: Aside from having the fire department test the atmosphere for carbon monoxide, is there any other way to test the patient in the prehospital setting?

Answer 5: Yes, there are some EMS agencies that have portable CO monitors that are similar to pulse oximeters and end-tidal carbon dioxide devices. Though relatively new to the market, these devices appear to be fairly dependable and are noninvasive.

Question 6: Why would it be a smart decision to do a 12-lead ECG on this patient?

Answer 6: Remember the situation of "silent" coronary ischemia, which can present as an otherwise ill patient who is not complaining of chest pain. This presentation, though not common, does tend to occur more in women, diabetics, and the elderly. All three of these "risk factors" were present in this patient. Also, the ECG is a helpful, noninvasive screening tool for evaluating the presence of arrhythmia or possible toxic/metabolic abnormalities.

Question 7: Is the sinus tachycardia a problem in Mrs. Alverez?

Answer 7: In the absence of any other significant symptoms (ie, decreasing mental status, paralysis, hypotension), a slightly tachycardic pulse is acceptable and an indicator that Mrs. Alverez is most likely suffering from some degree of physiologic stress, be it from dehydration, hypothermia, or hypoglycemia.

Question 8: Since Mrs. Alverez's blood glucose is 70 mg/dL, will you need to administer IV dextrose in addition to the oral dextrose [Glutose]?

Answer 8: Probably not, but if her mental status changes it would be easy enough to do provided the IV line is a good one. Remember that 25 grams of 50% dextrose ($D_{50}W$) should not be pushed into a tiny IV or one where it may be infiltrated since the leakage of the drug into the surrounding tissue can cause necrosis.

Case Study III Suspected Stroke

Question 1: What is the significance of the cartoons?

Answer 1: Many geriatric patients have very specific routines they follow every day (ie, going for a morning walk, driving to the news stand rather than having the paper delivered, getting up early and going to bed early, and watching the same TV shows every morning or evening). When there is something unusual to their typical routine that has been noticed by a family member in the context of medical symptoms, it may indicate an acute delirium or confusional state, which always has a pathophysiologic basis to it.

Question 2: What is the significance of the drooling?

Answer 2: That all depends on what he usually does. If it is unusual behavior for Mr. Jones to drool, it can be significant and might indicate an altered mental status, difficulty swallowing, or even a partial upper airway obstruction. If he always seems to mess up his clean shirts, it might just be the way Mr. Jones is these days! The observation of his son can be very helpful in this case to help the paramedics determine if there is any new behavior for the patient.

Case Study ANSWERS

Question 3: What does the Cincinnati Prehospital Stroke Scale involve?

Answer 3: As we all learned in our EMT course and again reviewed in our paramedic training, the Cincinnati Prehospital Stroke Scale is the assessment tool that involves asking the patient to smile, checking for pronator drift, and asking the patient to say a simple sentence so you can listen for slurred speech (or lack thereof).

Question 4: What is the significance of the medical history in this case (ie, hypertension, glaucoma, arthritis, and arteritis)?

Answer 4: Patients with a history of hypertension and glaucoma are likely candidates for stroke. The medications used to treat these conditions are known to cause problems in the geriatric patient.

Question 5: What is a major risk factor for stopping the use of corticosteroids?

Answer 5: One major risk factor for abruptly ending steroid treatment is developing adrenal crisis, a life-threatening state caused by insufficient circulating levels of cortisol.

Question 6: Can Mr. Jones' low blood glucose be associated with adrenal crises?

Answer 6: Yes, one of the signs of adrenal crises may be hypoglycemia. Hyperglycemia or diabetes may be a side effect of long-term corticosteroid use.

Question 7: What are some major side effects of taking NSAIDs?

Answer 7: GI bleeding/gastropathy, platelet inhibition, and renal toxicity.

Question 8: What are the primary organs for detoxifying and metabolizing most drugs?

Answer 8: The liver and kidneys are the primary organs for detoxifying and metabolizing most drugs.

Medication Review

Activated Charcoal (Liqui-Char)

Indications Most oral poisonings and medication overdoses; can be used after evacuation of poisons.

Contraindications Oral administration to comatose patient; after ingestion of corrosives, caustics, or petroleum distillates (ineffective and may induce vomiting); simultaneous administration with other oral drugs.

Dosage and administration Note: if not in premixed slurry, dilute with 1 part charcoal/4 parts water. Adult: 1–2 g/kg PO or via NGT.

Adenosine (Adenocard)

Indications Conversion of PSVT to sinus rhythm. May convert re-entry SVT due to Wolff-Parkinson-White syndrome. Not effective in converting atrial fibrillation/flutter or V-tach.

Contraindications Second- or third-degree block or sick sinus syndrome, atrial flutter/atrial fibrillation, ventricular tachycardia, hypersensitivity to adenosine, poison-induced tachycardia.

Dosage and administration Adult: 6 mg over 1–3 seconds, followed by a 20-mL saline flush and elevate extremity; if no response after 1–2 minutes, administer 12 mg over 1–3 seconds; if no response, repeat 12 mg again; maximum total dose, 30 mg.

Albuterol (Proventil, Ventolin)

Indications Treatment of bronchospasm in patients with reversible obstructive airway disease (COPD/asthma). Prevention of exercise-induced bronchospasm.

Contraindications Known prior hypersensitivity reactions to albuterol. Tachycardia arrhythmias, especially those caused by digitalis. Synergistic with other sympathomimetics.

Dosage and administration Adult: Administer 2.5 mg (0.5 mL of the 0.5% solution) added to 2 mL of normal saline for inhalation by nebulizer treatment and administer over 10–15 minutes. May repeat every 20 minutes up to three times. MDI: 1–2 inhalations (90–180 µg). Five minutes between inhalations. Pediatric: (between the ages of 2 and 12) administer 2.5 mg (0.5 mL of the 0.083% solution) added to 2 mL of normal saline for inhalation by nebulizer treatment and administer over 10–15 minutes. May repeat every 20 minutes up to three times.

Amiodarone (Cordarone, Pacerone)

Indications V-fib/pulseless V-tach and unstable V-tach in patients refractory to other therapy. Also persistent SVTs unresponsive to other treatment.

Contraindications Known hypersensitivity, cardiogenic shock, sinus bradycardia, and second- or third-degree AV block (unless a functional pacemaker is available).

Dosage and administration Adult: V-fib/pulseless V-tach unresponsive to CPR, defibrillation, and vasopressors: 300 mg IV/IO push (recommend dilution in 20–30 mL D_5W). Initial dose can be followed one time in 3–5 minutes at 150 mg IV/IO push. Recurrent life-threatening ventricular arrhythmias: Maximum cumulative dose is 2.2 g/24 hours, administered as follows: Rapid infusion: 150 mg IV/IO over 10 minutes (15 mg/min). May repeat rapid infusion (150 mg IV/IO) every 10 minutes as needed. Slow infusion: 360 mg IV/IO over 6 hours (1 mg/min). Maintenance infusion: 540 mg IV/IO over 18 hours (0.5 mg/min).

Aspirin

Indications New onset chest pain suggestive of acute myocardial infarction. Signs and symptoms suggestive of recent cerebrovascular accident.

Contraindications Hypersensitivity. Relatively contraindicated in patients with active ulcer disease or asthma.

Dosage and administration 160 mg to 325 mg PO (chewed if possible).

Medication Review

Atropine Sulfate

Indications Hemodynamically unstable bradycardia, asystole, bradycardic (< 60 beats/min) pulseless electrical activity (PEA), organophosphate poisoning, bronchospastic pulmonary disorders.

Contraindications Tachycardia, hypersensitivity, unstable cardiovascular status in acute hemorrhage and myocardial ischemia, narrow-angle glaucoma.

Dosage and administration Adult: Asystole or bradycardic PEA: 1 mg IV/IO push. May repeat every 3–5 minutes (if asystole or PEA persists) to a maximum of 0.04 mg/kg. Endotracheal administration: 2–3 mg diluted in 10 mL of water or normal saline. Unstable bradycardia: 0.5 mg IV/IO every 3–5 minutes as needed, not to exceed total dose of 0.04 mg/kg. Use shorter dosing interval (3 minutes) and higher doses in severe clinical conditions. Organophosphate poisoning: Extremely large doses (2–4 mg or higher) may be needed.

Benzocaine Spray (Hurricane)

Indications Used as a lubricant and topical anesthetic to facilitate passage of diagnostic and treatment devices. Suppresses the pharyngeal and tracheal gag reflex.

Contraindications Patients with a known hypersensitivity to benzocaine.

Dosage and administration Adult: 0.5–1.0 second spray, repeat as needed.

Calcium Chloride

Indications Hypocalcemia, hyperkalemia, magnesium sulfate overdose, calcium channel blocker overdose, adjunctive therapy in treatment of insect bites and stings.

Contraindications Hypercalcemia, V-fib, digitalis toxicity.

Dosage and administration Adult: 500 mg to 1,000 mg (5–10 mL of a 10% solution) IV/IO push for hyperkalemia and calcium channel blocker overdose. May be repeated as needed.

Dextrose

Indications Hypoglycemia, altered level of consciousness, coma of unknown etiology, seizure of unknown etiology, status epilepticus.

Contraindications Intracranial hemorrhage.

Dosage and administration Adult: 12.5–25 g slow IV; may be repeated as necessary.

Diazepam (Valium)

Indications Acute anxiety states, acute alcohol withdrawal (delirium tremens), muscle relaxant, seizure activity, agitation. Analgesia for medical procedures (fracture reduction, cardioversion).

Contraindications Hypersensitivity, glaucoma, coma, shock, substance abuse, head injury.

Dosage and administration Seizure activity: Adult: 5–10 mg IV every 10–15 minutes as needed (5 mg over 5 min)(maximum dose, 30 mg). Sedation for cardioversion: 5–15 mg IV over 5–10 minutes prior to cardioversion.

Digoxin (Lanoxin)

Indications Congestive heart failure, re-entry SVT, especially atrial flutter and atrial fibrillation.

Contraindications Ventricular fibrillation, ventricular tachycardia, digitalis toxicity, hypersensitivity to digoxin.

Dosage and administration Adult: Loading dose of 10 to 15 μg/kg.

Medication Review

Diltiazem Hydrochloride (Cardizem, Lyo-Ject)

Indications Control of rapid ventricular rates due to atrial flutter, atrial fibrillation, and re-entry SVT; angina pectoris.

Contraindications Hypotension, sick sinus syndrome, second- or third-degree AV block, cardiogenic shock, wide-complex tachycardias, poison/drug-induced tachycardia.

Dosage and administration Adult: Initial bolus: 0.25 mg/kg (average dose 15–20 mg) IV over 2 minutes. If inadequate response, may re-bolus in 15 minutes: 0.35 mg/kg (average dose 20–25 mg) IV over 2 minutes. Maintenance infusion of 5–15 mg/h.

Diphenhydramine (Benadryl)

Indications Symptomatic relief of allergies, allergic reactions, anaphylaxis, acute dystonic reactions (phenothiazines). Blood administration reactions; used for motion sickness, hay fever.

Contraindications Asthma, glaucoma, pregnancy, hypertension, narrow-angle glaucoma, infants, patients taking monoamine oxidase inhibitors (MAOIs).

Dosage and administration Adult: 25–50 mg IM or IV or PO.

Dobutamine (Dobutrex)

Indications Cardiogenic shock, CHF, left ventricular dysfunction. Often used in conjunction with other drugs.

Contraindications Tachyarrhythmias, IHSS, severe hypotension.

Dosage and administration Adult: IV infusion at 2–20 µg/kg/min titrated to desired effect.

Dopamine (Intropin)

Indications Cardiogenic, septic or spinal shock, hypotension with low cardiac output states, distributive shock.

Contraindications Hypovolemic shock, pheochromocytoma, tachyarrhythmias, V-fib.

Dosage and administration Adult: 2–20 µg/kg/min titrated to patient response.

Epinephrine (Adrenalin)

Indications Cardiac arrest (V-fib/pulseless V-tach, asystole, PEA), symptomatic bradycardia as an alternative infusion to dopamine, severe hypotension secondary to bradycardia when atropine and transcutaneous pacing are unsuccessful, allergic reactions, anaphylaxis, asthma.

Contraindications Hypertension, hypothermia, pulmonary edema, myocardial ischemia, hypovolemic shock.

Dosage and administration Adult: Mild allergic reactions and asthma: 0.3–0.5 mg (0.3–0.5 mL of 1:1,000) SC. Anaphylaxis: 0.1 mg (1 mL of 1:10,000) IV/IO over 5 minutes. Cardiac arrest: IV/IO dose: 1 mg (10 mL of 1:10,000 solution) every 3–5 minutes during resuscitation. Follow each dose with 20 mL flush and elevate arm for 10 to 20 seconds after dose. Higher dose: Higher doses (up to 0.2 mg/kg) may be used for specific indications (beta-blocker or calcium channel blocker overdose). Continuous infusion: Add 1 mg (1 mL of 1:1,000 solution) to 500 mL normal saline or D_5W. Initial infusion rate of 1 µg/min titrated to effect (typical dose: 2–10 µg/min). Endotracheal (ET) dose: 2–2.5 mg diluted in 10 mL normal saline. Profound bradycardia or hypotension: 2–10 µg/min; titrate to patient response.

Medication Review

Fentanyl Citrate (Sublimase)

Indications This drug is used to treat severe pain and is used with anesthesia.

Contraindications Myasthenia gravis, children under 2 years old. May cause life-threatening hypoventilation so naloxone hydrochloride [Narcan] should be readily available.

Dosage and administration Adult: 25–100 μg (0.5–1 mcg/kg) IM, IO, IVP or atomized intranasal.

Flumazenil (Romazicon)

Indications Reversal of respiratory depression and sedative effects from pure benzodiazepine overdose.

Contraindications Hypersensitivity, tricyclic antidepressant overdose, seizure-prone patients, coma of unknown etiology.

Dosage and administration Adult: First dose: 0.2 mg IV/IO over 15 seconds. Second dose: 0.3 mg IV/IO over 30 seconds. If no response, give third dose. Third dose: 0.5 mg IV/IO over 30 seconds. If no response, repeat once every minute until adequate response or a total of 3 mg is given.

Furosemide (Lasix)

Indications CHF, pulmonary edema, hypertensive crisis.

Contraindications Hypovolemia, anuria, hypotension (relative contraindication); hypersensitivity, hepatic coma.

Dosage and administration Adult: 0.5–1.0 mg/kg injected IV over 1 to 2 minutes. If no response, double the dose to 2 mg/kg over 1 to 2 minutes.

Glucagon

Indications Altered level of consciousness when hypoglycemia is suspected. May be used as inotropic agent in beta-blocker overdose.

Contraindications Hyperglycemia, hypersensitivity.

Dosage and administration Adult: Hypoglycemia: 0.5–1 mg IM; may repeat in 7–10 minutes. Calcium channel blocker or beta-blocker overdose: 3 mg initially, followed by infusion at 3 mg/h as necessary.

Haloperidol (Haldol)

Indications Acute psychotic episodes.

Contraindications Agitation secondary to shock or hypoxia. Hypersensitivity.

Dosage and administration Adult: 2–5 mg IM every 30–60 minutes until sedation achieved.

Hydroxyzine Hydrochloride (Atarax, Vistaril)

Indications To potentiate the effects of analgesics; to control nausea and vomiting, anxiety reactions, and motion sickness; preoperative and postoperative sedation.

Contraindications Hypersensitivity.

Dosage and administration Adult: 25–100 mg IM.

Isoetharine (Bronchosol, Bronkometer)

Indications Acute bronchial asthma, bronchospasm (especially in COPD patient).

Contraindications Use with caution in patients with diabetes, hyperthyroidism, cardiovascular and cerebrovascular disease.

Dosage and administration Adult: 1–2 inhalations with MDI. COPD: 2.5–5.0 mg (0.25 mL–0.5 mL) diluted in 3 mL normal saline (NS) and nebulized.

Ketorolac Tromethamine (Toradol IM)

Indications Short-term management of moderate to severe pain.

Contraindications Allergy to salicylates or other NSAIDs; patients with history of asthma; bleeding disorders, especially gastrointestinal (GI) related (peptic ulcer disease); renal failure.

Dosage and administration Adult: 30–60 mg IM.

Medication Review

Labetalol (Normodyne, Trandate)

Indications Moderate to severe hypertension.

Contraindications Bronchial asthma, CHF, cardiogenic shock, second- and third-degree heart block, bradycardia.

Dosage and administration Adult: 5–20 mg slow IV over 2 minutes (additional injections of 10–40 mg can be given at 10-minute intervals). Infusion: 2 mg/min titrated to acceptable supine blood pressure.

Lidocaine Hydrochloride (Xylocaine)

Indications Alternative to amiodarone in cardiac arrest from V-fib/pulseless V-tach, stable monomorphic V-tach, stable polymorphic V-tach with normal baseline QT interval.

Contraindications Hypersensitivity, second- and third-degree AV blocks in the absence of artificial pacemaker, Stokes-Adams syndrome, prophylactic use in AMI, wide-complex ventricular escape beats with bradycardia.

Dosage and administration Adult: Cardiac arrest from V-fib/pulseless V-tach: Initial dose: 1–1.5 mg/kg IV/IO. Repeat dose: 0.5–0.75 mg/kg, repeated in 5–10 minutes to maximum dose of 3 mg/kg. Endotracheal (ET) dose: 2–4 mg/kg. Stable V-tach, wide-complex tachycardia of uncertain type, significant ectopy: Doses ranging from 0.5–0.75 mg/kg and up to 1–1.5 mg/kg may be used. Repeat 0.5–0.75 mg/kg every 5–10 minutes. Maximum total dose is 3 mg/kg. Maintenance infusion: 1–4 mg/min (30–50 µg/kg/min); can dilute in D_5W or normal saline.

Lorazepam (Ativan)

Indications Initial control of status epilepticus or severe recurrent seizures, severe anxiety, sedation.

Contraindications Acute narrow-angle glaucoma. Coma, shock, or suspected drug abuse.

Dosage and administration Note: When given IV or IO, must dilute with equal volume of sterile water or sterile saline; When given IM, lorazepam is not to be diluted. Adult: 2–4 mg slow IV at 2 mg/min or IM; may repeat in 15–20 minutes to maximum dose of 8 mg. For sedation: 0.05 mg/kg up to 4 mg IM.

Magnesium Sulfate

Indications Seizures of eclampsia (toxemia of pregnancy), torsade de pointes, hypomagnesemia, Class IIa agent for V-fib/pulseless V-tach that is refractory to lidocaine.

Contraindications Heart blocks, myocardial damage.

Dosage and administration Adult: Cardiac arrest due to hypomagnesemia or torsade de pointes: 1–2 g (2–4 mL of a 50% solution) diluted in 10 mL of D_5W IV/IO over 5–20 minutes. Torsade de pointes with a pulse or AMI with hypomagnesemia: Loading dose of 1–2 g mixed in 50–100 mL D_5W over 5–60 minutes IV. Follow with 0.5–1 g/h IV (titrate to control torsade de pointes).

Meperidine Hydrochloride (Demerol)

Indications Analgesia for moderate to severe pain.

Contraindications Hypersensitivity to narcotic agents, diarrhea caused by poisoning, patients taking MAOIs, during labor or delivery of a premature infant, undiagnosed abdominal pain or head injury.

Dosage and administration Adult: 50–100 mg IM, SC or 25–50 mg slowly IV.

Metaproterenol 5% (Alupent)

Indications Bronchial asthma, reversible bronchospasm secondary to bronchitis, COPD.

Contraindications Tachyarrhythmias, hypersensitivity, tachycardias due to digitalis toxicity.

Dosage and administration Adult: MDI: 2–3 inhalations every 3–4 hours (2 minutes between inhalations). Inhalation solution 5%: via hand-held nebulizer 0.2–0.3 mL diluted in 2.5 mL saline. Inhalation solution unit-dose 0.4% or 0.6% vials: intermittent positive-pressure breathing device only: one vial/treatment.

Medication Review

Methylprednisolone Sodium Succinate (Solu-Medrol)

Indications Acute spinal cord trauma, anaphylaxis, bronchodilator for unresponsive asthma.

Contraindications Premature infants, systemic fungal infections; use with caution in patients with gastrointestinal bleeding, sepsis, local infection.

Dosage and administration Adult: Acute spinal cord injury: 30 mg/kg IV over 30 minutes followed by infusion: 5.4 mg/kg/h. Asthma, COPD: 1–2 mg/kg IV.

Midazolam (Versed)

Indications Sedation, anxiolytic prior to endotracheal or nasotracheal intubation; administer for conscious sedation.

Contraindications Glaucoma, shock, coma, alcohol intoxication, overdose, depressed vital signs, concomitant use with other CNS depressants, barbiturates, alcohol, narcotics.

Dosage and administration Adult: 2.0–2.5 mg slow IV over 2–3 minutes; may be repeated to total maximum: 0.1 mg/kg.

Morphine Sulfate (Astramorph/PF and others)

Indications Severe CHF, pulmonary edema, chest pain associated with acute MI, analgesia for moderate to severe acute and chronic pain (use with caution).

Contraindications Head injury, exacerbated COPD, depressed respiratory drive, hypotension, undiagnosed abdominal pain, decreased level of consciousness, suspected hypovolemia, patients who have taken MAOIs within the past 14 days.

Dosage and administration Adult: Initial dose: 2–4 mg IV (over 1–5 minutes) every 5–30 minutes. Repeat dose: 2–8 mg at 5- to 15-minute intervals.

Nalbuphine (Nubain)

Indications Chest pain associated with acute MI; moderate to severe acute pain; pulmonary edema, with or without associated chest pain (morphine remains first line).

Contraindications Head injury or undiagnosed abdominal pain, diarrhea caused by poisoning, hypovolemia, hypotension.

Dosage and administration Adult: 2–5 mg slowly IV; may repeat 2-mg doses as needed to maximum dose of 10 mg.

Naloxone Hydrochloride (Narcan)

Indications Opiate overdose, coma; complete or partial reversal of CNS and respiratory depression induced by opioids; decreased level of consciousness; coma of unknown origin; narcotic agonist for the following: morphine, heroin, hydromorphone (Dilaudid), methadone, meperidine (Demerol), paregoric, fentanyl citrate (Sublimase), oxycodone (Percodan), codeine, propoxyphene (Darvon); narcotic agonist and antagonist for the following: Butorphanol (Stadol), pentazocine (Talwin), nalbuphine (Nubain).

Contraindications Use with caution in narcotic-dependent patients.

Dosage and administration Adult: 0.4–2.0 mg IV, IM, SC, or ET (diluted); minimum recommended dose, 0.4 mg/kg; repeat at 5-minute intervals to a maximum dose of 10 mg (medical control may request higher amounts). Infusion: 2 mg in 500 mL of D_5W (4 µg/mL), infuse at 0.4 mg/h (100 mL/h).

Nitroglycerin (Nitrostat, Tridil, and others)

Indications Acute angina pectoris, ischemic chest pain, hypertension, CHF, pulmonary edema.

Contraindications Hypotension, hypovolemia; intracranial bleeding or head injury; previous administration of Viagra, Revatio, Levitra, Cialis, or similar agents within past 24 hours.

Dosage and administration Adult: Tablets: 0.3–0.4 mg SL; may repeat in 3–5 minutes to maximum of 3 doses. NTG spray: 0.4 mg under the tongue; 1–2 sprays. NTG IV infusion: begin at 10 to 20 µg/min; increase by 5–10 µg/min every 5 minutes until desired effect.

Medication Review

Nitropaste (Nitro-Bid Ointment)

Indications Angina pectoris and chest pain associated with acute MI.

Contraindications Same as NTG.

Dosage and administration Adult: Paste: Apply ½-inch to ¾-inch (1–2 cm), 15–30 mg, cover with wrap and secure with tape; maximum, 5-inch (75 mg) per application. Transdermal: Apply unit to intact skin (usually chest wall) in varying doses.

Norepinephrine Bitrartrate (Levophed, Levarterenol)

Indications Cardiogenic shock, significant hypotensive (< 70 mm Hg) states.

Contraindications Hypotensive patients with hypovolemia, pregnancy (relative contraindication).

Dosage and administration Adult: Dilute 8 mg in 500 mL of D_5W or 4 mg in 250 mL of D_5W (16 mg/mL); infuse by IV piggyback at 0.5–1.0 µg/min, titrated to improve blood pressure (up to 30 µg/min).

Ondansetron Hydrochloride (Zofran)

Indications For the prevention or control of nausea or vomiting. Also used in the hospital setting for patients undergoing chemotherapy or surgical procedures.

Contraindications Known allergy to this medicine or other 5-HT3 receptor antagonists.

Dosage and administration Adult: 4 mg IV or IM (may repeat in 10 minutes).

Oral Glucose (Insta-Glucose)

Indications Conscious patients with suspected hypoglycemia.

Contraindications Decreased level of consciousness, nausea, vomiting.

Dosage and administration Adult: Should be sipped slowly by patient until clinical improvement noted.

Oxygen

Indications Confirmed or expected hypoxemia, ischemic chest pain, respiratory insufficiency, prophylactically during air transport, confirmed or suspected carbon monoxide poisoning, all other causes of decreased tissue oxygenation, decreased level of consciousness.

Contraindications Certain patients with COPD or emphysema who will not tolerate oxygen concentrations over 35%, hyperventilation. Oxygen should never be withheld from a patient who needs it, however. Be prepared to assist with ventilations in a patient with COPD who requires high concentration, as apnea may result.

Dosage and administration Adult: Cardiac arrest and carbon monoxide poisoning: 100%. Hypoxemia: 10–15 L/min via nonrebreathing mask. COPD: 1–6 L/min via nasal cannula or 28%–35% Venturi mask. Be prepared to provide ventilatory support if higher concentrations of oxygen are needed.

Pancuronium Bromide (Pavulon)

Indications Induction or maintenance of paralysis after intubation to assist ventilations.

Contraindications Hypersensitivity, inability to control airway and support ventilations with oxygen and positive pressure, neuromuscular disease (myasthenia gravis), hepatic or renal failure.

Dosage and administration Adult: 0.1 mg/kg slow IV; repeat every 30–60 minutes as needed.

Phenobarbital (Luminal)

Indications Prevention and treatment of seizure activity; prophylaxis for febrile seizures; anxiety, apprehension; status epilepticus.

Contraindications Patients with porphyria, hypersensitivity, severe liver or respiratory diseases.

Dosage and administration Adult: 100–250 mg slow IV, or IM; may repeat as needed in 20–30 minutes.

Medication Review

Phenytoin (Dilantin)

Indications Prophylaxis and treatment of major motor seizures, digitalis-induced arrhythmias.

Contraindications Hypersensitivity, bradycardia, second- and third-degree heart block.

Dosage and administration Adult: Seizures: 10–20 mg/kg slow IV, not to exceed 1 g or rate of 50 mg/min). Arrhythmias: 50–100 mg (diluted) slow IV every 5–15 min as needed; maximum, 1 g.

Procainamide Hydrochloride (Pronestyl, Procanbid)

Indications Stable monomorphic V-tach with normal QT interval, reentry SVT uncontrolled by vagal maneuvers and adenosine, stable wide-complex tachycardia of unknown origin, atrial fibrillation with rapid ventricular rate in patients with Wolff-Parkinson-White syndrome.

Contraindications Torsade de pointes, second- and third-degree AV block (without functional artificial pacemaker), digitalis toxicity, tricyclic antidepressant overdose.

Dosage and administration Adult: Recurrent V-fib/pulseless V-tach: 20 mg/min IV infusion (maximum dose: 17 mg/kg). In urgent situations, up to 50 mg/min may be administered (maximum dose of 17 mg/kg). Other indications: 20 mg/min IV infusion until any one of the following occurs: arrhythmia suppression, hypotension, QRS widens by > 50% of its pretreatment width, or total dose of 17 mg/kg has been given. Maintenance infusion: 1–4 mg/min (dilute in D_5W or normal saline).

Promethazine Hydrochloride (Phenergan)

Indications Nausea, vomiting, motion sickness; sedation for patients in labor; potentiation of analgesic effects of narcotics.

Contraindications Hypersensitivity, coma, CNS-depressed patients from alcohol, barbiturates, narcotics, Reye's syndrome.

Dosage and administration Adult: 12.5–25 mg IV, deep IM, PO, rectally.

Propranolol Hydrochloride (Inderal)

Indications Hypertension, angina pectoris, V-tach and V-fib refractory to lidocaine; selected supraventricular tachycardias.

Contraindications Sinus bradycardia, second- or third-degree AV block, asthma, CHF, COPD.

Dosage and administration Adult: Dilute 1–3 mg in 10–30 mL of D_5W; administer slowly IV at rate of 1 mg/min; maximum, 5 mg.

Streptokinase (Streptase)

Indications Acute evolving MI, massive pulmonary emboli, arterial thrombosis and embolism, to clear arteriovenous cannulas.

Contraindications Hypersensitivity; active bleeding, recent surgery (within 2–4 weeks), recent CVA; prolonged CPR; intracranial or intraspinal neoplasm, arteriovenous malformation, or surgery; recent significant trauma (particularly head trauma); uncontrolled hypertension.

Dosage and administration Note: Reconstitute by slowly adding 5 mL of sodium chloride or D_5W, directing stream to side of vial instead of into powder. Gently roll and tilt vial for reconstitution; dilute slowly to 45 mL total. Adult: 500,000–1,500,000 IU diluted to 45 mL IV over 1 hour.

Succinylcholine Chloride (Anectine, Quelicin)

Indications To facilitate intubation, to terminate laryngospasm, to promote muscle relaxation, to facilitate electroconvulsive shock therapy.

Contraindications Acute narrow-angle glaucoma, penetrating eye injuries, inability to control airway or support ventilations with oxygen and positive pressure.

Dosage and administration Adult: 1–2 mg/kg rapid IV; repeat once if needed.

Medication Review

Terbutaline Sulfate (Brethine, Bricanyl)

Indications Bronchial asthma, reversible bronchospasm associated with exercise, chronic bronchitis, and emphysema.

Contraindications Hypersensitivity, tachyarrhythmias.

Dosage and administration Adult: 0.25 mg SC; may repeat in 15–30 minutes to maximum dose of 0.5 mg in 4-hour period. 400 µg (two inhalations by MDI) every 4–6 hours; allow 1–2 minutes between inhalations.

Thiamine Hydrochloride (Vitamin B-1)

Indications Coma of unknown origin, delirium tremens, beriberi, Wernicke's encephalopathy.

Contraindications None.

Dosage and administration Adult: 100 mg slow IV or IM.

Tissue Plasminogen Activator (TPA)

Indications Acute evolving myocardial infarction, massive pulmonary emboli, arterial thrombosis and embolism, to clear arteriovenous cannulas.

Contraindications Recent surgery (within 3 weeks), active bleeding, recent CVA, prolonged CPR, intracranial or intraspinal surgery; recent significant trauma, especially head trauma; uncontrolled hypertension (generally BP over 200 mm Hg).

Dosage and administration Adult: 10-mg bolus IV over 2 minutes; then 50 mg over 1 hour, then 20 mg over the second hour and 20 mg over the third hour, for a total dose of 100 mg (other doses may be prescribed through Medical Direction).

Vasopressin (Pitressin synthetic)

Indications Alternate vasopressor to the first or second dose of epinephrine in cardiac arrest, may be useful in cases of vasodilatory shock (ie, septic shock).

Contraindications Responsive patients with coronary artery disease.

Dosage and administration Adult: 40-unit one-time dose IV/IO to replace the first or second dose of epinephrine in cardiac arrest.

Vecuronium Bromide (Norcuron)

Indications To facilitate intubation, to terminate laryngospasm, to promote muscle relaxation, to facilitate electroconvulsive shock therapy.

Contraindications Acute narrow-angle glaucoma, penetrating eye injuries, inability to control airway or support ventilations with oxygen and positive pressure, myasthenia gravis, hepatic or renal failure.

Dosage and administration Adult: 0.1 mg/kg IV push; maintenance dose within 25–40 minutes: 0.01–0.05 mg/kg IV push.

Verapamil (Calan, Isoptin)

Indications PSVT, PAT, atrial fibrillation and atrial flutter with rapid ventricular response.

Contraindications Wolff-Parkinson-White syndrome, second-degree or third-degree AV block, sick sinus syndrome (unless patient has functioning pacemaker), hypotension, cardiogenic shock, severe CHF, pulmonary edema, patients receiving IV beta-blockers, wide-complex tachycardias, children less than 12 months of age.

Dosage and administration Adult: 2.5–5.0 mg IV bolus over 2 minutes (over 3 minutes in older patients). Repeat doses of 5–10 mg may be given every 15–30 minutes to a maximum of 20 mg.

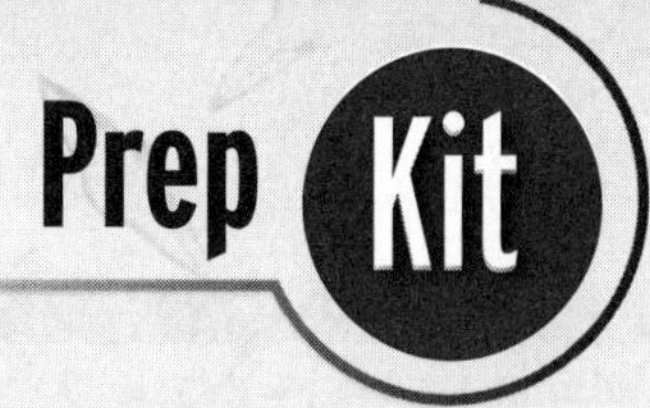

Chapter Summary

- The geriatric patient becomes more susceptible to an adverse response to drug therapy when they develop a decline in liver and kidney functions and cannot eliminate drugs at the same rate as a younger person might.
- When a geriatric patient is taking medications, it could be a contributing factor to nearly any health problem.
- The issues of concern with geriatric medication administration involve polypharmacy, medication non-compliance, potential dosing errors, and increased sensitivity.
- Geriatric patients that have decreased cardiac functions, circulation, or renal and liver functions will have a slower metabolic rate that decreases medication clearance efficiency and leads to toxic or adverse reactions.
- There are certain medications that are associated with falls in the geriatric patient and should be used with caution or, if possible, substituted with another drug.
- Some of the conditions affecting various body systems in the geriatric population include pneumonia, myocardial infarction, delirium, and diabetes.
- NSAIDs are nonopioid pain reliever drugs that treat mild to moderate pain. NSAIDs do not produce physical dependence but are strongly associated with GI bleeding.
- Opioids are highly effective for managing severe pain, but carry the risk of dependence in the long-term treatment of chronic pain, and geriatric patients have increased sensitivity to opioids and tend to require smaller doses than younger patients.

Vital Vocabulary

Adrenal crisis Also known as Addisonian crisis and acute adrenal insufficiency, it is a potentially life-threatening state caused by insufficient levels of cortisol.

Corneal diseases Conditions affecting the transparent part of the cover of the eyeball which covers the iris and pupil and admits light into the interior of the eye.

Encephalopathy Degeneration of brain function, caused by any of various acquired disorders, including metabolic disease, organ failure, inflammation, and chronic infection.

Nonopioid Medications designed to relieve pain without the side effects of opioids.

Opioid Effective for managing severe pain but carry the risk of dependence.

Polypharmacy Simultaneous use of multiple medications.

Presbyopia A visual condition which becomes apparent in middle age. Due to defective elasticity of the lens, the eye's ability to accommodate and focus sharply for near vision becomes diminished.

Syncope Fainting; brief loss of consciousness caused by transiently inadequate blood flow to the brain.

Temporal arteritis An inflammatory condition that involves the arteries of the external carotid system, causing them to become inflamed and possibly obstructed, with associated headache and potential visual loss.

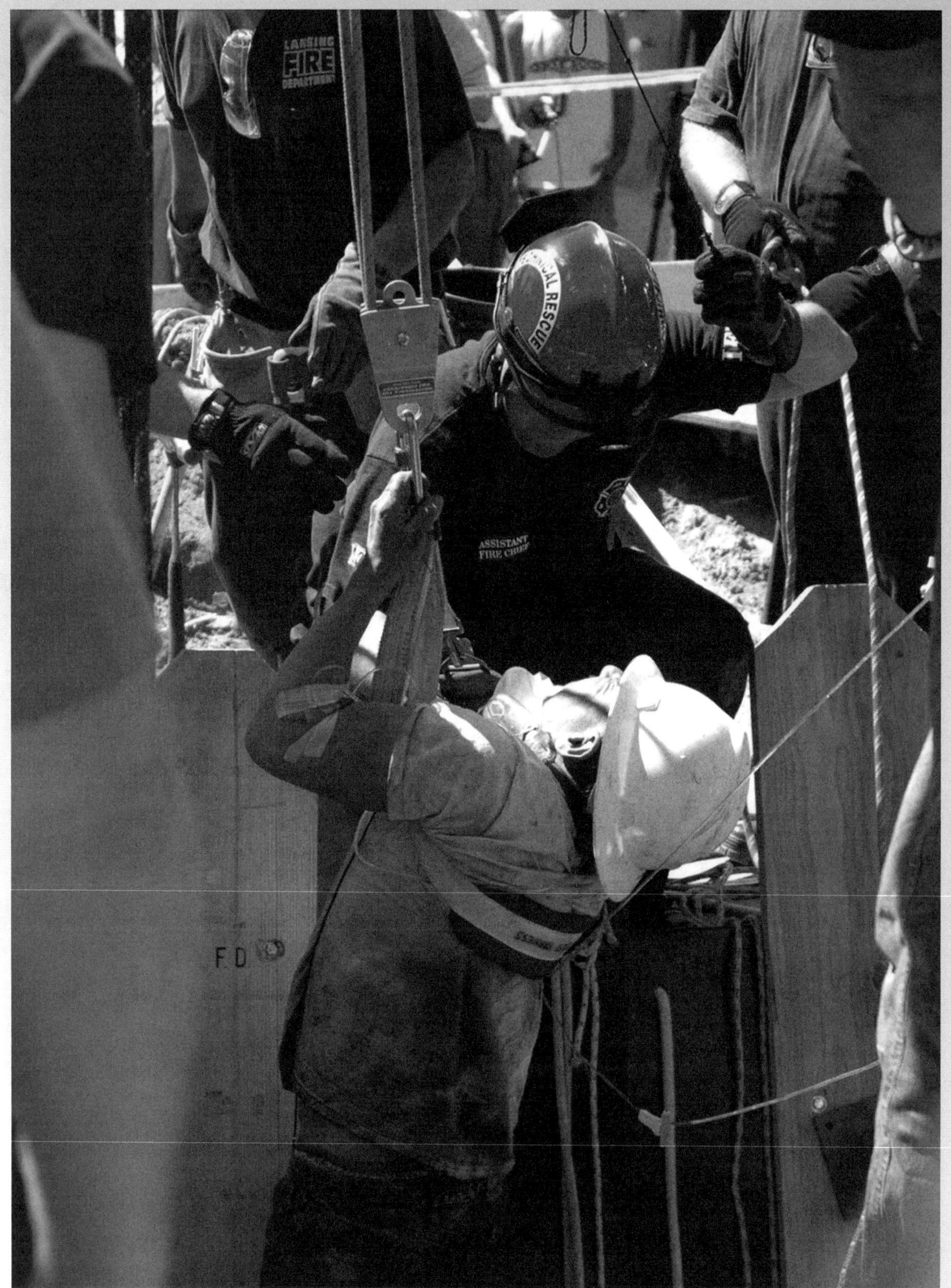
LANSING
FIRE
DEPARTMENT
ASSISTANT
F.D

Rescue Awareness, Operations, and Terrorism Response

15

Objectives

Cognitive

8-3.38 Explain the indications, contraindications and methods of pain control for entrapped patients. (pages 440–448)

Affective

None

Psychomotor

None

Additional Objectives

15-1 List nuclear/chemical/biological/explosive agents that may be used by a terrorist. (pages 449–450)

15-2 Describe the treatment to be rendered to a victim of a nuclear/chemical/biological/explosive attack. (pages 450–455)

15-3 Discuss the following medications used in the prehospital setting for the unique problems encountered during rescue operations: morphine sulfate (Astramorph/PF), fentanyl citrate (Sublimase), sodium bicarbonate, naloxone hydrochloride (Narcan), ondansetron hydrochloride (Zofran), promethazine (Phenergan), and the Mark I kits (Atropine and 2-PAM). (pages 444–447, 453)

The Rescue Process

Paramedics respond to rescue calls all the time. Most commonly a patient has been involved in a motor vehicle crash and that is why every community has an agency, usually the fire department, trained in the discipline of vehicle rescue (**Figure 15-1 ▸**).

The process of rescuing a patient can be as simple as opening a door to as complicated as disentangling a patient who is severely entrapped. The process of rescue is usually taught from a systems approach involving a series of phases including arrival and size-up, hazard control, gaining access to the patient, medical treatment, disentanglement, patient packaging, and transportation.

This chapter discusses some of the unique rescue situations and the impact on the patient (**Figure 15-2 ▸**).

Wherever it pertains we also discuss the specific pharmacological interventions that are a part of the patient's management in the prehospital environment. Simply stated, there are not many rescue operations or terrorist threats that are managed with new and unique medications aside from those that have already been discussed in other chapters of this book (ie, oxygen, analgesics, sodium bicarbonate, atropine sulphate, etc).

Rather than focus on the routine rescues (if there ever is such a thing as a routine rescue), we will try to stick to the unique situations. One essential part of training for rescue is to become aware of the hazards and know who in your region has the appropriate rescue training to mitigate the situation. Take the time now to think seriously about who should be called to assist with a high-angle rescue, a confined space rescue, a trench rescue, a hazardous materials incident, or a swift water or ice rescue.

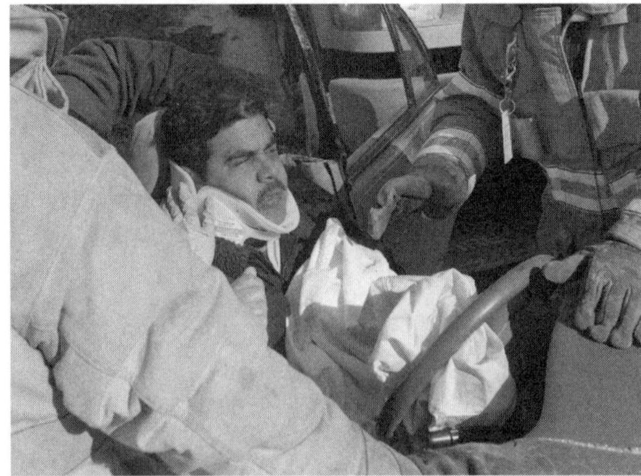

Figure 15-1 This patient is trapped between the steering wheel and the seat.

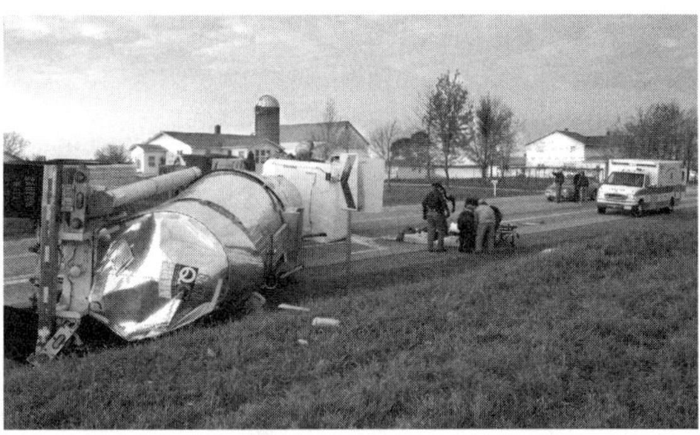

Figure 15-2 This unique rescue situation involves hazardous materials with the potential of the patient having a crush injury.

Crush Syndrome

<u>Crush syndrome</u> can occur when an area of the body is trapped for longer than 4 hours and arterial blood flow is compromised. In some cases, it may be difficult to gauge the extent of internal injury. In other cases it will be quite apparent (**Figure 15-3 ▸**). It can lead to life-threatening arrhythmias or severe acidosis and electrolyte imbalance, particularly on release from entrapment.

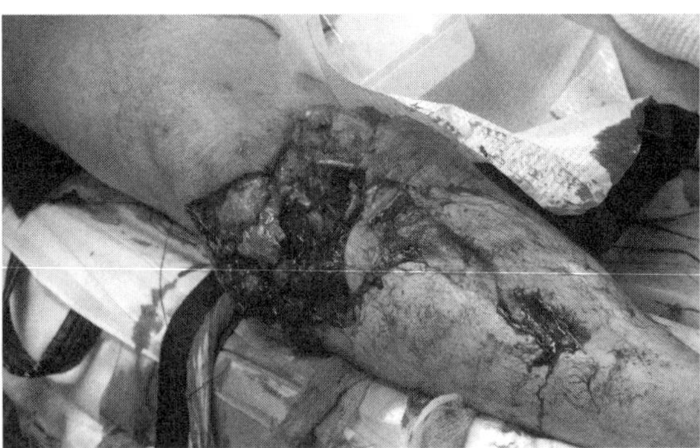

Figure 15-3 This crush injury reveals extensive tissue damage and deformity. Swelling and blood loss are also apparent.

When EMS providers and rescue workers work for hours to extricate the patient from whatever it is that is crushing them, they can easily get an impression of the patient's condition. The rescuer and the crushed patient often carry on a conversation for long periods of time and usually in close quarters. When the trapped patient is alert and conversing, this is often referred to as "smiling death." The patient appears to be "stable" up to the point of when the weight is lifted off of them. The sudden release of prolonged high pressure on compressed myofascial compartments and traumatized soft tissue allows built-up lactic acid and potassium to wash into the central circulation. This phenomenon has been known to provoke cardiac arrest in a subject who moments before appeared to be relatively stable. The term for destruction of muscle and subsequent release of breakdown products and toxins into the systemic circulation from a crushing type injury is **rhabdomyolysis**. The consequences of rhabdomyolysis can contribute to acute renal failure as well as hypocalcemia, hypovolemia, and hyperkalemia, all of which can result in cardiotoxic states.

Crush Syndrome Management

The goals of crush syndrome management include prevention of sudden death, prevention of renal failure, and optimizing the long-term limb salvage by instituting care as early as possible in the prehospital environment. Pain medication may also be appropriate with the patient who is pinned down. When considering pharmacology for analgesia, it is important to constantly monitor the vital signs because some analgesics are contraindicated in hypotension. **Table 15-1** lists some of the medications that are considered in the pain management of patients during rescue efforts.

Maintaining the patient's urine output is important and is considered a sensitive indicator that will help you monitor and make sure that treatment for hypovolemia, acidosis, and hyperkalemia are proceeding appropriately, all of which goes toward preventing sudden cardiac arrest.

If unable to control the hyperkalemia, the resulting risk of hyperkalemic arrhythmia would dictate the need for treatment with calcium chloride. As an alternative, 5% dextrose in 0.45% sodium chloride [D_5½NS] would also be considered compared to the use of straight calcium chloride because it may help maintain the urine output better. Of course, this all assumes that the patient who is becoming hypovolemic is being managed with oxygenation, ventilation, and fluid therapy as well as being kept warm. Hyperbaric therapy may be another option in some EMS systems.

The time to manage crush syndrome is early on. Do not wait until the patient has been extricated or until the patient has been moved to the ambulance. Ventricular ectopy, resulting in cardiac arrest, can occur even with the most gentle handling.

To prevent renal failure, it is not uncommon for the patient to receive an initial crystalloid fluid bolus of 1 to 2 liters followed by more than 12 additional liters in the first 24 hours of care. Renal protection from rhabdomyolysis is enhanced by alkalinizing the urine and blood. Although this is primarily an

Table 15-1 Medications for Pain Management in Rescue Situations

Medication	Characteristics
Morphine sulfate	Narcotic analgesic and central nervous system depressant often used in the treatment of myocardial infarction, kidney stones, and pulmonary edema. It is contraindicated in patients who are volume-depleted or suffering from severe hypotension.
Meperidine Hydrochloride (Demerol)	Narcotic analgesic and central nervous system depressant primarily used for the treatment of moderate to severe pain. It is relatively contraindicated in patients with undiagnosed abdominal pain and head injuries.
Nitrous oxide (Nitronox, Entonox)	This central nervous system depressant with analgesic properties is used for musculoskeletal pain, fractures, and burns. It should not be used in patients who cannot follow verbal instructions, those with head injuries, COPD patients, and patients with thoracic injuries or possible pneumothorax. Use caution in environments with temperatures of less than 21°F, which could make administration difficult to impossible.
Fentanyl citrate (Sublimase)	Unrelated to morphine but with similar analgesic effects, it is considered 50 to 100 times more potent than morphine; however, its duration of action is much shorter. It can be used for rapid-sequence intubation and severe pain, but is contraindicated with severe hemorrhage, shock, or known hypersensitivity.
Butorphanol tartrate (Stadol)	This synthetic analgesic, with effects equal to a large dose of morphine, is indicated for the treatment of moderate to severe pain, but is contraindicated in patients with undiagnosed abdominal pain and head injuries.
Nalbuphine (Nubain)	Synthetic analgesic with the same effects as morphine. Nubain has the hemodynamic effects of morphine and is used in patients with moderate to severe pain. Like morphine, Nubain is contraindicated in patients with undiagnosed abdominal pain and head injuries.
Ketorolac (Toradol)	Classified as a nonsteroidal anti-inflammatory drug (NSAID), ketorolac has analgesic, anti-inflammatory, and antipyretic effects. It is considered in controlling moderate to severe pain. Its only true contraindication is in patients with a known hypersensitivity to the drug and patients with reported allergies to aspirin or NSAIDs.

in-hospital intervention, the goal is to maintain a urine pH of greater than 7.0. Sodium bicarbonate is often given in the prehospital setting as either an IV push or drip to begin to achieve this goal. Most regions have a protocol or will contact medical control in the crushing situation for consideration of sodium bicarbonate. Some experts suggest that mannitol [Osmitrol] (10 g or 20% solution added to each liter of IV fluid) will promote an osmotic diuresis that may be helpful in keeping the kidneys clear. Loop diuretics, such as furosemide [Lasix] are not initially recommended because they further acidify the urine. The most appropriate medications are not normally carried on a paramedic unit so they would need to be taken to the scene if a surgical team is deployed (ie, 10 units of regular insulin IV for hyperkalemia).

If a surgeon is requested to respond to the scene for a possible field amputation, the surgeon may want to consider bringing a liter of 5% dextrose in water [D_5W], 3 ampules of sodium bicarbonate, and 10 g of 20% solution of mannitol [Osmitrol]. Another option would be to administer a bolus line of normal saline plus a sodium bicarbonate drip after a sodium bicarbonate bolus (the mannitol [Osmitrol] would be an in-hospital consideration).

Case Study 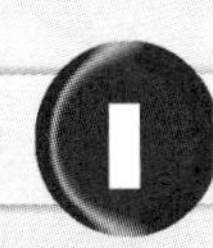 Crush Syndrome

Part 1

You are responding to a call for a structural collapse in the older section of town. Multiple calls are coming in and police, fire, and rescue are arriving. The incident commander established a command post across the street from the structure. The building that collapsed is an old three-story brick structure with a restaurant on the first two floors and an apartment on the third floor. Fortunately it is 7:00 a.m. so there were no customers in the restaurant.

The scene is not yet safe so you are assigned to report to the command post to work in the treatment sector. All of the necessary components of the EMS branch of the Incident Command structure are quickly falling into place as supervisory personnel are arriving. Since you were not the first ambulance to arrive at the scene, other personnel have already assumed the role of Triage/Treatment and Transportation sector officers.

As the scene is quickly becoming congested with emergency vehicles, the medical commander has determined that a staging sector will be set up for additional units to await further reports from the scene as to their need. Staging has been set up in the parking lot of the strip mall three blocks away. The police have already begun to set up a perimeter since many of the neighbors are out in the street.

According to a neighbor who was out walking his dog, there was a rumble and suddenly the side brick wall of the building collapsed. The family of five who lived upstairs is being removed from the rubble by fire fighters. They all seem to have relatively minor injuries (ie, lacerations, contusions, and covered with dust) since their beds seemed to have slid out of their bedrooms onto the piles of bricks.

As you attend to the family's bumps and bruises you can hear over the radio that one of the fire fighters hears screaming from under the pile of rubble. The neighbor states that it is probably Joey the cook who sometimes stays there overnight after he has had a few drinks, rather than drive home. The fire fighters begin to carefully remove bricks from the pile in the area where Joey's voice can be heard. This will take some time.

After about 40 minutes, the family has been attended to and transported to the ED, and the Medical Branch of the ICS structure has been "geared down" a bit since there is only one suspected patient. With this reorganization you are now assigned to the ambulance that will attend to Joey once he is removed. There is also plenty of help on the scene should his condition be critical.

You and your partner have your PPE on and are nearby Joey so you can begin to talk to him. Mean-

Case Study I Continued

while, the fire fighters have determined that a concrete slab is on top of his legs. According to the rescue sector officer, they may be able to get a camera in there with a light so you can see what Joey's condition is. In the meantime, you are doing your best to try to get a general impression and perform the initial assessment from simply talking to Joey (see **Table 1**).

Once you have better access to the patient he will need a rapid trauma examination. The rescue sector officer informs you that they have found a support beam that they are shoring up to allow them access to the patient. It will still take some time to remove the slab from his legs but at least you will be able to evaluate him and begin treatment.

Question 1: Is there any significance to the statement by the neighbor that Joey sleeps over when he has had too many drinks to drive?

Question 2: Once you have access to the patient, what will the priority be?

Table 1 Initial Assessment

Initial Assessment	Recording Time: 40 Minutes
General Impression/ Appearance	In good spirits considering he is crushed under a slab of concrete
Mental Status	"V" verbal (knows his name, day of the week but is confused about where he was before the collapse). He is able to carry on a conversation.
Airway	Open although the patient says he is very dry probably due to inhaling dust
Breathing	Based on his speech it is within normal range
Circulation	He obviously has a pulse. He says he is not sure if he is bleeding but can feel the pulse in his wrist which is very fast.
Priority/Plan	High due to the extent of the potential injury and MOI

Part 2

After another 20 minutes of shoring up the structure, it is now possible for you and your partner to get right into the area where the patient is confined. Most of the bricks have been removed and special low pressure air bags and cribbing have been brought in. The patient is in good spirits considering his legs are crushed under a heavy slab of concrete.

Your partner is obtaining a set of vital signs while you begin to ask Joey some of the "OPQRST" questions to elaborate on the chief complaint. You are glad to hear that the patient is not a diabetic and he is not taking blood thinners. These are two examples of serious complicating factors. The diabetic patient often has neuropathy and may not be able to express the sensation of pain well and the patient on a blood thinner (ie, post stroke or TIA) will bleed considerably from a crushing injury. You will do the best you can to complete the focused history and physical examination given the circumstances (see **Table 2**).

Table 2 Focused History and Physical Examination

Baseline Vital Signs	Recording Time: 60 Minutes
Skin CTC (color, temperature, condition)	Pale, cool, and diaphoretic (clammy)
Pulse	Rapid, regular, and thready
Blood Pressure	96/68 mm Hg
Respirations	22 breaths/min and normal

You are able to place the patient on a nonrebreathing mask to supplement his oxygen.

Question 3: If the patient states he is taking a blood thinner, how would that be relevant?

Question 4: If the patient states he is a diabetic, how would that affect your management?

Part 3

The rescue sector officer notifies you that they are less than 5 minutes away from lifting the concrete slab off the patient. Your partner has been on the radio with medical control who would like you to add 50 mEq of sodium bicarbonate to a liter of normal saline and run it wide open into a large bore IV. This should help neutralize the acids and manage shock as well as flush out the toxins with the fluids (normal saline). They are also considering sending a surgeon to the scene in case an emergency field amputation is the only way to save Joey's life.

Case Study I Continued

At this point you have the following additional information from Joey (see **Table 3**).

Table 3 SAMPLE History

SAMPLE History	Comments
Signs/symptoms	Extreme pain, nausea, diaphoretic
Allergies	Penicillin and codeine
Medications	Vitamins (C and E), zolpidem tartrate [Ambien]
Pertinent past medical history	Basically in good health
Last oral intake	A few beers about 4 hours ago
Events leading up to the incident	Suddenly covered in debris and a heavy concrete slab

Treatment Plan

1. Ensure an open and clear airway.
2. Assess ventilations and assist as needed, otherwise administer supplemental oxygen via nonrebreathing mask.
3. Obtain baseline vital signs.
4. Start an IV and obtain bloods for the ED.
5. Administer 1 liter IV normal saline bolus followed by a sodium bicarbonate drip and reevaluate (see **Table 4**).This should help to neutralize the acids and flush out the toxins as well as manage the impending shock.
6. As soon as possible obtain an ECG.
7. Administer the following medications, as needed:
   a. Fentanyl citrate [Sublimase] 0.5–2 mcg/kg IV, IM, or atomized intranasal for pain relief (see **Table 5**).
   b. Morphine sulfate [Astramorph/PF] 2–4 mg IV or IM (may repeat per medical control) (see **Table 6**) for pain relief. Also, it is always appropriate to have naloxone hydrochloride [Narcan] available whenever a narcotic is being administered in case the patient's respirations become depressed (see **Table 7**).
   c. Ondansetron hydrochloride [Zofran] 4 mg IV/IM for nausea (some regions may choose to administer 12.5 to 25 mg IV/IM promethazine hydrochloride [Phenergan] for nausea) (see **Table 8** and **Table 9**).
   d. Mannitol [Osmitrol] 25 grams IV push (easier than the drip method). Give it after at least a liter of IV fluid, if infused. Since mannitol [Osmitrol] is generally an in-hospital medicine and not routinely carried on the paramedic unit, it is listed here because a surgical team may be called to the scene due to the criticality of the situation and length of time of extrication.
8. Splint and immobilize the patient.
9. Transport to the ED with notification and serial vital signs and a 12-lead ECG.

Table 4 Sodium Bicarbonate

Do you know?	Comments
Right drug? Generic name: **[Sodium Bicarbonate]** Trade name: [Citrocarbonate, Neut]	This drug is an alkalinizing agent, antacid, and electrolyte. It is used to treat acute metabolic acidosis caused by shock, severe dehydration, anoxia, uncontrolled diabetes, renal disease, cardiac arrest, and severe lactic acidosis. It is also used to treat hyperacidity, and prophylaxis for renal calculi.
Right patient?	In this case it can be used for prolonged acidosis in the affected tissues.
Right dose?	1 mEq/kg.
Right route?	IV bolus in a secondary line.
Right time?	Just prior to removing the object crushing the tissues in an effort to neutralize the acids. After vasopressors, antiarrhythmics, and any other drugs. It is typically used as a last option drug in cardiac arrest.
Right documentation?	Dose, route, time administered, and reassessment should be clearly documented on the patient care report.
Expected action	Relief of metabolic acidosis.
Side effects	Hypernatremia, alkalosis, tetany, and fluid overload.

continues

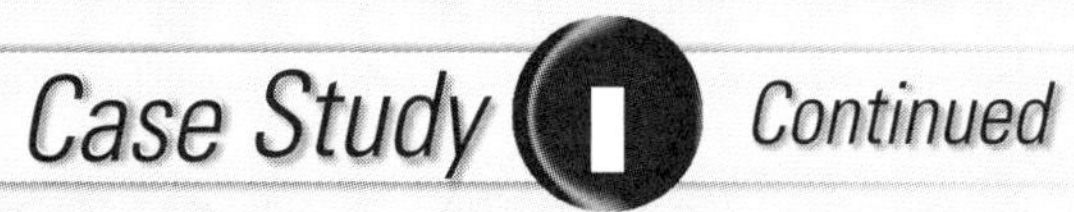

Table 4 **Sodium Bicarbonate (*Continued*)**

Do you know?	Comments
Contraindications	Metabolic and respiratory alkalosis, hypertension, convulsions, and congestive heart failure (CHF).
Precautions	Used with caution in patients with impaired renal and hepatic function, and cardiovascular insufficiency with or without CHF.
Pharmacokinetics	Rapidly metabolized to carbonic acid which rapidly dissociates into water and carbon dioxide. The carbon dioxide is excreted via the lungs.

Table 5 **Fentanyl Citrate**

Do you know?	Comments
Right drug? Generic name: [**Fentanyl Citrate**] Trade name: [Sublimase]	This is drug is a narcotic analgesic (schedule II narcotic). It is used to treat severe pain and is used with anesthesia. It has actions similar to morphine sulfate and meperidine hydrochloride.
Right patient?	Relief of severe pain.
Right dose?	0.5–2 mcg/kg IV, IM, or atomized intranasal.
Right route?	IV/IM.
Right time?	After assessment and contraindications for use have been considered.
Right documentation?	Always document how and when the drug was administered as well as the patient's response to the medication on your patient care report.
Expected action	Pain relief.
Side effects	Skeletal and thoracic muscle rigidity, bradycardia, seizures, and diaphoresis.
Contraindications	Myasthenia gravis.
Precautions	May cause life-threatening hypoventilation.
Pharmacokinetics	Onset immediate IV, 2–7 minutes IM; peak 30 minutes; duration 30–60 minutes IV, 1–2 hours IM; metabolized in the liver and excreted in urine.

Table 6 **Morphine Sulfate**

Do you know?	Comments
Right drug? Generic name: [**Morphine Sulfate**] Trade name: [Astramorph/PF]	This drug is an opioid analgesic (schedule II narcotic). It is used for relief of severe pain, anxiety, sedation, reduces left ventricular work, and for treating dyspnea caused by left ventricular failure and pulmonary edema.
Right patient?	For severe CHF, pulmonary edema, chest pain associated with acute MI, analgesia for moderate to severe acute and chronic pain (as in this case). *However, this patient's BP may be a concern so monitor it very closely or consider another pain reliever.*
Right dose?	Initial dose of 2–4 mg IV (over 1–5 minutes) every 5–30 minutes. Repeat dose 2–8 mg at 5- to 15-minute intervals.
Right route?	Slow IV, IM/SC.
Right time?	When the patient has severe pain as long as their vital signs are stable.
Right documentation?	Always document how and when the drug was administered as well as the patient's response to the medication on your patient care report.
Expected action	It should alleviate pain through CNS action, suppress fear and anxiety centers in the brain, depress brain stem respiratory centers, increase peripheral venous capacitance and decrease venous return, decrease preload and afterload, which decreases myocardial oxygen demand.

continues

Case Study 1 Continued

Table 6 Morphine Sulfate (*Continued*)

Do you know?	Comments
Side effects	Respiratory depression, hypotension, decreased level of consciousness, nausea, vomiting, bradycardia, tachycardia, syncope, facial flushing, euphoria, bronchospasm, and dry mouth.
Contraindications	Head injury, exacerbated COPD, depressed respiratory drive, hypotension, undiagnosed abdominal pain, decreased level of consciousness, suspected hypovolemia, patients who have taken MAOIs within the past 14 days.
Precautions	Potentiates sedative effects of phenothiazines. CNS depressant may potentiate effects of morphine sulfate. MAOIs may cause paradoxical excitation.
Pharmacokinetics	Onset: immediate; peak effect: 20 minutes; duration: 2–7 hours, metabolized in the liver and excreted in urine.

Table 7 Naloxone Hydrochloride

Do you know?	Comments
Right drug? Generic name: [**Naloxone Hydrochloride**] Trade name: [Narcan]	This drug is a narcotic antagonist. When the paramedic suspects that the patient's respiratory depression is due to an overdose of a narcotic or opiate, such as morphine, heroin, or methadone, the drug of choice to reverse the effects of the narcotic or opiate is naloxone hydrochloride [Narcan].
Right patient?	Patients who have depressed respirations or an altered mental status from too high a dose of a narcotic or opiate.
Right dose?	The dose is 0.4 mg to 2 mg and is best to titrate to desirable effect of improved respirations.
Right route?	Can be given by IV, IO, IM, or ET routes although the ET route is the least effective and not generally recommended if other routes are available.
Right time?	If the patient has respiratory depression, assist the ventilations with your bag-mask device while properly positioning and restraining the patient on your stretcher. Then it is time to administer the naloxone hydrochloride [Narcan] just in case the patient wakes up in an argumentative or violent mood.
Right documentation?	Always document how and when the drug was administered as well as the patient's response to the medication on your patient care report. Also document if humane restraint was applied prior to the administration of the drug.
Expected action	Antagonistic to narcotic or opiate medications. Expect it to reverse the effect of the overdose. Small doses should improve the patient's ventilations. Larger doses may cause the patient to actually wake up which is generally not necessary since they wake up in an argumentative or violent mood.
Side effects	Nausea, upset stomach, or drowsiness can occur. More serious side effects from naloxone hydrochloride [Narcan] include withdrawal symptoms including vomiting, sweating, tremors, seizures, rapid and pounding irregular pulse.
Contraindications	None aside from the precautions.
Precautions	Administer this drug slowly and only administer enough to lighten up the patient and improve their respirations. If you give the entire dose the patient is likely to be awakened with withdrawal symptoms and be very aggressive. You just spoiled his high!
Pharmacokinetics	Onset: within 2 minutes; peak effect: variable; duration is dependent on dose and route, usually 30–60 minutes; metabolized in the liver and excreted in urine.

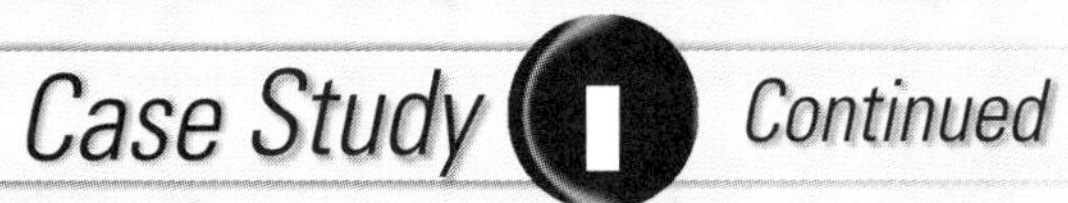

Case Study 1 Continued

Table 8 Ondansetron Hydrochloride

Do you know?	Comments
Right drug? Generic name: [**Ondansetron Hydrochloride**] Trade name: [Zofran]	This drug is an antiemetic. It is used to relieve or prevent nausea and vomiting in a variety of situations. (Although a number of EMS systems are using this drug, it is important to note that at this time, ondansetron hydrochloride [Zofran] for anything other than chemotherapy-induced symptoms is considered off-label use by the FDA.)
Right patient?	Nausea and vomiting.
Right dose?	4 mg initial dose; may be repeated—follow local protocol.
Right route?	IV.
Right time?	Adjunct treatment in suspected ACS after treating with aspirin (ASA), nitrates, and/or morphine.
Right documentation?	Document the administration of the medication as well as the ongoing assessment findings, including lung sounds on the patient care report.
Expected action	Relief of nausea.
Side effects	Seizures, tachycardia, bradycardia, headache, sedation, chest pain, bronchospasm, acute dystonic reactions, blurred vision, hypokalemia, fever.
Contraindications	Known sensitivity.
Precautions	May worsen preexisting symptoms.
Pharmacokinetics	Onset: 30 minutes IV; peak effect: 2 hours; duration: 3–6 hours, metabolized in the liver, excreted in urine.

Table 9 Promethazine Hydrochloride

Do you know?	Comments
Right drug? Generic name: [**Promethazine Hydrochloride**] Trade name: [Phenergan]	This drug is an antihistamine (H1 antagonist). It is a mild anticholinergic, antiemetic, and potentiates the actions of analgesics. It is commonly used to relieve or prevent nausea and vomiting.
Right patient?	Nausea and vomiting.
Right dose?	12.5–25 mg.
Right route?	IV or IM.
Right time?	Adjunct treatment when morphine sulfate [Astramorph] is being administered. May be used for most patients with nausea or vomiting provided they are not in a coma and do not have large amounts of depressants (ie, alcohol) in their system.
Right documentation?	Document the administration of the medication as well as the ongoing assessment findings, including lung sounds on the patient care report.
Expected action	Relief of nausea and enhanced effects of morphine sulfate [Astramorph].
Side effects	Drowsiness, sedation, blurred vision, tachycardia, bradycardia, and dizziness.
Contraindications	Known sensitivity, comatose states, patients with large amounts of depressants in their system.
Precautions	Avoid accidental intra-arterial injection.
Pharmacokinetics	Onset: immediate; peak effect: 30–60 minutes; duration: 4–6 hours, metabolized in the liver, excreted in urine.

Question 5: If it is helpful to get the patient moving fluids, why not give him furosemide [Lasix]?

Question 6: What is meant by "smiling death?"

Case Study 1 Continued

Part 4

Just prior to the lifting of the concrete slab, the patient's condition is reevaluated and it has been decided that a surgeon will not be needed at the scene. You completed a rapid trauma examination as well as a detailed physical examination on Joey and found that he may have a cracked rib or two, numerous contusions, and a few lacerations. As a precaution, you had tied a tourniquet loosely on each of the legs prior to removing the concrete slab. Fortunately the tourniquets did not have to be tightened because the bleeding was controlled by other means. For the most part he looks pretty good considering the extent of the trauma sustained. Of course both of his legs are completely immobilized under the slab at this point so they cannot be evaluated. His pelvis still has sensation and is not injured.

You have administered a liter of normal saline and sodium bicarbonate to alkalinize the patient. Everything is ready to carefully but quickly slide him onto a long backboard and remove him with a Stokes basket out to the ambulance.

One of the EMT-Basics will be driving your medic unit to the hospital so your partner can work with you in the back of the ambulance en route to the ED. You will reassess the patient en route (see **Table 10**). The hospital is in close contact with the scene so they have been able to mobilize the surgical team and everyone is ready on their end.

Table 10 Reassessment and Ongoing Assessment of the Patient

Serial Vital Signs and Relevant Data	Recording Time: 90 Minutes
Skin CTC	Pale, cool, and diaphoretic (clammy and covered with concrete dust)
Pulse	118 beats/min and regular
Blood Pressure	98/70 mm Hg
Respirations	22 breaths/min and shallow
Mental Status	"A" alert (oriented to person, place, and day)
ECG	Sinus tachycardia
SpO_2	97% on nonrebreathing mask
Lung Sounds	Clear bilaterally
Other (ie glucose, core body temperature)	Glucose was normal range

Question 7: If it was clear that the patient's condition was deteriorating, what option would you have?

Question 8: Should a tourniquet be applied to both legs?

Part 5

When Joey was removed from under the concrete slab, both of his legs were severely crushed. There were multiple open fractures evident in the long bones of the leg, and there were associated massive soft-tissue injuries. You moved him to the long backboard, and you noted little in the way of external bleeding so the tourniquets were not tightened. Fluid resuscitation was continued and pain medication was given while en route to the ED. On arrival the surgical team was waiting, and after reassessment of the ABCs, Joey was quickly taken to the surgical suite. Five hours into surgery it was clear that both of his legs would require above-knee amputation. A couple of days later, after all the media coverage surrounding the event dies down, you and your partner stop by the hospital to visit with Joey. As you would have expected from those hours of conversation with Joey during the incident, he is a real survivor and you find him in great spirits. He is already discussing getting fitted for those special jogging legs so he can stay fit. It will be a long time before his body will be ready to run in new legs but it certainly will help that he has the strength and will to deal with the challenges that his extended recovery will bring.

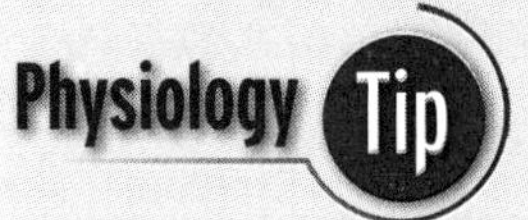

The crush syndrome scenario can be life-threatening because the acids and toxins produced in the crushed legs are suddenly released to the systemic circulation, thus changing the pH. Let's review the relationship between an acid, a base, and the pH in the body.

An **acid** is a substance that increases the concentration of hydrogen ions in a water solution. A **base** is a substance that decreases the concentration of hydrogen ions. The concentration of dissolved hydrogen (H+) is the main determinant of whether the body fluid is acidic, basic, or neutral. Since hydrogen is an acid, the more hydrogen present, the more acidic the body fluid. If the H+ concentration is lower, the body fluid will be more basic. Homeostasis maintains H+ concentration in a restricted range.

pH is a value calculated from the H+ concentration. Due to the mathematics, there is an inverse relationship between pH and the H+ concentration where higher H+ levels (more acidic) lead to lower pH and lower H+ levels (more basic) lead to higher pH. The pH of 7.0 is neutral. The blood pH in humans is normally 7.35 to 7.45, slightly basic (alkaline). If the value is lower, blood is considered to be acidotic. If the value is higher, blood is considered alkalotic.

Response to Terrorism

The FBI defines terrorism as "the unlawful use of force against person or property to intimidate or coerce a government, the civilian population, or any segment thereof, in the furtherance of political or social objectives." Although certainly not the first act of terrorism against the United States, the events of September 11, 2001 have caused EMS, rescue, and law enforcement communities to have a heightened awareness to the potential threats to our citizens posed by terrorists. What sets these incidents apart from those explosions or hazardous material spills that rescue workers respond to on a regular basis are three key elements. Terrorist activities are illegal and involve the use of force, the actions intend to intimidate or coerce, and the actions are committed in support of political or social objectives.

There are five categories of terrorist incidents that can be remembered by using the acronym B-NICE (**Table 15-2** ▸).

Nerve Agents

Nerve agents are a class of chemicals called organophosphates and are among the most deadly to which the body can be exposed. Organophosphates are found in agricultural pesticides, bug spray, and in some industrial chemicals. Organophosphate chemicals can enter the body through the air or on contact with the skin. Examples of organophosphates are listed in **Table 15-3** ▴.

All HAZMAT scenes are a scene safety hazard to the EMS personnel before they are properly evaluated by the individuals who have the appropriate training to assess and manage a HAZMAT incident. Do not proceed into a HAZMAT scene until you have the appropriate PPE and training. The NFPA 704, *Standard System for the Identification of the Hazards of Materials for Emergency Response* placard system outlines five toxicity levels.

Toxicity Levels

Toxicity Level	Health Hazard	Required Protection
0	Little or no hazard	None
1	Slightly hazardous	SCBA (level C suit) only
2	Slightly hazardous	SCBA (level C suit) only
3	Extremely hazardous	Full protection, with no exposed skin (level A or B suit)
4	Minimal exposure causes death	Special hazardous materials gear (level A suit)

Table 15-2 The Categories of Terrorist Incidents

B	Biological
N	Nuclear
I	Incendiary
C	Chemical
E	Explosives

Table 15-3 Examples of Organophosphate Pesticides

• Disulfoton	• Runnel
• Phorate	• Coumaphos
• Dimethoate	• Diazinon
• Ciodrin	• Trichlorfon
• Dichlorvos	• Paraoxon
• Ioxathion	• Potasan
• Ruelene	• Dimefox
• Carbophenothion	• Mipafox
• Supona	• Schradan
• TEPP, EPN, HETP	• Sevin
• Parathion	• Chlorpyrifos
• Malathion	• Dimeton

Table 15-4 Nerve Agents

Name	Code Name	Odor	Special Features	Onset of Symptoms	Volatility	Route of Exposure
Tabun	GA	Fruity	Easy to manufacture	Immediate	Low	Both contact and vapor hazard
Sarin	GB	None (if pure) or strong	Will off-gas while on victim's clothing	Immediate	High	Primarily respiratory vapor hazard; extremely lethal if skin contact is made
Soman	GD	Fruity	Ages rapidly, making it difficult to treat	Immediate	Moderate	Contact with skin; minimal vapor hazard
V agent	VX	None	Most lethal chemical agent; difficult to decontaminate	Immediate	Very low	Contact with skin; no vapor hazard (unless aerosolized)

When the strength of the organophosphate is increased to an amount beyond what is needed for its intended uses, the chemical becomes a nerve agent and is capable of harming humans and animals (**Table 15-4**▲).

Nerve agents can exist as liquids, sprays, or vapors and block the essential nervous system enzyme, **cholinesterase**. This causes the body's organs to become overstimulated and eventually burn out. Nerve agents can cause cardiac arrest within seconds or minutes following exposure.

Nerve transmission occurs when **acetylcholine (ACh)** is released by the nerve ending and stimulates the muscle or gland that the nerve controls. The nerve impulse is stopped as acetylcholine is deactivated by **acetylcholinesterase (AChE)**. Nerve agents like organophosphates interfere with normal nerve transmission by blocking the activity of AChE, preventing the breakdown of ACh in the synapse, and resulting in continued stimulation of the nerves, glands, and muscles by ACh that accumulates throughout the central and autonomic nervous systems. Signs and symptoms of cholinergic poisoning manifest with neuromuscular, autonomic nervous system (ANS), and central nervous system (CNS) effects (**Table 15-5**▶).

To help the paramedic remember the symptoms of exposure to nerve agents, there are two commonly used mnemonics (**Table 15-6**▶).

Before approaching a patient who you suspect has been exposed to a nerve agent, ask yourself if you have on the appropriate PPE. You do not want to become a patient yourself.

Table 15-5 Signs and Symptoms of Cholinergic Poisoning

Autonomic Nervous System Effects
• Abdominal pain • Drooling • Diarrhea • Dilated pupils • Nausea and vomiting • Reduced vision • Sweating
Central Nervous System Effects
• Coma • Confusion • Headache • Respiratory depression and arrest • Seizures • Slurred speech
Neuromuscular Effects
• Muscle twitching • Paralysis • Respiratory failure • Weakness

Antidotes for Nerve Agents

In addition to treating the patient with airway and ventilatory support, atropine sulfate and pralidoxime chloride [2-PAM] are two drugs that are used effectively as antidotes for nerve agent poisoning. Atropine sulfate works by blocking one type of acetylcholine (ACh) receptor so that the acetylcholine that is already in the synapse cannot work. It blocks the effects of glands (ie, watering eyes, drooling, diarrhea, bronchorrhea, seizures). Pralidoxime chloride works by blocking the binding of the nerve agent to the acetylcholinesterase. It acts to sever the bond between the enzyme acetylcholinesterase and the nerve agent that prevents synapse functioning. Both of these drugs were issued to U.S. troops during the Persian Gulf War in the form of an antidote kit called the Mark I, or the Nerve Agent Antidote Kit (NAAK). The Mark I kit

Table 15-6 Symptoms of Nerve Agent Exposure

Military Mnemonic: SLUDGEM
S—salivation
L—lacrimation
U—urination
D—defecation
G—GI distress
E—emesis
M—miosis
Or the Medical Mnemonic: DUMBELS
D—defecation
U—urination
M—miosis
B—bradycardia, bronchorrhea
E—emesis
L—lacrimation
S—salivation

usually contains the following: an atropine sulfate [Atropine] auto-injector (2-mg total dose per injection) and a pralidoxime chloride [2-PAM, 2-PAM CL] auto-injector (600-mg total dose per injection). Diazepam [Valium] may be used to treat seizures brought on by nerve agent exposure. Bronchodilators (albuterol and ipratropium [Atrovent]) may also be used for bronchorrhea-associated bronchospasm.

The identity of a substance, level of PPE to use, and treatment options can be made on scene or en route using resources such as the *Emergency Response Guidebook*, consulting with CHEMTREC (CHEMical TRansportation Emergency Center), contacting medical control, obtaining material safety data sheets (MSDS), or using dispatch.

Case Study II Organophosphate Exposure

Part 1

You are responding with the fire department and HAZMAT team to a farm near a small airport on the outskirts of town for multiple unresponsive adults with a possible exposure to pesticides. The police have arrived first and your unit is ahead of the fire department and HAZMAT truck. There is another ambulance en route since there are multiple patients involved. You cautiously make your way into the property. A couple of men are talking with the police and wave you down; you stop to get the information. They first tell you that there is a locked storage area near the last barn that contains chemicals including fertilizers and pesticides, and it appears that it was broken into. They go on to say that there are rumors that a clandestine methamphetamine lab is operating in the area and that their boss has been watching for a possible break-in to the storage area by the individuals that are running the lab. While making a check on the locked storage area, the boss found two men who are unconscious and possibly overcome by an insecticide product.

You pass this information on to dispatch and request two more ambulances, one for the second patient and one for a stand-by for the rescuers, and then you prepare to talk to the fire department and HAZMAT crew that are arriving now. You recall that pesticides are typically organophosphate-based, and have properties similar to those found in nerve agents. These attack neuro-neuro and neuro-muscular junctions (synapses) that use acetylcholine as their neurotransmitter. Thus both the central and peripheral nervous systems are affected. The HAZMAT entry teams are getting right to work. It takes time to set up a decontamination area, but the teams are experienced and the process is moving along. The second ambulance has arrived so you update them on what you know. They will be assessing and managing the second patient. The first rescue team has reached the patients and confirms that there are two unresponsive males that appear to be in their early twenties. They are breathing and will be moved into the decontamination area. The team also confirms that the organophosphate methyl parathion is the product the patients were exposed to. Methyl parathion is a liquid chemical and inhalation is likely the route of exposure.

Before you can assess and begin treatment on the patients they will need immediate and complete washing of the skin and eyes with water and a soapy solution. That will be part of the role of those doing the decontamination. Once this is completed, you will complete your initial assessment (see **Table 1**). A diluted (0.5%) bleach solution could be considered after the soap and water. If the patients were unconscious, this step may be skipped.

Case Study II Continued

Table 1 Initial Assessment

Initial Assessment	Recording Time: 10 Minutes
General Impression/ Appearance	Unresponsive at the site of a chemical storage area. An organophosphate exposure has been confirmed.
Mental Status	Unresponsive
Airway	Unknown
Breathing	Breathing, unknown how effective
Circulation	Unknown how effective
Priority/Plan	High priority with decontamination first using the most appropriate solution per the resources

At this point we do not know if trauma is a factor. The priority plan is high due to the unresponsiveness of the patients and the chemical exposure.

Question 1: How do nerve agents affect humans?

Question 2: What measures must be taken to remove the chemical from the patients?

Part 2

The first patient is coming out on a backboard in the treatment sector. He has a nonrebreathing mask on his face, is unresponsive, has secretions in his airway, his breathing is slow and shallow, he has a distal pulse that is slow and regular, skin is cool, wet, and pale, and his pupils are each 8 mm in diameter. The second ambulance crew on the scene quickly suctions his airway, obtains vital signs, and starts an IV. A focused history and physical examination reveal facial abrasions, small lacerations on the right hand, and lungs sounds are diminished with shallow respirations so ventilations are assisted with a bag-mask device and high concentration oxygen (see **Table 2**). The EMS supervisor has arrived on scene with Mark I kits and extra atropine. On her way to the scene she learned from dispatch that the police are investigating methamphetamine labs in the area. Apparently drug dealers have been stealing anhydrous ammonia from farms to be used in cooking up methamphetamine. The two patients are likely to be drug dealers and/or manufacturers of methamphetamine that were looking for anhydrous ammonia but got into parathion by accident.

Table 2 Focused History and Physical Examination

Baseline Vital Signs	Recording Time: 30 Minutes
Skin CTC (color, temperature, condition)	Pale, cool, and diaphoretic (wet)
Pulse	68 beats/min and regular
Blood Pressure	110/50 mm Hg
Respirations	12 breaths/min and shallow, diminished lung sounds

Question 3: What resources can you use at the scene of a HAZMAT incident to help you decide the appropriate treatment options?

Question 4: What was the most likely route of exposure of the organophosphate?

Part 3

Just as the first patient was intubated and placed on a transport ventilator, the second patient arrives on a backboard. He is also unresponsive and breathing slow and shallow. Your partner begins the initial assessment while you begin the SAMPLE history of the first patient (see **Table 3**). The second HAZMAT team is containing the chemical spill; the first team has exited the hot zone without any problems. One EMT stays available for the HAZMAT team while the paramedic assists you with your patient.

Treatment Plan

1. Remove the patient(s) from the source.
2. Make sure that the patient has been decontaminated. This involves removing clothing, and using soap and water to completely wash the poison off. Be sure to irrigate the eyes if the exposure potentially warrants it.
3. Support and maintain the ABCs; ensure adequate oxygenation prior to instituting atropine sulfate therapy (see **Table 4**).
4. Start an IV.

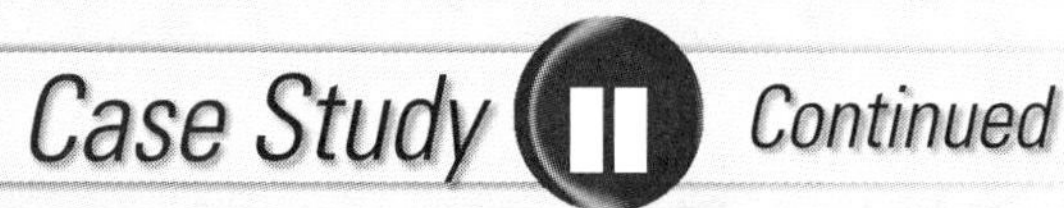

Table 3 SAMPLE History

SAMPLE History	Comments
Signs/symptoms	Unresponsive, with clinical evidence of cholinergic poisoning likely the result of an organophosphate exposure
Allergies	Unknown
Medications	Unknown
Pertinent past medical history	Unknown
Last oral intake	Unknown
Events leading up to the incident	Unknown length of exposure

5. Administer atropine sulfate 2 to 4 mg for secretions (see **Table 5**).
6. Administer pralidoxime chloride 1 g for muscle weakness.
7. Administer diazepam [Valium] for seizures.
8. Repeat if necessary in 5–10 minutes.
9. Administer albuterol or another available bronchodilator for severe bronchospasm.

Table 4 Atropine-Pralidoxime

Do you know?	Comments
Right drug? Generic name: [**Atropine–Pralidoxime**] (2-PAM CL) Trade name: [Mark I Kit]	This kit contains two drugs, atropine sulfate and pralidoxime chloride (2-PAM CL). When a patient has been exposed to an organophosphate pesticide or nerve agent, the chemical causes ACh overstimulation at the synapse and associated signs and symptoms of cholinergic poisoning. Think: SLUDGE+ Respiration-CNS.
Right patient?	Patient exposed to an organophosphate or nerve agent with signs and symptoms of SLUDGE+ Respiration-CNS (remember SLUDGE stands for salivation, lacrimation, urination, defecation, gastrointestinal cramping, and emesis [vomiting]).
Right dose?	2 g atropine, 600 mg pralidoxime chloride. Repeat dosing will vary depending on the severity and persistence of symptoms.
Right route?	Auto-injectors, IV.
Right time?	As soon as possible after assessment and recognition of exposure to organophosphate or nerve agent in the context of evidence of cholinergic toxicity.
Right documentation?	Always document how and when the drug was administered and the patient's response to the medication on your patient care report.
Expected action	Atropine competitively inhibits the uptake of excess ACh in the synapse, effectively blocking cholinergic overstimulation of the synapse. This results in relaxation of smooth muscle in the lungs and GI tract, and dries respiratory secretions. 2-PAM-CL works to bind the organophosphate molecule and allows AChE to regenerate, effectively enhancing the action of atropine.
Side effects	Atropine: tachycardia, dizziness, dilated pupils, blurred vision, dry mouth, urinary retention; pralidoxime chloride: tachycardia, dizziness, blurred vision, speech problems, muscle weakness or stiffness.
Contraindications	No contraindications when exposure produces moderate to severe symptoms.
Precautions	Do not use prophylactically.
Pharmacokinetics	Onset rapid; metabolism rapid; potentiates the effects of atropine.

Case Study II Continued

Table 5 Atropine Sulfate

Do you know?	Comments
Right drug? Generic name: [**Atropine Sulfate**] Trade name: [Atropine]	This drug is an anticholinergic agent. It is used to restore cardiac rate and arterial pressure. It is also used as an antidote for toxicity due to organophosphate or nerve agents, cholinergic drugs, pilocarpine, physostigmine, or isoflurophate.
Right patient?	Known or suspected organophosphate poisoning with signs and symptoms.
Right dose?	2 mg every 5–10 minutes until secretions dry. Remarkably high doses may be required in significant cases of organophosphate toxicity.
Right route?	IV/IM/IO.
Right time?	As soon as possible after organophosphate exposure has been recognized and the patient is experiencing signs and symptoms.
Right documentation?	Dose, route, time administered, and reassessment should be clearly documented on the patient care report.
Expected action	Parasympatholytic reaction that inhibits the action of acetylcholine at the postganglionic parasympathetic neuroeffector sites.
Side effects	Headache, dizziness, palpitations, nausea and vomiting, tachycardia, arrhythmias, anticholinergic effects (blurred vision, dry mouth, urinary retention), paradoxical bradycardia when pushed slowly or at low doses, flushed, hot, dry skin.
Contraindications	Tachycardia, hypertension, unstable cardiovascular status in acute hemorrhage and myocardial ischemia, narrow-angle glaucoma.
Precautions	Potential adverse effects when administered with digoxin, cholinergics, physostigmine. Effects enhanced by antihistamines, procainamide, quinidine, antipsychotics, benzodiazepines, and antidepressants.
Pharmacokinetics	Onset: immediate; peak effect: 1–2 minutes; duration: 2–6 hours; metabolized by the liver, excreted through urine unchanged. About 30% to 50% is excreted unchanged in urine and the rest as metabolites; half-life 4 hours.

Question 5: How does atropine sulfate work to reverse the effects of organophosphate poisoning?

Question 6: How does 2-PAM work to reverse the effects of organophosphate poisoning?

Part 4

At this point the first patient is still unresponsive and is being ventilated with high concentration oxygen (see **Table 6**). He seems to be maintaining his low blood pressure and is still bradycardic. As you prepare to transport him to the ED, you recall reading that the inhalation route of exposure is the quickest to develop symptoms, followed by ingestion and then absorption through the skin.

The second patient is more critical than the first. He has signs of pulmonary edema in addition to unstable vital signs. You recall from reviewing the resource materials that the muscarinic effects of acetylcholine cause bronchoconstriction and a marked increase in bronchial secretions. Increased length or dose of exposure is the likely cause of the bronchorrhea, manifesting as pulmonary edema. He will need

Table 6 Reassessment and Ongoing Assessment of the Patient

Serial Vital Signs and Relevant Data	Recording Time: 25 Minutes
Skin CTC	Pale, cool, diaphoretic (wet)
Pulse	50 beats/min and regular
Blood Pressure	102/48 mm Hg
Respirations	10 breaths/min and shallow
Mental Status	Unresponsive
ECG	Sinus bradycardia
SpO_2	90%
Lung Sounds	Rales
Other (ie, blood glucose, core body temperature)	Pupils are both 8 mm, not reactive

Case Study II Continued

to be intubated as soon as possible. IV access looks to be challenging in this patient so an IO is established and the first doses of atropine and 2-PAM are administered. En route to the hospital, medical control is established and additional orders are received. Nebulized albuterol and ipratropium bromide [Atrovent] will be administered through the ET tube; he will receive 2 mg of atropine every 5 minutes until the secretions clear and one additional dose of 2-PAM while en route. Seizures are a possibility so an order for diazepam [Valium] as needed is received.

Question 7: Why did the second patient develop pulmonary edema?

Question 8: What route of exposure is associated with the quickest onset of symptoms?

Part 5

Chronic exposure to organophosphate pesticides produces symptoms over time due to the cumulative effect causing progressive inhibition of cholinesterase. Acute signs can develop within 1–12 hours following inhalation or cutaneous absorption and more rapidly following ingestion. The excess acetylcholine at nerve endings, which mimics hyperactivity of the parasympathetic nervous system, produces signs and symptoms relative to the GI tract including excess salivation, lacrimation, abdominal pain, vomiting, intestinal hypermotility, and diarrhea. The nicotinic effects of acetylcholine consist of involuntary irregular, violent muscle contractions and weakness of the skeletal muscles. The muscarinic effects of acetylcholine cause bronchoconstriction and a marked increase in bronchial secretions. Death occurs as a result of respiratory failure.

Treatment begins with removing the patient from the source of exposure and decontamination. Two drugs that are effective as antidotes for nerve agent poisoning are atropine and pralidoxime chloride. Atropine works by blocking one type of acetylcholine receptor so that the acetylcholine that is already in the synapse cannot work. Pralidoxime works by blocking the binding of the nerve agent to the acetylcholinesterase, allowing the AChE to regenerate. Diazepam [Valium] may be used to treat seizures brought on by exposure to nerve agents, and bronchodilators (albuterol and ipratropium [Atrovent] may be used to manage any associated bronchospasm.

Methyl Parathion

Methyl parathion is a manufactured nerve agent made in the United States. Since 1952 it has been used to kill insects on many types of crops. It is considered an organophosphate. The technical-grade solution of parathion is a brownish liquid, which contains methyl parathion (80%) and inactive ingredients in a solvent. The technical-grade methyl parathion smells like rotten eggs or garlic. Because methyl parathion can be dangerous to humans, the EPA has restricted how it can be used and applied. Methyl parathion must be sprayed on crops from the air or from the ground in certain ways to minimize the danger of exposure, and only trained people are allowed to spray methyl parathion.

Anhydrous Ammonia

The agricultural community has used anhydrous ammonia as a low cost, highly effective nitrogen-based fertilizer for many years. However, drug dealers have discovered that it can also be used to manufacture the illegal drug, methamphetamine, and have targeted farm tanks as a source for this material. This organophosphate chemical can be extremely dangerous when it is not properly handled.

Case Study ANSWERS

Case Study 1 Crush Syndrome

Question 1: Is there any significance to the statement by the neighbor that Joey sleeps over when he has had too many drinks to drive?

Answer 1: If he had enough drinks, he may still be a little intoxicated which might dilate his blood vessels.

Question 2: Once you have access to the patient, what will the priority be?

Answer 2: The first priority should be to obtain a set of baseline vital signs.

Question 3: If the patient states he is taking a blood thinner, how would that be relevant?

Answer 3: It would lead you to predict that the patient has already had a significant amount of blood loss and there will be more when the slab is lifted from the patient.

Question 4: If the patient states he is a diabetic, how would that affect your management?

Answer 4: Diabetics do not always feel pain in the periphery and he may have an irregular blood glucose level. Actually, with all the excitement and trauma, the patient's glucose level is likely to be high, but it is a good idea to check his glucose as a part of the prehospital management.

Question 5: If it is helpful to get the patient moving fluids, why not give him furosemide [Lasix]?

Answer 5: Furosemide [Lasix] is a loop diuretic that tends to increase the acidity of the blood. In this instance, it would not be appropriate to increase the acidity (lowering the pH); rather, it is important to consider managing the pH in an effort to alkalinize the urine and protect the kidneys, as well as help prepare for potential hyperkalemia after the crushing force is released.

Question 6: What is meant by "smiling death?"

Answer 6: "Smiling death" is a reference to sudden death associated with release of protracted crushing forces. The patient seems to be "stable" up to the point when the weight is lifted when suddenly all accumulated toxic products from compressed and badly traumatized soft-tissue compartments are able to rapidly infuse into the systemic circulation. This phenomenon will often result in sudden cardiac arrest.

Question 7: If it was clear that the patient's condition was deteriorating, what option would you have?

Answer 7: With the advisement of medical control, a trauma surgeon could be brought to the scene to perform an emergency field amputation of one or both of Joey's legs (if this was going to be a situation where the extrication will simply take too long for him to survive the rescue effort).

Question 8: Should a tourniquet be applied to both legs?

Answer 8: If you have enough access to the top of each leg, it may be wise to tie a loose tourniquet on each leg and as the patient is removed make a quick decision, based on the blood loss (trickle versus steady flow), on the need for the tourniquet to control the blood loss from the crushed extremities.

Case Study ANSWERS

Case Study II Organophosphate Exposure

Question 1: How do nerve agents affect humans?

Answer 1: All nerve agents are cholinesterase inhibitors. They block ACh breakdown which results in increased levels of ACh and subsequent overstimulation of the nerves and glands.

Question 2: What measures must be taken to remove the chemical from the patients?

Answer 2: The patient must be removed from the source, clothing removed, and then the patient must be totally washed with soap and water. The eyes must be irrigated as well. A light concentration of bleach may also be used after the soap and water if the patient is stable.

Question 3: What resources can you use at the scene of a HAZMAT incident to help you decide the appropriate treatment options?

Answer 3: Possible treatment options can be obtained using resources such as the *Emergency Response Guidebook*, consulting with CHEMTREC, obtaining MSDSs, on-line medical control, or using dispatch.

Question 4: What was the most likely route of exposure of the organophosphate?

Answer 4: Parathion is stored in a liquid form and inhalation is most likely. The container may have been broken during the attempted theft, leaking fumes and overwhelming the victims.

Question 5: How does atropine sulfate work to reverse the effects of organophosphate poisoning?

Answer 5: Atropine sulfate works by outcompeting ACh at the receptor within the synapse, so that the acetylcholine that is already in the synapse cannot work. It works rapidly to reverse glandular secretions (watering eyes, drooling, diarrhea, bronchospasm) and neuromuscular and CNS effects (seizures, tremors).

Question 6: How does 2-PAM work to reverse the effects of organophosphate poisoning?

Answer 6: Pralidoxime (2-PAM) works by blocking the binding of the nerve agent to the acetylcholinesterase. It acts like a breaker bar to sever the bond between the enzyme acetylcholinesterase, allowing the AChE to regenerate and restore normal synapse functioning. This process occurs over a considerably longer time frame than that of atropine.

Question 7: Why did the second patient develop pulmonary edema?

Answer 7: The muscarinic effects of acetylcholine cause bronchoconstriction and a marked increase in bronchial secretions. Increased length or dose of exposure is the likely cause of the bronchorrhea, manifesting as pulmonary edema.

Question 8: What route of exposure is associated with the quickest onset of symptoms?

Answer 8: The inhalation route is associated with the quickest onset of symptoms, followed by GI absorption and then skin exposure.

Medication Review

Amyl Nitrite, Sodium Nitrite, Sodium Thiosulfate (Cyanide Antidote Kit)

Indications Cyanide or hydrocyanic acid poisoning.

Contraindications Not applicable.

Dosage and administration Adult: Amyl nitrite: breathe 30 seconds out of every minute. Sodium thiosulfate and sodium nitrite: IV per antidote kit directions. Pediatric: Same as adult.

Atropine Sulfate

Indications Hemodynamically unstable bradycardia, asystole, bradycardic (< 60 beats/min) pulseless electrical activity (PEA), organophosphate poisoning, bronchospastic pulmonary disorders.

Contraindications Tachycardia, hypersensitivity, unstable cardiovascular status in acute hemorrhage and myocardial ischemia, narrow-angle glaucoma.

Dosage and administration Adult: Asystole or bradycardic PEA: 1 mg IV/IO push. May repeat every 3–5 minutes (if asystole or PEA persists) to a maximum of 0.04 mg/kg. Endotracheal administration: 2–3 mg diluted in 10 mL of water or normal saline. Unstable bradycardia: 0.5 mg IV/IO every 3–5 minutes as needed, not to exceed total dose of 0.04 mg/kg. Use shorter dosing interval (3 minutes) and higher doses in severe clinical conditions. Organophosphate poisoning: Extremely large doses (2–4 mg or higher) may be needed. Pediatric: 0.02 mg/kg via IV/IO push; may double this dose for second IV/IO dose. Minimum single dose: 0.1 mg. Maximum doses: child single dose: 0.5 mg, child total dose: 1 mg, adolescent single dose: 1 mg, adolescent total dose: 2 mg. Endotracheal administration: 0.03 mg/kg (absorption may be unreliable).

Calcium Chloride

Indications Hypocalcemia, hyperkalemia, magnesium sulfate overdose, calcium channel blocker overdose, adjunctive therapy in treatment of insect bites and stings.

Contraindications Hypercalcemia, V-fib, digitalis toxicity.

Dosage and administration Adult: 500 mg to 1,000 mg (5–10 mL of a 10% solution) IV/IO push for hyperkalemia and calcium channel blocker overdose. May be repeated as needed. Pediatric: 20 mg/kg (0.2 mL/kg) slow IV/IO push. Maximum 1 g dose; may repeat in 10 minutes.

Diazepam (Valium)

Indications Acute anxiety states, acute alcohol withdrawal (delirium tremens), muscle relaxant, seizure activity, agitation. Analgesia for medical procedures (fracture reduction, cardioversion).

Contraindications Hypersensitivity, glaucoma, coma, shock, substance abuse, head injury.

Dosage and administration Seizure activity: Adult: 5–10 mg IV every 10–15 minutes as needed (5 mg over 5 min) (maximum dose, 30 mg). Seizure activity: Pediatric: 0.2–0.5 mg slowly every 2–5 minutes up to 5 mg (maximum dose, 10 mg/kg). Rectal diazepam: 0.5 mg/kg via rectal catheter and flush with 2–3 mL air after administration. Sedation for cardioversion: 5–15 mg IV over 5–10 minutes prior to cardioversion.

Fentanyl Citrate (Sublimase)

Indications This drug is used to treat severe pain and is used with anesthesia.

Contraindications Myasthenia gravis, children under 2 years old. May cause life-threatening hypoventilation so naloxone hydrochloride [Narcan] should be readily available.

Dosage and administration Adult dose is 25–100 µg (0.5–1 µg/kg) IM, IO, IVP or atomized intranasal. Pediatric 2–12 years old: 1.7–3.3 µg/kg IM, IO, IVP.

Meperidine Hydrochloride (Demerol)

Indications Analgesia for moderate to severe pain.

Contraindications Hypersensitivity to narcotic agents, diarrhea caused by poisoning, patients taking MAOIs, during labor or delivery of a premature infant, undiagnosed abdominal pain or head injury.

Dosage and administration Adult: 50–100 mg IM, SC or 25–50 mg slowly IV. Pediatric: 1–2 mg/kg/dose IV, IO, IM, SC.

Medication Review

Midazolam (Versed)

Indications Sedation, anxiolytic prior to endotracheal or nasotracheal intubation; administer for conscious sedation.

Contraindications Glaucoma, shock, coma, alcohol intoxication, overdose, depressed vital signs, concomitant use with other CNS depressants, barbiturates, alcohol, narcotics.

Dosage and administration Adult: 2.0–2.5 mg slow IV over 2–3 minutes; may be repeated to total maximum: 0.1 mg/kg. Pediatric: Not recommended.

Morphine Sulfate (Astramorph/PF and others)

Indications Severe CHF, pulmonary edema, chest pain associated with acute MI, analgesia for moderate to severe acute and chronic pain (use with caution).

Contraindications Head injury, exacerbated COPD, depressed respiratory drive, hypotension, undiagnosed abdominal pain, decreased level of consciousness, suspected hypovolemia, patients who have taken MAOIs within the past 14 days.

Dosage and administration Adult: Initial dose: 2–4 mg IV (over 1–5 minutes) every 5–30 minutes. Repeat dose: 2–8 mg at 5- to 15-minute intervals. Pediatric: 0.1–0.2 mg/kg per dose via IV, IO, IM, or SC; maximum dose of 5 mg.

Naloxone Hydrochloride (Narcan)

Indications Opiate overdose, coma; complete or partial reversal of CNS and respiratory depression induced by opioids; decreased level of consciousness; coma of unknown origin; narcotic agonist for the following: morphine, heroin, hydromorphone (Dilaudid), methadone, meperidine (Demerol), paregoric, fentanyl citrate (Sublimase), oxycodone (Percodan), codeine, propoxyphene (Darvon); narcotic agonist and antagonist for the following: Butorphanol (Stadol), pentazocine (Talwin), nalbuphine (Nubain).

Contraindications Use with caution in narcotic-dependent patients; use with caution in neonates of narcotic-addicted mothers.

Dosage and administration Adult: 0.4–2.0 mg IV, IM, SC, or ET (diluted); minimum recommended dose, 0.4 mg/kg; repeat at 5-minute intervals to a maximum dose of 10 mg (medical control may request higher amounts). Infusion: 2 mg in 500 mL of D_5W (4 µg/mL), infuse at 0.4 mg/h (100 mL/h). Pediatric: 0.1 mg/kg/dose IV, IM, SC, ET (diluted); maximum dose of 0.8 mg; if no response in 10 minutes, administer an additional 0.1 mg/kg/dose.

Nitrous Oxide: Oxygen (50:50) (Nitronox)

Indications Moderate to severe pain, anxiety, apprehension.

Contraindications Impaired level of consciousness, head injury, inability to comply with instructions; decompression sickness (nitrogen narcosis, air embolism, air transport); undiagnosed abdominal pain or marked distention, bowel obstruction; hypotension, shock, COPD (with history/suspicion of carbon dioxide retention); cyanosis; chest trauma with pneumothorax.

Dosage and administration Adult: (Note: Invert cylinder several times before use) Instruct the patient to inhale deeply through demand valve and mask or mouthpiece. Pediatric: Same as adult.

Ondansetron Hydrochloride (Zofran)

Indications For the prevention or control of nausea or vomiting. Also used in the hospital setting for patients undergoing chemotherapy or surgical procedures.

Contraindications Known allergy to this medicine or other 5-HT3 receptor antagonists.

Dosage and administration Adult: 4 mg IV or IM (may repeat in 10 minutes). Pediatric: 0.1 mg/kg IV or IM.

Medication Review

Oxygen

Indications Confirmed or expected hypoxemia, ischemic chest pain, respiratory insufficiency, prophylactically during air transport, confirmed or suspected carbon monoxide poisoning, all other causes of decreased tissue oxygenation, decreased level of consciousness.

Contraindications Certain patients with COPD or emphysema who will not tolerate oxygen concentrations over 35%, hyperventilation. Oxygen should never be withheld from a patient who needs it, however. Be prepared to assist with ventilations in a patient with COPD who requires high concentration, as apnea may result.

Dosage and administration Adult: Cardiac arrest and carbon monoxide poisoning: 100%. Hypoxemia: 10–15 L/min via nonrebreathing mask. COPD: 1–6 L/min via nasal cannula or 28%–35% Venturi mask. Be prepared to provide ventilatory support if higher concentrations of oxygen needed. Pediatric: Same as for adult with exception of premature infant.

Pralidoxime Chloride (2-PAM Chloride, Protopam)

Indications As an antidote in the treatment of poisoning by organophosphate pesticides and chemicals. In the prehospital arena, is used when atropine is or has become ineffective in management of organophosphate poisoning.

Contraindications Use with caution in patients with reduced renal function; patients with myasthenia gravis and organophosphate poisoning.

Dosage and administration Note: If Protopam is to be used, it should be administered almost simultaneously with atropine. Adult: Initial dose of 1–2 g as an IV infusion with 100 mL saline over 15–30 minutes. Pediatric: 20–40 mg/kg as IV infusion over 15–30 minutes. Doses may be repeated every 1 hour if muscle weakness persists. If IV administration is not feasible, IM or SC injection may be utilized.

Promethazine Hydrochloride (Phenergan)

Indications Nausea, vomiting, motion sickness; sedation for patients in labor; potentiation of analgesic effects of narcotics.

Contraindications Hypersensitivity, coma, CNS-depressed patients from alcohol, barbiturates, narcotics, Reye's syndrome.

Dosage and administration Adult: 12.5–25 mg IV, deep IM, PO, rectally. Pediatric: (greater than 2 years old) 0.25–0.5 mg/kg dose IM.

Sodium Bicarbonate

Indications Mild or moderate metabolic acidosis due to shock, severe dehydration, anoxia, uncontrolled diabetes, renal disease, cardiac arrest, and severe primary lactic acidosis. To treat overdose of aspirin and cyclic-antidepressants.

Contraindications Metabolic and respiratory alkalosis, hypertension, convulsions, CHF, and other situations where sodium can be dangerous.

Dosage and administration 1 mEq per kg IV bolus (may repeat every 10 minutes at ½ initial dose).

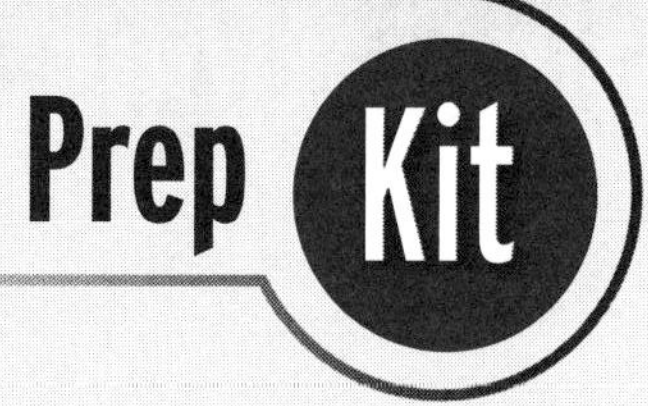

Chapter Summary

- Pain medication or analgesia such as fentanyl citrate (Sublimase) and morphine sulfate (Astramorph/PF) may be indicated for a patient who has experienced crush syndrome.
- When considering pharmacology for analgesia, it is important to constantly monitor the vital signs because some analgesics are contraindicated in hypotension.
- In a crushing situation, most regions have a protocol or would contact medical control for consideration of sodium bicarbonate. This would help to neutralize the acids and flush out the toxins as well as manage the impending shock.
- Nerve agents are a class of chemicals called organophosphates. Organophosphates are found in agricultural pesticides, bug spray, and in some industrial chemicals.
- Nerve agents can exist as liquids, sprays, or vapors and block the essential nervous system enzyme, cholinesterase.
- To help the paramedic remember the symptoms of exposure to nerve agents, there are two commonly used mnemonics: SLUDGEM and DUMBELS.
- In addition to treating the patient with airway and ventilatory support, atropine sulfate and pralidoxime chloride (2-PAM) are two drugs that are used effectively as antidotes for nerve agent poisoning.
- Atropine sulfate works by blocking one type of acetylcholine (ACh) receptor so that the acetylcholine that is already in the synapse cannot work. It blocks the effects of glands (ie, watering eyes, drooling, diarrhea, bronchorrhea, seizures).
- Pralidoxime chloride works by blocking the binding of the nerve agent to the acetylcholinesterase. It acts to sever the bond between the enzyme acetylcholinesterase and the nerve agent that prevents synapse functioning.
- Diazepam [Valium] may be used to treat seizures brought on by nerve agent exposure.

Vital Vocabulary

Acetylcholine (ACh) A neurotransmitter secreted by the autonomic nervous system.

Acetylcholinesterase (AChE) An enzyme that rapidly destroys acetylcholine once it has reached the target tissue.

Acid A substance that increases the concentration of hydrogen ions in a water solution.

Base A substance that decreases the concentration of hydrogen ions.

Cholinesterase An enzyme that causes the body's organs to be overstimulated.

Crush syndrome Occurs when an area of the body is trapped for longer than 4 hours and the arterial blood flow is compromised. It can lead to life-threatening arrhythmias, acidosis, and electrolyte imbalance.

Nerve agents Chemicals that are designed to affect the normal chemical neurotransmission in the body's autonomic nervous system.

Organophosphates Nerve agents or chemicals that are found in agricultural pesticides, insecticides, and other industrial chemicals.

Rhabdomyolysis Destruction of muscle and the subsequent release of breakdown products and toxins into the systemic circulation from a crushing injury.

The Metric System and Drug Calculations

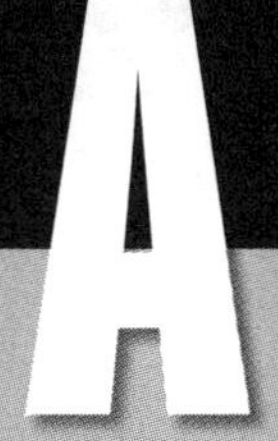

Objectives

Cognitive

1-8.2 Review mathematical principles. (pages 463–465)

1-8.3 Review mathematical equivalents. (pages 464–465)

1-8.4 Differentiate temperature readings between the Centigrade and Fahrenheit scales. (page 464)

1-8.5 Discuss formulas as a basis for performing drug calculations. (page 465)

1-8.6 Discuss applying basic principles of mathematics to the calculation of problems associated with medication dosages. (page 465)

1-8.7 Describe how to perform mathematical conversions from the household system to the metric system. (page 465)

Affective

None

Psychomotor

None

Introduction

Pharmacology is a medical science and the measurement system used in science is the metric system. Since the metric system may not be the system you have traditionally used it may be necessary to review the common medical abbreviations as they relate to pharmacology (**Table A-1**▼), review common metric conversions, and practice conversions to the metric system so that you can be prepared to calculate drug doses. All of the drug doses you will be given by medical control will use the metric system.

The metric system is an international decimal system of weights and measures representing the basic unit of weight (**Table A-2**▶), volume (**Table A-3**▶), length (**Table A-4**▶), and temperature (**Table A-5**▶). The metric system is based on multiples of 10, and all measurements are expressed in decimals (**Figure A-1**▶).

Table A-1 Common Medical Abbreviations Related to Pharmacology

$\bar{a}$	before	nitro	nitroglycerin
α	alpha	NKA	no known allergies
amp.	ampule	NKDA	non known diagnosed allergies
APAP	acetaminophen	NTG	nitroglycerin
ASA	aspirin	o	null or none
β	beta	$\bar{p}$	after
bid	Bis in die (twice a day)	pc	post cibos (after eating)
c–	with	pedi	pediatric
caps	capsules	po	per os (by mouth)
cc	cubic centimeter	pr	per rectus (by rectum)
D/C	discontinue	prn	per re nata (when necessary)
dig	digitails	$\bar{q}$	quisque (every)
ET	endotracheal	qh	quisque hora (every hour)
ETOH	ethyl alcohol	qid	quarter in die (four times a day)
g or gr	gram	god	every other day
gtt	gutta (drop)	RL	Ringer's lactate
gtts	guttae (drops)	$\bar{s}$	sine (without)
HHN	hand-held nebulizer	SC	subcutaneous
Hs	hor a somni (at bedtime)	sol	solution
IC	intracardiac	SQ	subcutaneous
IM	intramuscular	stat	statim (now or immediately)
IO	intraosseous	SVN	small volume nebulizer
IV	intravenous	tid	ter in die (three times a day)
IVP	intravenous push	TKO	to keep open
IVPB	intravenous piggyback	u	unit
kg	kilogram	ut dict	ut dictum (as directed)
KO	keep open	®	registered trademark
KVO	keep vein open	/	female
L or l	liter	?	male
lb	pound	>	greater than
LR	lactated Ringer's	<	less than
MAX	maximum	≥	greater than or equal to
MDI	metered dose inhaler	≤	less than or equal to
μ	micro	~	approximately
μgtt	microdrop	=	equal
μg or mcg	microgram	≠	not equal
mEq	milliequivalent	Δ	change(s)
mg	milligram	±	plus or minus
min	minute	°	degree(s)
mL	milliliter	™	trademark

Table A-2 Metric Units of Weight

1 kilogram (kg)	2.2 pounds (lb)
1 kilogram (kg)	1,000 grams (g)
1 hectogram (hg)	100 grams (g)
1 decagram (dkg or dag)	10 grams (g)
1 gram (g)	1,000 milligrams (mg)
1 decigram (dg)	0.1 grams (g)
1 centigram (cg)	0.01 grams (g)
1 milligram (mg)	0.001 grams (g)
1 milligram (mg)	1,000 micrograms (μg or mcg)
1 microgram (μg or mcg)	0.001 milligram (mg)

Table A-3 Metric Units of Volume

1 liter (L)	1,000 milliliters (mL)
1 milliliter (mL)	0.001 liter (L)
1 microliter (μL or mcL)	0.001 milliliter (mL)

Why Are Weight and Volume Conversion Necessary?

In order to prepare the appropriate dose of medication for your patient, you need to know how to convert larger units of weight to smaller units of weight (for example, g to mg) and smaller units of weight to larger units of weight (for example, mg to g). You will also need to know how to convert larger units of volume to smaller units of volume (for example L to mL) and smaller units of volume to larger units of volume (for example, mL to L). These conversions are particularly important because paramedics receive medication orders in metric system volumes and weights. If your patient is to receive 1 mg/kg it becomes necessary to first convert the patient's weight from pounds to kilograms (2.2 lb = 1 kg) and then determine how much medication (in kg) the patient should be receiving (ie, 100-kg patient would receive 100 mg of the medication).

In some situations it will be necessary for you to withdraw the determined dose from a multiple-dose vial. Let's say that the multiple-dose vial has 1 g in it. Following with our example of the 100 mg required to administer to our patient, it will be necessary to know that 1 g = 1,000 mg so we will need to draw out 1/10 of the volume in the multiple-dose vial. Then, of course, you should recheck to be sure that the dose you have collected into the syringe is absolutely correct prior to administering it. Let's say the medication was packaged as 1 g in a 50-mL multiple-dose vial. In this situation, you would be drawing off 1/10 (5.0 mL) which is expected to contain 100 mg of the medication. To confirm, if 1 g = 1,000 mg, then the 50-mL multiple-dose vial (when unopened) contains 1,000 mg. Therefore, 1/10 of 1,000 mg = 100 mg as well as 1/10 of 50 mL = 5.0 mL. Some paramedics believe they can do this math in their head. We strongly recommend that you find the formulas that work for you, practice them, and always do the math

Table A-4 Metric Units of Length

1 centimeter (cm)	0.01 meter (m)
1 millimeter (mm)	0.001 meter (m)
1 centimeter (cm)	10 millimeters (mm)

Table A-5 Temperature Conversion

37 degrees Celsius (°C)	98.6 degrees Fahrenheit (°F)

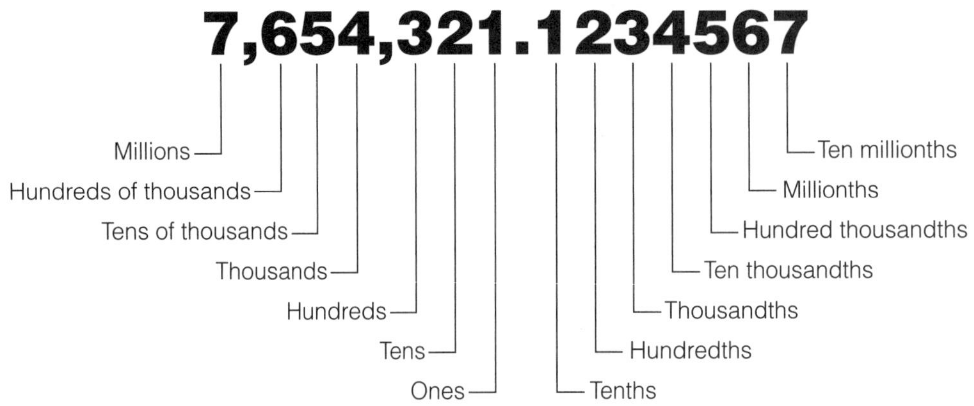

Figure A-1 Decimal Scale

on paper and recheck it prior to administering medication to your patient.

Weight and Volume Conversion

To convert weight or volume, you need to multiply or divide by 1,000 or move the decimal point three places to the right or left.

To convert a larger unit of weight or volume to a smaller unit of weight or volume, multiply the larger unit of weight or volume by 1,000 or move the decimal point three places to the right. For example, to convert grams (g) to milligrams (mg) or liters (L) to milliliters (mL), move the decimal point three places to the right [0.1 g = 100 mg] or [1 L = 1,000 mL].

To convert a smaller unit of weight or volume to a larger unit of weight or volume, divide the smaller unit of weight or volume by 1,000 or move the decimal point three places to the left. For example, to convert milligrams (mg) to grams (g) or milliliters (mL) to liters (L), move the decimal point three places to the left [1 mg = 0.001 g] or [1 mL = 0.001 L].

To review your understanding of weight and volume conversions, complete the following questions and check your answers. The answers can be found at the end of this appendix.

Question 1: Convert 2.5 L to mL.

Question 2: Convert 4,500 mg to g.

Question 3: Convert 800 μg or mcg to g.

Question 4: Convert 2 g to mg.

Question 5: Convert 750 mL to L.

Converting a Patient's Weight from Pounds to Kilograms

When calculating drugs it is important to convert a patient's weight in pounds (lb) to kilograms (kg) since standard medication orders are calculated in the "mg per kg" of patient body weight. The conversion factor is 2.2 pounds equals one kilogram. Divide the number of pounds by 2.2 to get the number of kilograms. For example, a patient who weighs 220 lb would be 100 kg (220 divided by 2.2 = 100).

Calculating Medication Doses

Since the drug dose is generally in "mg" and not in liquid form, yet you actually infuse a fluid or volume, it is necessary to determine the concentration of a medication you have on hand. The concentration on hand is the amount of medication that is present in the ampule or vial. This is usually expressed in milligrams (mg), or grams (g).

The volume of the medication on hand is the amount of fluid that is present in the ampule or vial in which the medication was dissolved.

You will need to use the following formula:

$$\text{concentration on hand} = \frac{(\text{concentration on hand in mg})}{(\text{volume on hand in mL})}$$

For example, if you have 2 g of lidocaine in a 500-mL bag of saline, that means you have a concentration on hand of 4 mg/mL.

Concentration on hand = 2,000 mg/500 mL (the same as 4 mg/mL)

In some situations, the dose you receive may be a range. That means that it is appropriate for a patient of a certain weight to receive between 4 mg to 6 mg of the drug. To be most accurate, you should calculate both the low dose (4 mg) and the high dose (6 mg). If the dose is specifically related to the patient's weight, you may be asked to administer 4 mg/kg to 6 mg/kg. Once again, calculate the dose range. So assuming you have a 220-lb or 100-kg patient, the low dose would be 400 mg and the high dose would be 600 mg of the drug.

Dose and Rate for a Medication Infusion

To calculate a drip or infusion, use the formula below (drops per minute is abbreviated as (gtt/min).

$$(\text{gtt/min}) = \frac{(\text{total fluid to be administered in mL}) \times (\text{drop factor})}{(\text{total time in minutes})}$$

The "drop factor" is a function of the type of IV administration set where the number of drops that equals 1 mL appears on the packaging. The abbreviation for drops is "gtt." This is important to know because the administration sets used to infuse fluids and mix medication drips come in various standards of numbers of gtt/mL. For example, if it is a 15 gtt administration set, that would mean if you count the drops dripping into the administration set's drip chamber, for every 15 you see, another mL of fluid has been administered. Many medication doses that are infused are given in gtt/min. A typical administration set would be 60 gtt/mL and this is also referred to as a "mini drip" or a "micro drip." They also come in 20, 15, and 10 gtt/mL; these are larger drops that take less to add up to a mL. These are usually used for fluid administration, although they can be used sometimes for medication administration, and are referred to as "macro drips."

To review your understanding of calculating medication doses, complete the following questions and check your answers. The answers can be found at the end of this appendix.

Question 6: You receive a drug order to administer activated charcoal [Liquid-Char] to an 18-lb child who ingested a non-corrosive toxic substance. The dose is 1-2 g/kg. How much should the child receive?

Question 7: You receive a drug order to administer adenosine [Adenocard] to a 20-lb child with a symptomatic supraventricular tachycardia (SVT). The dose is 0.1-0.2 mg/kg. How much should the child receive?

Question 8: You receive a drug order to administer morphine sulfate [Astramorph/PF] to a 30-lb child who sustained partial- and full-thickness scalding burns. The child has a stable blood pressure but is in severe pain. The dose is 0.1-0.2 mg/kg. How much should the child receive?

Question 9: You receive a drug order to administer albuterol [Proventil] to a 15-lb child who has a history of asthma. The child is wheezing. The dose is 0.05-0.15 mg/kg (diluted in 2 mL saline). How much should the child receive?

Question 10: You receive a drug order to administer amiodarone [Cordarone] to a 13-lb child during a resuscitation. The initial rhythm was ventricular fibrillation and the child has already received shocks and vasopressor agents according to the ACLS algorithm. The dose is 5 mg/kg. How much should the child receive?

Question 11: You receive a drug order to administer atropine sulfate [Atropine] to a 22-lb child who has a symptomatic bradycardia. The dose is 0.02 mg/kg. How much should the child receive?

Question 12: You receive a drug order to administer Calcium Chloride to a 30-lb child. The physician suspects the cardiac arrest may have been due to a calcium channel blocker overdose since the child is in PEA. The dose is 20 mg/kg. How much should the child receive?

Question 13: You receive a drug order to administer diazepam [Valium] to a 26-lb child in an effort to stop an ongoing seizure. The dose is 0.2 mg/kg. How much should the child receive?

Question 14: You receive a drug order to administer diphenhydramine [Benadryl] to an 18-lb child who has had a mild allergic reaction. The dose is 1-2 mg/kg. How much should the child receive?

Question 15: You receive a drug order to administer activated charcoal [Liquid-Char] to a 45-lb child who still has a gag reflex. The child apparently drank what was left in all the plastic cups after a party involving cocktails and a keg of beer. The dose is 1-2 g/kg. How much should the child receive?

Question 16: You receive a drug order to administer adenosine [Adenocard] to a 70-lb child who has paroxysmal atrial tachycardia (PAT). The dose is 0.1-0.2 mg/kg. How much should the child receive?

Question 17: You receive a drug order to administer morphine sulfate [Astramorph/PF] to an 85-lb child who has a severe ulna and radius fracture after a fall on an outstretched arm. The dose is 0.1-0.2 mg/kg. How much should the child receive?

Question 18: You receive a drug order to administer albuterol [Proventil] to a 70-lb child in respiratory distress. The dose is 0.05-0.15 mg/kg (diluted in 2 mL saline). How much should the child receive?

Question 19: You receive a drug order to administer amiodarone [Cordarone] to a 65-lb child during a resuscitation. The dose is 5 mg/kg. How much should the child receive?

Question 20: You receive a drug order to administer atropine sulfate [Atropine] to a 50-lb child who has symptoms and a second-degree type one heart block. The dose is 0.02 mg/kg. How much should the child receive?

Question 21: You receive a drug order to administer Calcium Chloride to a 60-lb child during a resuscitation. The dose is 20 mg/kg. How much should the child receive?

Question 22: You receive a drug order to administer diazepam [Valium] to an 88-lb child in status epilepticus. The dose is 0.2 mg/kg. How much should the child receive?

Question 23: You receive a drug order to administer diphenhydramine [Benadryl] to a 45-lb child who is having a mild reaction to hay at the circus. The dose is 1-2 mg/kg. How much should the child receive?

Question 24: You receive a drug order to administer methylprednisolone sodium succinate [Solu-Medrol] to a 55-lb child as a part of the care for an asthma attack. The dose is 1-2 mg/kg. How much should the child receive?

Question 25: You receive a drug order to administer epinephrine [Adrenalin] to a 40-lb child in cardiac arrest. The dose is 0.01 mg/kg of 1:10,000. How much should the child receive?

Question 26: You receive a drug order to administer furosemide [Lasix] to a 58-lb child with pitting edema and acute pulmonary edema. The dose is 1 mg/kg. How much should the child receive?

Question 27: You receive a drug order to administer lidocaine hydrochloride [Xylocaine] to a 65-lb child during a resuscitation. The dose is 1 mg/kg. How much should the child receive?

Question 28: You receive a drug order to administer hydroxyzine [Atarax] to a 53-lb child to potentiate the effect of an analgesic. The dose is 0.5-1 mg/kg. How much should the child receive?

Question 29: You receive a drug order to administer lorazepam [Ativan] to a 75-lb child for recurrent seizure activity. The dose is 0.05-0.20 mg/kg. How much should the child receive?

Question 30: You receive a drug order to administer magnesium sulfate to an 85-lb child with congenital cardiac defects causing torsades de pointes. The dose is 25-50 mg/kg. How much should the child receive?

Question 31: You receive a drug order to administer pralidoxime chloride [2-PAM Chloride] to a 70-lb child who was exposed to an overdose of an organophosphate. The dose is 20-40 mg/kg. How much should the child receive?

Question 32: You receive a drug order to administer methylprednisolone sodium succinate [Solu-Medrol] to a 13-lb child who is having an asthma attack. The dose is 1-2 mg/kg. How much should the child receive?

Question 33: You receive a drug order to administer epinephrine [Adrenalin] to a 20-lb child during resuscitation. The dose is 0.01 mg/kg of 1:10,000. How much should the child receive?

Question 34: You receive a drug order to administer furosemide [Lasix] to a 35-lb child in acute pulmonary edema. The dose is 1 mg/kg. How much should the child receive?

Question 35: You receive a drug order to administer lidocaine hydrochloride [Xylocaine] to a 15-lb child during resuscitation. The dose is 1 mg/kg. How much should the child receive?

Question 36: You receive a drug order to administer hydroxyzine [Atarax] to a 25-lb child to calm him down without impairing his mental alertness. The dose is 0.5-1 mg/kg. How much should the child receive?

Question 37: You receive a drug order to administer naloxone hydrochloride [Narcan] to an 11-lb child who may have accidentally overdosed on a narcotic. The dose is 0.1 mg/kg. How much should the child receive?

Question 38: You receive a drug order to administer lorazepam [Ativan] to a 33-lb child to stop a seizure. The dose is 0.05-0.20 mg/kg. How much should the child receive?

Question 39: You receive a drug order to administer magnesium sulfate to a 30-lb child who has severe hypomagnesemia. The dose is 25-50 mg/kg. How much should the child receive?

Question 40: You receive a drug order to administer pralidoxime chloride [2-PAM Chloride] to a 10-lb child who was exposed to a nerve agent. The dose is 20-40 mg/kg. How much should the child receive?

Question 41: You receive a drug order to start a dopamine [Intropin] drip to be run in at 10 μg/kg/min. You have 400 mg of dopamine in 5 mL, a 250-mL bag of normal saline, a 60-gtt/mL microdrip set, and your patient weighs 220 lb. What is the concentration in mg/mL of the drip and how many gtt/min will the patient receive?

Question 42: You receive a drug order for a lidocaine drip to be run in at 2 mg/min. You have 200 mg in 10 mL, 50 mL of normal saline, and a 60-gtt/mL microdrip set. What is the concentration in mg/mL of the drip and how many gtt/min will the patient receive?

Question 43: You receive a drug order to administer 150 mg amiodarone [Cordarone] via slow IV drip over 10 minutes. You have 150 mg of amiodarone, a 50-mL bag of normal saline, and a 10-gtt/mL macrodrip set. Determine the concentration and calculate the drip rate.

Question 44: You receive a drug order to run an oxytocin [Pitocin] drip 10 milliunits/min. You have 10 units of oxytocin, 1 L of normal saline, and a 60-gtt/mL microdrip set. Determine the concentration and calculate the drip rate.

Question 45: You receive a drug order to run an epinephrine [Adrenalin] drip at 4 μg/min. You have 1 mg epinephrine, 250 mL of normal saline, and a 15-gtt/mL macrodrip set. Determine the concentration and calculate the drip rate.

Answers

NOTE: In these exercises the dose or dose range may vary slightly from your local protocols. Remember these are exercises for you to practice the concepts and calculations. Always follow your local protocols for the exact doses to administer to your patients!

Answer 1: A milliliter is 1/1,000 of a liter so (× 1,000).
2.5 L × 1,000 = 2,500 mL

Answer 2: A milligram is smaller than a gram so (÷ 1,000).
4,500 mg ÷ 1,000 = 4.5 g

Answer 3: A microgram is 1/1,000,000 of a gram so you can do this in one or two steps:
800 µg or ÷ 1,000,000 = **0.0008**
or 800 µg ÷ 1,000 = 0.8 mg
0.8 mg ÷ 1,000 = **0.0008 g**

Answer 4: A milligram is 1/1,000 of a liter so (× 1,000).
2.0 g × 1,000 = 2,000 mg

Answer 5: A milliliter is smaller than a liter so (÷ 1,000).
750 mL ÷ 1,000 = 0.75 L

Answer 6: First convert the 18 lb to kg using the 2.2 rule. This means that 18 lb is approximately 8 kg. To give the child 1-2 g/kg, simply multiply 8 kg by 1 and then 2 for the dose range. Your answer should be **8 to 16 g** of activated charcoal [Liquid-Char].

Answer 7: First convert the 20 lb to kg using the 2.2 rule. This means that 20 lb is approximately 9 kg. To give the child 0.1-0.2 mg/kg, simply multiply 9 kg by 0.1 and then 0.2 for the dose range. Your answer should be **0.9 to 1.8 mg** of adenosine [Adenocard].

Answer 8: First convert the 30 lb to kg using the 2.2 rule. This means that 30 lb is approximately 14 kg. To give the child 0.1-0.2 mg/kg, simply multiply 14 kg by 0.1 and then 0.2 for the dose range. Your answer should be **1.4 to 2.8 mg** of morphine sulfate [Astramorph/PF].

Answer 9: First convert the 15 lb to kg using the 2.2 rule. This means that 15 lb is approximately 7 kg. To give the child 0.05-0.15 mg/kg, simply multiply 7 kg by 0.05 and then 0.15 for the dose range. Your answer should be **0.35 to 1.05 mg** of albuterol [Proventil].

Answer 10: First convert the 13 lb to kg using the 2.2 rule. This means that 13 lb is approximately 6 kg. To give the child 5 mg/kg, simply multiply 6 kg by 5 for the dose. Your answer should be **30 mg** of amiodarone [Cordarone].

Answer 11: First convert the 22 lb to kg using the 2.2 rule. This means that 22 lb is approximately 10 kg. To give the child 0.02 mg/kg, simply multiply 10 kg by 0.02 for the dose. Your answer should be **0.2 mg** of atropine sulfate [Atropine].

Answer 12: First convert the 30 lb to kg using the 2.2 rule. This means that 30 lb is approximately 14 kg. To give the child 20 mg/kg, simply multiply 14 kg by 20 for the dose. Your answer should be **280 mg** of Calcium Chloride.

Answer 13: First convert the 26 lb to kg using the 2.2 rule. This means that 26 lb is approximately 12 kg. To give the child 0.2 mg/kg, simply multiply 12 kg by 0.2 for the dose. Your answer should be **2.4 mg** of diazepam [Valium].

Answer 14: First convert the 18 lb to kg using the 2.2 rule. This means that 18 lb is approximately 8 kg. To give the child 1-2 mg/kg, simply multiply 8 kg by 1 and then 2 for the dose range. Your answer should be **8 to 16 mg** of diphenhydramine [Benadryl].

Answer 15: First convert the 45 lb to kg using the 2.2 rule. This means that 45 lb is approximately 20 kg. To give the child 1-2 g/kg, simply multiply 20 kg by 1 and then 2 for the dose range. Your answer should be **20 to 40 g** of activated charcoal [Liqui-Char].

Answer 16: First convert the 70 lb to kg using the 2.2 rule. This means that 70 lb is approximately 32 kg. To give the child 0.1-0.2 mg/kg, simply multiply 32 kg by 0.1 and then 0.2 for the dose range. Your answer should be **3.2 to 6.4 mg** of adenosine [Adenocard].

Answer 17: First convert the 85 lb to kg using the 2.2 rule. This means that 85 lb is approximately 39 kg. To give the child 0.1-0.2 mg/kg, simply multiply 39 kg by 0.1 and then 0.2 for the dose range. Your answer should be **3.9 to 7.8 mg** of morphine sulfate [Astramorph/PF].

Answer 18: First convert the 70 lb to kg using the 2.2 rule. This means that 70 lb is approximately 32 kg. To give the child 0.05-0.15 mg/kg, simply multiply 32 kg by 0.05 and then 0.15 for the dose range. Your answer should be **1.6 to 4.8 mg** of albuterol [Proventil].

Answer 19: First convert the 65 lb to kg using the 2.2 rule. This means that 65 lb is approximately 30 kg. To give the child 5 mg/kg, simply multiply 30 kg by 5 for the dose. Your answer should be **150 mg** of amiodarone [Cordarone].

Answer 20: First convert the 50 lb to kg using the 2.2 rule. This means that 50 lb is approximately 23 kg. To give the child 0.02 mg/kg, simply multiply 23 kg by 0.02 for the dose. Your answer should be **0.46 mg** of atropine sulfate [Atropine].

Answer 21: First convert the 60 lb to kg using the 2.2 rule. This means that 60 lb is approximately 27 kg. To give the child 20 mg/kg, simply multiply 27 kg by 20 for the dose. Your answer should be **540 mg** of Calcium Chloride.

Answer 22: First convert the 88 lb to kg using the 2.2 rule. This means that 88 lb is approximately 40 kg. To give the child 0.2 mg/kg, simply multiply 40 kg by 0.2 for the dose. Your answer should be **8 mg** of diazepam [Valium].

Answer 23: First convert the 45 lb to kg using the 2.2 rule. This means that 45 lb is approximately 20 kg. To give the child 1-2 mg/kg, simply multiply 20 kg by 1 and then 2 for the dose range. Your answer should be **20 to 40 mg** of diphenhydramine [Benadryl].

Answer 24: First convert the 55 lb to kg using the 2.2 rule. This means that 55 lb is approximately 25 kg. To give the child 1-2 mg/kg, simply multiply 25 kg by 1 and then 2 for the dose range. Your answer should be **25 to 50 mg** of methylprednisolone sodium succinate[Solu-Medrol].

Answer 25: First convert the 40 lb to kg using the 2.2 rule. This means that 40 lb is approximately 18 kg. To give the child 0.01 mg/kg of 1:10,000, simply multiply 18 kg by 0.01 for the dose. Your answer should be **0.18 mg** of epinephrine [Adrenalin].

Answer 26: First convert the 58 lb to kg using the 2.2 rule. This means that 58 lb is approximately 26 kg. To give the child 1 mg/kg, simply multiply 26 kg by 1 for the dose. Your answer should be **26 mg** of furosemide [Lasix].

Answer 27: First convert the 65 lb to kg using the 2.2 rule. This means that 65 lb is approximately 30 kg. To give the child 1 mg/kg, simply multiply 30 kg by 1 for the dose. Your answer should be **30 mg** of lidocaine hydrochloride [Xylocaine].

Answer 28: First convert the 53 lb to kg using the 2.2 rule. This means that 53 lb is approximately 24 kg. To give the child 0.5-1 mg/kg, simply multiply 24 kg by 0.5 and then 1 for the dose range. Your answer should be **12 to 24 mg** of hydroxyzine [Atarax].

Answer 29: First convert the 75 lb to kg using the 2.2 rule. This means that 75 lb is approximately 34 kg. To give the child 0.05-0.20 mg/kg, simply multiply 34 kg by 0.05 and then 0.20 for the dose range. Your answer should be **1.7 to 6.8 mg** of lorazepam [Ativan].

Answer 30: First convert the 85 lbs to kg using the 2.2 rule. This means that 85 lb is approximately 39 kg. To give the child 25-50 mg/kg, simply multiply 39 kg by 25 and then 50 for the dose range. Your answer should be **975 to 1,950 mg** of magnesium sulfate.

Answer 31: First convert the 70 lb to kg using the 2.2 rule. This means that 70 lb is approximately 32 kg. To give the child 20-40 mg/kg, simply multiply 32 kg by 20 and then 40 for the dose range. Your answer should be **640 to 1,280 mg** of pralidoxime chloride [2-PAM Chloride].

Answer 32: First convert the 13 lb to kg using the 2.2 rule. This means that 13 lb is approximately 6 kg. To give the child 1-2 mg/kg, simply multiply 6 kg by 1 and then 2 for the dose range. Your answer should be **6 to 12 mg** of methylprednisolone sodium succinate [Solu-Medrol].

Answer 33: First convert the 20 lb to kg using the 2.2 rule. This means that 20 lb is approximately 9 kg. To give the child 0.01 mg/kg of 1:10,000, simply multiply 9 kg by 0.01 for the dose. Your answer should be **0.09 mg** of epinephrine [Adrenalin].

Answer 34: First convert the 35 lb to kg using the 2.2 rule. This means that 35 lb is approximately 16 kg. To give the child 1 mg/kg, simply multiply 16 kg by 1 for the dose. Your answer should be **16 mg** of furosemide [Lasix].

Answer 35: First convert the 15 lb to kg using the 2.2 rule. This means that 15 lb is approximately 7 kg. To give the child 1 mg/kg, simply multiply 7 kg by 1 for the dose. Your answer should be **7 mg** of lidocaine hydrochloride [Xylocaine].

Answer 36: First convert the 25 lb to kg using the 2.2 rule. This means that 25 lb is approximately 11 kg. To give the child 0.5-1 mg/kg, simply multiply 11 kg by 0.5 and then 1 for the dose range. Your answer should be **5.5 to 11 mg** of hydroxyzine [Atarax].

Answer 37: First convert the 11 lb to kg using the 2.2 rule. This means that 11 lb is approximately 5 kg. To give the child 0.1 mg/kg, simply multiply 5 kg by 0.1 for the dose. Your answer should be **0.5 mg** of naloxone hydrochloride [Narcan].

Answer 38: First convert the 33 lb to kg using the 2.2 rule. This means that 33 lb is approximately 15 kg. To give the child 0.05-0.20 mg/kg, simply multiply 15 kg by 0.05 and then 0.20 for the dose range. Your answer should be **0.75 to 3 mg** of lorazepam [Ativan].

Answer 39: First convert the 30 lb to kg using the 2.2 rule. This means that 30 lb is approximately 14 kg. To give the child 25-50 mg/kg, simply multiply 14 kg by 25 and then 50 for the dose range. Your answer should be **350 to 700 mg** of magnesium sulfate.

Answer 40: First convert the 10 lb to kg using the 2.2 rule. This means that 10 lb is approximately 5 kg. To give the child 20-40 mg/kg, simply multiply 5 kg by 20 and then 40 for the dose range. Your answer should be **100 to 200 mg** of pralidoxime chloride [2-PAM Chloride].

Answer 41: This problem requires several steps:
Step 1. Determine the concentration after mixing the drug in the IV solution 250-mL bag.

$$\frac{\text{400 mg (total weight of dopamine)}}{\text{250 mL (total volume normal saline)}} =$$

1.6 mg/mL (concentration) = 1,600 μg/mL

{NOTE: you will actually remove 5 mL from the bag to make room for the fluid you inject into the bag}

Step 2. Convert the patient's weight from pounds to kilograms.
220 lb ÷ 2.2 = 100 kg

Step 3. Calculate the drip rate. Multiply the patient's weight (100 kg) times the desired dose or drug order (10 μg/kg) times the drip set (60 gtt/mL) and divide this into the IV solution you have mixed (1,600 μg/mL).

$$\frac{\text{(100 kg) (10 μg/kg) (60 gtt/mL)}}{\text{1,600 μg/mL}} = \frac{60{,}000}{1{,}600} =$$

37.5 gtt/min (round up 38 gtt/min)

NOTE: If you do not have a calculator handy, you could convert the 60,000/1,600 to 600/16 and then divide.

Answer 42: Step 1. Determine the concentration after mixing the drug in the IV solution.

$$\frac{\text{200 mg (total weight of lidocaine) in 50 mL}}{\text{50 mL (total volume normal saline)}} = \textbf{4 mg/mL}$$

NOTE: Remove 10 mL of normal saline then add the 10 mL of lidocaine for a total of 50 mL.

Step 2. Calculate the drip rate. Multiply the order (2 mg/min) times the drip set (60 gtt/mL) and divide this into the IV solution you have mixed (4 mg/mL).

$$\frac{\text{(2 mg/min) (60 gtt/mL)}}{\text{4 mg/mL}} = \textbf{30 gtt/min}$$

Answer 43: Step 1. Determine the concentration after mixing the drug in the IV solution.

$$\frac{\text{150 mg (amiodarone)}}{\text{50 mL (IV solution)}} = \textbf{3 mg/mL}$$

Step 2. Calculate the drip rate. Multiply the drip order (15 mg/min) times the drip set (10 gtt/min) and divide this into the IV solution you have mixed (3 mg/mL).

$$\frac{\text{15 mg/min (10 gtt/min)}}{\text{3 mg/mL}} = \text{50 gtt/min}$$

Answer 44: Step 1. Determine the concentration after mixing the drug in the IV solution.

$$\frac{\text{10 units (oxytocin)}}{\text{1 L or 1,000 mL}} = \frac{\text{10,000 mu}}{\text{1,000}} = \textbf{10 mu/mL}$$

NOTE: mu = units

Step 2. Calculate the drip rate. Multiply the order (10 mu/min) times the drip set (60 gtt/mL) and divide this into the IV solution you have mixed (10 mu/mL).

$$\frac{\text{(10 mu/min) (60 gtt/min)}}{\text{10 mu/mL}} = \textbf{60 gtt/min}$$

Answer 45: Step 1. Determine the concentration after mixing the drug in the IV solution.

$$\frac{\text{1 mg or 1,000 μg (epinephrine)}}{\text{250 mL (IV solution)}} = \textbf{4 μg/mL}$$

Step 2. Calculate the drip rate. Multiply the order (4 μg/min) times the drip set (15 gtt/mL) and divide this into the IV solution you have mixed (4 μg/mL).

$$\frac{\text{(4 μg/min) (15 gtt/mL)}}{\text{4 μg/mL}} = \textbf{15 gtt/min}$$

Rapid Sequence Intubation

B

Sample Procedure For Rapid Sequence Intubation

Rapid sequence intubation (RSI) or medication facilitated intubation (MFI) is used to provide definitive airway control in the unstable patient with a potentially full stomach to negate the extreme risks attendant with the induction of general anesthesia. This procedure is performed on critically ill or injured patients in need of definitive airway support or mechanical ventilation who are not flaccidly unconscious. RSI uses a combination of medications and techniques performed in rapid succession. The use of certain medications (ie, neuromuscular blockers or paralytic agents) during RSI is absolutely contraindicated in the prehospital setting if the patient cannot be ventilated with a bag-mask device due to their anatomy, significantly complicating facial or airway trauma, or other physiologic reasons (ie, morbid obesity).

A typical RSI protocol includes the following steps:

1. Evaluate the airway and position the patient appropriately to optimize "first-pass" placement of the endotracheal tube.
2. Make sure that the patient is attached to all appropriate monitors prior to the RSI procedure, including SpO_2, waveform $EtCO_2$, NIBP, and ECG monitor.
3. Always preoxygenate the patient via a high-concentration face mask (**Figure B-1** ▾). If the SpO_2 is below 95% and the patient is apneic, use a bag-mask device attached to high-concentration oxygen.
4. Assemble and test all basic and advanced airway equipment (ie, suction, oropharyngeal airway, intubation equipment, $EtCO_2$ detector, etc).
5. Draw up the medications as specified in your protocols and label the syringes clearly.
6. Consider pre-treatment with the paralytic vecuronium bromide [Norcuron] 0.01 mg/kg for defasciculation.
7. Consider the possibility of elevated intracranial pressure and administer lidocaine [Xylocaine] 1.5 mg/kg (max dose of 100 mg) if indicated, to decrease the risk of a spike in ICP associated with stimulation of the upper airway.
8. Have a second rescuer apply and maintain gentle cricoid pressure.
9. Administer etomidate [Amidate] 0.3 mg/kg rapid IV/IO push for sedation.
10. Perform laryngoscopy and proceed with intubation if ideal intubating conditions are achieved.
    - If ideal intubation conditions do not exist, administer succinylcholine [Anectine] 1.5 mg/kg IV/IO which will paralyze the patient.
    - If the intubation fails, maintain an open airway, ventilate with a bag-mask device, place a rescue airway, and proceed accordingly.
    - If not already done, assess for the presence of end-tidal CO_2 monitor, confirm endotracheal tube placement, and secure the endotracheal tube.
11. Administer continued sedation with:
    - Midazolam [Versed] 0.03-0.05 mg/kg IV every 15 minutes if hemodynamically stable, or:
    - Etomidate [Amidate] 0.3 mg/kg repeated every 5–10 minutes if the systolic blood pressure < 100 mm Hg.
12. Administer vercuronium bromide [Norcuron] 0.1 mg/kg as an intermediate-acting neuromuscular blocking agent, and only if necessary for patient and crew safety.
13. Continuously monitor ETT placement including effectiveness of oxygenation and ventilation.

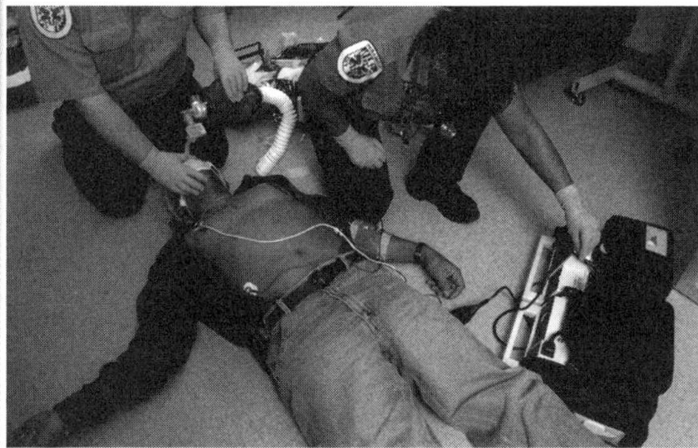

Figure B-1

RSI or MFI is a procedure not without risk or the potential for serious complications, including death. There are several situations when a patient with an altered mental status needs advanced airway management because he/she is not alert enough to protect his/her own airway. In these cases, sedation without paralytics and alternative advanced airway management (ie, nasal intubation, laryngeal mask airway or LMA) may be an option. Consider sedation first and the fact that sometimes "less is more." The more medications administered, the more chances exist for errors in dosage and adverse medication reactions. Complications with difficult or unexpected airway anatomy can occur during RSI procedures, and avoiding paralysis allows patients to potentially continue to breathe on their own if intubation attempts are unsuccessful.

A number of other agents are used for induction of sedation/anesthesia and induction/maintenance of neuromuscular blockade. They are chosen based on patient parameters including underlying problem and physiology, as well as anticipated needs of treatment.

It is extremely important to realize that although a patient who has been given neuromuscular blocking agents is effectively paralyzed, he/she may be completely awake and able to perceive all manner of sensory input including pain. BE SURE to employ sedative agents for all patients who have been given neuromuscular blockers. It is cruel and unethical to use neuromuscular blockers without associated sedative/anesthetic agents, as there is immeasurable pain and fear associated with procedures like endotracheal intubation and line placement. Performing these procedures with the knowledge that the patient perceives all manner of noxious stimuli and dyspnea, but cannot move or speak in response to such stimuli, is inhumane and inappropriate. You should pay strict attention to vital signs in these patients. Sudden tachycardia/hypertension or tearing in a chemically paralyzed patient is often the only sign that a patient has "woken up" beneath their neuromuscular blockade. In that case, a dose of high-potency, fast-acting sedative (such as midazolam, etiomidate, or propofol) must be promptly administered.

C Medication Review

Reference for Medication Listings

Name of Medication (Other Common Names)

Class How the medication is categorized as compared to other medications. This is usually done by grouping those medications with similar characteristics, traits, or primary components.

Mechanism of action The manner of combination of parts, processes, etc., which form a common function.

Indications A circumstance that points to or shows the cause, pathology, treatment, or issue of an attack of disease; that which points out; that which serves as a guide or warning.

Contraindications Any condition, especially any condition of disease, which renders some particular line of treatment improper or undesirable.

Adverse reactions This is an abnormal or harmful effect to an organism caused by exposure to a chemical. It is indicated by some result such as death, a change in food or water consumption, altered body and organ weights, altered enzyme levels, or visible illness. An effect may be classed as adverse if it causes functional or anatomic damage, causes irreversible change in the homeostasis of the organism, or increases the susceptibility of the organism to other chemical or biologic stress. A nonadverse effect will usually be reversed when the organism is no longer being exposed to the chemical.

Drug interactions This refers to any potential effects that a medication may have when administered in conjunction or in the presence of another medication already in the patient's system, a medication delivery device, or fluid.

How supplied This is how the manufacturer packages the medication for distribution and sale. Typical methods of packaging are prefilled syringes, vials, or ampules.

Dosage and administration This is the typical or average volume of the medication that is to be administered to the patient and the route of introduction of the medication to the patient.

Duration of action Three values are given; (1) Onset: the estimated amount of time it will take for the medication to enter the body/system and begin to take effect, (2) Peak effect: the estimated amount of time it will take for the medication to have its greatest effect on the patient/system, and (3) Duration: the estimated amount of time that the medication will have any effect on the patient/system.

Special considerations Additional pertinent information concerning a medication.

Activated Charcoal (Liqui-Char)

Class Adsorbent.

Mechanism of action Adsorbs toxic substances from the gastrointestinal tract; onset of action is immediate.

Indications Most oral poisonings and medication overdoses; can be used after evacuation of poisons.

Contraindications Oral administration to comatose patient; after ingestion of corrosives, caustics, or petroleum distillates (ineffective and may induce vomiting); simultaneous administration with other oral drugs.

Adverse reactions May induce nausea and vomiting; may cause constipation; may cause black stools.

Drug interactions Bonds with and generally inactivates whatever it is mixed with, eg, syrup of ipecac.

How supplied 25 g (black powder)/125-mL bottle (200 mg/mL); 50 g (black powder)/250-mL bottle (200 mg/mL)

Dosage and administration Note: if not in premixed slurry, dilute with 1 part charcoal/4 parts water. Adult: 1–2 g/kg PO or via NGT. Pediatric: 1–2 g/kg PO or via NGT.

Duration of action Depends on gastrointestinal function; will act until excreted.

Special considerations Often used in conjunction with magnesium citrate. Must be stored in a closed container. Does not adsorb cyanide, lithium, iron, lead, or arsenic.

Adenosine (Adenocard)

Class Endogenous nucleotide.

Mechanism of action Slows conduction time through the AV node; can interrupt re-entrant pathways; slows heart rate; acts directly on sinus pacemaker cells. Is drug of choice for re-entry SVT. Can be used diagnostically for stable, wide-complex tachycardias of unknown type after two doses of lidocaine.

Indications Conversion of PSVT to sinus rhythm. May convert re-entry SVT due to Wolff-Parkinson-White syndrome. Not effective in converting atrial fibrillation/flutter or V-tach.

Contraindications Second- or third-degree block or sick sinus syndrome, atrial flutter/atrial fibrillation, ventricular tachycardia, hypersensitivity to adenosine, poison-induced tachycardia.

Adverse reactions Facial flushing, shortness of breath, chest pain, headache, paresthesia, diaphoresis, palpitations, hypotension, nausea, metallic taste.

Drug interactions Methylxanthines (theophylline-like drugs) antagonize the effects of adenosine. Dipyridamole (Persantine) potentiates the effects of adenosine. Carbamazepine (Tegretol) may potentiate the AV node, blocking the effects of adenosine. May cause bronchoconstriction in asthmatic patients.

How supplied 3 mg/mL in 2-mL flip-top vials for IV injection.

Dosage and administration Adult: 6 mg over 1–3 seconds, followed by a 20 mL saline flush and elevate extremity; if no response after 1–2 minutes, administer 12 mg over 1–3 seconds; if no response repeat 12 mg again. Maximum total dose, 30 mg; Pediatric: 0.1–0.2 mg/kg rapid IV; maximum single dose, 12 mg.

Duration of action Onset and peak effects in seconds; duration, 12 seconds.

Special considerations Short half-life limits side effects in most patients. Pregnancy safety: Category C.

Albuterol (Proventil, Ventolin)

Class Sympathomimetic, bronchodilator.

Mechanism of action Selective beta-2 agonist that stimulates adrenergic receptors of the sympathomimetic nervous system resulting in smooth muscle relaxation in the bronchial tree and peripheral vasculature.

Indications Treatment of bronchospasm in patients with reversible obstructive airway disease (COPD/asthma). Prevention of exercise-induced bronchospasm.

Contraindications Known prior hypersensitivity reactions to albuterol. Tachycardia arrhythmias, especially those caused by digitalis. Synergistic with other sympathomimetics.

Adverse reactions Often dose-related and include restlessness, tremors, dizziness, palpitations, tachycardia, nervousness, peripheral vasodilatation, nausea, vomiting, hyperglycemia, increased blood pressure, and paradoxical bronchospasm.

Drug interactions Tricyclic antidepressants may potentiate vasculature effects. Beta-blockers are antagonistic. May potentiate hypokalemia caused by diuretics.

How supplied Solution for aerosolization: 0.5% (5 mg/mL). Metered dose inhaler: 90 µg/metered spray (17-g canister with 200 inhalations). Syrup: 2 mg/5 mL.

Dosage and administration Adult: Administer 2.5 mg (0.5 mL of the 0.5% solution) added to 2 mL of normal saline for inhalation by nebulizer treatment and administer over 10–15 minutes. May repeat every 20 minutes up to three times. MDI: 1–2 inhalations (90–180 µg). Five minutes between inhalations. Pediatric: (between the ages of 2 and 12) administer 2.5 mg (0.5 mL of the 0.083% solution) added to 2 mL of normal saline for inhalation by nebulizer treatment and administer over 10–15 minutes. May repeat every 20 minutes up to three times.

Duration of action Onset in 5–15 minutes with peak effect in 30 minutes to 2 hours and duration of 3–4 hours.

Special considerations Pregnancy safety: Category C. Antagonized by beta-blockers (eg, Inderal, Lopressor). May precipitate angina pectoris and arrhythmias. Should only be administered by inhalation methodology in prehospital management.

Amiodarone (Cordarone, Pacerone)

Class Antiarrhythmic.

Mechanism of action Blocks sodium channels and myocardial potassium channels.

Indications V-fib/pulseless V-tach and unstable V-tach in patients refractory to other therapy. Also persistent SVTs unresponsive to other treatment.

Contraindications Known hypersensitivity, cardiogenic shock, sinus bradycardia, and second- or third-degree AV block (unless a functional pacemaker is available).

Adverse reactions Hypotension, bradycardia, prolongation of the P-R, QRS, and Q-T intervals.

Drug interactions Use with digoxin may cause digitalis toxicity. Antiarrhythmics may cause increased serum levels. Beta-blockers and calcium channel blockers may potentiate bradycardia, sinus arrest, and AV heart blocks.

How supplied Ampules containing 150 mg/3 mL (50 mg/mL) and prefilled syringes containing 150 mg/3 mL (50 mg/mL).

Dosage and administration Adult: V-fib/pulseless V-tach unresponsive to CPR, defibrillation, and vasopressors: 300 mg IV/IO push (recommend dilution in 20–30 mL D_5W). Initial dose can be followed one time in 3–5 minutes at 150 mg IV/IO push. Recurrent life-threatening ventricular arrhythmias: Maximum cumulative dose is 2.2 g/24 hours, administered as follows: Rapid infusion: 150 mg IV/IO over 10 minutes (15 mg/min). May repeat rapid infusion (150 mg IV/IO) every 10 minutes as necessary. Slow infusion: 360 mg IV/IO over 6 hours (1 mg/min). Maintenance infusion: 540 mg IV/IO over 18 hours (0.5 mg/min). Pediatric: Refractory V-fib/pulseless V-tach: 5 mg/kg IV/IO bolus. Can repeat the 5 mg/kg IV/IO bolus up to a total dose of 15 mg/kg per 24 hours. Maximum single dose is 300 mg. Perfusing supraventricular and ventricular tachycardias: Loading dose of 5 mg/kg IV/IO over 20–60 minutes (maximum single dose of 300 mg). Can repeat to maximum of 15 mg/kg per day.

Duration of action Onset: immediate with peak effect in 10–15 minutes. Duration of action: 30–45 minutes.

Special considerations Pregnancy safety: Category D. Monitor patient for hypotension. May worsen arrhythmias or precipitate new arrhythmias.

Amyl Nitrite, Sodium Nitrite, Sodium Thiosulfate (Cyanide Antidote Kit)

Class Antidote.

Mechanism of action Amyl nitrite: affinity for cyanide ions; reacts with hemoglobin to form methemoglobin (low toxicity); sodium nitrite: same as amyl nitrite; sodium thiosulfate: produces thiocyanate, which is then excreted.

Indications Cyanide or hydrocyanic acid poisoning.

Contraindications Not applicable.

Adverse reactions Excessive doses of amyl nitrite and sodium nitrite can produce severe, life-threatening methemoglobinemia. Use only recommended doses.

Drug interactions None.

How supplied Amyl nitrite: in capsules similar to ammonia capsules.

Dosage and administration Adult: Amyl nitrite: breathe 30 seconds out of every minute. Sodium thiosulfate and sodium nitrite: IV per antidote kit directions. Pediatric: Same as adult.

Duration of action Variable.

Special considerations Cyanide poisoning must be recognized quickly and treated quickly; if pulse persists, even in presence of apnea, prognosis is good with treatment. The antidote kit must be used in conjunction with administration of oxygen.

Aspirin

Class Platelet inhibitor, anti-inflammatory agent.

Mechanism of action Prostaglandin inhibition.

Indications New onset chest pain suggestive of acute myocardial infarction. Signs and symptoms suggestive of recent cerebrovascular accident.

Contraindications Hypersensitivity. Relatively contraindicated in patients with active ulcer disease or asthma.

Adverse reactions Heartburn, GI bleeding, prolonged bleeding, nausea, and vomiting. Wheezing in allergic patients.

Drug interactions Use with caution in patients allergic to NSAIDs.

How supplied 81-mg, 160-mg, or 325-mg tablets (chewable and standard).

Dosage and administration 160 mg to 325 mg PO (chewed if possible).

Duration of action Onset: 30–45 minutes. Peak effect: variable. Duration: variable.

Special considerations Pregnancy safety: Category D. Not recommended in pediatric population.

Atropine Sulfate

Class Anticholinergic agent.

Mechanism of action Parasympatholytic: inhibits action of acetylcholine at postganglionic parasympathetic neuroeffector sites. Increases heart rate in life-threatening bradyarrhythmias.

Indications Hemodynamically unstable bradycardia, asystole, bradycardic (< 60 beats/min) pulseless electrical activity (PEA), organophosphate poisoning, bronchospastic pulmonary disorders.

Contraindications Tachycardia, hypersensitivity, unstable cardiovascular status in acute hemorrhage and myocardial ischemia, narrow-angle glaucoma.

Adverse reactions Headache; dizziness; palpitations; nausea and vomiting; tachycardia; arrhythmias; anticholinergic effects (blurred vision, dry mouth, urinary retention); paradoxical bradycardia when pushed slowly or at low doses; flushed, hot, dry skin.

Drug interactions Potential adverse effects when administered with digoxin, cholinergics, physostigmine. Effects enhanced by antihistamines, procainamide, quinidine, antipsychotics, benzodiazepines, and antidepressants.

How supplied Prefilled syringes: 1 mg in 10 mL (0.1 mg/mL). Nebulizer: 0.2% (1 mg in 0.5 mL) and 0.5% (2.5 mg in 0.5 mL).

Dosage and administration Adult: Asystole or bradycardic PEA: 1 mg IV/IO push. May repeat every 3–5 minutes (if asystole or PEA persists) to a maximum dose of 0.04 mg/kg. Endotracheal administration: 2–3 mg diluted in 10 mL of water or normal saline. Unstable bradycardia: 0.5 mg IV/IO every 3–5 minutes as necessary, not to exceed total dose of 0.04 mg/kg. Use shorter dosing interval (3 minutes) and higher doses in severe clinical conditions. Organophosphate poisoning: Extremely large doses (2–4 mg or higher) may be needed. Pediatric: 0.02 mg/kg via IV/IO push; may double this dose for second IV/IO dose. Minimum single dose: 0.1 mg. Maximum doses: child single dose: 0.5 mg, child total dose: 1 mg, adolescent single dose: 1 mg, adolescent total dose: 2 mg. Endotracheal administration: 0.03 mg/kg (absorption may be unreliable).

Duration of action Onset: immediate. Peak effect: rapid to 1–2 minutes. Duration: 2–6 hours.

Special considerations Pregnancy safety: Category C. Moderate doses may cause pupillary dilation.

Benzocaine Spray (Hurricane)

Class Topical anesthetic.

Mechanism of action Stabilizes neuronal membrane.

Indications Used as a lubricant and topical anesthetic to facilitate passage of diagnostic and treatment devices. Suppresses the pharyngeal and tracheal gag reflex.

Contraindications Patients with a known hypersensitivity to benzocaine.

Adverse reactions Methemoglobinemia has been reported following the use of benzocaine on extremely rare occasions.

Drug interactions No significant interactions found or known.

How supplied Multidose aerosol can, 20% benzocaine.

Dosage and administration Adult: 0.5–1.0 second spray, repeat as necessary. Pediatric: 0.25–0.5 second spray, repeat as necessary.

Duration of action Onset: Immediate. Peak effect: 30 seconds. Duration: 15 minutes.

Special considerations Pregnancy safety: Category A. Topical use only, not for ocular use or injection.

Calcium Chloride

Class Electrolyte.

Mechanism of action Increases cardiac contractile state (positive inotropic effect). May enhance ventricular automaticity.

Indications Hypocalcemia, hyperkalemia, magnesium sulfate overdose, calcium channel blocker overdose, adjunctive therapy in treatment of insect bites and stings.

Contraindications Hypercalcemia, V-fib, digitalis toxicity.

Adverse reactions Bradycardia, asystole, hypotension, peripheral vasodilation, metallic taste, local necrosis, coronary and cerebral artery spasm, nausea and vomiting.

Drug interactions May worsen arrhythmias secondary to digitalis toxicity. May antagonize the effects of verapamil. Do not mix with or infuse immediately before or after sodium bicarbonate without intervening flush.

How supplied Prefilled syringes containing a 10% solution in 10 mL (100 mg/mL).

Dosage and administration Adult: 500 mg to 1,000 mg (5–10 mL of a 10% solution) IV/IO push for hyperkalemia and calcium channel blocker overdose. May be repeated as necessary. Pediatric: 20 mg/kg (0.2 mL/kg) slow IV/IO push. Maximum 1 g dose; may repeat in 10 minutes.

Duration of action Onset: 5–15 minutes. Peak effect: 3–5 minutes. Duration: 15–30 minutes, but may persist for 4 hours (dose dependent).

Special considerations Pregnancy safety: Category C. Do not use routinely in cardiac arrest.

Dexamethasone Sodium Phosphate (Decadron, Hexadrol)

Class Corticosteroid.

Mechanism of action Suppresses acute and chronic inflammation; immunosuppressive effects.

Indications Anaphylaxis, asthma, croup.

Contraindications Hypersensitivity to product, systemic sepsis, bacterial infection.

Adverse reactions Hypertension, sodium and water retention, gastrointestinal bleeding, TB. None from single dose.

Drug interactions Calcium, metaraminol.

How supplied 100 mg/5-mL vials or 20 mg/1-mL vials.

Dosage and administration Adult: 10–100 mg IV (1 mg/kg slow IV bolus) (considerable variance through medical control). Pediatric: 0.25–1.0 mg/kg/dose IV, IO, IM.

Duration of action Onset: Hours. Peak effects: 8–12 hours. Duration: 24–72 hours.

Special considerations Pregnancy safety: unknown. Protect medication from heat. Toxicity and side effects with long-term use.

Dextrose

Class Carbohydrate, hypertonic solution.

Mechanism of action Rapidly increases serum glucose levels. Short-term osmotic diuresis.

Indications Hypoglycemia, altered level of consciousness, coma of unknown etiology, seizure of unknown etiology, status epilepticus.

Contraindications Intracranial hemorrhage.

Adverse reactions Extravasation leads to tissue necrosis. Warmth, pain, burning, thrombophlebitis, rhabdomyolysis, hyperglycemia.

Drug interactions Sodium bicarbonate, Coumadin.

How supplied 25 g/50-mL prefilled syringes (500 mg/mL).

Dosage and administration Adult: 12.5–25 g slow IV; may be repeated as necessary. Pediatric: 0.5–1 g/kg/dose slow IV; may be repeated as necessary.

Duration of action Onset: less than 1 minute. Peak effects: variable. Duration: variable.

Special considerations Administer thiamine prior to D_{50} in known alcoholic patients. Draw blood to determine glucose level before administering. Do not administer to patients with known CVA unless hypoglycemia documented.

Diazepam (Valium)

Class Benzodiazepine, sedative-hypnotic, anticonvulsant.

Mechanism of action Potentiates effects of inhibitory neurotransmitters. Raises seizure threshold. Induces amnesia and sedation.

Indications Acute anxiety states, acute alcohol withdrawal (delirium tremens), muscle relaxant, seizure activity, agitation. Analgesia for medical procedures (fracture reduction, cardioversion).

Contraindications Hypersensitivity, glaucoma, coma, shock, substance abuse, head injury.

Adverse reactions Respiratory depression, hypotension, drowsiness, ataxia, reflex tachycardia, nausea, confusion, thrombosis, and phlebitis.

Drug interactions Incompatible with most drugs, fluids.

How supplied 10 mg/5-mL prefilled syringes, ampules, vials, and Tubex.

Dosage and administration Seizure activity: Adult: 5–10 mg IV every 10–15 minutes as necessary (5 mg over 5 min)(maximum dose, 30 mg). Seizure activity: Pediatric: 0.2–0.5 mg slowly every 2–5 minutes up to 5 mg (maximum dose, 10 mg/kg). Rectal diazepam: 0.5 mg/kg via rectal catheter and flush with 2–3 mL air after administration. Sedation for cardioversion: 5–15 mg IV over 5–10 minutes prior to cardioversion.

Duration of action Onset: 1–5 minutes. Peak effect: Minutes. Duration: 20–50 minutes.

Special considerations Pregnancy safety: Category D. Short duration of anticonvulsant effect. Reduce dose 50% in elderly patient.

Diltiazem Hydrochloride (Cardizem, Lyo-Ject)

Class Calcium channel blocker.

Mechanism of action Block influx of calcium ions into cardiac muscle; prevents spasm of coronary arteries. Arterial and venous vasodilator. Reduces preload and afterload. Reduces myocardial oxygen demand.

Indications Control of rapid ventricular rates due to atrial flutter, atrial fibrillation, and re-entry SVT; angina pectoris.

Contraindications Hypotension, sick sinus syndrome, second- or third-degree AV block, cardiogenic shock, wide-complex tachycardias, poison/drug-induced tachycardia.

Adverse reactions Bradycardia, second- or third-degree AV blocks, chest pain, CHF, syncope. V-Fib, V-tach, nausea, vomiting, dizziness, dry mouth, dyspnea, headache.

Drug interactions Caution in patients using medications that affect cardiac contractility. In general, should not be used in patients on beta-blockers.

How supplied 25 mg/5-mL vial; 50 mg/10-mL vial. Nonrefrigerated: Lyo-Ject syringe.

Dosage and administration Adult: Initial bolus: 0.25 mg/kg (average dose 15–20 mg) IV over 2 minutes. If inadequate response, may re-bolus in 15 minutes: 0.35 mg/kg (average dose 20–25 mg) IV over 2 minutes. Maintenance infusion of 5–15 mg/h. Pediatric: Not recommended.

Duration of action Onset: 2–5 minutes. Peak effect: variable. Duration: 1–3 hours.

Special considerations Pregnancy safety: Category C. Use with caution in patients with renal or hepatic dysfunction. PVCs may be noted at time of conversion of PSVT to sinus rhythm.

Diphenhydramine (Benadryl)

Class Antihistamine; anticholinergic.

Mechanism of action Blocks cellular histamine receptors; decreases vasodilation; decreases motion sickness. Reverses extrapyramidal reactions.

Indications Symptomatic relief of allergies, allergic reactions, anaphylaxis, acute dystonic reactions (phenothiazines). Blood administration reactions; used for motion sickness, hay fever.

Contraindications Asthma, glaucoma, pregnancy, hypertension, narrow-angle glaucoma, infants, patients taking monoamine oxidase inhibitors (MAOIs).

Adverse reactions Sedation, hypotension, seizures, visual disturbances, vomiting, urinary retention, palpitations, arrhythmias, dry mouth and throat, and paradoxical CNS excitation in children.

Drug interactions Potentiates effects of alcohol and other anticholinergics, may inhibit corticosteroid activity; MAOIs prolong anticholinergic effects of diphenhydramine.

How supplied Tablets: 25, 50 mg; Capsules: 25, 50 mg; Prefilled syringes: 50- or 100-mg vials (IV or IM); elixir, 12.5 mg/5 mL.

Dosage and administration Adult: 25–50 mg IM or IV or PO. Pediatric: 1–2 mg/kg IV, IO slowly or IM. If given PO: 5 mg/kg/24 hours.

Duration of action Onset: 15–30 minutes. Peak effect: 1 hour. Duration: 3–12 hours.

Special considerations Not used in infants or in pregnancy: Category B. If used in anaphylaxis, will be in conjunction with epinephrine, corticosteroids.

Dobutamine (Dobutrex)

Class Sympathomimetic, inotropic agent.

Mechanism of action Synthetic catecholamine. Increased myocardial contractility and stroke volume, increased cardiac output. Minimal chronotropic activity. Increases renal blood flow.

Indications Cardiogenic shock, CHF, left ventricular dysfunction. Often used in conjunction with other drugs.

Contraindications Tachyarrhythmias, IHSS, severe hypotension.

Adverse reactions May increase infarct size in patient with MI, headache, arrhythmias, hypertension, PVCs.

Drug interactions Incompatible with sodium bicarbonate and furosemide. Beta-blockers may blunt inotropic effects.

How supplied 250 mg/20-mL vials.

Dosage and administration Adult: IV infusion at 2–20 µg/kg/min titrated to desired effect. Pediatric: 2–20 µg/kg/min titrated to desired effect.

Duration of action Onset: 2 minutes. Peak effect: 10 minutes. Duration: 1–2 minutes after infusion discontinued.

Special considerations Pregnancy safety: not well established. Monitor blood pressure closely.

Dopamine (Intropin)

Class Sympathomimetic, inotropic agent.

Mechanism of action Immediate metabolic precursor to norepinephrine. Increases systemic vascular resistance, dilates renal and splanchnic vasculature. Increases myocardial contractility and stroke volume.

Indications Cardiogenic, septic or spinal shock, hypotension with low cardiac output states, distributive shock.

Contraindications Hypovolemic shock, pheochromocytoma, tachyarrhythmias, V-fib.

Adverse reactions Cardiac arrhythmias, hypertension, increased myocardial oxygen demand; extravasation may cause tissue necrosis.

Drug interactions Incompatible in alkaline solutions. MAOIs will enhance effects of dopamine. Bretylium may potentiate effect of dopamine. Beta-blockers may antagonize effects of dopamine. When administered with phenytoin: may cause hypotension, bradycardia, and seizures.

How supplied 200 mg/5 mL–400 mg/5 mL prefilled syringes, ampules for IV infusion; 400 mg in 250-mL D_5W premixed solutions.

Dosage and administration Adult: 2–20 µg/kg/min titrated to patient response; Pediatric: 2–20 µg/kg/min titrated to patient response.

Duration of action Onset: 1–4 minutes. Peak effect: 5–10 minutes. Duration: Effects cease almost immediately after infusion is shut off.

Special considerations Pregnancy safety not established. Effects are dose-dependent. Dopaminergic response: 2–4 µg/kg/min: dilates vessels in kidneys; increased urine output. Beta-adrenergic response: 4–10 µg/kg/min: positive chronotropic and inotropic adrenergic response: 10–20 µg/kg/min: primarily alpha stimulant/vasoconstriction. Greater than 20 µg/kg/min: reversal of renal effects/override alpha effects. Always monitor drip rate. Avoid extravasation injury.

Epinephrine (Adrenalin)

Class Sympathomimetic.

Mechanism of action Direct-acting alpha- and beta-agonist. Alpha: vasoconstriction. Beta-1: positive inotropic, chronotropic, and dromotropic effects. Beta-2: bronchial smooth muscle relaxation and dilation of skeletal vasculature.

Indications Cardiac arrest (V-fib/pulseless V-tach, asystole, PEA), symptomatic bradycardia as an alternative infusion to dopamine, severe hypotension secondary to bradycardia when atropine and transcutaneous pacing are unsuccessful, allergic reactions, anaphylaxis, asthma.

Contraindications Hypertension, hypothermia, pulmonary edema, myocardial ischemia, hypovolemic shock.

Adverse reactions Hypertension, tachycardia, arrhythmias, pulmonary edema, anxiety, restlessness, psychomotor agitation, nausea, headache, angina.

Drug interactions Potentiates other sympathomimetics, deactivated by alkaline solutions (ie, sodium bicarbonate), monamine oxidase inhibitors (MAOIs) may potentiate effects, beta-blockers may blunt effects.

How supplied 1:1,000 solution: ampules and vials containing 1 mg/mL. 1:10,000 solution: prefilled syringes containing 1 mg in 10 mL (0.1 mg/mL). Auto-injector (EpiPen): 0.5 mg/mL (1:2,000).

Dosage and administration Adult: Mild allergic reactions and asthma: 0.3–0.5 mg (0.3–0.5 mL of 1:1,000) SC. Anaphylaxis: 0.1 mg (1 mL of 1:10,000) IV/IO over 5 minutes. Cardiac arrest: IV/IO dose: 1 mg (10 mL of 1:10,000 solution) every 3–5 minutes during resuscitation. Follow each dose with 20 mL flush and elevate arm for 10 to 20 seconds after dose. Higher dose: Higher doses (up to 0.2 mg/kg) may be used for specific indications (beta-blocker or calcium channel blocker overdose). Continuous infusion: Add 1 mg (1 mL of 1:1,000 solution) to 500 mL normal saline or D_5W. Initial infusion rate of 1 µg/min titrated to effect (typical dose: 2–10 µg/min). Endotracheal (ET) dose: 2–2.5 mg diluted in 10 mL normal saline. Profound bradycardia or hypotension: 2–10 µg/min; titrate to patient response. Pediatric: Mild allergic reactions and asthma: 0.01 mg/kg (0.01 mL/kg) of 1:1,000 solution SC (maximum of 0.3 mL). Cardiac arrest: IV/IO dose: 0.01 mg/kg (0.1 mL/kg) of 1:10,000 solution every 3–5 minutes during arrest. All endotracheal (ET) doses: 0.1 mg/kg (0.1 mL/kg) of 1:1,000 solution. Symptomatic bradycardia: IV/IO dose: 0.01 mg/kg (0.1 mL/kg) of 1:10,000 solution. Continuous IV/IO infusion: Begin with rapid infusion, then titrate to response. Typical initial infusion: 0.1–1 µg/min. Higher doses may be effective.

Duration of action Onset: immediate. Peak effect: minutes. Duration: several minutes.

Special considerations Pregnancy safety: Category C. May cause syncope in asthmatic children. May increase myocardial oxygen demand.

Epinephrine Racemic (microNefrin, Vaponefrin)

Class Sympathomimetic.

Mechanism of action Stimulates beta-2 receptors in lungs: bronchodilatation with relaxation of bronchial smooth muscles. Reduces airway resistance. Useful in treating laryngeal edema; inhibits histamine release.

Indications Bronchial asthma, prevention of bronchospasm. Croup, laryngotracheobronchitis, laryngeal edema.

Contraindications Hypertension, underlying cardiovascular disease, epiglottitis.

Adverse reactions Tachycardia, arrhythmias.

Drug interactions MAOIs and bretylium may potentiate effects. Beta-blockers may blunt effects.

How supplied MDI: 0.16–0.25 mg/spray. Solution: 7.5, 15, 30 mL in 1%, 2.25% solutions.

Dosage and administration Adult: MDI: 2–3 inhalations, repeated every 5 minutes as necessary. Solution: dilute 5 mL (1%) in 5.0 mL NS, administer over 15 minutes. Pediatric: Solution: dilute 0.25 mL (0.1%) in 2.5 mL NS (if less than 20 kg); dilute 0.5 mL in 2.5 mL NS (if 20–40 kg); dilute 0.75 mL in 2.5 mL NS (if greater than 40 kg). Administer by aerosolization.

Duration of action Onset: within 5 minutes. Peak effect: 5–15 minutes. Duration: 1–3 hours.

Special considerations May cause tachycardia and other arrhythmias. Monitor vital signs. Excessive use may cause bronchospasm.

Fentanyl Citrate (Sublimase)

Class Narcotic Analgesic (schedule II)

Mechanism of Action Agonist actions at the body's opioid (eg, morphine) receptor. Increases tone and decreases smooth muscles of the GI tract.

Indications This drug is used to treat severe pain, used as an anesthetic or for procedural sedation.

Contraindications Myasthenia gravis, children under 2 years old.

Adverse reactions Skeletal and thoracic muscular rigidity, bradycardia, seizures, and diaphoresis.

Drug interactions May interact with alcohol or any CNS depressants.

How supplied 50 µg/mL ampules

Dosage and administration Adult dose is 25-100 µg (0.5–2 µg/kg) IM, IO, IVP or atomized intranasal. (varies considerably by protocols). Pediatric 2–12 years old: 1.7–3.3 µg/kg IM, IO, IVP.

Duration of action Onset: immediate IV, 7–15 minutes IM, peak effect 3–5 minutes IV, 30 minutes IM, Duration: 30–60 minutes IV, 1–2 hours IM.

Special considerations Pregnancy safety: Category C. May cause life-threatening hypoventilation, naloxone hydrochloride [Narcan] should be readily available.

Flumazenil (Romazicon)

Class Benzodiazepine receptor antagonist.

Mechanism of action Antagonizes the actions of benzodiazepines on the CNS.

Indications Reversal of respiratory depression and sedative effects from pure benzodiazepine overdose.

Contraindications Hypersensitivity, tricyclic antidepressant overdose, seizure-prone patients, coma of unknown etiology, benzodiazepine dependence.

Adverse reactions Nausea, vomiting, agitation, injection site pain, visual disturbances, seizures, cutaneous vasodilation.

Drug interactions Toxic effects of mixed-drug overdose (especially tricyclics).

How supplied 5- and 10-mL vials (0.1 mg/mL).

Dosage and administration Adult: First dose: 0.2 mg IV/IO over 15 seconds. Second dose: 0.3 mg IV/IO over 30 seconds. If no response, give third dose. Third dose: 0.5 mg IV/IO over 30 seconds. If no response, repeat once every minute until adequate response or a total of 3 mg is given. Pediatric: Not recommended.

Duration of action Onset: 1–2 minutes. Peak effect and duration: related to plasma concentration of benzodiazepines.

Special considerations Pregnancy safety: Category C. Be prepared to manage seizures in patients who are physically dependent on benzodiazepines or who have ingested large doses of other drugs. Romazicon may precipitate withdrawal syndromes in patients dependent on benzodiazepines. Monitor patients for re-sedation and respiratory depression. Be prepared to assist ventilations.

Furosemide (Lasix)

Class Loop diuretic.

Mechanism of action Inhibits electrolyte reabsorption and promotes excretion of sodium, potassium, chloride.

Indications CHF, pulmonary edema, hypertensive crisis.

Contraindications Hypovolemia, anuria, hypotension (relative contraindication); hypersensitivity, hepatic coma.

Adverse reactions May exacerbate hypovolemia, hypokalemia, ECG changes, dry mouth, hypochloremia, hyponatremia, hyperglycemia (due to hemoconcentration).

Drug interactions Lithium toxicity may be potentiated by sodium depletion. Digitalis toxicity may be potentiated by potassium depletion.

How supplied 100 mg/5 mL, 20 mg/2 mL, 40 mg/4-mL vials.

Dosage and administration Adult: 0.5–1.0 mg/kg injected IV over 1 to 2 minutes. If no response, double the dose to 2 mg/kg over 1 to 2 minutes. Pediatric: 1 mg/kg/dose IV, IO.

Duration of action Onset: 5 minutes. Peak effects: 20–60 minutes. Duration: 4–6 hours.

Special considerations Pregnancy safety: Category C. Ototoxicity and deafness can occur with rapid administration. Should be protected from light.

Glucagon

Class Hyperglycemic agent, pancreatic hormone, insulin antagonist.

Mechanism of action Increases blood glucose level by increasing glycogenolysis. Unknown mechanism of stabilizing cardiac rhythm in beta-blocker overdose. Minimal positive inotropic and chronotropic response. Decreases gastrointestinal motility and secretions.

Indications Altered level of consciousness when hypoglycemia is suspected. May be used as inotropic agent in beta-blocker overdose.

Contraindications Hyperglycemia, hypersensitivity.

Adverse reactions Nausea, vomiting, tachycardia, hypertension.

Drug interactions Incompatible in solution with most other substances. No significant drug interactions with other emergency medications.

How supplied 1-mg ampules (requires reconstitution with diluent provided).

Dosage and administration Adult: Hypoglycemia: 0.5–1 mg IM; may repeat in 7–10 minutes. Calcium channel blocker or beta-blocker overdose: 3 mg initially, followed by infusion at 3 mg/h as necessary. Pediatric: Hypoglycemia: 0.5–1 mg IM (for children < 20 kg). Calcium channel blocker or beta-blocker overdose: not recommended.

Duration of action Onset: 1 minute. Peak effect: 30 minutes. Duration: variable (generally 9–17 minutes).

Special considerations Pregnancy safety: Category C. Ineffective if glycogen stores depleted. Should always be used in conjunction with 50% dextrose whenever possible. If patient does not respond to second dose glucagon, 50% dextrose must be administered.

Haloperidol (Haldol)

Class Tranquilizer, antipsychotic.

Mechanism of action Inhibits central nervous system (CNS) catecholamine receptors: strong antidopaminergic and weak anticholinergic. Acts on CNS to depress subcortical areas, mid-brain and ascending reticular activating system in the brain.

Indications Acute psychotic episodes.

Contraindications Agitation secondary to shock or hypoxia. Hypersensitivity.

Adverse reactions Extrapyramidal signs and symptoms, restlessness, spasms, Parkinson-like symptoms, drooling, dystonia, hypotension, orthostatic, hypotension, nausea, vomiting, blurred vision.

Drug interactions Enhanced CNS depression and hypotension in combination with alcohol. Antagonized amphetamines and epinephrine. Other CNS depressants may potentiate effects.

How supplied 5 mg/mL ampule.

Dosage and administration Adult: 2–5 mg IM every 30–60 minutes until sedation achieved. Pediatric: Not recommended.

Duration of action Onset: 10 minutes. Peak effect: 30–45 minutes. Duration: variable (generally 12–24 hours).

Special considerations Pregnancy safety: not established. Treat hypotension secondary to Haldol with fluids and norepinephrine, not epinephrine. Patient may also be taking Cogentin (benztropine mesylate) if on long-term therapy with Haldol.

Hydrocortisone Sodium Succinate (Solu-Cortef)

Class Corticosteroid

Mechanism of action Anti-inflammatory and immunosuppressive with salt-retaining actions.

Indications Shock due to acute adrenocortical insufficiency.

Contraindications None if given as single dose.

Adverse reactions Only for long-term use.

Drug interactions Incompatible with heparin and metaraminol.

How supplied 100-mg, 250-mg, or 500-mg vials.

Dosage and administration Adult: 4 mg/kg slow IV bolus. Pediatric: 0.16–1.0 mg/kg slow IV bolus.

Duration of action Onset: 1 hour. Peak effect: variable. Duration: 8–12 hours.

Special considerations May be used in status asthmaticus as a second-line drug.

Hydroxyzine Hydrochloride (Atarax, Vistaril)

Class Antihistamine, antiemetic, antianxiety agent.

Mechanism of action Potentiates effects of analgesics; calming effect without impairing mental alertness.

Indications To potentiate the effects of analgesics; to control nausea and vomiting, anxiety reactions, and motion sickness; preoperative and postoperative sedation.

Contraindications Hypersensitivity.

Adverse reactions Dry mouth and drowsiness.

Drug interactions Potentiates the effects of CNS depressants such as narcotics, barbiturates, and alcohol.

How supplied 25 mg/mL or 50 mg/mL in 1-mL vials.

Dosage and administration Adult: 25–100 mg IM. Pediatric: 0.5–1.0 mg/kg/dose IM.

Duration of action Onset: IM: 15–30 minutes. Peak effect: 45 minutes to 1.5 hours. Duration: 4–6 hours.

Special considerations Should be given by IM injection only. Localized burning at injection site is common complaint.

Ipratropium Bromide (Atrovent)

Class Anticholinergic.

Mechanism of action Antagonizes action of acetylcholine on bronchial smooth muscle in the lungs causing bronchodilation.

Indications Maintenance treatment of bronchospasm in patients with reversible obstructive airway disease (COPD/asthma). Can be used alone or in combination with other bronchodilators (especially beta-adrenergics).

Contraindications Known prior hypersensitivity reactions to ipratropium bromide. Hypersensitivity to atropine or any anticholinergic derivatives or to soya lecithin or related food products.

Adverse reactions Palpitations, aggravates hypertension, exacerbates cough symptoms, nervousness, dizziness, and headache. Can also cause blurred vision; local irritation; epistaxis, nasal dryness, nasal congestion, taste perversion, nasal burning, conjunctivitis, hoarseness, pharyngitis (0.06% nasal spray formulation only).

Drug interactions Ipratropium bromide has been shown to be a safe and effective bronchodilator when used in conjunction with beta adrenergic bronchodilators. Ipratropium bromide has also been used with other pulmonary medications, including methylxanthines and corticosteroids, without adverse reactions.

How supplied Solution for aerosolization: a clear, colorless solution in 2.5-mL unit dose vials.

Dosage and administration Adult: Administer 500 μg (1 Unit-Dose vial) administered three to four times a day by oral nebulization, with doses 6 to 8 hours apart. Ipratropium Bromide Inhalation Solution Unit-Dose vials contain 500 μg Ipratropium bromide anhydrous in 2.5 mL normal saline. Ipratropium Bromide Inhalation Solution can be mixed in the nebulizer with albuterol or metaproterenol if used within one hour. Pediatric: Safety and effectiveness in the pediatric population below the age of 12 have not been established.

Duration of action Onset: 15–30 minutes; peak effect: 1–2 hours; duration of action: 4–5 hours.

Special considerations Pregnancy safety: Category B. Safety and efficacy in children younger than 12 yr of age not established for aerosol and solution; younger than 6 yr of age for 0.03% nasal spray; younger than 5 yr of age for 0.06% nasal spray.

Isoetharine (Bronchosol, Bronkometer)

Class Sympathomimetic.

Mechanism of action Beta-2 agonist; relaxes smooth muscle of bronchioles.

Indications Acute bronchial asthma, bronchospasm (especially in COPD patient).

Contraindications Use with caution in patients with diabetes, hyperthyroidism, cardiovascular and cerebrovascular disease.

Adverse reactions Dose-related tachycardia, palpitations, tremors, nervousness, nausea. Multiple doses can cause paradoxical bronchoconstriction.

Drug interactions Additive adverse effects if given with other beta-2 agonist drugs.

How supplied MDI; 2 mL unit dose of 1% solution.

Dosage and administration Adult: 1–2 inhalations with MDI. COPD: 2.5–5.0 mg (0.25 mL–0.5 mL) diluted in 3 mL normal saline (NS) and nebulized. Pediatric: 0.01 mL/kg; maximum dose: 0.5 mL diluted in 3 mL NS and nebulized.

Duration of action Onset: immediate. Peak effect: 5–15 minutes. Duration: 1–4 hours.

Special considerations None.

Ketorolac Tromethamine (Toradol IM)

Class Nonsteroidal anti-inflammatory (NSAID) analgesic.

Mechanism of action NSAID that also exhibits peripherally acting nonnarcotic analgesic activity by inhibiting prostaglandin synthesis.

Indications Short-term management of moderate to severe pain.

Contraindications Allergy to salicylates or other NSAIDs; patients with history of asthma; bleeding disorders, especially gastrointestinal (GI) related (peptic ulcer disease); renal failure.

Adverse reactions Anaphylaxis due to hypersensitivity, nausea, GI bleeding, sedation, hypotension or hypertension, rash, headache, edema.

Drug interactions May increase bleeding time in patients taking anticoagulants.

How supplied 15 or 30 mg in 1 mL or 60 mg in 2-mL vials.

Dosage and administration Adult: 30–60 mg IM. Pediatric: Not recommended.

Duration of action Onset: 10 minutes. Peak effect: 1–2 hours. Duration: 2–6 hours.

Special considerations Pregnancy safety: Category C. Use with caution in elderly patient. May be given IV in lower dosage (15–30 mg).

Labetalol (Normodyne, Trandate)

Class Selective alpha and nonselective beta-adrenergic blocker.

Mechanism of action Blood pressure reduced without reflex tachycardia; total peripheral resistance reduced without significant alteration in cardiac output.

Indications Moderate to severe hypertension.

Contraindications Bronchial asthma, CHF, cardiogenic shock, second- and third-degree heart block, bradycardia.

Adverse reactions Headache, dizziness, ventricular arrhythmias, hypotension, dyspnea, facial flushing, postural hypotension, diaphoresis, allergic reaction.

Drug interactions Trandate may block bronchodilator effects of beta-adrenergic agonists. NTG may augment hypotensive effects of Labetalol.

How supplied Trandate injection 5 mg/mL, 20 mL (100 mg) and 40 mL (200 mg) vials.

Dosage and administration Adult: 5–20 mg slow IV over 2 minutes (additional injections of 10–40 mg can be given at 10-minute intervals). Infusion: 2 mg/min titrated to acceptable supine blood pressure. Pediatric: safety not established.

Duration of action Onset: less than 5 minutes. Peak effect: variable. Duration: 3–6 hours.

Special considerations Pregnancy safety: Category C. Continuous monitoring of BP, pulse rate, and ECG. Observe for signs of CHF, bradycardia, bronchospasm. Should only be administered with patient in supine position.

Levalbuterol (Xopenex)

Class Bronchodilator, adrenergic Beta-2 agonist.

Mechanism of Action Causes bronchodilation by action on the Beta-2 pulmonary receptors to relax smooth muscle as well as produce CNS and cardiac stimulation.

Indications Used to treat or prevent bronchospasm in patients 6 years or older. Relaxes the smooth muscles of the lower airways.

Contraindications Known sensitivity to the drug. Hypersensitivity to sympathomimetics, tachyarrhythmias, and severe cardiac disease.

Adverse reactions Tremors, anxiety, insomnia, headache, dizziness, restlessness, hallucinations, flushing, irritability, vomiting, nausea, palpitations, tachycardia, hypertension, angina, hypotension, and arrhythmias.

Drug interactions Increased actions of aerosol bronchodilators, tricyclic antidepressants, MAOIs, and other adrenergics.

How supplied Solution for inhalation 0.63 mg, 1.25 mg/3 mL.

Dosage and administration For adults and pediatrics over 6 years old: 1.25 mg in 3 mL administered by the nebulizer route. For adults only: 2 puffs by MDI.

Duration of action Onset: 5–15 minutes, peak effect: 60–90 minutes, duration: 6–8 hours. Metabolized in the liver.

Special considerations Crosses the placenta, breast milk, blood-brain barrier. Precautions should be taken with lactation, pregnancy (Class C), cardiac disorders, hyperthyroidism, diabetes mellitus, hypertension, prostatic hypertrophy, narrow-angle glaucoma, and seizures.

Lidocaine Hydrochloride (Xylocaine)

Class Antiarrhythmic.

Mechanism of action Decreases automaticity by slowing the rate of phase 4 depolarization.

Indications Alternative to amiodarone in cardiac arrest from V-fib/pulseless V-tach, stable monomorphic V-tach, stable polymorphic V-tach with normal baseline QT interval.

Contraindications Hypersensitivity, second- and third-degree AV blocks in the absence of artificial pacemaker, Stokes-Adams syndrome, prophylactic use in AMI, wide-complex ventricular escape beats with bradycardia.

Adverse reactions Slurred speech, seizures (with high doses), altered mental status, confusion, lightheadedness, blurred vision, bradycardia.

Drug interactions Apnea induced with succinylcholine may be prolonged with high doses of lidocaine. Cardiac depression may occur in conjunction with IV phenytoin (Dilantin). Procainamide may exacerbate CNS effects. Metabolic clearance is decreased in patients with liver disease or in patients taking beta-blockers.

How supplied 100 mg in 5-mL prefilled syringes and ampules (20 mg/mL), 1-g and 2-g additive syringes, 1-g and 2-g vials in 30 mL of solution.

Dosage and administration Adult: Cardiac arrest from V-fib/pulseless V-tach: Initial dose: 1–1.5 mg/kg IV/IO. Repeat dose: 0.5–0.75 mg/kg, repeated in 5–10 minutes to maximum dose of 3 mg/kg. Endotracheal (ET) dose: 2–4 mg/kg. Stable V-tach, wide-complex tachycardia of uncertain type, significant ectopy: Doses ranging from 0.5–0.75 mg/kg and up to 1–1.5 mg/kg may be used. Repeat 0.5–0.75 mg/kg every 5–10 minutes. Maximum total dose is 3 mg/kg. Maintenance infusion: 1–4 mg/min (30–50 µg/kg/min); can dilute in D_5W or normal saline. Pediatric: IV/IO dose: 1 mg/kg rapid IV/IO push. Maximum dose: 100 mg. Continuous IV/IO infusion: 20–50 µg/kg/min. Administer bolus dose (1 mg/kg) when infusion is initiated if bolus has not been given within previous 15 minutes. Endotracheal (ET) dose: 2–3 mg/kg.

Duration of action Onset: 1–3 minutes. Peak effect: 5–10 minutes. Duration: variable (15 minutes–2 hours).

Special considerations Pregnancy safety: Category B. Reduce maintenance infusions by 50% if patient is over 70 years of age, has liver or renal disease, or is in CHF or shock. A 75–100 mg bolus maintains blood levels for only 20 minutes (if not in shock). Exceedingly high doses of lidocaine can result in coma or death. Avoid lidocaine for reperfusion arrhythmias after fibrinolytic therapy. Cross-reactivity with other forms of local anesthetics.

Lorazepam (Ativan)

Class Benzodiazepine; sedative; anticonvulsant.

Mechanism of action Anxiolytic, anticonvulsant, and sedative effects; suppresses propagation of seizure activity produced by foci in cortex, thalamus, and limbic areas.

Indications Initial control of status epilepticus or severe recurrent seizures, severe anxiety, sedation.

Contraindications Acute narrow-angle glaucoma. Coma, shock, or suspected drug abuse.

Adverse reactions Respiratory depression, apnea, drowsiness, sedation, ataxia, psychomotor impairment, confusion, restlessness, delirium, hypotension, bradycardia.

Drug interactions May precipitate CNS depression if patient is already taking CNS depressant medications.

How supplied 2 and 4 mg/mL concentrations in 1-mL vials.

Dosage and administration Note: When given IV or IO, must dilute with equal volume of sterile water or sterile saline; When given IM, lorazepam is not to be diluted. Adult: 2–4 mg slow IV at 2 mg/min or IM; may repeat in 15–20 minutes to maximum dose of 8 mg. For sedation: 0.05 mg/kg up to 4 mg IM. Pediatric: 0.05–0.20 mg/kg slow IV, IO slowly over 2 minutes or IM; may repeat in 15–20 minutes to maximum dose of 0.2 mg/kg.

Duration of action Onset: 1–5 minutes. Peak effect: variable. Duration: 6–8 hours.

Special considerations Pregnancy safety: Category D. Monitor BP and respiratory rate during administration. Have advanced airway equipment readily available. Inadvertent arterial injection may result in vasospasm and gangrene. Lorazepam expires in 6 weeks if not refrigerated.

Magnesium Sulfate

Class Electrolyte.

Mechanism of action Reduces striated muscle contractions and blocks peripheral neuromuscular transmission by reducing acetylcholine release at the myoneural junction, manages seizures in toxemia of pregnancy, induces uterine relaxation, can cause bronchodilation after beta-agonists and anticholinergics have been used.

Indications Seizures of eclampsia (toxemia of pregnancy), torsade de pointes, hypomagnesemia, Class IIa agent for V-fib/pulseless V-tach that is refractory to lidocaine.

Contraindications Heart blocks, myocardial damage.

Adverse reactions CNS depression, facial flushing, diaphoresis, depressed reflexes, circulatory collapse, hypotension.

Drug interactions May enhance effects of other CNS depressants, serious changes in overall cardiac function may occur with cardiac glycosides.

How supplied 10%, 12.5%, 50% solution in 40, 80, 100, and 125 mg/mL.

Dosage and administration Adult: Seizure activity associated with pregnancy: 1–4 g IV/IO over 3 minutes; maximum dose of 30–40 g/day. Cardiac arrest due to hypomagnesemia or torsade de pointes: 1–2 g (2–4 mL of a 50% solution) diluted in 10 mL of D_5W IV/IO over 5–20 minutes. Torsade de pointes with a pulse or AMI with hypomagnesemia: Loading dose of 1–2 g mixed in 50–100 mL D_5W over 5–60 minutes IV. Follow with 0.5–1 g/hr IV (titrate to control torsade de pointes). Pediatric: IV/IO infusion: 25–50 mg/kg (maximum dose: 2 g) over 10–20 minutes; faster for torsade de pointes. For asthma: 25–50 mg/kg (maximum dose: 2 g) over 10–20 minutes.

Duration of action Onset: IV/IO: immediate, IM: 3–4 hours, Duration: 30 minutes (IV/IO), 3–4 hours (IM).

Special considerations Pregnancy safety: Category B. Recommended that the drug not be given in the 2 hours before delivery, if possible. IV calcium chloride or calcium gluconate should be available as a magnesium antagonist if needed. Use with caution in patients with renal failure.

Meperidine Hydrochloride (Demerol)

Class Opioid analgesic.

Mechanism of action Synthetic opioid agonist that acts on opioid receptors to produce analgesia, euphoria, respiratory and physical depression; a schedule II drug with potential for physical dependency and abuse.

Indications Analgesia for moderate to severe pain.

Contraindications Hypersensitivity to narcotic agents, diarrhea caused by poisoning, patients taking MAOIs, during labor or delivery of a premature infant, undiagnosed abdominal pain or head injury.

Adverse reactions Respiratory depression, sedation, apnea, circulatory depression, arrhythmias, shock, euphoria, delirium, agitation, hallucinations, visual disturbances, coma, seizures, headache, facial flushing, increased ICP, nausea, vomiting.

Drug interactions Do not give concurrently with MAOIs (even with a dose in the last 14 days!). Exacerbates CNS depression when given with these medications.

How supplied 50 mL in 1-mL prefilled syringes and Tubex.

Dosage and administration Adult: 50–100 mg IM, SC or 25–50 mg slowly IV. Pediatric: 1–2 mg/kg/dose IV, IO, IM, SC.

Duration of action Onset: IM: 10–45 minutes; IV: immediate. Peak effect: 30–60 minutes. Duration: 2–4 hours.

Special considerations Pregnancy safety: Category C. Use with caution in patients with asthma and COPD. May aggravate seizures in patients with known convulsive disorders. Naloxone hydrochloride (Narcan) should be readily available as antagonist.

Metaproterenol 5% (Alupent)

Class Sympathomimetic bronchodilator.

Mechanism of action Beta-2 agonist acts directly on bronchial smooth muscle causing relaxation of the bronchial tree and peripheral vasculature.

Indications Bronchial asthma, reversible bronchospasm secondary to bronchitis, COPD.

Contraindications Tachyarrhythmias, hypersensitivity, tachycardias due to digitalis toxicity.

Adverse reactions Tachyarrhythmias, anxiety, nausea, vomiting, restlessness, apprehension, palpitations, hypotension, coughing, facial flushing, diaphoresis.

Drug interactions Other sympathomimetics may exacerbate cardiovascular effects. MAOIs may potentiate hypotensive effects. Beta-blockers may antagonize metaproterenol.

How supplied MDI: 0.65 mg/dose/spray (15-mL inhaler). Solution: 5% solution in bottles of 10 and 30 mL with calibrated dropper; Alupent inhalation solution unit-dose vial, 0.4% or 0.6%.

Dosage and administration Adult: MDI: 2–3 inhalations every 3–4 hours (2 minutes between inhalations). Inhalation solution 5%: via hand-held nebulizer 0.2–0.3 mL diluted in 2.5 mL saline. Inhalation solution unit-dose 0.4% or 0.6% vials: intermittent positive-pressure breathing device only: one vial/treatment. Pediatric: MDI: not recommended. Inhalation solution 5%: age 6–12 years: 0.1–0.2 mL diluted in 3 mL saline.

Duration of action Onset: 1 minute after inhalation. Peak effect: 45 minutes. Duration: 3–6 hours.

Special considerations Pregnancy safety: Category C. Monitor for hypotension or tachycardia. Use with caution in patients with diabetes mellitus and coronary artery disease.

Methylprednisolone Sodium Succinate (Solu-Medrol)

Class Anti-inflammatory glucocorticoid.

Mechanism of action Synthetic corticosteroid that suppresses acute and chronic inflammation; potentiates vascular smooth muscle relaxation by beta-adrenergic agonists.

Indications Acute spinal cord trauma, anaphylaxis, bronchodilator for unresponsive asthma.

Contraindications Premature infants, systemic fungal infections; use with caution in patients with gastrointestinal bleeding, sepsis, local infection.

Adverse reactions Headache, hypertension, sodium and water retention. CHF, hypokalemia, alkalosis, peptic ulcer disease, nausea, vomiting.

Drug interactions Hypoglycemic responses to insulin and hypoglycemic agents may be blunted. Potassium-depleting agents may exacerbate hypokalemic effects.

How supplied 40-, 125-, 500- and 1,000-mg vials.

Dosage and administration Adult: Acute spinal cord injury: 30 mg/kg IV over 30 minutes followed by infusion: 5.4 mg/kg/h. Asthma, COPD: 1–2 mg/kg IV. Pediatric: Acute spinal cord trauma: 30 mg/kg IV over 30 minutes; infusion: 5.4 mg/kg/h. Asthma: 1–2 mg/kg/dose IV.

Duration of action Onset of action: 1–2 hours. Peak effects: variable. Duration of action: 8–24 hours.

Special considerations Pregnancy safety: not established. Not effective if spinal cord injury greater than 8 hours. Crosses the placenta and may cause fetal harm.

Metoprolol Tartrate (Lopressor)

Class Beta-adrenergic receptor blocking agent

Mechanism of action Exerts mostly beta-1 adrenergic blocking activity although beta-2 receptors are blocked at high doses. The precise action in patients with suspected ACS is not known.

Indications Suspected ACS provided heart rate is > 80 beats/min and systolic blood pressure is > 120 mm Hg. Patients may be taking the tablet form for hypertension or angina. The usual tablet initial dose is 100 mg and effective dose is between 100 and 400 mg daily. Has also been used for ventricular arrhythmias and migraine headaches. Paramedic protocols are usually for the IV dose of the drug.

Contraindications In the context of a suspected MI, the drug is contraindicated in patients with a heart rate < 45 beats/min; second- and third-degree heart block; significant first-degree heart block (P-R interval ≥ 0.24 sec); systolic blood pressure < 100 mm Hg; or moderate to severe cardiac failure. Hypersensitivity to the drug, related derivatives, or other beta-blockers (cross sensitivity between beta-blockers can occur).

Adverse reactions For suspected MI include: CNS symptoms: tiredness, vertigo, sleep disturbances, hallucinations, headache, dizziness, visual disturbances, and confusion. Respiratory symptoms: dyspnea. Gastrointestinal symptoms: nausea and abdominal pain. Dermatologic symptoms: rash and worsened psoriasis.

Drug interactions Catecholamine-depleting drugs may have an additive effect when given with beta-blocking agents. Patients treated with Lopressor plus a catecholamine depletor should be closely observed for evidence of hypotension or marked bradycardia, which may produce vertigo, syncope, or postural hypotension. Risk of anaphylactic reaction. While taking beta-blockers, patients with a history of severe anaphylactic reaction to a variety of allergens may be more reactive to repeated challenge, either accidental, diagnostic, or therapeutic. Such patients may be unresponsive to the usual doses of epinephrine used to treat allergic reaction.

How supplied Metoprolol tartrate (for injection) comes in 5-mL ampules containing 5 mg.

Dosage and administration Adult: 5 mg slow IV bolus, may be repeated every 2 minutes up to maximum of 15 mg. Pediatric: Not recommended.

Duration of action Onset: 1–5 minutes. Peak effect: 90 minutes. Metabolized in the liver, excreted in the urine.

Special considerations Pregnancy safety: Category C. Precautions with patients who have impaired hepatic function.

Midazolam (Versed)

Class Short-acting benzodiazepine CNS depressant.

Mechanism of action Anxiolytic and sedative properties similar to other benzodiazepines, memory impairment.

Indications Sedation, anxiolytic prior to endotracheal or nasotracheal intubation; administer for conscious sedation.

Contraindications Glaucoma, shock, coma, alcohol intoxication, overdose, depressed vital signs, concomitant use with other CNS depressants, barbiturates, alcohol, narcotics.

Adverse reactions Hiccough, cough, oversedation, nausea, vomiting, injection site pain, headache, blurred vision, hypotension, respiratory depression, and arrest.

Drug interactions Should not be used in patients who have taken a CNS depressant.

How supplied 2-, 5-, 10-mL vials (1 mg/mL); 1-, 2- , 5-, 10-mL vials (5 mg/mL).

Dosage and administration Adult: 2.0–2.5 mg slow IV over 2–3 minutes; may be repeated to total maximum: 0.1 mg/kg. Pediatric: Not recommended.

Duration of action Onset: 1–3 minutes, IV and dose dependent. Peak effect: variable. Duration: 2–6 hours, dose dependent.

Special considerations Pregnancy safety: Category D. Administer immediately prior to intubation procedure. Requires continuous monitoring of respiratory and cardiac function. Never administer as IV bolus.

Morphine Sulfate (Astramorph/PF and others)

Class Opioid analgesic (schedule II narcotic).

Mechanism of action Alleviates pain through CNS action, suppresses fear and anxiety centers in brain; depresses brain stem respiratory centers, increases peripheral venous capacitance and decreases venous return, decreases preload and afterload, which decreases myocardial oxygen demand.

Indications Severe CHF, pulmonary edema, chest pain associated with acute MI, analgesia for moderate to severe acute and chronic pain (use with caution).

Contraindications Head injury, exacerbated COPD, depressed respiratory drive, hypotension, undiagnosed abdominal pain, decreased level of consciousness, suspected hypovolemia, patients who have taken MAOIs within the past 14 days.

Adverse reactions Respiratory depression, hypotension, decreased level of consciousness, nausea, vomiting, bradycardia, tachycardia, syncope, facial flushing, euphoria, bronchospasm, dry mouth.

Drug interactions Potentiates sedative effects of phenothiazines. CNS depressant may potentiate effects of morphine. MAOIs may cause paradoxical excitation.

How supplied 10 mg in 1 mL of solution, ampules, and Tubex syringes.

Dosage and administration Adult: Initial dose: 2–4 mg IV (over 1–5 minutes) every 5–30 minutes. Repeat dose: 2–8 mg at 5- to 15-minute intervals. Pediatric: 0.1–0.2 mg/kg per dose via IV, IO, IM, or SC; maximum dose of 5 mg.

Duration of action Onset: immediate. Peak effect: 20 minutes. Duration: 2–7 hours.

Special considerations Pregnancy safety: Category C. Morphine rapidly crosses the placenta. Safety in neonate not established. Use with caution in geriatric population and those with COPD, asthma. Vagotonic effect in patient with acute inferior MI (bradycardia, heart block). Naloxone hydrochloride (Narcan) should be readily available as an antidote.

Nalbuphine Hydrochloride (Nubain)

Class Opioid analgesic.

Mechanism of action Activates opiate receptor in limbic system of CNS, analgesic similar to morphine on a milligram for milligram basis, agonist and antagonist properties; may be preferred for chest pain in setting of acute MI as it reduces the myocardial oxygen demand without reducing the blood pressure.

Indications Chest pain associated with acute MI; moderate to severe acute pain; pulmonary edema, with or without associated chest pain (morphine remains first line).

Contraindications Head injury or undiagnosed abdominal pain, diarrhea caused by poisoning, hypovolemia, hypotension.

Adverse reactions Hypotension, bradycardia, facial flushing, respiratory depression, CNS depression, euphoria, paradoxical CNS stimulation, blurred vision.

Drug interactions CNS depressants may potentiate effects.

How supplied 10 mg in 1-mL ampule (10 mg/mL), 20 mg in 1-mL ampule.

Dosage and administration Adult: 2–5 mg slowly IV; may repeat 2-mg doses as necessary to maximum dose of 10 mg. Pediatric: Not recommended.

Duration of action Onset: 2–3 minutes. Peak effect: variable. Duration: 3–6 hours.

Special considerations Pregnancy safety: Category B. Use with caution in patients with impaired respiratory function. May precipitate withdrawal syndromes in narcotic-dependent patients. Naloxone hydrochloride (Narcan) should be readily available.

Naloxone Hydrochloride (Narcan)

Class Narcotic antagonist.

Mechanism of action Competitive inhibition at narcotic receptor sites, reverse respiratory depression secondary to opiate drugs, completely inhibits the effect of morphine.

Indications Opiate overdose, coma; complete or partial reversal of CNS and respiratory depression induced by opioids; decreased level of consciousness; coma of unknown origin; narcotic agonist for the following: morphine, heroin, hydromorphone (Dilaudid), methadone, meperidine (Demerol), paregoric, fentanyl citrate (Sublimase), oxycodone (Percodan), codeine, propoxyphene (Darvon); narcotic agonist and antagonist for the following: Butorphanol (Stadol), pentazocine (Talwin), nalbuphine (Nubain).

Contraindications Use with caution in narcotic-dependent patients; use with caution in neonates of narcotic-addicted mothers.

Adverse reactions Withdrawal symptoms in the addicted patient, tachycardia, hypertension, arrhythmias, nausea, vomiting, diaphoresis.

Drug interactions Incompatible with bisulfite and alkaline solutions.

How supplied 0.02 mg/mL (neonate); 0.4 mg/mL, 1 mg/mL; 2.0 mg/5-mL ampules; 2 mg/5-mL prefilled syringe.

Dosage and administration Adult: 0.4–2.0 mg IV, IM, SC, or ET (diluted); minimum recommended dose, 0.4 mg; repeat at 5-minute intervals to a maximum dose of 10 mg (medical control may request higher amounts). Infusion: 2 mg in 500 mL of D_5W (4 µg/mL), infuse at 0.4 mg/h (100 mL/h). Pediatric: 0.1 mg/kg/dose IV, IM, SC, ET (diluted); maximum dose of 0.8 mg; if no response in 10 minutes, administer an additional 0.1 mg/kg/dose.

Duration of action Onset: within 2 minutes. Peak effect: variable. Duration: 30–60 minutes.

Special considerations Pregnancy safety: Category B. Seizures without causal relationship have been reported. May not reverse hypotension. Use caution when administering to narcotic addicts (potential violent behavior).

Nifedipine (Procardia)

Class Calcium channel blocker.

Mechanism of action Inhibits movement of calcium ions across cell membranes; calcium channel blocker, arterial and venous vasodilator; reduces preload and afterload; prevents coronary artery spasm and decreases total peripheral resistance; reduces myocardial oxygen demand; does not prolong AV nodal conduction.

Indications Hypertensive crisis, angina pectoris, pulmonary edema (investigational).

Contraindications Compensatory hypertension, hypotension, hypersensitivity.

Adverse reactions Hypotension, CHF, headache, dizziness, lightheadedness, facial flushing, heat sensation, weakness, nausea, muscle cramps, mood changes, peripheral edema, myocardial infarction.

Drug interactions Beta-blockers may potentiate effects. Effects of theophylline may be increased. Antihypertensives may potentiate hypotensive effects.

How supplied Soft gelatin capsules, 10–20 mg. Extended-release tablets, 30, 60, 90 mg.

Dosage and administration Adult: 10 mg SL or buccal (puncture end of capsule with needle and squeeze; may administer SL or buccally or may have patient bite and swallow); may repeat in 30 minutes. Pediatric: Not recommended.

Duration of action Onset: 15–30 minutes. Peak effect: 1–3 hours. Duration: 6–8 hours.

Special considerations Pregnancy safety: Category C. Does not slow AV nodal activity. Have beta-blocker available for control of reflex tachycardia. Use with caution in geriatric population; hypotension and angina pectoris may occur.

Nitroglycerin (Nitrostat, Tridil, and others)

Class Vasodilator.

Mechanism of action Smooth muscle relaxant acting on vascular, bronchial, uterine, and intestinal smooth muscle; dilation of arterioles and veins in the periphery; reduces preload and afterload; decreases the work load of the heart and, thereby, myocardial oxygen demand.

Indications Acute angina pectoris, ischemic chest pain, hypertension, CHF, pulmonary edema.

Contraindications Hyptension, hypovolemia; intracranial bleeding or head injury; previous administration of Viagra, Revatio, Levitra, Cialis, or similar agents within past 24 hours.

Adverse reactions Headache, hypotension, syncope, reflex tachycardia, flushing, nausea, vomiting, diaphoresis, muscle twitching.

Drug interactions Additive effects with other vasodilators; incompatible with other drugs IV.

How supplied Tablets: 0.15 mg (1/400 grain); 0.3 mg (1/200 grain); 0.4 mg (1/150 grain); 0.6 mg (1/100 grain). NTG spray: 0.4 mg–0.8 mg under the tongue. NTG IV (Tridil).

Dosage and administration Adult: Tablets: 0.3–0.4 mg SL; may repeat in 3–5 minutes to maximum of 3 doses. NTG spray: 0.4 mg under the tongue; 1–2 sprays. NTG IV infusion: begin at 10 to 20 µg/min; increase by 5–10 µg/min every 5 minutes until desired effect. Pediatric: Not recommended.

Duration of action Onset: 1–3 minutes. Peak effect: 5–10 minutes. Duration: 20–30 minutes or if IV, 1–10 minutes after discontinuation of infusion.

Special considerations Pregnancy safety: Category C. Hypotension more common in geriatric population. NTG decomposes if exposed to light or heat. Must be kept in airtight containers. Active ingredient may have a stinging effect when administered.

Nitropaste (Nitro-Bid Ointment)

Class Vasodilator.

Mechanism of action Same as NTG.

Indications Angina pectoris and chest pain associated with acute MI.

Contraindications Same as NTG.

Adverse reactions Same as NTG.

Drug interactions Same as NTG.

How supplied 2% solution of NTG in absorbent paste; 20-, 60-g tubes of paste with measuring applicators; transdermal units of varying doses.

Dosage and administration Adult: Paste: Apply ½-inch to ¾-inch (1–2 cm), 15–30 mg, cover with wrap and secure with tape; maximum, 5-inch (75 mg) per application. Transdermal: Apply unit to intact skin (usually chest wall) in varying doses. Pediatric: Not recommended.

Duration of action Onset: 30 minutes. Peak effect: variable. Duration: 18–24 hours.

Special considerations Pregnancy safety: Category C. Not of great value in prehospital arena. Avoid using fingers to spread paste. Store paste in cool place with tube tightly capped. Erratic absorption rates quite common.

Nitrous Oxide: Oxygen (50:50) (Nitronox)

Class Gaseous analgesic and anesthetic.

Mechanism of action Exact mechanism unknown; affects central nervous system phospholipids.

Indications Moderate to severe pain, anxiety, apprehension.

Contraindications Impaired level of consciousness, head injury, inability to comply with instructions; decompression sickness (nitrogen narcosis, air embolism, air transport); undiagnosed abdominal pain or marked distention, bowel obstruction; hypotension, shock, COPD (with history/suspicion of carbon dioxide retention); cyanosis; chest trauma with pneumothorax.

Adverse reactions Dizziness, apnea, expansion of gas-filled pockets, cyanosis, nausea, vomiting, malignant hyperthermia, drowsiness, euphoria.

Drug interactions None of significance.

How supplied D and E cylinders (blue and green); of 50% nitrous oxide and 50% oxygen compressed gas.

Dosage and administration Adult: (Note: Invert cylinder several times before use) Instruct the patient to inhale deeply through demand valve and mask or mouthpiece. Pediatric: Same as adult.

Duration of action Onset: 2–5 minutes. Peak effect: variable. Duration: 2–5 minutes.

Special considerations Pregnancy safety: Nitrous oxide increases the incidence of spontaneous abortion. Ventilate patient area during use. Nitrous oxide is a nonflammable and nonexplosive gas. Nitrous oxide is ineffective in 20% of the population.

Norepinephrine Bitartrate (Levophed, Levarterenol)

Class Sympathomimetic.

Mechanism of action Potent alpha-agonist resulting in intense vasoconstriction; positive chronotropic and increased inotropic effect (from 10% beta effects) with increased cardiac output.

Indications Cardiogenic shock, significant hypotensive (< 70 mm Hg) states.

Contraindications Hypotensive patients with hypovolemia, pregnancy (relative contraindication).

Adverse reactions Headache, arrhythmias, tachycardia, reflex bradycardia; angina pectoris, hypertension; decreased blood flow to gastrointestinal tract, kidneys, skeletal muscle, and skin.

Drug interactions Can be deactivated by alkaline solutions. Sympathomimetics and phosphodiesterase inhibitors may exacerbate arrhythmias. Bretylium may potentiate the effects of catecholamines.

How supplied 1-mg/mL, 4-mL ampules.

Dosage and administration Adult: Dilute 8 mg in 500 mL of D_5W or 4 mg in 250 mL of D_5W (16 mg/mL); infuse by IV piggyback at 0.5–1.0 µg/min, titrated to improve blood pressure (up to 30 µg/min). Pediatric: 0.1–1.0 µg/min IV infusion, titrated to patient response.

Duration of action Onset: 1–3 minutes. Peak effect: variable. Duration: 5–10 minutes and lasts only 1 minute after infusion discontinued.

Special considerations Pregnancy safety: not established. May cause fetal anoxia when used in pregnancy. Must be infused through large stable vein to avoid tissue necrosis (antidote: local phentolamine injection). Often used with low-dose dopamine to spare renal and mesenteric blood flow.

Ondansetron Hydrochloride (Zofran)

Class 5-HT3 receptor antagonist.

Mechanism of action Blocks action of serotonin, which is a natural substance that causes nausea or vomiting.

Indications For the prevention or control of nausea or vomiting. Also used in the hospital setting for patients undergoing chemotherapy or surgical procedures.

Contraindications Known allergy to this medicine or other 5-HT3 receptor antagonists.

Adverse reactions Chest pain, wheezing or hives/skin rash.

Drug interactions Not recommended if the patient is taking: apomorphine, mesoridazine, pimozide, or thioridazine.

How supplied Tablets (not for emergency use) and injectable solution in 2-mL single dose vial containing 2 mg/mL.

Dosage and administration Adult: 4 mg IV or IM (may repeat in 10 minutes). Pediatric: 0.1 mg/kg IV or IM.

Duration of action Onset: 30 minutes. Peak effect: 2 hours. Duration: 3–6 hours.

Special considerations Pregnancy safety: Category B.

Oral Glucose (Insta-Glucose)

Class Hyperglycemic.

Mechanism of action Provides quickly absorbed glucose to increase blood glucose levels.

Indications Conscious patients with suspected hypoglycemia.

Contraindications Decreased level of consciousness, nausea, vomiting.

Adverse reactions Nausea, vomiting.

Drug interactions None.

How supplied Glucola: 300-mL bottles. Glucose pastes and gels in various forms.

Dosage and administration Adult: Should be sipped slowly by patient until clinical improvement noted. Pediatric: Same as adult.

Duration of action Onset: immediate. Peak effect: variable. Duration: variable.

Special considerations As noted in indications section.

Oxygen

Class Naturally occurring atmospheric gas.

Mechanism of action Reverses hypoxemia.

Indications Confirmed or expected hypoxemia, ischemic chest pain, respiratory insufficiency, prophylactically during air transport, confirmed or suspected carbon monoxide poisoning, all other causes of decreased tissue oxygenation, decreased level of consciousness.

Contraindications Certain patients with COPD or emphysema who will not tolerate oxygen concentrations over 35%, hyperventilation. Oxygen should never be withheld from a patient who needs it however. Be prepared to assist with ventilations in a patient with COPD who requires high concentration, as apnea may result.

Adverse reactions Decreased level of consciousness and respiratory depression in patients with chronic carbon dioxide retention. Retrolental fibroplasia if giving high concentrations to premature infants (maintain 30%-40% oxygen).

Drug interactions None.

How supplied Oxygen cylinders (usually green and white) of 100% compressed oxygen gas.

Dosage and administration Adult: Cardiac arrest and carbon monoxide poisoning: 100%. Hypoxemia: 10–15 L/min via nonrebreathing mask. COPD: 1–6 L/min via nasal cannula or 28%–35% Venturi mask. Be prepared to provide ventilatory support if higher concentrations of oxygen needed. Pediatric: Same as for adult with exception of premature infant.

Duration of action Onset: immediate. Peak effect: not applicable. Duration: Less than 2 minutes.

Special considerations Be familiar with liter flow and each type of delivery device used. Supports possibility of combustion.

Oxytocin (Pitocin)

Class Hormone.

Mechanism of action Increases uterine contractions.

Indications Postpartum hemorrhage after infant and placental delivery.

Contraindications Presence of second fetus, unfavorable fetal position, hypersensitivity.

Adverse reactions Hypotension, hypertension, tachycardia, arrhythmias, angina pectoris; anxiety, seizures, nausea, vomiting, uterine rupture; anaphylaxis.

Drug interactions Other vasopressors may potentiate hypertension.

How supplied 10 USP units/1-mL ampule (10 U/mL) and prefilled syringe. 5 USP units/1-mL ampule (5 U/mL) and prefilled syringe.

Dosage and administration IM administration: 3–10 units after delivery of placenta. IV administration: Mix 10–40 units in 1,000 mL of a nonhydrating diluent: Infused at 20–40 milliunits/min, titrated to severity of bleeding and uterine response.

Duration of action Onset: IM: 3–5 minutes; IV: immediate. Peak effect: variable. Duration: IM; 30–60 minutes; IV: 20 minutes after infusion discontinued.

Special considerations Pregnancy safety: not applicable. Monitor vital signs, including fetal heart rate and uterine tone closely.

Pancuronium Bromide (Pavulon)

Class Nondepolarizing neuromuscular blocker/paralytic.

Mechanism of action Binds to the receptor for acetylcholine at the neuromuscular junction.

Indications Induction or maintenance of paralysis after intubation to assist ventilations.

Contraindications Hypersensitivity, inability to control airway and support ventilations with oxygen and positive pressure, neuromuscular disease (myasthenia gravis), hepatic or renal failure.

Adverse reactions Apnea, weakness, salivation, premature ventricular contractions, tachycardia; transient hypotension, increased blood pressure; pain, burning at injection site.

Drug interactions Positive chronotropic drugs may potentiate tachycardia.

How supplied 4-mg/2-mL ampule.

Dosage and administration Adult: 0.1 mg/kg slow IV; repeat every 30–60 minutes as necessary. Pediatric: 0.1 mg/kg slow IV, IO.

Duration of action Onset: 30 seconds. Peak effect: paralysis in 3–5 minutes. Duration: 45–60 minutes.

Special considerations Pregnancy safety: not established. If patient is conscious, explain the effect of the medication before administration and always sedate the patient before using pancuronium. Intubation and ventilatory support must be readily available. Monitor the patient carefully. Effects may be reversed with neostigmine (Prostigmin) 0.05 mg/kg and should be accompanied by atropine sulfate (0.5–1.2 mg IV). Pancuronium has no effect on consciousness or pain. Will not stop neuronal seizure activity. Pulse rate, cardiac output are increased. Decrease doses for patients with renal disease.

Phenobarbital (Luminal)

Class Barbiturate, anticonvulsant.

Mechanism of action Generally unknown but believed to reduce neuronal excitability by increasing the motor cortex threshold to electrical stimulation.

Indications Prevention and treatment of seizure activity; prophylaxis for febrile seizures; anxiety, apprehension; status epilepticus.

Contraindications Patients with porphyria, hypersensitivity, severe liver or respiratory diseases.

Adverse reactions Respiratory depression, hypotension, coma, bradycardia, nausea, vomiting; central nervous system (CNS) depression, ataxia, nystagmus, pupillary constriction; burning at injection site.

Drug interactions Effects potentiated by other CNS depressants, anticonvulsants, and MAOIs; incompatible with all other drugs; flush line before and after use.

How supplied Elixir: 20 mg/5 mL. Tablets: 8, 15, 30, 60, 90, 100 mg. Parenteral: 30, 60, 65 mg, 130 mg/mL ampule; dose may be diluted with 9 mL of D_5W (6.5, 13 mg/mL).

Dosage and administration Adult: 100–250 mg slow IV, or IM; may repeat as necessary in 20–30 minutes. Pediatric: 10–20 mg/kg IV, IO (less than 1 mg/kg/min) or IM; repeat as necessary in 20–30 minutes.

Duration of action Onset: 3–30 minutes. Peak effect: 30 minutes. Duration: 4–6 hours.

Special considerations Pregnancy safety: Category B. Potential for abuse. Carefully monitor vital signs. Use with caution in patients with pulmonary, cardiovascular, hepatic, or renal insufficiency. Use a large, stable vein for injection.

Phenytoin (Dilantin)

Class Anticonvulsant.

Mechanism of action Promotes sodium efflux from neurons, thereby stabilizing the neuron's threshold against excitability caused by excess stimulation; in similar fashion, decreases abnormal ventricular automaticity and decreases the refractory period in the myocardial conduction system.

Indications Prophylaxis and treatment of major motor seizures, digitalis-induced arrhythmias.

Contraindications Hypersensitivity, bradycardia, second- and third-degree heart block.

Adverse reactions Hypotension with too rapid IV push, heart block, arrhythmias, cardiovascular collapse, nausea, vomiting, ataxia, central nervous system depression, nystagmus, pain at injection site, respiratory depression.

Drug interactions Serum Dilantin levels increased by: anticoagulants, Tagamet, sulfonamides, salicylates. Metabolism increased by chronic alcohol use. Cardiac depressant effects increased by lidocaine, propranolol, and other beta-blockers. Precipitation may occur when mixed with D_5W. Incompatible with many solutions and medications.

How supplied 50 mg/mL in 2- and 5-mL ampules, 2-mL prefilled syringes. May be diluted in normal saline (NS) (1–10 mg/mL); use in-line filter. Note: IV line should be flushed with 0.9% NS before and after drug administration.

Dosage and administration Adult: Seizures: 10–20 mg/kg slow IV, not to exceed 1 g or rate of 50 mg/min). Arrhythmias: 50–100 mg (diluted) slow IV every 5–15 min as necessary; maximum, 1 g. Pediatric: Seizures: 10–20 mg/kg slow IV (1–3 mg/kg/min). Arrhythmias: 5 mg/kg slow IV; maximum, 1 g.

Duration of action Onset: 20–30 minutes for seizure disorder. Peak effect: 1–3 hours. Duration: 18–24 hours but as long as 15 days reported.

Special considerations Pregnancy safety: not established. Carefully monitor vital signs. Venous irritation may occur (use large stable vein).

Pralidoxime Chloride (2-PAM Chloride, Protopam)

Class Cholinesterase reactivator.

Mechanism of action Reactivation of cholinesterase to effectively act as an antidote to organophosphate pesticide poisoning. This action allows for destruction of accumulated acetylcholine at the neuromuscular junction.

Indications As an antidote in the treatment of poisoning by organophosphate pesticides and chemicals. In the prehospital arena, is used when atropine is or has become ineffective in management of organophosphate poisoning.

Contraindications Use with caution in patients with reduced renal function; patients with myasthenia gravis and organophosphate poisoning.

Adverse reactions Dizziness, blurred vision, diplopia, headache, drowsiness, nausea, tachycardia, hyperventilation, muscular weakness, excitement, and manic behavior.

Drug interactions No direct drug interactions; however, patients with organophosphate poisoning should not be given barbiturates, morphine, theophylline, aminophylline, succinylcholine, reserpine, and phenothiazines.

How supplied Emergency Single Dose Kit containing: One 20-mL vial of 1 g sterile Protopam chloride. One 20-mL ampule of sterile diluent. Sterile, disposable 20-mL syringe. Needle and alcohol swab.

Dosage and administration Note: If Protopam is to be used, it should be administered almost simultaneously with atropine. Adult: Initial dose of 1–2 g as an IV infusion with 100 mL saline over 15–30 minutes. Pediatric: 20–40 mg/kg as IV infusion over 15–30 minutes. Doses may be repeated every 1 hour if muscle weakness persists. If IV administration is not feasible, IM or SC injection may be utilized.

Duration of action Onset: minutes. Peak effects: variable. Duration: variable.

Special considerations Pregnancy safety: unknown. Treatment will be most effective if given within a few hours after poisoning. Cardiac monitoring should be considered in all cases of severe organophosphate poisoning.

Procainamide Hydrochloride (Pronestyl, Procanbid)

Class Antiarrhythmic.

Mechanism of action Suppresses phase 4 depolarization in normal ventricular muscle and Purkinje fibers, reducing ectopic pacemaker automaticity; suppresses intraventricular conduction.

Indications Stable monomorphic V-tach with normal QT interval, re-entry SVT uncontrolled by vagal maneuvers and adenosine, stable wide-complex tachycardia of unknown origin, atrial fibrillation with rapid ventricular rate in patients with Wolff-Parkinson-White syndrome.

Contraindications Torsade de pointes, second- and third-degree AV block (without functional artificial pacemaker), digitalis toxicity, tricyclic antidepressant overdose.

Adverse reactions Widening of the PR, QRS, and QT intervals, AV heart block, hypotension, reflex tachycardia, bradycardia, nausea and vomiting.

Drug interactions May increase plasma levels of amiodarone and quinidine.

How supplied 1 g in 10-mL vials (100 mg/mL); 1 g in 2-mL vials (500 mg/mL) for infusion.

Dosage and administration Adult: Recurrent V-fib/pulseless V-tach: 20 mg/min IV infusion (maximum dose: 17 mg/kg). In urgent situations, up to 50 mg/min may be administered (maximum dose of 17 mg/kg). Other indications: 20 mg/min IV infusion until any one of the following occurs: arrhythmia suppression, hypotension, QRS widens by > 50% of its pretreatment width, or total dose of 17 mg/kg has been given. Maintenance infusion: 1–4 mg/min (dilute in D_5W or normal saline). Pediatric: Loading dose of 15 mg/kg IV/IO over 30–60 minutes.

Duration of action Onset: 10–30 minutes. Peak effect: variable. Duration: 3–6 hours.

Special considerations Pregnancy safety: Category C. Potent vasodilating and negative inotropic effects. Hypotension may occur with rapid infusion. Administer cautiously to patients with renal, hepatic, or cardiac insufficiency. Administer cautiously to patients with asthma or digitalis-induced arrhythmias.

Promethazine Hydrochloride (Phenergan)

Class Antihistamine.

Mechanism of action H-1 receptor antagonist; blocks action of histamine; possesses sedative, antimotion, antiemetic and anticholinergic activity; potentiates the effects of narcotics to induce analgesia.

Indications Nausea, vomiting, motion sickness; sedation for patients in labor; potentiation of analgesic effects of narcotics.

Contraindications Hypersensitivity, coma, CNS-depressed patients from alcohol, barbiturates, narcotics, Reye's syndrome.

Adverse reactions Sedation, dizziness, impairment of mental and physical ability, arrhythmias, nausea, vomiting, hyperexcitability; hallucinations, convulsions, and sudden death when used in children.

Drug interactions Additive with other CNS depressants. Increased extrapyramidal effects with MAOIs.

How supplied 25 and 50 mg/mL in 1-mL ampules and Tubex syringes.

Dosage and administration Adult: 12.5–25 mg IV, deep IM, PO, rectally. Pediatric: (greater than 2 years old) 0.25–0.5 mg/kg dose IM.

Duration of action Onset: IV: immediate. Peak effect: 30–60 minutes. Duration: 4–6 hours.

Special considerations Pregnancy safety: Category C. Use cautiously in patients with asthma, peptic ulcer disease, and bone marrow suppression. Do not use in children with vomiting of unknown etiology. Avoid intra-arterial injection. IM injection is preferred route.

Propranolol Hydrochloride (Inderal)

Class Beta-adrenergic blocker, antiarrhythmic (Class II).

Mechanism of action Nonselective beta-adrenergic blocker that inhibits chronotropic, inotropic, and vasodilator response to beta-adrenergic stimulation.

Indications Hypertension, angina pectoris, V-tach and V-fib refractory to lidocaine; selected supraventricular tachycardias.

Contraindications Sinus bradycardia, second- or third-degree AV block, asthma, CHF, COPD.

Adverse reactions Bradycardia, heart blocks, angina pectoris, palpitations, syncope. Bronchospasm, dyspnea, hallucinations, anxiety, nausea, vomiting, visual disturbances.

Drug interactions Verapamil may worsen AV conduction abnormalities. Succinylcholine effects may be enhanced. Effects may be reversed by isoproterenol (Isuprel), norepinephrine, dopamine.

How supplied Solution of 1-mg/mL vials.

Dosage and administration Adult: Dilute 1–3 mg in 10–30 mL of D_5W; administer slowly IV at rate of 1 mg/min; maximum, 5 mg. Pediatric: 0.01–0.05 mg/kg/dose slow IV over 10 minutes; maximum, 3 mg.

Duration of action Onset: 15–60 minutes. Peak effect: variable. Duration: 6–12 hours.

Special considerations Pregnancy safety: Category C. Closely monitor patient during administration. Use cautiously in geriatric population. Atropine sulfate should be readily available.

Sodium Bicarbonate

Class Alkalizing agent, electrolyte, and an antacid.

Mechanism of action Neutralizes hydrochloric acid. Systemic and urinary alkalinizer.

Indications Mild or moderate metabolic acidosis due to shock, severe dehydration, anoxia, uncontrolled diabetes, renal disease, cardiac arrest, and severe primary lactic acidosis. To treat overdose of aspirin and cyclic-antidepressants.

Contraindications Metabolic and respiratory alkalosis, hypertension, convulsions, CHF, and other situations where sodium can be dangerous.

Adverse reactions Gastric distension, hypercalcemia, metabolic acidosis, extravasation following IV use may cause tissue sloughing, cellulitis, or necrosis at the site.

Drug interactions Increases amphetamine effects, increases renal tubular reabsorption (tricyclic antidepressants) decreases benzodiazepine effects, decreases iron effects, increases urine alkalinity, decreases the effects of tetracycline.

How supplied Paramedics use the 8.4% solution; (50 mEg in 50 mL) preload syringe

Dosage and administration Adult and pediatric: 1 mEq per kg IV bolus (may repeat every 10 minutes at ½ initial dose).

Duration of action Onset is seconds; Peak effect 1–2 minutes, Duration is 10 minutes. Metabolized in the kidneys and through respiration.

Special considerations Pregnancy safety: Category C. Do not mix in the same IV line as Calcium Chloride without first flushing the line or the drugs may precipitate.

Streptokinase (Streptase)

Class Thrombolytic agent.

Mechanism of action Combines with plasminogen to produce an activator complex that converts free plasminogen to the proteolytic enzyme plasmin. Plasmin degrades fibrin threads as well as fibrinogen, causing clot lysis.

Indications Acute evolving MI, massive pulmonary emboli, arterial thrombosis and embolism, to clear arteriovenous cannulas.

Contraindications Hypersensitivity; active bleeding, recent surgery (within 2–4 weeks), recent CVA; prolonged CPR; intracranial or intraspinal neoplasm, arteriovenous malformation, or surgery; recent significant trauma (particularly head trauma); uncontrolled hypertension.

Adverse reactions Bleeding (GU, GI, intracranial, other sites), allergic reactions, hypotension, chest pain, reperfusion arrhythmias, abdominal pain.

Drug interactions Aspirin may increase risk of bleeding as well as improve outcome. Heparin and other anticoagulants may increase risk of bleeding as well as improve outcome.

How supplied 250,000, 750,000, 1.5 million IU vials.

Dosage and administration Note: Reconstitute by slowly adding 5 mL of sodium chloride or D_5W, directing stream to side of vial instead of into powder. Gently roll and tilt vial for reconstitution; dilute slowly to 45 mL total. Adult: 500,000–1,500,000 IU diluted to 45 mL IV over 1 hour. Pediatric: safety not established.

Duration of action Onset: 10–20 minutes (fibrinolysis: 10–20 minutes; clot lysis: 60–90 minutes). Peak effects: variable. Duration: 3–4 hours (prolonged bleeding times up to 24 hours).

Special considerations Pregnancy safety: Category A. Do not administer IM injections to patients receiving thrombolytics. Obtain blood sample for coagulation studies prior to administration. Carefully monitor vital signs. Observe patient for bleeding.

Succinylcholine Chloride (Anectine, Quelicin)

Class Depolarizing neuromuscular blocker, paralyzing agent.

Mechanism of action Bind to the receptors for acetylcholine.

Indications To facilitate intubation, to terminate laryngospasm, to promote muscle relaxation, to facilitate electroconvulsive shock therapy.

Contraindications Acute narrow-angle glaucoma, penetrating eye injuries, inability to control airway or support ventilations with oxygen and positive pressure.

Adverse reactions Apnea, malignant hyperthermia, arrhythmias, bradycardia, hypertension, hypotension, cardiac arrest, hyperkalemia, increased intraocular pressure, fasciculations, exacerbation of hyperkalemia in trauma patients.

Drug interactions Effects potentiated by oxytocin, beta-blockers, and organophosphates. Diazepam may reduce duration of action.

How supplied 40 mg in 2-mL ampule (20 mg/mL). 100 mg in 5-mL ampule (20 mg/mL). Multidose vial.

Dosage and administration Adult: 1–2 mg/kg rapid IV; repeat once if needed. Pediatric: 1–1.5 mg/kg dose rapid IV, IO; repeat once if needed.

Duration of action Onset: 1 minute. Peak effect: 1–3 minutes. Duration: 5 minutes.

Special considerations Pregnancy safety: Category C. EMS use primarily to facilitate endotracheal intubation. If the patient is conscious, explain the effects of the drug before administration. Consider premedication with atropine sulfate, particularly in pediatric age group. Premedication with lidocaine may blunt any increase in intracranial pressure during intubation. Diazepam or midazolam should be used in any conscious patient undergoing neuromuscular blockade.

Terbutaline Sulfate (Brethine, Bricanyl)

Class Sympathomimetic bronchodilator.

Mechanism of action Selective beta-2 adrenergic receptor activity resulting in relaxation of smooth muscles of the bronchial tree and peripheral vasculature. Minimal cardiac effects.

Indications Bronchial asthma, reversible bronchospasm associated with exercise, chronic bronchitis, and emphysema.

Contraindications Hypersensitivity, tachyarrhythmias.

Adverse reactions Usually transient and dose-related, restlessness, apprehension, palpitations, tachycardia, chest pain, coughing, bronchospasm, nausea, facial flushing.

Drug interactions Cardiovascular effects exacerbated by other sympathomimetics. MAOIs may potentiate arrhythmias. Beta-blockers may antagonize terbutaline.

How supplied MDI: 200-µg/metered spray. Parenteral: 1-mg/mL ampule.

Dosage and administration Adult: 0.25 mg SC; may repeat in 15–30 minutes to maximum dose of 0.5 mg in 4-hour period. 400 µg (two inhalations by MDI) every 4–6 hours; allow 1–2 minutes between inhalations. Pediatric: Not recommended for children under 12 years of age; 0.01 mg/kg/dose SC every 15–20 minutes as necessary to maximum 0.25 mg dose. 0.03–0.05 mg/kg in 1.25 mL saline for aerosolization every 4 hours.

Duration of action Onset: SC: 15–30 minutes; MDI, 5–30 minutes. Peak effect: variable. Duration: SC: 1.5–4 hours; MDI: 3–6 hours.

Special considerations Pregnancy safety: Category B. Carefully monitor vital signs. Use with caution in patients with cardiovascular disease or hypertension. Patient should receive oxygen before and during bronchodilator administration.

Tetracaine HCL (ophthalmic) (Pontocaine, Supracaine)

Class Ophthalmic anesthetic.

Mechanism of action Decreased ion permeability by stabilizing the neuronal membrane.

Indications Cataract extraction, tonometry, gonioscopy, removal of foreign objects, corneal suture removal, glaucoma surgery. Also used in conjunction with the Morgan Lens for flushing the eyes.

Contraindications Known allergy to this medicine or hypersensitivity para-aminobenzoic acid (PABA).

Adverse reactions Blurred vision, stinging, burning, lacrimination, photophobia, conjunctival redness.

Drug interactions Decreases the antibacterial action of sulfonamides.

How supplied Solution (drops) and ointment.

Dosage and administration Adult and pediatric: 1 to 2 gtt before the procedure.

Duration of action Onset: 15–30 seconds. Peak effect: minutes. Duration: 15 to 20 minutes.

Special considerations Use with caution in patients who have hyperthyroidism, hypertension, and cardiac disease. Pregnancy safety: Category C.

Thiamine Hydrochloride (Vitamin B-1)

Class Vitamin (B-1).

Mechanism of action Combines with ATP to form thiamine pyrophosphate coenzyme, a necessary component for carbohydrate metabolism. The brain is extremely sensitive to thiamine deficiency.

Indications Coma of unknown origin, delirium tremens, beriberi, Wernicke's encephalopathy.

Contraindications None.

Adverse reactions Hypotension from too rapid of an injection or too high a dose, anxiety, diaphoresis, nausea, vomiting, allergy (rare).

Drug interactions Give thiamine before glucose under all circumstances.

How supplied 1,000 mg in 10-mL vial (100 mg/mL).

Dosage and administration Adult: 100 mg slow IV or IM. Pediatric: 10–25 mg slow IV or IM.

Duration of action Onset: rapid. Peak effects: variable. Duration: dependent upon degree of deficiency.

Special considerations Pregnancy safety: Category A. Large IV doses may cause respiratory difficulties. Anaphylaxis reactions reported.

Tissue Plasminogen Activator (TPA)

Class Thrombolytic agent.

Mechanism of action Binds to fibrin-bound plasminogen at the clot site, converting plasminogen to plasmin; plasmin digests the fibrin strands of the clot, restoring perfusion.

Indications Acute evolving myocardial infarction, massive pulmonary emboli, arterial thrombosis and embolism, to clear arteriovenous cannulas.

Contraindications Recent surgery (within 3 weeks), active bleeding, recent CVA, prolonged CPR, intracranial or intraspinal surgery; recent significant trauma, especially head trauma; uncontrolled hypertension (generally BP over 200 mm Hg).

Adverse reactions GI, GU, intracranial, and other site bleeding; hypotension, allergic reactions, chest pain, abdominal pain, CVA, reperfusion arrhythmias.

Drug interactions Acetylsalicylic acid may increase risk of hemorrhage. Heparin and other anticoagulants may increase risk of hemorrhage.

How supplied 20 mg with 20-mL diluent vial. 50 mg with 50-mL diluent vial.

Dosage and administration Adult: 10-mg bolus IV over 2 minutes; then 50 mg over 1 hour, then 20 mg over the second hour and 20 mg over the third hour, for a total dose of 100 mg (other doses may be prescribed through Medical Direction). Pediatric: safety not established.

Duration of action Onset: clot lysis most often within 60–90 minutes. Peak effect: variable. Duration: 30 minutes with 80% cleared within 10 minutes.

Special considerations Pregnancy safety: contraindicated. Closely monitor vital signs. Observe for bleeding. Do not give IM injection to patient receiving tissue plasminogen activator.

Vasopressin (Pitressin synthetic)

Class Antidiuretic hormone.

Mechanism of action Stimulation of V_1 smooth muscle receptors, potent vasoconstrictor when given in high doses.

Indications Alternate vasopressor to the first or second dose of epinephrine in cardiac arrest, may be useful in cases of vasodilatory shock (ie, septic shock).

Contraindications Responsive patients with coronary artery disease.

Adverse reactions Bronchoconstriction, ischemic chest pain, nausea and vomiting, abdominal pain.

Drug interactions None reported.

How supplied 1-mL vials containing 20 units (20 U/mL).

Dosage and administration Adult: 40-unit one-time dose IV/IO to replace the first or second dose of epinephrine in cardiac arrest. Pediatric: Not recommended.

Duration of action Onset: immediate. Duration of action: variable.

Special considerations Pregnancy safety: Category C. May increase peripheral vascular resistance and provoke cardiac ischemia and angina.

Vecuronium Bromide (Norcuron)

Class Paralytic agent.

Mechanism of action Nondepolarizing neuromuscular blocking agent, paralytic.

Indications To facilitate intubation, to terminate laryngospasm, to promote muscle relaxation, to facilitate electroconvulsive shock therapy.

Contraindications Acute narrow-angle glaucoma, penetrating eye injuries, inability to control airway or support ventilations with oxygen and positive pressure, newborns, myasthenia gravis, hepatic or renal failure.

Adverse reactions Apnea, weakness, salivation, premature ventricular contractions, tachycardia, transient hypotension, increased blood pressure.

Drug interactions Use of inhalational anesthetics will enhance neuromuscular blockade.

How supplied 10 mg/10 mL vecuronium bromide vials with diluent. 20-mL vials (20 mg vecuronium) without diluent.

Dosage and administration Adult: 0.1 mg/kg IV push; maintenance dose within 25–40 minutes: 0.01–0.05 mg/kg IV push. Pediatric: 0.1 mg/kg IV, IO; maintenance dose within 20–35 minutes: 0.01–0.05 mg/kg IV push.

Duration of action Onset: 30 seconds. Peak effects: 2.5–3 minutes. Duration: 25–30 minutes.

Special considerations Pregnancy safety: Category C. If patient is conscious, explain the effect of the medication before administration and always sedate the patient before using vecuronium. Intubation and ventilatory support must be readily available. Monitor the patient carefully. Vecuronium has no effect on consciousness or pain. Will not stop neuronal seizure activity. Pulse rate, cardiac output are increased. Decrease doses for patients with renal disease.

Verapamil (Calan, Isoptin)

Class Antiarrhythmic.

Mechanism of action Calcium channel blocker, class IV antiarrhythmic, prolongs AV nodal refractory period, dilates coronary arteries and arterioles.

Indications PSVT, PAT, atrial fibrillation and atrial flutter with rapid ventricular response.

Contraindications Wolff-Parkinson-White syndrome, second-degree or third-degree AV block, sick sinus syndrome (unless patient has functioning pacemaker), hypotension, cardiogenic shock, severe CHF, pulmonary edema, patients receiving IV beta-blockers, wide-complex tachycardias, children less than 12 months of age.

Adverse reactions Hypotension, AV block, bradycardia, asystole, dizziness, headache, nausea, vomiting, complete AV block, peripheral edema.

Drug interactions Increases serum concentration of digoxin. Beta-adrenergic blockers may have additive negative inotropic and chronotropic effects. Antihypertensives may potentiate hypotensive effects.

How supplied 5 mg/2 mL in 2-, 4-, 5-mL vials or 2-, 4-mL ampules.

Dosage and administration Adult: 2.5–5.0 mg IV bolus over 2 minutes (over 3 minutes in older patients). Repeat doses of 5–10 mg may be given every 15–30 minutes to a maximum of 20 mg. Pediatric: 0.1–0.2 mg/kg/dose IV, IO push over 2 minutes. Repeat dose in 30 minutes if not effective. (Note: not to be used in children less than 12 months of age.).

Duration of action Onset: 2–5 minutes. Peak effect: variable. Duration: 30–60 minutes.

Special considerations Pregnancy safety: Category C. Closely monitor patient's vital signs. Be prepared to resuscitate. AV block or asystole may occur as result of slowed AV conduction.

IV Solutions (Colloids and Crystalloids)

Colloids expand plasma volume by colloidal osmotic pressure. Colloids are most often used in hypovolemic shock states. Crystalloids are substances in solution that can diffuse through the intravascular compartment. Crystalloid solutions are used for electrolyte replacement, a route for medication, and short-term intravascular volume expansion.

Plasma Protein Fraction (Plasmanate)

Class Natural colloid.

Mechanism of action Plasmanate is a protein-containing colloid that remains in the intravascular compartment. It increases intravascular volume by attracting water from other fluid compartments by virtue of its colloid osmotic pressure.

Indications Hypovolemic shock, especially burn shock; hypoproteinemia (low protein states).

Contraindications There are no major contraindications to plasma protein fraction when used in the treatment of life-threatening hypovolemic states.

Adverse reactions Chills, fever, urticaria (hives), nausea, and vomiting have all been reported with plasma protein fraction use.

Drug interactions Solutions should not be mixed with or administered through the same administration sets as other intravenous fluids.

How supplied Plasma protein fraction is supplied in 250- and 500-mL bottles of a 5% solution. An administration set is usually attached.

Dosage and administration The plasma protein fraction infusion rate should be titrated according to the patient's hemodynamic response. In the management of shock secondary to burns, the physician's orders regarding the rate of administration must be closely followed. Standard formulas for IV fluid administration have been developed. The medical control physician will use these in judging the correct rate of intravenous administration.

Duration of action 24–36 hours.

Special considerations Do not use if the solution is cloudy or if you see sedimentation.

Dextran

Class Artificial colloid.

Mechanism of action Dextran is a sugar-containing colloid used as an intravascular volume expander. It remains in the intravascular compartment for approximately 12 hours. It increases intravascular volume by attracting water from other fluid compartments by virtue of its colloid osmotic pressure.

Indications Hypovolemic shock.

Contraindications Dextran should not be administered to patients who have a known hypersensitivity to the drug. It should not be administered to patients suffering congestive heart failure, renal failure, or known bleeding disorders.

Adverse reactions Rash, itching, dyspnea, chest tightness, and mild hypotension have all been reported with dextran use. The incidence of these side effects is, however, very low, and reactions are generally mild. Increased bleeding time has also been reported with dextran use due to its interference with platelet function.

Drug interactions Dextran should not be administered to patients who are receiving anticoagulants as it significantly retards blood clotting.

How supplied Dextran 40 and Dextran 70 are supplied in 250- and 500-mL bottles.

Dosage and administration The dosage of dextran is titrated according to the patient's physiologic response.

Duration of action 8–12 hours.

Special considerations In the management of burn shock, it is especially important to follow standard fluid resuscitation regimens to prevent possible circulatory overload.

Hetastarch (Hespan)

Class Artificial colloid.

Mechanism of action Hetastarch is a starch-containing colloid used as an intravascular volume expander. Following administration, the plasma volume is expanded slightly in excess of the volume of hetastarch administered. This effect has been observed for up to 24 to 36 hours. Hetastarch increases intravascular volume by virtue of its colloid osmotic pressure.

Indications Hypovolemic shock, especially burn shock; septic shock.

Contraindications There are no major contraindications to hetastarch when used in the management of life-threatening hypovolemic states.

Adverse reactions Nausea, vomiting, mild febrile reactions, chills, itching, and urticaria (hives) have been reported with hetastarch administration. Severe anaphylactic reactions have been rarely reported.

Drug interactions Hetastarch should not be administered to patients who are receiving anticoagulants.

How supplied Sterile 6% hetastarch in 0.9% sodium chloride is supplied in 500-mL bottles.

Dosage and administration The dosage of hetastarch is titrated according to the patient's physiologic response.

Duration of action 24–36 hours.

Special considerations Pregnancy safety: Category C. Patients allergic to corn may be allergic to hetastarch.

Lactated Ringer's (Hartman's Solution)

Class Isotonic crystalloid solution.

Mechanism of action Lactated Ringer's replaces water and electrolytes.

Indications Hypovolemic shock; keep open IV.

Contraindications Lactated Ringer's should not be used in patients with congestive heart failure or renal failure.

Adverse reactions Rare in therapeutic dosages.

Drug interactions Few in the emergency setting.

How supplied Lactated Ringer's is supplied in 250-, 500-, and 1,000-mL bags, IV infusion.

Dosage and administration Hypovolemic shock; titrate according to patient's physiologic response.

Duration of action Short-term therapy.

Special considerations None.

5% Dextrose in Water (D_5W)

Class Hypotonic dextrose-containing solution.

Mechanism of action D_5W provides nutrients in the form of dextrose as well as free water.

Indications IV access for emergency drugs; for dilution of concentrated drugs for intravenous infusion.

Contraindications D_5W should not be used as a fluid replacement for hypovolemic states.

Adverse reactions Rare in therapeutic dosages.

Drug interactions D_5W should not be used with phenytoin (Dilantin) or amrinone (Inocor).

How supplied D_5W is supplied in bags of 50, 100, 150, 250, 500, and 1,000 mL.

Dosage and administration D_5W is usually administered through a minidrip (60 gtt/mL) set at a rate of "to keep open" (TKO).

Duration of action Short-term therapy.

Special considerations None.

10% Dextrose in Water ($D_{10}W$)

Class Hypertonic dextrose-containing solution.

Mechanism of action $D_{10}W$ provides nutrients in the form of dextrose as well as free water.

Indications Neonatal resuscitation, hypoglycemia.

Contraindications $D_{10}W$ should not be used as a fluid replacement for hypovolemic states.

Adverse reactions Rare in therapeutic dosages.

Drug interactions Should not be used with phenytoin (Dilantin) or amrinone (Inocor).

How supplied $D_{10}W$ is supplied in bags of 50, 100, 150, 250, 500, and 1,000 mL.

Dosage and administration The administration rate of $D_{10}W$ will usually be dependent on the patient's condition.

Duration of action Short-term therapy.

Special considerations None.

0.9% Sodium Chloride (Normal Saline)

Class Isotonic crystalloid solution.

Mechanism of action Normal saline replaces water and electrolytes.

Indications Heat-related problems (heat exhaustion, heat stroke), freshwater drowning, hypovolemia, diabetic ketoacidosis, keep open IV.

Contraindications The use of 0.9% sodium chloride should not be considered in patients with congestive heart failure as circulatory overload can be easily induced.

Adverse reactions Rare in therapeutic dosages.

Drug interactions Few in the emergency setting.

How supplied Normal saline is supplied in 250-, 500-, and 1,000-mL bags. Sterile normal saline for irrigation should not be confused with that designed for intravenous administration.

Dosage and administration The specific situation being treated will dictate the rate in which normal saline will be administered. In severe heat stroke, diabetic ketoacidosis, and freshwater drowning, it is likely that you will be called on to administer the fluid quite rapidly. In other cases, it is advisable to administer the fluid at a moderate rate (for example, 100 mL/h).

Duration of action Short-term therapy.

Special considerations None.

0.45% Sodium Chloride (½ Normal Saline)

Class Hypotonic crystalloid solution.

Mechanism of action One-half normal saline replaces free water and electrolytes.

Indications Patients with diminished renal or cardiovascular function for which rapid rehydration is not indicated.

Contraindications Cases in which rapid rehydration is indicated.

Adverse reactions Rare in therapeutic dosages.

Drug interactions Few in the emergency setting.

How supplied One-half normal saline is supplied in 250-, 500-, and 1,000-mL bags.

Dosage and administration The specific situation and patient condition will dictate the rate at which one-half normal saline will be administered.

Duration of action Short-term therapy.

Special considerations None.

5% Dextrose in 0.45% Sodium Chloride (D_5½NS)

Class Hypertonic dextrose-containing crystalloid solution.

Mechanism of action D_5½NS replaces free water and electrolytes and provides nutrients in the form of dextrose.

Indications Heat exhaustion, diabetic disorders; for use as a way to keep open solution in patients with impaired renal or cardiovascular function.

Contraindications D_5½NS should not be used when rapid fluid resuscitation is indicated.

Adverse reactions Rare in therapeutic dosages.

Drug interactions D_5½NS should not be used with phenytoin (Dilantin) or amrinone (Inocor).

How supplied D_5½NS is supplied in bags containing 250, 500, and 1,000 mL of the fluid.

Dosage and administration The specific situation and patient condition will dictate the rate at which D_5½NS should be administered.

Duration of action Short-term therapy.

Special considerations None.

5% Dextrose in 0.9% Sodium Chloride (D_5NS)

Class Hypertonic dextrose-containing crystalloid solution.

Mechanism of action D_5NS replaces free water and electrolytes and provides nutrients in the form of dextrose.

Indications Heat-related disorders, freshwater drowning, hypovolemia, peritonitis.

Contraindications D_5NS should not be administered to patients with impaired cardiac or renal function.

Adverse reactions Rare in therapeutic dosages.

Drug interactions D_5NS should not be used with phenytoin (Dilantin) or amrinone (Inocor).

How supplied D_5NS is supplied in bags containing 250, 500, and 1,000 mL of the solution.

Dosage and administration The specific situation and patient condition will dictate the rate at which D_5NS is given.

Duration of action Short-term therapy.

Special considerations None.

5% Dextrose in Lactated Ringer's (D_5LR)

Class Hypertonic dextrose-containing crystalloid solution.

Mechanism of action D_5LR replaces water and electrolytes and provides nutrients in the form of dextrose.

Indications Hypovolemic shock, hemorrhagic shock, certain cases of acidosis.

Contraindications D_5LR should not be administered to patients with decreased renal or cardiovascular function.

Adverse reactions Rare in therapeutic dosages.

Drug interactions D_5LR should not be used with phenytoin (Dilantin) or amrinone (Inocor).

How supplied D_5LR is supplied in bags containing 250, 500, and 1,000 mL of the fluid.

Dosage and administration In severe hypovolemic shock D_5LR should be infused through a large-bore catheter (14 or 16 gauge). This infusion should be administered "wide open" until a blood pressure of 100 mm Hg is achieved. When the blood pressure is attained, the infusions should be reduced to 100 mL/h. In other cases, the specific situation and patient condition will dictate the rate of administration.

Duration of action Short-term therapy.

Special considerations None.

Numbers and Symbols

A

C

D

E

F

G

H

O

P

Q

R

T

U

W

X

Z

Photo Credits

Chapter 1
1-1a: © Stephen Aaron Rees/ShutterStock, Inc.; 1.1b: © Photos.com; 1.1c: Courtesy of Yellowstone National Park; 1.1d: Courtesy of Linda Bartlett/National Cancer Institute; 1.4: Courtesy of Wolfe Tory Medical, Inc.; 1.5: Courtesy of Engel USA; 1.6: Courtesy of The Harloff Company; 1.12: Courtesy of Rhonda Beck; 1.13: Courtesy of Pyng Medical Corporation; 1.14: Courtesy of Persys Medical/Waismed; 1.15: Courtesy of VidaCare® Corporation; Skill Drill 10.1: Courtesy of Wolfe Tory Medical, Inc.

Chapter 2
2.2: © J. Yakwichuk/Custom Medical Stock Photo; 2.4a-b: © Charles Stewart & Associates; 2.6a: © Amy Walters/ShutterStock, Inc.; 2.6b: © E. M. Singletary, M.D. Used with permission; 2.7: Courtesy of Rhonda Beck; 2.12: © Charles Stewart & Associates.

Chapter 3
3.2b: Courtesy of Stuart Mirvis, MD; 3.3: © Scott Rothstein/ShutterStock, Inc.; 3.4: Courtesy of Respironics, Inc., Murrysville, PA. All rights reserved.

Chapter 4
4.4: Courtesy of Advanced Circulatory Systems, Inc.; 4.5: Courtesy of ZOLL Medical Corporation; 4.6: Courtesy of Michigan Instruments, Inc.; 4.7, 4.10, 4.11, 4.12, 4.13: Reproduced from *Arrhythmia Recognition: The Art of Interpretation,* courtesy of Tomas B. Garcia, MD; Case Study 4.3a-b, 4: Reproduced from *Arrhythmia Recognition: The Art of Interpretation,* courtesy of Tomas B. Garcia, MD.

Chapter 7
7.2: Courtesy of Dey, L.P.

Chapter 8
Opener: © Chris Priest/Photo Researchers, Inc.; 8.3: Courtesy of Dornier MedTech America, Inc.

Chapter 9
Opener: © Comstock Images/Getty Images; 9.1: © Anne Kitzman/ShutterStock, Inc.

Chapter 10
Opener: © Robert Harding Picture Library Ltd/Alamy Images; 10.4: © Alan Heartfield/ShutterStock, Inc.

Chapter 12
Opener, 12.3: Courtesy of Marianne Gausche-Hill, MD, FACEP, FAAP.

Chapter 13
Opener: © Eddie M. Sperling; 13.2: © Scott Rothstein/ShutterStock, Inc.

Chapter 14
14.3: © Archetype/ShutterStock, Inc.; 14.4: © Cheryl Casey/ShutterStock, Inc.

Chapter 15
Opener: Courtesy of Captain David Jackson, Saginaw Township Fire Department; 15.1: © Mark C. Ide; 15.2: © Dennis MacDonald/Alamy Images; 15.3: © Mark C. Ide.

Unless otherwise indicated, photographs are under copyright of Jones and Bartlett Publishers, courtesy of Maryland Institute for Emergency Medical Services Systems, or provided by the American Academy of Orthopaedic Surgeons.